中国中成药大典

（汉英版）

Collection of Chinese Patent Medicines

(Chinese-English Edition)

赖小平　苏子仁　李远志　主编

羊城晚报出版社

·广州·

图书在版编目（CIP）数据

中国中成药大典：汉英版 / 赖小平，苏子仁，李远志主编. -- 广州：羊城晚报出版社，2011.3
ISBN 978-7-80651-877-9

Ⅰ.①中… Ⅱ.①赖… ②苏… ③李… Ⅲ.①中成药－汉、英 Ⅳ.①R286

中国版本图书馆CIP数据核字（2010）第205291号

中国中成药大典（汉英版）

Zhongguo Zhongchengyao Dadian (Hanyingban)

责任编辑 陈倩钜 黄捷生
责任技编 张广生
装帧设计 广东同文
责任校对 胡艺超
出版发行 羊城晚报出版社（广州市东风东路733号 邮编：510085）
发行部电话：（020）87133824
出 版 人 罗贻乐
经　　销 广东新华发行集团股份有限公司
印　　刷 广州市岭美彩印有限公司
（广州市荔湾区花地大道南海南工商贸易区A栋）
规　　格 889毫米×1194毫米 1/16 印张32.25 字数880千
版　　次 2011年3月第1版 2011年3月第1次印刷
书　　号 ISBN 978-7-80651-877-9/R·203
定　　价 120.00元

中国中成药大典

（汉英版）

Collection of Chinese Patent Medicines

（Chinese-English Edition）

主　　编　赖小平　苏子仁　李远志

副 主 编　晏亦林　何　柳　吴长海　王文楚
　　　　　陈建南

审　　订　李衍文

编　　委　（按姓氏拼音为序）
　　　　　陈　薇　冯耀文　赖志坚　黎　洪
　　　　　李光亮　欧阳强　苏碧茹　王德勤
　　　　　王建平　魏大华　温宪文　严志标
　　　　　曾惠芳

编写人员　（按姓氏拼音为序）
　　　　　暴梅佳　陈剑平　陈志维　何耀慧
　　　　　胡家敏　赖正权　黎玉翠　李一圣
　　　　　梁海春　梁远园　刘　尉　卢小凤
　　　　　彭绍忠　秦　臻　苏冀彦　武　文
　　　　　谢庆凤　易宇阳　周添浓

Collection of Chinese Patent Medicines
(Chinese-English Edition)

Editor-in-chief:

Lai Xiaoping Su Ziren Li Yuanzhi

Associate Chief Editors:

Yan Yilin He Liu Wu Changhai Wang Wenchu
Chen Jiannan

Reviser:

Li Yanwen

Editors:

Chen Wei Feng Yaowen Lai Zhijian Li Hong
Li Guangliang Ouyang Qiang Su Biru Wang Deqin
Wang Jianping Wei Dahua Wen Xianwen Yan Zhibiao
Zeng Huifang

Writers:

Bao Meijia Chen Jianping Chen Zhiwei He Yaohui
Hu Jiamin Lai Zhengquan Li Yucui Li Yisheng
Liang Haichun Liang Yuanyuan Liu Wei Lu Xiaofeng
Peng Shaozhong Qin Zhen Su Jiyan Wu Wen
Xie Qingfeng Yi Yuyang Zhou Tiannong

内容简介

本书收录中国中成药药品 1412 种。每种中成药设有名称，汉语拼音文字名称，处方，功能主治和注意五个栏目，按中文原意进行英译。本书基本涵盖了内、外、妇、儿科常见病治疗的常用中成药。编写目的是方便国外读者了解相关中成药的信息，如组方的药物内容和使用范围等；在国内则为制药厂家编写出口中成药资料或说明书时提供参考。

本书可供中成药制药厂家的外贸部门，技术部门，宣传广告部门和中医药院校的师生参考。

Introduction

This book collects 1412 Chinese patent medicines, each of which contains five columns both in Chinese and English, namely the name, name in Chinese phonetic alphabet, formula, actions and indications and warning. The collected Chinese patent medicines here include the major ones for the treatment of commonly encountered diseases of internal medicine, surgery, gynecology and pediatrics. The book is aimed to provide readers abroad with information on the related Chinese patent medicines, such as the compositions and indications of their prescriptions. Hopefully, it may serve as a reference for domestic pharmaceutical enterprises in compiling information or instructions for their export patent medicines; and it may also meet some research needs of teachers and students in medical colleges.

序

中成药（Chinese Patent Medicine）是以中草药为原料，经制剂加工制成各种不同剂型的中药制品。中成药因其疗效确切且便于储存、携带和使用，在当代社会中深受医生和患者的欢迎，在中药现代化和国际化发展中扮演着越来越重要的角色。

中成药是中药资源深度开发的重要形式，系由中药饮片依据中医治病的原则配方制成，其药物配方、制备工艺及剂型历经历代医药学家临床反复使用与验证而演变成型，可谓浓缩了历代中医有效方剂的精华。中成药源远流长，其肇始可上溯到中医早期典籍，至汉唐之间已初具轮廓。如《黄帝内经》已记载9种成药，涉及丸、散、膏、丹、药酒等剂型，《神农本草经》也有“药有宜丸者、宜散者”之记载。东汉著名医学家张仲景所撰《伤寒杂病论》为中国方书之祖，全书收载成药达60余种。东晋著名医学家葛洪编著的《肘后备急方》，记载了铅硬膏、蜡丸、锭剂、条剂、灸剂、尿道栓、饼剂等不少中成药剂型。唐代孙思邈所著《备急千金要方》收集了东汉至唐代约6300个医方，并依“处方”、“用药”、“合和”、“服饼”、“藏药”等分叙，述及中成药的生产工艺和质量控制。至宋代，中成药生产和推广进入了一个大发展时期。宋朝设立了“太医局卖药所”，为中国历史上第一个官办药局(即中成药制药厂)，还由官方编印了《太平惠民和剂局方》，收方788个，剂型有汤、丸、散、膏、丹、饼子、砂、锭、香等13种，实际上是建立了国家中成药标准规范。当时的中成药品种至宝丹、牛黄清心丸、苏合香丸、紫雪丹（丸）等一直流传至今。明清时期，中成药创制、生产和应用进入鼎盛时期。一方面，由于中医基础理论和临床各科进一步发展成熟，许多医家从医疗实践中总结研制了新的中成药品种；另一方面，随着商品经济的发展，“前店后坊”式的药铺不断涌现，其中一些逐步演变为专业的中成药生产企业。如创立于明代的山西广盛号药铺、广州陈李济药铺，创立于清代的北京同仁堂、苏州雷允上涌芬堂、杭州胡庆余堂等，所推出的龟龄集、安宫牛黄丸、乌鸡白凤丸、六神丸等名牌产品至今享誉不衰。

我国中成药产业已成为中国现代生物医药产业中极具活力的一个新兴领域。中华人民共和国成立之后，在政府的高度重视和大力扶持下，中国中成药行业从手工业生产逐步改造、发展为现代工业化生产体系，中成药的研制、生产、应用的科技含量和规范化水平也得到巨大的提升，尤其是中国实行改革开放以来，中成药产业以前所未有的速度迅猛发展，成为中医药产业中的主导产业。中成药作为临床安全有效、制备工艺合理、质量稳定可控且经批准依法生产的成方中药制剂，现已有40多个剂型、5000多个品种。如今，中成药在我国医疗保健中的使用量已逐渐超越中药传统饮片配方，并且在中药出口中占有重要地位，有些中成药品种已经在欧洲、亚洲、非洲等不同国家和地区作为药品合法注册。

进入21世纪以来，世界各国政府和国际组织对以中医药为代表的传统医药愈加重视，国际间传统医药科技合作和交流不断深化，中医药在世界范围的传播与影响日益扩大。国家科技部等国务院十六个部委局共同发布的《中医药创新发展规划纲要（2006-2020年）》，明确将“继承、创新、现代化、国际化”作为今后一段时期内中医药发展的基本任务，中医药现代化发展正呈现加速发展的势头。在此背景下，中医药对外翻译作为中医药国际化的一项基础性工作，近年开始得到各方面的关注和支持。有关中医药翻译论文论著大量增加，汉英（英汉）对照中医药教材、工具书也陆续出版，特别是中医用语英译国际标准化工作取得建设性进展，对于促进中医药全球信息共享，增进国际社会对中医药的理解和以中医药为代表的传统医药的推广应用发挥了重要作用。

尽管如此，目前中成药对外翻译的标准或研究专著尚付阙如，而所见的中成药英文说明书，对中成药名称、中草药名称的翻译不尽规范、准确，甚至仅以汉语拼音代之，有关药物用途(功能主治)的英文译法莫衷一是，且专业术语英译尚不规范，常令国外人士不明所以、无所适从。有鉴于此，我们从便利国外读者的阅读理解着眼，组织编纂本书，以期为中成药厂商对外宣传提供参考工具，也可供国外读者了解我国中成药基本信息之需。

本书的主要特点有三：1. 代表性。本书以《国家基本药物》所载中成药制剂品种目录为依据，精选我国基本中成药1412种作中英文对照介绍，可以说体现了我国中成药品种的整体面貌，传统中成药“名方名药”也尽在其中。2. 规范性。全书内容力求严谨、规范。书中中文内容严格遵循国家标准，所采用的英文中医术语主要参照全国科学技术名词审定委员会公布的《中医药学名词》和世界卫生组织(WHO)亚太西区2007年所公布的《传统医学名词术语国际标准》，对中成药处方组成药物反复校订正品并依《中华人民共和国药典》写明拉丁名称。3. 实用性。这是本书最大的特色。本书所拟中成药的英文名称力求既能体现中文原名又能“以名见义”，尽量使国外读者能看得懂并从名称中获得药物主要功能的信息。书中对中成药功能主治的英文介绍采用“中西并举”，“功能”以中医病名、证名主之，“主治”则以现代医学病名、术语解说。本书介绍每一种中成药的基本框架是中成药中英文名称、处方组成药物中文/拉丁名称、功能主治中英对照、注意事项(禁忌或毒副作用)中英文对照，虽未包括药品说明书的全部栏目，但足以提供该中成药最核心的信息。另外，本书还提供了三个附录，方便读者检索全书中成药英文名称、中药拉丁学名、中药英文名称之用。

中成药是我国医坛药苑中的一枝奇葩，也是世界医药文化的瑰宝。中成药的命名、遣方、修制、功能主治等，不仅蕴含中医药理论的深厚内涵，往往还浸染了中国历史文化的特殊意涵，在英文翻译实践中寻求相同或相近的对应语有时近乎奢望，本书编者在处理中成药名称英译时尤费思量，此中甘苦有不足为外人道者。诚望我们的努力和探索可以对中医药同行提供参考或启发，对关心中医药的国外朋友有所帮助，更期待海内外读者不吝批评指教，共同促进中成药对外翻译水平的提高，让中医药更好地造福全人类。

赖小平

2010年秋于广州中医药大学

Preface

Chinese patent medicines (also CPMs) are Chinese medicinal products with various dosage forms made of materia medica by means of preparation processes. Because of their excellent effectiveness and convenience in terms of storage, carrying and administration, nowadays CPMs have been well received by doctors and patients and are playing an increasingly important role in the procedures of modernization and internationalization of Chinese medicinal.

Processed with special herbal decocting pieces according to the therapeutic principles of traditional Chinese medicine (also TCM), CPMs have been deemed an vital form of further exploitation of Chinese medicinal resources. With their formulae, processing techniques and dosage forms applied and tested repeatedly by physicians and pharmaceutical researchers at all times, there is no exaggeration to say they are the essence of the experimental prescriptions of TCM throughout the ages. The history of CPMs can be traced back to the early classics of TCM, and their rudiments appeared between the Han and Tang Dynasties. For example, 9 CPMs were recorded in *Huangdi's Internal Classic* in forms of pill, powder, paste preparation, pellet, and medicated wine. Similarly, *Shennong's Classic of Materia Medica* said that drugs should be prepared as pills or powder for their respective purposes. And in *Treatise on Cold Damage and Miscellaneous Diseases*, the earliest book on Chinese medicinal formulae, *Zhang Zhongjing*, a celebrated doctor in the *Eastern Han* dynasty, has collected over 60 CPMs. In his *Handbook of Prescriptions for Emergencies*, *Ge Hong*, a noted physician in the *Eastern Jin* dynasty, mentioned respectable preparation forms including lead-plaster, waxed pill, pastille, medicinal strip, moxa cone or roll, urethral medical insertion, and pie preparation. Furthermore, in the *Tang* dynasty *Sun Simiao's Essential Prescriptions Worth a Thousand Gold for Emergencies* collected approximately 6300 formulas whose processing techniques and quality controls were stated from the aspects of "prescription", "usage", "compatibility", "*Fubing*", "storage", etc. When it came to the *Song* dynasty, the production and promotion of CPMs entered a booming era. The authorities established the first national drug administration in Chinese history named Taiyiju Maiyaosuo and published the *Prescriptions from the Great Peace Imperial Grace Pharmacy* containing 788 formulas with 13 dosage forms including decoction, pill, powder, paste preparation, pellet, pie preparation, granular preparation, pastille, aromatic preparation, which actually set up the national standard for CPMs. Some of these medicines, such as *Zhibao* Pellet, Bezoar Pill for Clearing Heart-fire, Storax Bolus, Heat-clearing and Convulsion-relieving Powder, have been passed down hitherto. And during the *Ming* and *Qing* Dynasties, CPMs witnessed prosperity in terms of their innovation, manufacture and application. For one thing, basing on the theoretical and clinical improvements of TCM, many doctors had developed numbers of new CPMs. For the other, many pharmacies that had been operated in the business model of "herbal medicine store in front with workshop behind" evolved into professional CPMs manufacturing enterprises, such as Guangsheng's Herbal Medicine Pharmacy in Shanxi Province (since the *Ming* dynasty), Chenliji's Herbal Medicine Pharmacy in Guangzhou (since the *Ming* dynasty), Tongrentang in Beijing (since the *Qing* dynasty), Lei Yunshang Yongfentang in Suzhou (since the *Qing* dynasty), Hu Qing Yu Tang in Hangzhou (since the *Qing* dynasty). Furthermore, these time-honored pharmaceutical enterprises have introduced many brand-new medicines that are still enjoying an extensive popularity today, like *Guiling* Tonic Capsule, *Angong* Bezoar Pill, Silky Chicken Bolus, Miraculous Pill of Six Ingredients.

At the present time, CPM has become a most dynamic and burgeoning branch of China's modern bioengineering and pharmaceutical industry. With ample governmental support since the foundation of the People's Republic of China, CPM industry has been reformed and advanced gradually from manual work to modern industrialized system, which brings on a huge upgrade in the sense of its technology and standardization. In particular after China's reform and opening up, it has developed into the leading industry of TCM at an unprecedented pace. There are over 5000 varieties of CPMs in more than 40 dosage forms available on the market, all of which are produced with governmental authorizations and have been proved safe and effective in clinical applications owing to their reasonable processes as well as the stable and controllable quality. What's more, the usage of CPMs has surpassed that of the traditional Chinese herbal decocting pieces formulas, taking an important place in the export of Chinese medicines. Some of them have even been registered as legitimate drugs in some countries and regions of Europe, Asia, and Africa.

In the 21st century, governments and organizations around the world are attaching more and more attention to traditional medicine represented by Chinese medicine, and international cooperation and communication in this field are continually deepened, which has, in return, boosted the spread and influence of Chinese medicine. In *The Plan for Innovation and Development of Chinese Medicine* (2006-2009), it is clarified that the fundamental tasks for the development of Chinese medicine in the coming years will be "inheritance, innovation, modernization, and internationalization", and that modernization of Chinese medicine is in an accelerating trend. Against such a background, TCM translation, as a fundamental task for the internationalization of Chinese medicine, has received much attention and support in many ways. Plenty of works and books on it have come forth and numbers of Chinese-English/English-Chinese TCM textbooks and references have been published in the recent years. All these achievements, together with the constructive progress in the international standardization for Chinese-English translation of TCM terminologies, are playing a significant role in facilitating the worldwide sharing of TCM information, enhancing international communities' understanding of TCM, and popularizing traditional medicine represented by TCM.

However, the current monographs on CPM translation standard are still wanting. This may explain the phenomenon that the name translations of CPMs and Chinese herbs are nonstandard or inaccurate, sometimes even substituted by Chinese Pinyin in many English CPM specifications; the translations of products' actions and indications and terminologies are so diverse that foreign customers can neither understand them nor distinguish the right from the wrong. Herein we did our utmost to organize and compile this book aiming to supply a reference for CPM manufacturers and foreign customers who expect to understand basic information of CPMs.

This book boosts three specialties. First, it's typical. Choicely, 1412 CPMs from the catalog of *National Essential Drugs* are introduced both in Chinese and English, and the book may be considered a representation of the whole status of CPMs including the renowned prescriptions. Second, it's normative. The Chinese contents in the book are strictly in line with the national standard while the English interpretations of TCM terminologies are mainly selected from the *Chinese Terms in Traditional Chinese Medicine and Pharmacy* published by China National Committee for Terms in Sciences and Technologies and *WHO International Standard Terminologies on Traditional Medicine in the Western Pacific Region* published by WHO in 2007. We repeatedly revised every ingredient herb of each CPM and indicated their corresponding Latin names according to the *Pharmacopoeia of the People's Republic of China*. Third, this book also features practicability. We strived to make the English name of each CPM reflect not only its original Chinese name but also its meaning, so as to enable foreign customers realize the main functions of the medicine from its name. In the book, functions and indications of CPMs are explained by means of both TCM and modern medicine terms. To be specific, functions are expressed with TCM terminologies, while indications with modern medicine ones. The basic framework of each item is comprised of the Chinese and English names of the CPM, the Chinese and Latin names of ingredient medicines, functions and indications, contraindications, toxic or side-effects both in Chinese and English. The most essential information of CPMs is involved in this book, although it does not offer all of the dispensatory contents. Moreover, the book contains three appendixes, namely *Key of CPMs, Key of Scientific Names of Chinese Medicinal* and *Key of Chinese Medicinal Names in English* which facilitates the retrieval of the relevant objects.

If we compare TCM to a beautiful garden, then CPM is one of the most splendid flowers blooming in it, and has enriched the great treasure house of the world medicine-culture. Since the nomenclature, recipe construction, preparing method, function and indication of CPMs contain not only profound TCM theories but also the connotations of Chinese historical culture, probably it is an extravagant wish to find identical or similar English words or expressions in translating practice. All the time in compiling this book, the translation of CPM names has been an arduous job for us. We sincerely hope our work will provide some reference or enlightenment for people who participate in Chinese medicine industry, and give some help to those foreign friends who are interested in TCM. We also highly appreciate any suggestion and comment from customers home and abroad, so as to promote the development of CPM translation jointly and make TCM contribute more to human health.

Lai Xiaoping
at Guangzhou University of Chinese Medicine
in the Autumn of 2010

目录

Contents

使用说明

1. 本书共收录我国基本中成药1412种，收录的中成药品种以2002年版《国家基本药物》中成药制剂品种目录为依据，并据该书的中文内容作相应英译。

2. 全书的排列次序以药名中文的首字笔画多少为顺序，首字排列顺序则依《辞海》笔画查字表顺序。首字笔画数相同者，以第一笔笔形一（横），丨（竖），丿（撇），丶（点），乛（折）为序。

3. 每种中成药设名称、汉语拼音文字名称、处方（不标示每种中草药的剂量）、功能主治和注意五个栏目。

4. 名称一栏通译为英文，包括含有中草药名称者，亦采用通用英文名称。凡剂型为丸剂者，大丸剂译为Bolus，小丸剂译为Pill。

5. 处方一栏所用的中草药名称均为拉丁文名称。其中，属2010年版《中华人民共和国药典》已收载的中草药，引用《药典》所载的拉丁文名称，如属《药典》未收载的，则参照《药典》命名法则自拟该药名称。

6. 本书所采用的英文中医术语，主要参照全国科学技术名词审定委员会公布的《中医药学名词》（Chinese Terms in Traditional Chinese Medicine and Pharmacy，2005年版）和WHO Western Pacific Region公布的《WHO International Standard Terminologies on Traditional Medicine in the Western Pacific Region》（2007年版）。

7. 注意事项一栏扼要简介该中成药的禁忌或毒副作用。

8. 本书所收录的中成药，少数品种出现原料有原动（植）物属于国家珍稀和保护野生动（植）物，注意使用时应严格遵照国家的有关规定。

9. 本书设有三个附录，方便读者检索中成药英文名称、中药拉丁学名、中药英文名称。

Guide to the Use of the Book

1. In this book, 1412 Essential CPMs are collected, all of which are selected from the catalog of CPM preparations in *National Essential Drugs* (2002 Edition), and each of which is illustrated bilingually in Chinese and English.

2. The sorting of the entries are arranged by the numbers of strokes of the first Chinese character of each patent medicine. If the stroke numbers of the first Chinese character are the same, then see the first stroke. Basing on Ci Hai, the stokes of calligraphy form are arranged as follows: horizontal stroke (一), vertical stroke (丨), left falling stroke (丿), dot stroke (丶) and turning stroke (乛).

3. Each entry contains five columns, namely CPM name, name of Chinese phonetic alphabet, formula (not including the dosage of each ingredient), actions and indications and warning.

4. CPM names (including those named after some Chinese medicinal) are translated into English. Pilular medicines in this book are named boluses and pills according to different sizes of medicines.

5. Names of herbal medicines in columns of "formula" are Latin names. Generally the names are based upon *Pharmacopoeia of the People's Republic of China* (2010 Edition, also *Pharmacopoeia*); in case of those not collected by *Pharmacopoeia*, their names are proposed according to the nomenclature rules in *Pharmacopoeia.*

6. The TCM terms used in the book are mainly from *Chinese Terms in Traditional Chinese Medicine and Pharmacy* examined and approved by National Commission of Science and Technology terms (2005 Edition) and *WHO International Standard Terminologies on Traditional Medicine in the Western Pacific Region* issued by WHO Western Pacific Region (2007 Edition).

7. Contraindications and side effects of the CPMs are briefly introduced in the "warning" column.

8. Some medicines mentioned in the book are derived from the national rare and protected animals (or plants), and their clinical application should conform to the state relative laws and regulations strictly.

9. Three appendixes are provided for readers' convenience of reference, including *Key of CPMs, Key of Scientific Names of Chinese Medicinals* and *Key of Chinese Medicinal Names in English.*

中成药名称笔画索引

Index of Strokes Numbers of the 1st Chinese Character of Each Patent Medicine

一画

二画

三画

四画

五画

六画

七画

八画

九画

十画

十一画

十二画

十三画

十四画

十五画

十六画

十七画

十八画

十九画

二十画

二十一画

一画

一捻金

【处方】大黄、牵牛子（炒）、槟榔、人参、朱砂。

【功能主治】消食导滞，祛痰，通便。用于小儿停乳停食，腹胀便秘，痰盛喘咳。

Yi Nian Jin Powder for Children

Name of Chinese Phonetic Alphabet Yi Nian Jin

Formula Rhei Radix et Rhizoma, Pharbitidis Semen (fried), Arecae Semen, Ginseng Radix et Rhizoma and Cinnabaris.

Actions and Indications Promoting digestion and removing food stagnation, dispelling phlegm and relaxing the bowels. It is used for children stagnant milk and food, dyspepsia, abdominal distention, constipation and productive cough.

一清胶囊

【处方】黄连、大黄、黄芩。

【功能主治】清热燥湿，泻火解毒。用于火毒血热所致的身热烦躁，目赤口疮，咽喉、牙龈肿痛，大便秘结。

【注意】忌烟、酒及辛辣、油腻食物。高血压、心脏病、肝病、糖尿病、肾病等慢性病患者慎用。小儿、孕妇、年老体弱及脾胃虚寒者慎用。

Yi Qing Capsule

Name of Chinese Phonetic Alphabet Yi Qing Jiao Nang

Formula Coptidis Rhizoma, Rhei Radix et Rhizoma and Scutellariae Radix.

Actions and Indications Clearing heat, drying dampness, purging fire, detoxifying. It is used for vexation, conjunctival congestion, aphthae, sore-throat, gingivitis and constipation due to fire toxin and blood-heat.

Warning Smoking, drinking, pungent and oily foods should be avoided. It should be used cautiously for cases with hypertension, heart disease, hepatopathy, diabetes, nephrosis, children, pregnant women, physical debility, the aged, and deficiency-cold of the spleen and stomach.

乙肝宁冲剂

【处方】黄芪、白花蛇舌草、茵陈、金钱草、党参、蒲公英、制何首乌、牡丹皮、丹参、茯苓、白芍、白术、川楝子。

【功能主治】调气健脾，清热利胆，活血化瘀。用于慢性迁延性肝炎、慢性活动性肝炎属湿热内蕴、肝郁脾虚、气虚血瘀者，对急性肝炎属此证者亦有一定疗效。

【注意】服药期间忌食油腻、辛辣食品。

Hepatitis B Relieving Soluble Granules

Name of Chinese Phonetic Alphabet Yi Gan Ning Chong Ji

Formula Astragali Radix, Hedyotis Diffusae Herba, Artemisiae Scopariae Herba, Lysimachiae Herba, Codonopsis Radix, Taraxaci Herba, Polygoni Multiflori Radix Praeparata, Moutan Cortex, Salviae Miltiorrhizae Radix et Rhizoma, Poria, Paeoniae Radix Alba, Atractylodis Macrocephalae Rhizoma and Toosendan Fructus.

Actions and Indications Regulating *qi*, fortifying the spleen, clearing heat, soothing the gallbladder, activating blood, resolving stasis. It is used for chronic persistent hepatitis and chronic active hepatitis attributed to stagnation of damp-heat in the interior, depression of the liver, deficiency of the spleen, *qi*-deficiency and blood-stasis. The preparation possesses certain effect for acute hepatitis.

Warning During medication, oily and pungent foods should be avoided.

乙肝养阴活血冲剂

【处方】本品为地黄、北沙参、麦冬、女贞子（酒制）、黄芪、当归、白芍等药经加工制成的冲剂。

【功能主治】滋补肝肾，活血化瘀。用于肝肾阴虚性慢性肝炎。症见面色晦暗，头晕耳鸣，五心烦热，腰退酸软，齿鼻衄，胁下痞块，舌质红，少苔，脉沉弦，细涩。

【注意】忌烟、酒、油腻，肝胆湿热、脾虚气滞者忌用。

Relieving Chronic Hepatitis Soluble Granules

Name of Chinese Phonetic Alphabet Yi Gan Yang Yin Huo Xue Chong Ji

Formula Rehmanniae Radix, Glehniae Radix, Ophiopogoins Radix, Ligustri Lucidi Fructus (prepared with wine), Astragali Radix, Angelicae Sinensis Radix, Paeoniae Radix Alba, etc.

Actions and Indications Nourishing and tonifying the liver and kidney, activating blood, resolving stasis. It is used for chronic hepatitis due to dual *yin*-deficiency of the liver and kidney and manifested as gloomy complexion, dizziness, tinnitus, vexing heat in the chest, palms and soles, soreness and weakness of waist and legs, epistaxis, gingival bleeding, hypochondriac mass, red tongue body, few tongue fur, sunken and string-like, fine and rough pulse.

Warning It is contraindicated for cases due to accumulation of damp-heat in the liver and gallbladder, deficiency of the spleen and stagnation of *qi*. Smoking, alcohol and oily foods should be avoided.

乙肝健

【处方】本品为花锚草、黄芪、甘草经加工制成的片剂。

【功能主治】利胆退黄，改善肝功，调节免疫功能。用于急、慢性乙型肝炎及其他肝炎。

Hepatitis B Relieving Tablet

Name of Chinese Phonetic Alphabet Yi Gan Jian

Formula Haleniae Corniculatae Herba, Astragali Radix and Glycyrrhizae Radix et Rhizoma.

Actions and Indications Soothing the gallbladder, relieving jaundice, improving liver function, regulating immunologic function. It is used for acute and chronic hepatitis B and other hepatitides.

乙肝清热解毒胶囊

【处方】虎杖、白花蛇舌草、土茯苓、茜草、北豆根、拳参、茵陈等。

【功能主治】清肝利胆，解毒。用于肝胆湿热型急、慢性病毒性乙型肝炎初起或活动期，乙型肝炎病毒携带者。症见黄疸（或无黄疸），发热（或低热），舌质红，舌苔厚腻，脉弦滑数，口干苦或黏臭，厌油，胃肠不适。

Relieving Hepatitis B Capsule

Name of Chinese Phonetic Alphabet Yi Gan Qing Re Jie Du Jiao Nang

Formula Polygoni Cuspidati Rhizoma et Radix , Hedyotis Diffusae Herba, Smilacis Glabrae Rhizoma, Rubiae Radix et Rhizoma, Menispermi Rhizoma, Bistortae Rhizoma, Artemisiae Scopariae Herba, etc.

Actions and Indications Clearing the liver- and gallbladder-fire, detoxicating. It is indicated for initial or active stage of acute and chronic viral hepatitis B of damp-heat type, HBV carriers, manifested as jaundice (or anicteric), fever (or low fever), red tongue body, thick and greasy tongue fur, string-like and slippery pulse, dry and bitter taste, stickiness and halitosis in the mouth, disgust at oily foods, gastrointestinal disturbance.

乙肝解毒胶囊

【处方】黄柏、草河车、黄芩、大黄、胡黄连、土茯苓、黑矾、绵马贯众。

【功能主治】清热解毒，疏肝利胆。用于乙型肝炎，辨证属于肝胆湿热内蕴者。临床表现为：肝区热痛，全身乏力，口苦咽干，头晕耳鸣或面红耳赤，心烦易怒，大便干结，小便少而黄，舌苔黄腻，脉滑数或弦数。

Detoxicating Capsule for Hepatitis B

Name of Chinese Phonetic Alphabet Yi Gan Jie Du Jiao Nang

Formula Phellodendri Chinensis Cortex, Paridis Rhizoma, Scutellariae Radix, Rhei Radix et Rhizoma, Picrohizae Rhizoma, Smilacis Glabrae Rhizoma, Melanteritum and Dryopteridis Crassirhizomatis Rhizoma.

Actions and Indications Clearing heat and detoxicating, Soothing the liver and gallbladder. It is used for hepatitis B attributive to damp-heat syndrome of the liver and gallbladder. Clinical manifestation: hepatalgia, fatigue, bitter taste in the mouth, dry throat, dizziness, tinnitus, flushed complexion, vexation, hard bound stool, scanty and yellow urine, yellow and greasy tongue fur, rapid and slippery pulse, or string-like and rapid pulse.

二画

二十五味沉香丸

【处方】沉香、丁香、木瓜、肉豆蔻、红花、广枣、藏木香、鹿角、乳香、木香、珍珠母、马钱子、诃子、木棉花、降香、牛黄、兔心、余甘子等。

【功能主治】调和气血，安神镇静。用于偏瘫，高血压，神志紊乱，口眼歪斜，肢体麻木，失眠。

Chinese Eaglewood* Pill

Name of Chinese Phonetic Alphabet Er Shi Wu Wei Chen Xiang Wan

Formula Aquilariae Lignum Resinatum, Caryophylli Flos, Chaenomelis Fructus, Myristicae Semen, Carthami Flos, Choerospondiatis Fructus, Inulae Radix, Cervi Cornu, Olibanum, Aucklandiae Radix, Margaritifera Concha, Strychni Semen, Chebulae Fructus, Gossampini Flos., Dalbergiae Odoriferi Lignum, Bovis Calculus, Cuniculi Cor, Phyllanthi Fructus, etc.

Actions and Indications Harmonizing *qi* and blood, tranquilizing the mind. It is indicated for hemiplegia, hypertension, unconsciousness, deviated mouth and eyes, numbness of limbs, insomnia.

*沉香

二十五味松石丸

【处方】珍珠、珊瑚、朱砂、诃子（去核）、铁屑（诃子制）、余甘子、五灵脂膏、檀香、降香、马兜铃、鸭嘴花、牛黄、广木香、绿绒蒿、船形乌头、肉豆蔻、丁香、伞梗虎耳草、毛诃子（去核）、天竺黄、西红花、木棉花、麝香等。

【功能主治】清热解毒，疏肝利胆、化瘀。用于肝郁气滞、血瘀、肝痛、肝硬化及各种急、慢性肝炎和胆囊炎。

Song Shi Pill for Relieving Hepatic Disorder

Name of Chinese Phonetic Alphabet Er Shi Wu Wei Song Shi Wan

Formula Margarita, Corallii Japonici Sceletus Calx, Cinnabaris, Chebulae Fructus (removed nucleus), Ferum Squamae (prepared with Myrobalan), Phyllanthi Fructus, Trogopterori Extractum, Santali Albi Lignum, Dalbergiae Odoriferae Lignum, Aristolochiae Fructus, Adhatodae Vasicae Ramulus et Folium, Bovis Calculus, Saussureae Lappae Radix, Meconopsis Integrifoliae Herba, Aconiti Navicularis Herba, Myristicae Semen, Caryophylli Flos, Saxifragae Umbellulatae Herba, Terminaliae Belliricae Fructus (removed nucleus), Bambusae Concretio Silicea, Croci Stigma, Gossampini Flos., Moschus, etc.

Actions and Indications Clearing heat and detoxicating, soothing the liver and gallbladder, resolving stasis. It is indicated for blood-stasis, hepatalgia, cirrhosis, acute and chronic hepatitis and cholecystitis due to liver depression and *qi*-stagnation.

二十五味珍珠丸

【处方】珍珠、肉豆蔻、草果、丁香、降香、豆蔻、诃子、檀香、余甘子、沉香、肉桂、螃蟹甲、毛诃子、冬葵果、木香、荜茇、金礞石、牛黄、红花、黑种草子、麝香等。

【功能主治】安神开窍。用于中风，半身不遂，癫痫，口眼歪斜，昏迷不醒，神志紊乱，谵语发狂。

Pearl* Pill

Name of Chinese Phonetic Alphabet Er Shi Wu Wei Zhen Zhu Wan

Formula Margarita, Myristicae Semen, Tsaoko Fructus, Caryophylli Flos, Dalbergiae Odoriferae Lignum, Amomi Fructus Rotundus, Chebulae Fructus, Santali Albi Lignum, Phyllanthi Fructus, Aquilariae Lignum Resinatum, Cinnamomi Cortex, Phlomidis Younghusbandii Radix, Terminaliae Belliricae Fructus, Malvae Fructus, Aucklandiae Radix, Piperis Longi Fructus, Micae Lapis Aureus, Bovis Calculus, Carthami Flos, Nigellae Semen, Moschus, etc.

Actions and Indications Tranquilizing the mind, opening orifices. It is used for apoplexy, hemiparalysis, epilepsy, deviated mouth and eyes, coma, unconsciousness, delirium, mania.

* 珍珠

二十五味珊瑚丸

【处方】诃子、木香、藏菖蒲、铁棒锤、麝香、珍珠母、珊瑚、珍珠、丁香、肉豆蔻、磁石、沉香、紫菀、禹余粮、芝麻壳、獐牙菜、炉甘石、银朱、龙骨、红花、甘草等。

【功能主治】开窍，通络，止痛，调和血压。用于顽固性头痛，脑炎，头晕目眩，肢体麻木僵硬，神志不清，抽风痉挛。

Coral* Pill

Name of Chinese Phonetic Alphabet Er Shi Wu Wei Shan Hu Wan

Formula Chebulae Fructus, Aucklandiae Radix, Acori Calami Rhizoma, Aconiti Penduli Radix, Moschus, Margaritifera Concha, Corallii Japonici Sceletus Calx, Margarita, Caryophylli Flos, Myristicae Semen, Magnetitum, Aquilariae Lignum Resinatum, Asteris Radix et Rhizoma, Limonitum, Sesami Pericarpium, Swertiae Herba, Calamina, Mercuric Sulfide, Draconis Os, Carthami Flos, Glycyrrhizae Radix et Rhizoma, etc.

Actions and Indications Opening the orifices, dredging collaterals, alleviating pain, regulating blood pressure. It is used for obstinate headache, encephalitis, dizziness, dizzy vision, numbness and rigidity of limbs, obnubilation, spasm.

* 珊瑚

二仙膏

【处方】人参、枸杞子、鹿角胶、龟甲胶、牛鞭（干）、黄芪（蜜炙）、熟地黄（砂仁拌）、制何首乌、五味子（酒制）、沙苑子（盐炒）、牛膝、核桃仁、黑芝麻（炒）、山药（炒）、远志（制）、丹参。

【功能主治】滋阴助阳，益气养血。用于治疗气血两虚，神疲体倦，周身懒软，神经衰弱。

Deerhorn Glue* and Tortoise Shell Glue** Thick Paste

Name of Chinese Phonetic Alphabet Er Xian Gao

Formula Ginseng Radix et Rhizoma, Lycii Fructus, Cervi Cornus Colla, Testudinis Carapacis et Plastri Colla, Bovis Testis et Penis (dried), Astragali Radix (prepared with honey), Rehmanniae Radix Praeparata (mixed with villous amomum fruit***), Polygoni Multiflori Radix Praeparata, Schisandrae Chinensis Fructus (prepared with wine), Astragali Complanati Semen (fried with salt), Achyranthis Bidentatae Radix, Juglandis Semen , Sesami Semen Nigrum (fried), Dioscoreae Rhizoma (fried), Polygalae

Radix (prepared) and Salviae Miltiorrhizae Radix et Rhizoma.

Actions and Indications Enriching *yin* and *yang*, tonifying *qi* and nourishing blood. It is used for lassitude of spirit, tiredness and neurasthenia due to dual deficiency of *qi* and blood.

* 鹿角胶 ** 龟甲胶 *** 砂仁

二母宁嗽丸

【处方】川贝母、知母、石膏、栀子（炒）、黄芩、桑白皮（蜜炙）、茯苓、瓜蒌子（炒）、陈皮、枳实（麸炒）、甘草（蜜炙）、五味子（蒸）。

【功能主治】清肺润燥，化痰止咳。用于燥热蕴肺，痰黄而黏不易咳出，胸闷气促，久咳不止，声哑喉痛。

Honeyed Bolus of Sichuan Fritillary* and Common Anemarrhena** for Relieving Cough

Name of Chinese Phonetic Alphabet Er Mu Ning Sou Wan

Formula Fritillariae Cirrhosae Bulbus, Anemarrhenae Rhizoma, Gypsum Fibrosum, Gardeniae Fructus (fried), Scutellariae Radix, Mori Cortex (prepared with honey), Poria, Trichosanthis Semen (fried), Citri Reticulatae Pericarpium, Aurantii Fructus Immaturus (fried with bran), Glycyrrhizae Radix et Rhizoma (prepared with honey) and Schisandrae Chinensis Fructus (steamed).

Actions and Indications Clearing lung-heat and moistening dryness, resolving phlegm and relieving cough. It is indicated for chronic cough due to dryness-heat of the lung and marked by yellow and sticky phlegm, difficult expectoration, chest upset and panting, hoarseness and sore-throat.

* 川贝母 ** 知母

二母安嗽丸

【处方】知母、玄参、罂粟壳、麦冬、款冬花、紫菀、苦杏仁、百合、浙贝母。

【功能主治】清肺化痰，止嗽定喘。用于虚劳久嗽，春秋举发，咳嗽痰喘，骨蒸潮热，音哑声重，口燥舌干，痰涎壅盛。

Alleviating Cough Bolus

Name of Chinese Phonetic Alphabet Er Mu An Sou Wan

Formula Anemarrhenae Rhizoma, Scrophulariae Radix, Papaveris Pericarpium, Ophiopogonis Radix, Farfarae Flos, Asteris Radix et Rhizoma, Armeniacae Semen Amarum, Lilii Bulbus and Fritillariae Thunbergii Bulbus.

Actions and Indications Clearing lung-fire, resolving phlegm, alleviating cough and dyspnea. It is indicated for consumptive disease, marked by prolonged cough, dyspnea, tidal fever, hoarseness, deep turbid voice, dry tongue and mouth and excessive phlegm.

二至丸

【处方】女贞子（蒸）、墨旱莲。

【功能主治】补益肝肾，滋阴止血。用于肝肾阴虚，眩晕耳鸣，咽干鼻燥，腰膝酸痛，月经量多。

Chinese Privet* and Eclipta** Pill

Name of Chinese Phonetic Alphabet Er Zhi Wan

Formula Ligustri Lucidi Fructus (steamed) and Ecliptae Herba.

Actions and Indications Tonifying the liver and kidney, enriching *yin* and relieving bleeding. It is used for vertigo, tinnitus, dry throat and nose, soreness and pain of waist and knees and hypermenorrhea due to dual *yin*-deficiency of the liver and kidney.

* 女贞 ** 鳢肠（墨旱莲）

二陈丸

【处方】陈皮、半夏（制）、茯苓、甘草。

【功能主治】燥湿化痰，理气和胃。用于咳嗽痰多，胸脘胀闷，恶心呕吐。

Er Chen Pill for Relieving Productive Cough

Name of Chinese Phonetic Alphabet Er Chen Wan

Formula Citri Reticulatae Pericarpium, Pinelliae Rhizoma (prepared), Poria and Glycyrrhizae Radix et Rhizoma.

Actions and Indications Drying dampness and resolving phlegm, regulating *qi* and harmonizing the stomach. It is indicated for cough with profuse phlegm, distention and oppression in the chest, nausea and vomiting.

二妙丸

【处方】苍术（炒）、黄柏（炒）。

【功能主治】清热燥湿。用于湿热下注，足膝红肿热痛，下肢丹毒，白带，阴囊湿痒。

Two Wonderful Medicinals Pill

Name of Chinese Phonetic Alphabet Er Miao Wan

Formula Atractylodis Rhizoma (fried) and Phellodendri Chinensis Cortex (fried).

Actions and Indications Clearing heat and drying dampness. It is used for red, swelling and pain of the feet and knees, erysipelas of the lower limbs, white vaginal discharge and itching of the scrotum due to downward attack of damp-heat.

十五味黑药丸

【处方】寒水石、食盐（炒）、烈香杜鹃、肉豆蔻、芫荽果、芒硝、硇砂、藏木香、荜茇、黑胡椒、干姜等。

【功能主治】散寒消食，破瘀消积。用于慢性肠胃炎，胃出血，消化不良，食欲不振，呕吐泄泻，腹部有痞块及嗳气频作。

Containing Fifteen Medicinals Pill for Soothing Stomach

Name of Chinese Phonetic Alphabet Shi Wu Wei Hei Yao Wan

Formula Gypsum Rubrum, Sal (fried), Rhododendri Anthoponoidis Folium, Myristicae Semen, Coriandri Sativi Fructus, Natrii Sulfas, Sal Ammoniacum, Inulae Radix, Piperis Longi Fructus, Piperis Fructus Nigrum, Zingiberis Rhizoma, etc.

Actions and Indications Dissipating cold and promoting digestion, breaking blood-stasis and dispersing stagnation. It is indicated for chronic gastroenteritis, gastrorrhagia, dyspepsia, anorexia, vomiting and diarrhea, abdominal mass and frequent eructation.

十全大补丸

【处方】党参、白术（炒）、茯苓、肉桂、甘草（蜜炙）、当归、川芎、白芍（酒炒）、熟地黄、黄芪（蜜炙）。

【功能主治】温补气血。用于气血两虚，面色苍白，气短心悸，头晕自汗，体倦乏力，四肢不温，月经量多。

【注意】外感风寒、风热，阴虚阳亢者不宜服用。

Ten Powerful Tonics Bolus

Name of Chinese Phonetic Alphabet Shi Quan Da Bu Wan

Formula Codonopsis Radix, Atractylodis Macrocephalae Rhizoma (fried), Poria, Cinnamomi Cortex, Glycyrrhizae Radix et Rhizoma (prepared with honey), Angelicae Sinensis Radix, Chuanxiong Rhizoma, Paeoniae Radix Alba (fried with wine), Rehmanniae Radix Praeparata and Astragali Radix (prepared with honey).

Actions and Indications Warming and tonifying *qi* and blood. It is indicated for dual deficiency of *qi* and blood marked by pale complexion, shortness of breath, palpitation, dizziness, spontaneous sweating, fatigue, cold limbs and hypermenorrhea.

Warning It is contraindicated for cases with wind-cold or wind-heat external contraction and *yin*-deficiency with *yang*-hyperactivity.

十味龙胆花颗粒

【处方】龙胆花、烈香杜鹃、甘草、矮紫堇、川贝母、小檗皮、鸡蛋参、螃蟹甲、藏木香、马尿泡。

【功能主治】清热化痰，止咳平喘。用于痰热壅肺所致的咳嗽、喘鸣、痰黄，或兼发热，流涕，咽痛，口渴，尿黄，便干等症。也可用于急性支气管炎，慢性支气管炎急性发作见以上证候者。

Scabrous Gentian Flower* Soluble Granules for Relieving Cough and Bronchitis

Name of Chinese Phonetic Alphabet Shi Wei Long Dan Hua Ke Li

Formula Gentianae Flos, Rhododendri Anthoponoidis Folium, Glycyrrhizae Radix et Rhizoma, Corydalis Pygmaeae Herba, Fritillariae Cirrhosae Bulbus, Berberidis Amurensis Cortex, Codonopsis Radix Convolvulaceae, Phlomidis Younghusbandii Radix, Inulae Radix and Pedicularidis Resupinatae Folium seu Radix.

Actions and Indications Clearing heat and resolving phlegm, relieving cough and calming dyspnea. It is indicated for cough, dyspnea, yellow phlegm, or accompanied by fever, rhinorrhea, sore-throat, thirst, yellow urine and dry stools due to phlegm-heat accumulating in the lung, also for acute bronchitis, acute attack of chronic bronchitis with the above mentioned symptoms.

* 龙胆花

十味蒂达胶囊

【处方】獐芽菜、熊胆等。

【功能主治】舒肝理气，清热解毒，利胆溶石。用于慢性胆囊炎，胆石症。

Di Da Capsule for Relieving Chronic Cholecystitis

Name of Chinese Phonetic Alphabet Shi Wei Di Da Jiao Nang

Formula Swertiae Herba, Ursi Fel, etc.

Actions and Indications Soothing the liver and regulating *qi*, clearing heat and detoxicating, draining bile and dissolving stone. It is indicated for chronic cholecystitis, cholelithiasis.

十香丸

【处方】沉香、木香、丁香、小茴香（炒）、香附（制）、陈皮、乌药、泽泻（盐水炒）、荔枝核（炒）、猪牙皂。

【功能主治】疏肝行气，散寒止痛。用于气滞寒凝的疝气、腹痛。

【注意】孕妇慎用。

Ten Aromatic Medicinals Pill

Name of Chinese Phonetic Alphabet Shi Xiang Wan

Formula Aquilariae Lignum Resinatum, Aucklandiae Radix, Caryophylli Flos, Foeniculi Fructus (freid), Cyperi Rhizoma (prepared), Citri Reticulatae Pericarpium, Linderae Radix, Alismatis Rhizoma (fried with salt water), Litchi Semen (fried) and Gleditsiae Fructus Abnormalis.

Actions and Indications Soothing the liver, moving *qi*, dissipating cold, alleviating pain. It is indicated for hernia and abdominal pain due to stagnation of qi and cold.

Warning It should be used cautiously for pregnant women.

十香返生丸

【处方】沉香、丁香、檀香、青木香、香附（醋炙）、降香、广藿香、乳香（醋炙）、天麻、僵蚕（麸炒）、郁金、莲子心、瓜蒌子（蜜炙）、金礞石（煅）、诃子、甘草、苏合香、安息香、麝香、冰片、朱砂、琥珀、牛黄。

【功能主治】开窍化痰，镇静安神。用于中风痰迷心窍引起：言语不清，神志昏迷，痰涎壅盛，牙关紧闭。

【注意】孕妇忌服。

Promoting-resuscitation Bolus

Name of Chinese Phonetic Alphabet Shi Xiang Fan Sheng Wan

Formula Aquilariae Lignum Resinatum, Caryophylli Flos, Santali Albi Lignum, Aristolochiae Radix, Cyperi Rhizoma (prepared with vinegar), Dalbergiae Odoriferae Lignum, Pogostemonis Herba, Olibanum (prepared with vinegar), Gastrodiae Rhizoma, Bombyx Batryticatus (fried with bran), Curcumae Radix, Nelumbinis Plumula, Trichosanthis Semen (prepared with honey), Micae Lapis Aureus (calcined), Chebulae Fructus, Glycyrrbizae Radix et Rhizoma, Styrax, Benzoinum, Moschus, Borneolum Syntheticum, Cinnabaris, Succinum and Bovis Calculus.

Actions and Indications Inducing resuscitation, resolving phlegm, tranquilizing the mind. It is used for alalia, coma, obstruction of phlegm and lockjaw due to stroke and phlegm clouding the pericardium.

Warning It is contraindicated for pregnant women.

十香暖脐膏

【处方】八角茴香、小茴香（盐炙）、乌药、木香、香附、当归、白芷、母丁香、肉桂、沉香、乳香（醋炙）、没药（醋炙）。

【功能主治】用于脾肾虚寒引起的脘腹冷痛，腹胀腹泻，腰痛寒疝，宫寒带下。

【注意】孕妇忌贴。

Shi Xiang Soft Extract for Warming Middle Energizer

Name of Chinese Phonetic Alphabet Shi Xiang Nuan Qi Gao

Formula Anisi Stellati Fructus, Foeniculi Fructus (prepared with salt), Linderae Radix, Aucklandiae Radix, Cyperi Rhizoma, Angelicae Sinensis Radix, Angelicae Dahuricae Radix, Caryophylli Fructus, Cinnamomi Cortex, Aquilariae Lignum Resinatum, Olibanum (prepared with vinegar) and Myrrha (prepared with vinegar).

Actions and Indications It is indicated for abdominal cold-pain, abdominal distention, diarrhea, lumbago, colicky pain around the umbilicus and uterus-coldness with vaginal discharge due to deficiency-cold of the spleen and kidney.

Warning It is contraindicated for pregnant women.

十滴水

【处方】樟脑、干姜、大黄、小茴香、肉桂、辣椒、桉油。

【功能主治】健胃，祛风。用于因中暑而引起的头晕、恶心、腹痛、胃肠不适。

【注意】孕妇忌服。

Ten-drip Tincture

Name of Chinese Phonetic Alphabet Shi Di Shui

Formula Camphora, Zingiberis Rhizoma, Rhei Radix et Rhizoma, Foeniculi Fructus, Cinnamomi Cortex, Capsici Fructus and Eucalypti Oleum.

Actions and Indications Fortifying the stomach, dispelling wind. It is indicated for dizziness, nausea, abdominal pain, gastrointestinal disturbance due to summer-heat stroke.

Warning It is contraindicated for pregnant women.

丁蔻理中丸

【处方】丁香、豆蔻、党参、白术（炒）、干姜、甘草（蜜炙）。

【功能主治】温中散寒，补脾健胃。用于脾胃虚寒，脘腹挛痛，呕吐泄泻，消化不良。

【注意】忌食生冷油腻，感冒发热者忌服。

Clove* and Krervanh** Pill for Warming Middle Energizer

Name of Chinese Phonetic Alphabet Ding Kou Li Zhong Wan

Formula Caryophylli Flos, Amomi Fructus

Rotundus, Codonopsis Radix, Atractylodis Macrocephalae Rhizoma (fried), Zingiberis Rhizoma and Glycyrrhizae Radix et Rhizoma (prepared with honey).

Actions and Indications Warming the middle energizer and dissipating cold, tonifying the spleen and fortifying the stomach. It is indicated for abdominal pain and spasm, vomiting, diarrhea and indigestion due to deficiency-cold of the spleen and stomach.

Warning It is contraindicated for cases with common cold, and uncooked and oily foods should be avoided.

*丁香 **豆蔻

七十味珍珠丸

【处方】本品由珍珠、檀香、降香、西红花、牛黄、麝香等药加工制成的丸剂。

【功能主治】安神，镇静，通经活络，调和气血，醒脑开窍。用于中风、瘫痪、半身不遂、癫痫、脑出血、脑震荡、心脏病、高血压。

Seventy Medicinals Including Pearl* Pill

Name of Chinese Phonetic Alphabet Qi Shi Wei Zhen Zhu Wan

Formula Margarita, Santali Albi Lignum, Dalbergiae Odoriferae Lignum, Croci Stigma, Bovis Calculus, Moschus, etc.

Actions and Indications Tranquilizing the mind, dredging meridians, activating collaterals, harmonizing *qi* and blood, inducing resuscitation. It is used for apoplexy, paralysis, hemiparalysis, epilepsy, cerebral hemorrhage, concussion of brain, heart disease, hypertension.

*珍珠

七叶神安片

【处方】本品为三七叶提取的总皂苷。

【功能主治】益气安神，活血止痛，止血。用于心气不足，失眠、心悸、胸痹心痛，或肿瘤、痈肿疮毒及出血。

*Sanchi** Leaf Tablet

Name of Chinese Phonetic Alphabet Qi Ye Shen An Pian

Formula Total saponin from Notoginseng Folium.

Actions and Indications Tonifying *qi*, tranquilizing the mind, activating blood, alleviating pain and relieving bleeding. It is indicated for insomnia, palpitation, chest impediment syndrome, heart pain or tumor, abscess, sore and ulcer and hemorrhage due to insufficiency of heart-*qi*.

*三七

七味红花殊胜丸

【处方】红花、天竺黄、獐牙菜、诃子、麻黄、木香、马兜铃、五脉绿绒蒿。

【功能主治】清热消炎，保肝退黄。用于肝病、劳伤引起的肝肿大、巩膜黄染、食欲不振。

Safflower* Pill for Relieving Jaundice

Name of Chinese Phonetic Alphabet Qi Wei Hong Hua Shu Sheng Wan

Formula Carthami Flos, Bambusae Concretio Silicea, Swertiae Herba, Chebulae Fructus, Ephedrae Herba, Aucklandiae Radix, Aristolochiae Fructus and Meconopsidis Quintuplinerviae Flos.

Actions and Indications Clearing heat and antiphlogistic, protecting the liver and relieving jaundice. It is indicated for hepatomegaly, icteric sclera and anorexia due to hepatic diseases and over fatigue.

*红花

七制香附丸

【处方】香附（醋制）、鲜牛乳、地黄、茯苓、当归、熟地黄、川芎、白术（麸炒）、白芍、益母草、艾叶（炭）、黄芩、山茱萸（酒制）、天冬、阿胶、酸枣仁（炒）、小茴香（盐制）、人参、甘草、食盐。

【功能主治】开郁顺气，调经养血。用于气滞经闭，胸闷气郁，两胁胀满，饮食减少，四肢无力，腹内作痛，寒湿白带。

Nut-grass* Pill

Name of Chinese Phonetic Alphabet Qi Zhi Xiang Fu Wan

Formula Cyperi Rhizoma (prepared with vinegar), Vaccae Lac, Rehmanniae Radix, Poria, Angelicae Sinensis Radix, Rehmanniae Radix Praeparata, Chuanxiong Rhizoma, Atractylodis Macrocephalae Rhizoma (fried with bran), Paeoniae Radix Alba, Leonuri Herba, Artemisiae Argyi Folium Carbonisatus, Scutellariae Radix, Corni Fructus (prepared with wine), Asparagi Radix, Asini Corii Colla, Ziziphi Spinosae Semen (fried), Foeniculi Fructus (prepared with salt), Ginseng Radix et Rhizoma, Glycyrrhizae Radix et Rhizoma and Sal.

Actions and Indications Relieving depression, arranging *qi*, regulating menstruation, and nourishing blood. It is used for amenorrhea, depression in chest, fullness of hypochondrium, poor appetite, weakness of extremities, abdominal pain and white vaginal discharge due to stagnation of *qi*.

*莎草

七宝美髯颗粒

【处方】制何首乌、当归、补骨脂（黑芝麻炒）、枸杞子（酒蒸）、菟丝子（炒）、茯苓、牛膝（酒蒸）。

【功能主治】滋补肝肾。用于肝肾不足而引起的须发早白，遗精早泄，头眩耳鸣，腰酸背痛。

Blackening Beard and Hair Soluble Granules

Name of Chinese Phonetic Alphabet Qi Bao Mei Ran Ke Li

Formula Polygoni Multiflori Radix Praeparata, Angelicae Sinensis Radix, Psoraleae Fructus (fried with black sesame), Lycii Fructus (steamed by wine), Cuscutae Semen (fried), Poria and Achyranthis Bidentatae Radix (steamed by wine).

Actions and Indications Enriching the liver and kidney. It is indicated for premature graying of beard and hair, nocturnal emission, premature ejaculation, dizziness, tinnitus and soreness of waist due to dual insufficiency of liver and kidney.

七珍丸

【处方】僵蚕、全蝎、胆南星、天竺黄、麝香、朱砂、雄黄、巴豆霜等。

【功能主治】息风镇惊，豁痰开窍，消积通便。用于小儿饮食不节，食积伤中，积热内生，热极化风而致的惊风抽搐，面目红赤，高热神昏，痰涎壅盛，伴有呕吐、便秘者，常见舌苔厚腻，脉弦滑数。

【注意】体虚及泄泻者忌用。不宜久服。

Qi Zhen Pill

Name of Chinese Phonetic Alphabet Qi Zhen Wan

Formula Bombyx Batryticatus, Scorpio, Arisaema cum Bile, Bambusae Concretio Silicea, Moschus, Cinnabaris, Realgar, Crotonis Semen Pulveratum, etc.

Actions and Indications Extinguishing wind, settling fright, expelling phlegm, opening orifices, promoting digestion and bowels movement. It is used for improper diet of children, indigestion, accumulation of heat, convulsive tic, flushed complexion and congested eyes, high fever, obnubilation, excessive phlegm, vomiting, constipation, thick and greasy tongue coating, string-like, slippery and rapid pulse.

Warning It is contraindicated for physical debility and diarrhea. Long-term medication is prohibited.

七厘散

【处方】血竭、乳香（制）、没药（制）、红花、儿茶、冰片、麝香、朱砂。

【功能主治】化瘀消肿，止痛止血。用于跌扑损伤，血瘀疼痛，外伤出血。

【注意】孕妇禁用。

Qi Li Powder for Traumatic Injury

Name of Chinese Phonetic Alphabet Qi Li San

Formula Draconis Sanguis, Olibanum (prepared), Myrrha (prepared), Carthami Flos, Catechu, Borneolum Syntheticum, Moschus and Cinnabaris.

Actions and Indications Resolving stasis, reducing swelling, relieving pain and bleeding. It is used for traumatic injury with blood-stasis and pain, traumatic bleeding.

Warning It is contraindicated for pregnant women.

八正合剂

【处方】瞿麦、车前子（炒）、萹蓄、大黄、滑石、川木通、栀子、甘草、灯心草。

【功能主治】清热，通淋，通尿。用于湿热下注，小便短赤，淋沥涩痛，口燥咽干。

Ba Zheng Mixture for Relieving Strangury

Name of Chinese Phonetic Alphabet Ba Zheng He Ji

Formula Dianthi Herba, Plantaginis Semen (fried), Polygoni Avicularis Herba, Rhei Radix et Rhizoma, Talcum, Clematidis Armandii Caulis, Gardeniae Fructus, Glycyrrhizae Radix et Rhizoma and Junci Medulla.

Actions and Indications Clearing heat, relieving strangury and inducing urine. It is indicated for scanty dark urine, dribbling and painful urination, dry mouth and throat due to downward attack of damp-heat.

八宝丹

【处方】珍珠、象皮、龙骨、炉甘石、牛黄、冰片。

【功能主治】生肌敛疮，清热解毒。用于治疗疮疡溃后，脓毒不敛之症。

【注意】孕妇禁服。忌食辛辣。

Ba Bao Pill

Name of Chinese Phonetic Alphabet Ba Bao Dan

Formula Margarita, Elephantis Corium, Draconis Os, Calamina, Bovis Calculus and Borneolum Syntheticum.

Actions and Indications Promoting tissue regeneration and astringing, clearing heat and detoxicating. It is used for unconvergence of pus after diabrosis of sore.

Warning It is contraindicated for pregnant women and pungent foods should be avoided.

八珍丸

【处方】党参、白术（炒）、茯苓、甘草、当归、白芍、川芎、熟地黄。

【功能主治】补气益血。用于气血两虚，面色萎黄，食欲不振，四肢乏力，月经过多。

Eight Precious Medicinals Bolus

Name of Chinese Phonetic Alphabet Ba Zhen Wan

Formula Codonopsis Radix, Atractylodis Macrocephalae Rhizoma (fried), Poria, Glycyrrhizae Radix et Rhizoma, Angelicae Sinensis Radix, Paeoniae Radix Alba, Chuanxiong Rhizoma and Rehmanniae Radix Praeparata.

Actions and Indications Tonifying blood and *qi*. It is indicated for dual deficiency of *qi* and blood marked by sallow complexion, poor appetite, weakness of limbs and hypermenorrhea.

八珍益母丸

【处方】益母草、党参、白术（炒）、茯苓、甘草、当归、白芍（酒炒）、川芎、熟地黄。

【功能主治】补气血，调月经。用于妇女气血两虚，体弱无力，月经不调；又治行经腹痛，白带过多，腰酸倦怠，不思饮食。

Bolus of Chinese Motherwort* and Eight Medicinals

Name of Chinese Phonetic Alphabet Ba Zhen Yi Mu Wan

Formula Leonuri Herba, Codonopsis Radix, Atractylodis Macrocephalae Rhizoma (fried), Poria, Glycyrrhizae Radix et Rhizoma, Angelicae Sinensis Radix, Paeoniae Radix Alba (fried with wine), Chuanxiong Rhizoma and Rehmanniae Radix Praeparata.

Actions and Indications Tonifying *qi* and blood, regulating menstruation. It is indicated for debility and irregular menstruation of women due to dual deficiency of *qi* and blood, also for abdominal pain during menstruation, excessive white vaginal discharge, soreness of waist, tiredness and poor appetite.

* 益母草

人参归脾丸

【处方】人参、白术（麸炒）、茯苓、甘草（蜜炙）、黄芪（蜜炙）、当归、木香、远志（甘草炙）、龙眼肉、酸枣仁（炒）。

【功能主治】益气补血，健脾养心。用于心脾两虚，气血不足所致的心悸、怔忡，失眠健忘，食少体倦，面色萎黄以及脾不统血所致的便血、崩漏、带下诸症。

Ginseng*Bolus for Fortifying Spleen and Nourishing Blood

Name of Chinese Phonetic Alphabet Ren Shen Gui Pi Wan

Formula Ginseng Radix et Rhizoma, Atractylodis Macrocephalae Rhizoma (fried with bran), Poria, Glycyrrhizae Radix et Rhizoma (prepared with honey), Astragali Radix (prepared with honey), Angelicae Sinensis Radix, Aucklandiae Radix, Polygalae Radix (prepared with licorice root), Longan Arillus and Ziziphi Spinosae Semen (fried).

Actions and Indications Tonifying *qi* and blood, fortifying the spleen and nourishing the heart. It is indicated for palpitation, fearful throbbing, insomnia, amnesia, poor appetite, tiredness and sallow complexion due to dual deficiency of the heart and spleen, and insufficiency of *qi* and blood; hematochezia, metrorrhagia and vaginal discharge due to the spleen failing to control the blood.

* 人参

人参再造丸

【处方】人参（去芦）、广藿香、细辛、地龙、香附（醋制）、熟地黄、三七、青皮、乳香（醋制）、片姜黄、豆蔻、防风、没药（醋制）、甘草、川芎、黄芪、僵蚕（炒）、桑寄生、黄连、茯苓、骨碎补（炒）、制附子、赤芍、大黄、白术（麸炒）、威灵仙、葛根、麻黄、何首乌（制）、草豆蔻、全蝎、琥珀、蕲蛇（黄酒浸制）、天竺黄、沉香、天麻、六神曲（麸炒）、胆南星、绵萆薢、麝香、朱砂（水飞）、母丁香、檀香、玄参、豹骨（制）、肉桂、白芷、当归、水牛角浓缩粉、龟甲（制）、羌活、橘红、牛黄、乌药、冰片、血竭。

【功能主治】祛风化痰，活血通络。用于中风口眼歪斜，半身不遂，手足麻木，疼痛，拘挛，言语不清。

【注意】孕妇忌用。

Ginseng* Pill for Relieving Apoplexy

Name of Chinese Phonetic Alphabet Ren Shen Zai Zao Wan

Formula Ginseng Radix (removed rhizome), Pogostemonis Herba, Asari Radix et Rhizoma, Pheretima, Cyperi Rhizoma (prepared with vinegar), Rehmanniae Radix Praeparata, Notoginseng Radix et Rhizoma, Citri Reticulatae Pericarpium Viride, Olibanum (prepared with vinegar), Wenyujin Rhizoma Concisum, Amomi Fructus Rotundus, Saposhnikoviae Radix, Myrrha (prepared with vinegar), Glycyrrhziae Radix et Rhizoma, Chuanxiong Rhizoma, Astragali Radix, Bombyx Batryticatus (fried), Taxilli Herba, Coptidis Rhizoma, Poria, Drynariae Rhizoma (fried), Aconiti Lateralis Radix Praeparata, Paeoniae Radix Rubra, Rhei Radix et Rhizoma, Atractylodis

Macrocephalae Rhizoma (fried with bran), Clematidis Radix et Rhizoma, Puerariae Lobatae Radix, Ephedrae Herba, Polygoni Multiflori Radix Praeparata, Alpiniae Katsumadai Semen, Scorpio, Succinum, Agkistrodon (immersed in wine), Bambusae Concretio Silicea, Aquilariae Lignum Resinatum, Gastrodiae Rhizoma, Medicata Massa Fermentata (fried with bran), Arisaema cum Bile, Dioscoreae Spongiosae Rhizoma, Moschus, Cinnabaris (ground with water), Caryophylli Fructus, Santali Albi Lignum, Scrophulariae Radix, Pardi Os (prepared), Cinnamomi Cortex, Angelicae Dahuricae Radix, Angelicae Sinensis Radix, Bubali Cornu Pulvis Concentratio, Testudinis Carapax et Plastrum (prepared), Notopterygii Rhizoma et Radix, Citri Exocarpium Rubrum, Bovis Calculus, Linderae Radix, Borneolum Syntheticum and Draconis Sangui.

Actions and Indications Dispelling wind, resolving phlegm, activating blood, dredging collaterals. It is used for apoplexy, deviated eyes and mouth, hemiparalysis, pain, spasm and numbness of extremities, alalia.

Warning It is contraindicated for pregnant women.

*人参

人参固本丸

【处方】人参、地黄、熟地黄、山茱萸（酒炙）、山药、泽泻、牡丹皮、茯苓、麦冬、天冬。

【功能主治】滋阴益气，固本培元。用于阴虚气弱，虚劳咳嗽，心悸气短，骨蒸潮热，腰酸耳鸣，遗精盗汗，大便干燥。

Ginseng* Bolus for Strengthening Body Resistance

Name of Chinese Phonetic Alphabet Ren Shen Gu Ben Wan

Formula Ginseng Radix et Rhizoma, Rehmanniae Radix, Rehmanniae Radix Praeparata, Corni Fructus (prepared with wine), Dioscoreae Rhizoma, Alismatis Rhizoma, Moutan Cortex, Poria, Ophiopogonis Radix and Asparagi Radix.

Actions and Indications Enriching *yin* and tonifying *qi*, strengthening body resistance and source *qi*. It is indicated for consumptive disease, cough, palpitation, shortness of breath, tidal fever, soreness of waist, tinnitus, nocturnal emission, night sweating and dry stool due to deficiency of *qi* and *yin*.

*人参

人参保肺丸

【处方】人参、罂粟壳、五味子（醋制）、川贝母、陈皮、砂仁、枳实、麻黄、石膏、甘草、玄参、苦杏仁（去皮炒）。

【功能主治】益气补肺，止咳嗽定喘。用于肺气虚弱，津液亏损引起的虚痨久嗽，气短喘促等症。

【注意】感冒咳嗽者忌服。

Ginseng* Bolus for Improving Consumptive Disease

Name of Chinese Phonetic Alphabet Ren Shen Bao Fei Wan

Formula Ginseng Radix et Rhizoma, Papaveris Pericarpium, Schisandrae Chinensis Fructus (prepared with vinegar), Fritillariae Cirrhosae Bulbus, Citri Reticulatae Pericarpium, Amomi Fructus, Aurantii Fructus Immaturus, Ephedrae Herba, Gypsum Fibrosum, Glycyrrhizae Radix et Rhizoma, Scrophulariae Radix and Armeniacae Semen Amarum (removed seed coat and fried).

Actions and Indications Tonifying *qi* and the lung, relieving cough and calming dyspnea. It is used for consumptive disease, chronic cough, shortness of breath due to deficiency of lung-*qi* and body fluid depletion.

Warning It is contraindicated for cases with cough due to common cold.

*人参

人参首乌胶囊

【处方】红参、制何首乌。

【功能主治】补肝肾，益气血。用于气血虚弱，须发早白，神经衰弱，健忘失眠，食欲不振，疲劳过度。

【注意】高血压及动脉硬化等症忌服。

Ginseng★ and Chinese Knotweed★★ Capsule

Name of Chinese Phonetic Alphabet Ren Shen Shou Wu Jiao Nang

Formula Ginseng Radix et Rhizoma Rubra and Polygoni Multiflori Radix Praeparata.

Actions and Indications Tonifying the liver and kidney, *qi* and blood. It is indicated for deficiency of *qi* and blood, premature graying of hair, neurasthenia, amnesia, insomnia, poor appetite and over tiredness.

Warning It is contraindicated for hypertension and arteriosclerosis.

* 人参 ** 何首乌

人参养荣丸

【处方】人参、白术（土炒）、茯苓、甘草（蜜炙）、当归、熟地黄、白芍（麸炒）、黄芪（蜜炙）、陈皮、远志（制）、肉桂、五味子（酒蒸）。

【功能主治】温补气血。用于心脾不足，气血两亏，形瘦神疲，食少便溏，病后虚弱。

Ginseng★ Bolus for Tonifying *Qi* and Blood

Name of Chinese Phonetic Alphabet Ren Shen Yang Rong Wan

Formula Ginseng Radix et Rhizoma, Atractylodis Macrocephalae Rhizoma (fried with earth), Poria, Glycyrrhizae Radix et Rhizoma (prepared with honey), Angelicae Sinensis Radix, Rehmanniae Radix Praeparata, Paeoniae Radix Alba (fried with bran), Astragali Radix (prepared with honey), Citri Reticulatae Pericarpium, Polygalae Radix (prepared), Cinnamomi Cortex and Schisandrae Chinensis Fructus (steamed by wine).

Actions and Indications Warming and tonifying *qi* and blood. It is indicated for emaciation, lassitude of spirit, poor appetite, sloppy stool and copos due to dual insufficiency of the heart and spleen and dual deficiency of *qi* and blood.

* 人参

人参健脾丸

【处方】人参、白术（麸炒）、茯苓、山药、陈皮、木香、砂仁、黄芪（蜜炙）、当归、酸枣仁（炒）、远志（制）。

【功能主治】健脾益气，和胃止泻。用于脾胃虚弱引起的饮食不化，倒饱嘈杂，恶心呕吐，腹痛便溏，不思饮食，体弱倦怠。

Ginseng★ Bolus for Fortifying Spleen

Name of Chinese Phonetic Alphabet Ren Shen Jian Pi Wan

Formula Ginseng Radix et Rhizoma, Atractylodis Macrocephalae Rhizoma (fried with bran), Poria, Dioscoreae Rhizoma, Citri Reticulatae Pericarpium, Aucklandiae Radix, Amomi Fructus, Astragali Radix (prepared with honey), Angelicae Sinensis Radix, Ziziphi Spinosae Semen (fried) and Polygalae Radix (prepared).

Actions and Indications Fortifying the spleen and tonifying *qi*, harmonizing the stomach and relieving diarrhea. It is used for indigestion, gastric upset, nausea, vomiting, abdominal pain, sloppy stool, anorexia, debility and tiredness due to dual deficiency of the spleen and stomach.

* 人参

儿宝颗粒

【处方】太子参、北沙参、茯苓、山药、山楂（炒）、麦芽（炒）、陈皮、白芍（炒）、白扁豆（炒）、麦冬、葛根（煨）。

【功能主治】健脾益气，生津开胃。用于小儿面黄体弱，纳呆厌食，脾虚久泻，精神不振，口干燥渴，盗汗等症。

Children Precious Soluble Granules

Name of Chinese Phonetic Alphabet Er Bao Ke Li

Formula Pseudostellariae Radix, Glehniae Radix, Poria, Dioscoreae Rhizoma, Crataegi Fructus (fried), Hordei Fructus Germinatus (fried), Citri Reticulatae Pericarpium, Paeoniae Radix Alba (fried), Lablab Semen Album (fried), Ophiopogonis Radix and Puerariae Lobatae Radix (roasted).

Actions and Indications Fortifying the spleen and tonifying *qi*, engendering fluid and promoting appetite. It is used for children with sallow complexion and physical debility, loss of appetite and anorexia, chronic diarrhea due to deficiency of the spleen; lassitude, dry mouth and thirst, night sweating.

儿康宁

【处方】党参、黄芪、白术、茯苓、山药、薏苡仁、麦冬、制首乌、大枣、焦山楂、炒麦芽、桑枝。

【功能主治】益气健脾，和中开胃。用于儿童身体瘦弱，消化不良，食欲不佳。

Appetite-promoving Oral Liquid for Children

Name of Chinese Phonetic Alphabet Er Kang Ning

Formula Codonopsis Radix, Astragali Radix, Atractylodis Macrocephalae Rhizoma, Poria, Dioscoreae Rhizoma, Coicis Semen, Ophiopogonis Radix, Polygoni Multiflori Radix Praeparata, Jujubae Fructus, Crataegi Fructus (charred), Hordei Fructus Germinatus (fried) and Cinnamomi Ramulus.

Actions and Indications Tonifying *qi* and fortifying the spleen, harmonizing the middle and promoting appetite. It is used for children thinness, dyspepsia and poor appetite.

儿童咳液

【处方】紫菀、百部、枇杷叶、前胡、甘草、苦杏仁、桔梗、麻黄、蓼大青叶。

【功能主治】清热润肺，宣降肺气，祛痰止咳。用于咳嗽气喘，吐痰黄稠或咳痰不爽，咽干喉痛，急、慢性气管炎。

Oral Liquid for Relieving Children Cough

Name of Chinese Phonetic Alphabet Er Tong Ke Ye

Formula Asteris Radix et Rhizoma, Stemonae Radix, Eriobotryae Folium, Peucedani Radix, Glycyrrhizae Radix et Rhizoma, Armeniacae Semen Amarum, Platycodonis Radix, Ephedrae Herba and Polygoni Tinctorii Folium.

Actions and Indications Clearing heat and moistening the lung, diffusing and downbearing lung-*qi*, dispelling phlegm and alleviating cough. It is indicated for cough and dyspnea, yellow and thick phlegm or difficult expectoration, dry throat, sore-throat, acute, chronic trachitis.

儿童清肺口服液

【处方】麻黄、苦杏仁（炒）、石膏、甘草、桑白皮（蜜炙）、瓜蒌皮、黄芩、板蓝根、橘红、法半夏、紫苏子（炒）、葶苈子、浙贝母、紫苏叶、细辛、薄荷、枇杷叶（蜜炙）、白前、前胡、石菖蒲、天花粉、青礞石（煅）。

【功能主治】清肺，化痰，止嗽。用于小儿肺经痰热，面赤身热，咳嗽气促，痰多黏稠，咽痛声哑。

Children Oral Liquid for Resolving Phlegm and Relieving Cough

Name of Chinese Phonetic Alphabet Er Tong Qing Fei Kou Fu Ye

Formula Ephedrae Herba, Armeniacae Semen Amarum (fried), Gypsum Fibrosum, Glycyrrhizae Radix et Rhizoma, Mori Cortex (prepared with honey), Trichosanthis Pericarpium, Scutellariae Radix, Isatidis Radix, Citri Exocarpium Rubrum, Pinelliae Rhizoma Praeparatum, Perillae Fructus (fried), Lepidii Semen, Fritillariae Thunbergii Bulbus, Perillae Folium, Asari Radix et Rhizoma, Menthae Haplocalycis Herba, Eriobotryae Folium (prepared with honey), Cynanchi

Stauntonii Rhizoma et Radix, Peucedani Radix, Acori Tatarinowii Rhizoma, Trichosanthis Radix and Chloriti Lapis (calcined).

Actions and Indications Clearing lung-heat resolving phlegm and allevating cough. It is used for infantile phlegm-heat of lung meridian, red face and fever, cough and dyspnea, profuse thick and sticky phlegm, sore-throat and hoarseness .

儿童清热口服液

【处方】金银花、蝉蜕、石膏、滑石、黄芩、大黄、赤芍、板蓝根、广藿香、羚羊角。

【功能主治】清热解毒，解肌退热。用于内蕴伏热、外感时邪引起的咽喉肿痛、大便秘结等症。

Heat-clearing Oral Liquid for Children

Name of Chinese Phonetic Alphabet Er Tong Qing Re Kou Fu Ye

Formula Lonicerae Japonicae Flos, Cicadae Periostracum, Gypsum Fibrosum, Talcum, Scutellariae Radix, Rhei Radix et Rhizoma, Paeoniae Radix Rubra, Isatidis Radix, Pogostemonis Herba and Saigae Tataricae Cornu .

Actions and Indications Clearing heat and detoxicating, releasing the muscles and reducing fever. It is used for sore-throat, constipation due to internal accumulation of heat and invasion of exogenous seasonal pathogens.

儿童清热导滞丸

【处方】鸡内金（醋制）、莪术（醋制）、厚朴（姜制）、枳实、山楂（焦）、青皮（醋制）、半夏（制）、六神曲（焦）、麦芽（焦）、槟榔（焦）、榧子、使君子（仁）、胡黄连、苦楝皮、知母、青蒿、黄芩（酒制）、薄荷、车前子（盐制）、钩藤。

【功能主治】健胃导滞，消积化虫。用于小儿蓄乳宿食引起的胸膈满闷，积聚痞块，虫积腹痛，面黄肌瘦，消化不良，烦躁口渴，不思饮食。

Fortifying Stomach Pill for Dyspepsia

Name of Chinese Phonetic Alphabet Er Tong Qing Re Dao Zhi Wan

Formula Galli Gigerii Endothelium Corneum (prepared with vinegar), Curcumae Rhizoma (prepared with vinegar), Magnoliae Officinalis Cortex (prepared with ginger), Aurantii Fructus Immaturus, Crataegi Fructus (charred), Citri Reticulatae Pericarpium Viride (prepared with vinegar), Pinelliae Rhizoma (prepared), Medicata Massa Fermentata (charred), Hordei Fructus Germinatus (charred), Arecae Semen (charred), Torreyae Semen, Quisqualis Semen, Picrorhizae Rhizoma, Meliae Cortex, Anemarrhenae Rhizoma, Artemisiae Annuae Herba, Scutellariae Radix (prepared with wine), Menthae Haplocalycis Herba, Plantaginis Semen (prepared with salt) and Uncariae Ramulus cum Uncis.

Actions and Indications Fortifying the stomach and removing food stagnation, expelling worms. It is used for children hypochondriac fullness, parasite, abdominal pain, sallow complexion, emaciation, dyspepsia, vexation, thirst and anorexia due to milk and food accumulation.

九气拈痛丸

【处方】香附（醋制）、木香、高良姜、陈皮、郁金、莪术（醋制）、延胡索（醋制）、槟榔、甘草、五灵脂（醋炒）。

【功能主治】理气，活血，止痛。用于胸胁胀满疼痛，痛经。

【注意】孕妇禁用。

Dysmenorrhea-relieving Pill

Name of Chinese Phonetic Alphabet Jiu Qi Nian Tong Wan

Formula Cyperi Rhizoma (prepared with vinegar), Aucklandiae Radix, Alpiniae Officinarum Rhizoma, Citri Reticulatae Pericarpium, Curcumae Radix, Curcumae Rhizoma (prepared with vinegar), Corydalis Rhizoma (prepared with vinegar), Arecea Semen, Glycyrrhizae Radix et Rhizoma and

Trogopterori Faeces (fried with vinegar).

Actions and Indications Regulating *qi*, activating blood, alleviating pain. It is indicated for fullness and pain in hypochondrium, dysmenorrhea.

Warning It is contraindicated for pregnant women.

九分散

【处方】马钱子粉（制）、麻黄、乳香（制）、没药（制）。

【功能主治】活血散瘀，消肿止痛。用于跌扑损伤，瘀血肿痛。

【注意】本品含剧毒药，不可多服；孕妇禁用。

Jiu Fen Powder for Traumatic Injury

Name of Chinese Phonetic Alphabet Jiu Fen San

Formula Strychni Semen Pulvis (prepared), Ephedrae Herba, Olibanum (prepared), and Myrrha (prepared).

Actions and Indications Activating blood, dissipating stasis, reducing swelling, alleviating pain. It is used for traumatic injury marked by blood-stasis, swelling and pain.

Warning The preparation contains hypertoxicity, over dosage is prohibited; and it is contraindicated for pregnant women.

九味羌活冲剂

【处方】羌活、防风、苍术、细辛、川芎、白芷、黄芩、甘草、地黄。

【功能主治】解表除湿。用于恶寒发热，无汗，头痛口干，肢体酸痛。

Incised Notopterygium* Soluble Granules

Name of Chinese Phonetic Alphabet Jiu Wei Qiang Huo Chong Ji

Formula Notopterygii Rhizoma et Radix, Saposhnikoviae Radix, Atractylodis Rhizoma, Asari Radix et Rhizoma, Chuanxiong Rhizoma, Angelicae Dahuricae Radix, Scutellariae Radix, Glycyrrhizae Radix et Rhizoma and Rehmanniae Radix.

Actions and Indications Releasing the exterior and eliminating dampness. It is used for cases with aversion to cold, fever, anhidrosis, headache, dry mouth, soreness and pain of limbs.

* 羌活

九制大黄丸

【处方】大黄。

【功能主治】通便润燥，消食化滞。用于胃肠积滞，湿热下痢，口渴不休，胸热心烦，大便燥结，小便赤黄。

【注意】孕妇忌服，久病体弱者慎用。

Prepared Rhubarb* Pill

Name of Chinese Phonetic Alphabet Jiu Zhi Da Huang Wan

Formula Rhei Radix et Rhizoma (The rhubarb prepared with yellow millet wine and the concentrative extract of Platycladi Cacumen, Sophorae Fructus, Plantaginis Semen, Magnoliae Officinalis Cortex, Citri Reticulatae Pericarpium, etc).

Actions and Indications Relaxing the bowels, moistening dryness, promoting digestion to relieve food retention. It is indicated for gastrointestinal stagnation and dysentery due to damp-heat; thirst, dysphoria, hard and bound stool and yellow dark urine.

Warning It is contraindicated for pregnant women and should be used carefully for cases with chronic disease and debility.

* 大黄

九宝丸

【处方】麻黄、紫苏叶、葛根、前胡、桔梗、陈皮、枳壳（去瓤麸炒）、枳实、木香、法半夏、六神曲（麸炒）、麦芽、甘草。

【功能主治】解表止嗽，消食化痰。用于小儿肺热宿滞，外感风寒引起的头痛身热，鼻流清涕，咳嗽痰盛，呕吐食水，夜卧不安。

Jiu Bao Pill

Name of Chinese Phonetic Alphabet Jiu Bao Wan

Formula Ephedrae Herba, Perillae Folium, Puerariae Lobatae Radix, Peucedani Radix, Platycodonis Radix, Citri Reticulatae Pericarpium, Aurantii Fructus (removed pulp and fried with bran), Aurantii Fructus Immaturus, Aucklandiae Radix, Pinelliae Rhizoma Praeparatum, Medicata Massa Fermentata (fried with bran), Hordei Fructus Germinatus and Glycyrrhizae Radix et Rhizoma.

Actions and Indications Releasing the exterior and relieving cough, promoting digestion and resolving phlegm. It is indicated for children headache and generalized fever, clear nasal discharge, productive cough, watery vomitus and disturbed sleep due to stagnation of lung-heat and exogenous wind-cold.

三画

三十五味沉香丸

【处方】沉香、香樟、白沉香、檀香、丁香、诃子（去核）、降香、天竺黄、红花、肉豆蔻、豆蔻、草果、毛诃子（去核）、余甘子（去核）、木香、广枣、藏木香、悬钩木、宽筋藤、山柰、木棉花、马钱子、乳香、安息香、石榴子、铁棒锤、牛心、麝香等。

【功能主治】清瘟热，祛风，益肺，利痹。用于疠、热相搏引起的疾病，热病初起，肺痼疾，咳嗽气逆，痹症，疑难的气血上壅。

Thirty-five Medicinals Including Chinese Eaglewood* Pill

Name of Chinese Phonetic Alphabet San Shi Wu Wei Chen Xiang Wan

Formula Aquilariae Lignum Resinatum, Cinnamomi Camphorae Radix, Ilicis Rotundae Cortex, Santali Albi Lignum, Caryophylli Flos, Chebulae Fructus (removed nucleus), Dalbergiae Odoriferae Lignum, Bambusae Concretio Silicea, Carthami Flos, Myristicae Semen, Amomi Fructus Rotundus, Tsaoko Fructus, Terminaliae Belliricae Fructus (removed nucleus), Phyllanthi Fructus (removed nucleus), Aucklandiae Radix, Choerospondiatis Fructus, Inulae Radix, Rubi Corchorifolii Caulis, Cissi Hexangularis Caulis, Kaempferiae Rhizoma, Gossampini Flos, Strychni Semen, Olibanum, Benzoinum, Granati Semen, Aconiti Penduli Radix, Bovis Cor, Moschus, etc.

Actions and Indications Clearing pestilential heat, dispelling wind, tonifying the lung, relieving impediment disease. It is used for initial stage of heat syndrome, stubborn chronic disease of lung, cough, impediment syndrome, diseases of upward adverse flow of qi and blood.

*沉香

三七伤药片

【处方】三七、草乌（蒸）、雪上一枝蒿、冰片、骨碎补、红花、接骨木、赤芍。

【功能主治】舒筋活血，散瘀止痛。用于急慢性挫伤、扭伤、关节痛、神经痛、跌打损伤。

【注意】本品药性强烈，应按规定量服用。孕妇忌用。有心血管疾病患者慎用。

Sanchi* Tablet for Traumatic Injury

Name of Chinese Phonetic Alphabet San Qi Shang Yao Pian

Formula Notoginseng Radix et Rhizoma, Aconiti Kusnezoffii Radix (steamed), Aconiti Kongboensis Radix, Borneolum Syntheticum, Drynariae Rhizoma, Carthami Flos, Sambuci Williamsii Ramulus and Paeoniae Radix Rubra.

Actions and Indications Relaxing sinews, activating blood, dissipating stasis, alleviating pain. It is indicated for acute, chronic sprain and contusion, arthralgia, neuralgia, traumatic injury.

Warning It is contraindicated for pregnant women and should be used cautiously for cases with angiocardiopathy. Over dosage is prohibited.

＊三七

三七血伤宁胶囊

【处方】三七、重楼、山药、冰片、生草乌、朱砂、藜芦、大叶紫珠及提取物。

【功能主治】止血镇痛，祛瘀生新。用于瘀血阻滞、血不归经之各种血证及瘀血肿痛，如胃、十二指肠溃疡出血，支气管扩张出血，肺结核咯血，功能性子宫出血，外伤及痔疮出血，妇女月经不调，经痛，经闭及月经血量过多，产后瘀血，胃痛，肋间神经痛。

【注意】服药期间忌食蚕豆、鱼类和酸冷食物。孕妇忌服。

Sanchi⋆ Capsule for Hemorrhagic Syndrome

Name of Chinese Phonetic Alphabet San Qi Xue Shang Ning Jiao Nang

Formula Notoginseng Radix et Rhizoma, Paridis Rhizoma, Dioscoreae Rhizoma, Borneolum Syntheticum, Aconiti Kusnezoffii Radix (fresh), Cinnabaris, Veratri Radix et Rhizoma and Callicarpae Macrophyllae Folium (extract).

Actions and Indications Relieving bleeding, settling pain, dispelling stasis, promoting tissue regeneration. It is used for various hemorrhagic syndromes such as bleeding due to gastric and duodenal ulcer, bleeding due to bronchiectasis, hemoptysis due to pulmonary tuberculosis, dysfunctional uterine bleeding, traumatic bleeding, hemorrhoidal bleeding, irregular menstruation, dysmenorrhea, amenorrhea, menorrhagia, puerperal blood-stasis, stomach pain and intercostal neuralgia due to blood failing to stay in the merdian.

Warning It is contraindicated for pregnant women. During medication, broad bean, fish, sour and cold foods should be avoided.

＊三七

三七冠心宁胶囊

【处方】本品为三七浸膏制成的胶囊。

【功能主治】活血益气，宣畅心阳，疏通心脉，蠲除淤阻。用于胸痹或心脉淤阻所致之胸闷、心痛、气促、心悸。

【注意】本品不适用于心绞痛急性发作。

Sanchi⋆ Capsule for Chest Impediment

Name of Chinese Phonetic Alphabet San Qi Guan Xin Ning Jiao Nang

Formula Notoginseng Extractum.

Actions and Indications Activating blood, tonifying *qi*, diffusing heart-*yang*, dredging heart vessels, eliminating stasis. It is used for chest distress, cardialgia, shortness of breath and palpitation due to stagnation of heart vessels.

Warning The preparation is unsuitable for acute attack of angina pectoris.

＊三七

三七胶囊

【处方】三七。

【功能主治】散瘀止血，消肿定痛。用于咯血，吐血，衄血，便血，崩漏，外伤出血，胸腹刺痛，跌扑肿痛。

【注意】孕妇忌服。

Sanchi⋆ Capsule for Relieving Hemorrhage

Name of Chinese Phonetic Alphabet San Qi Jiao Nang

Formula Notoginseng Radix et Rhizoma.

Actions and Indications Dissipating stasis, relieving hemorrhage, reducing swelling, alleviating pain. It is used for hemoptysis, spitting blood, epistaxis, hematochezia, metrorrhagia, traumatic bleeding, stabbing pain of chest and abdomen, traumatic injury with swelling and pain.

Warning It is contraindicated for pregnant

women.

*三七

三九胃泰颗粒

【处方】三叉苦、九里香、两面针、木香、黄芩、茯苓、地黄、白芍。

【功能主治】消炎止痛，理气健胃。用于浅表性胃炎，糜烂性胃炎。

【注意】胃寒患者慎用。

San Jiu Soluble Granules for Relieving Gastritis

Name of Chinese Phonetic Alphabet San Jiu Wei Tai Ke Li

Formula Euodiae Leptae Folium, Murrayae Folium et Cacumen, Zanthoxyli Radix, Aucklandiae Radix, Scutellariae Radix, Poria, Rehmanniae Radix and Paeoniae Radix Alba.

Actions and Indications Antiphlogistic and alleviating pain, regulating *qi* and fortifying the stomach. It is indicated for superficial gastritis and erosive gastritis.

Warning It should be used carefully for cases with stomach-cold.

三号蛇胆川贝片

【处方】蛇胆（干）、川贝母、法半夏、黄连、甘草。

【功能主治】清热，祛痰，止咳。用于邪热蕴肺，肺失宣降所致的咳嗽咯痰，或久咳痰多，咯吐不利。

Forest Cobra Gall* and Sichuan Fritillary** Tablet

Name of Chinese Phonetic Alphabet San Hao She Dan Chuan Bei Pian

Formula Naja Fel (dried), Fritillariae Cirrhosae Bulbus, Pinelliae Rhizoma Praeparatum, Coptidis Rhizoma and Glycyrrhizae Radix et Rhizoma.

Actions and Indications Clearing heat, dispelling phlegm and relieving cough. It is indicated for productive cough, or chronic cough with profuse phlegm and difficult expectoration due to stagnation of heat pathogen in the lung, and the lung failing to purification.

*蛇胆 **川贝母

三妙丸

【处方】苍术（炒）、黄柏（炒）、牛膝。

【功能主治】燥湿清热。用于湿热下注，足膝红肿热痛，下肢沉重，小便黄少。

【注意】孕妇慎用。

Three Wonderful Medicinals Pill

Name of Chinese Phonetic Alphabet San Miao Wan

Formula Atractylodis Rhizoma (fried), Phellodendri Chinensis Cortex (fried) and Achyranthis Bidentatae Radix.

Actions and Indications Drying dampness and clearing heat. It is used for red, swelling, and pain of the feet and knees, heavy sensation of the lower limbs, scanty and yellow urine due to downward attack of damp-heat.

Warning It should be used carefully for pregnant women.

三金片

【处方】金樱根、菝葜、羊开口、金沙藤、积雪草。

【功能主治】清热解毒，利湿通淋，益肾。用于热淋，小便短赤，淋沥涩痛；急、慢性肾盂肾炎，膀胱炎，尿路感染属肾虚湿热下注证者。

San Jin Tablet for Relieving Strangury

Name of Chinese Phonetic Alphabet San Jin Pian

Formula Rosae Laevigatae Radix, Smilacis Chinae Rhizoma, Akebiae Fructus, Lygodii Flexuosi

Herba and Centellae Herba.

Actions and Indications Clearing heat and detoxicating, draining dampness and relieving strangury, replenishing the kidney. It is indicated for heat strangury, scanty dark urine, dribbling and painful urination, acute, chronic pyelonephritis, cystitis, urinary tract infection due to downward attack of damp-heat and kidney defficiency.

三黄片

【处方】大黄、盐酸黄连素、黄芩总苷。

【功能主治】清热解毒，泻火通便。用于三焦热盛，目赤肿痛，口鼻生疮，咽喉肿痛，牙龈出血，心烦口渴，尿黄便秘，急性胃肠炎，痢疾。

【注意】孕妇慎用。

Three-yellow Tablet for Purging Fire

Name of Chinese Phonetic Alphabet San Huang Pian

Formula Rhei Radix et Rhizoma, Berberine Hydrochloride and Total Saponins of Scutellariae Radix.

Actions and Indications Clearing heat and detoxicating, purging fire and relaxing the bowels. It is indicated for conjunctival congestion, aphthae, sore-throat, gingival bleeding, vexation, thirst, yellow urine, constipation, acute gastroenteritis and dysentery due to exuberant heat in triple energizers.

Warning It should be used cautiously for pregnant women.

三蛇胆川贝糖浆

【处方】蛇胆汁、川贝母、桑白皮、麻黄、枇杷叶、桔梗、牛白藤、白薇、肿节风、百部、薄荷油。

【功能主治】清热润肺，化痰止咳。用于痰热咳嗽。

Syrup of Forest Cobra Bile* and Sichuan Fritillary**

Name of Chinese Phonetic Alphabet San She Dan Chuan Bei Tang Jiang

Formula Naja Bilis, Fritillariae Cirrhosae Bulbus, Mori Cortex, Ephedrae Herba, Eriobotryae Folium, Platycodonis Radix, Hedyotidis Hedyotideae Caulis et Folium, Cynanchi Atrati Radix et Rhizoma, Sarcandrae Herba, Stemonae Radix, Menthae Haplocalycis Oleum.

Actions and Indications Clearing heat and moistening the lung, resolving phlegm and alleviating cough. It is indicated for cough due to phlegm-heat.

* 蛇胆汁 ** 川贝母

三鞭参茸固本丸

【处方】鹿鞭（烫）、驴鞭、狗鞭（烫）、鹿茸、人参、淫羊藿、枸杞子、山茱萸、菟丝子、杜仲、女贞子、制何首乌、茯苓。

【功能主治】补气养血，助阳添精，强筋壮骨。用于身体虚弱，气血双亏，腰腿酸软，阳痿，遗精早泄。

【注意】有外感实热者忌服。

Ginseng* and Pilose Deerhorn** Pill

Name of Chinese Phonetic Alphabet San Bian Shen Rong Gu Ben Wan

Formula Cervi Penis (scalded), Asini Testis et Penis (scalded), Canis Testis et Penis (scalded), Cervi Cornu Pantotrichum, Ginseng Radix et Rhizoma, Epimedii Folium, Lycii Fructrs, Corni Fructus, Cuscutae Semen, Eucommiae Cortex, Ligustri Lucidi Fructus, Polygoni Multiflori Radix Praeparata and Poria.

Actions and Indications Tonifying *qi*, nourishing blood, supporting *yang* and essence, strengthening the sinews and bone. It is used for debility of constitution, soreness and weakness of waist and legs, impotence, nocturnal emission and ejaculation praecox due to dual depletion of *qi* and blood.

Warning It is contraindicated for cases with exogenous excess heat.

* 人参 ** 鹿茸

下乳涌泉散

【处方】当归、白芍、桔梗、川芎、地黄、白芷、天花粉、甘草、柴胡、通草、漏芦、麦芽、穿山甲（烫）、王不留行（炒）。

【功能主治】养血催乳。用于产后少乳。

Lactation-promoting Powder

Name of Chinese Phonetic Alphabet Xia Ru Yong Quan San

Formula Angelicae Sinensis Radix, Paeoniae Radix Alba, Platycodonis Radix, Chuanxiong Rhizoma, Rehmanniae Radix, Angelicae Dahuricae Radix, Trichosanthis Radix, Glycyrrhizae Radix et Rhizoma, Bupleuri Radix, Tetrapanacis Medulla, Rhapontici Radix, Hordei Fructus Germinatus, Manis Squma (scalded) and Vaccariae Semen (fried).

Actions and Indications Nourishing blood and promoting lactation. It is indicated for puerperal oligogalactia.

大七厘散

【处方】大黄（酒制）、骨碎补、硼砂（煅）、血竭、当归尾（酒制）、乳香（煅）、没药（煅）、三七、冰片、自然铜（煅，醋淬）、土鳖虫（甘草制）。

【功能主治】化瘀消肿，止痛止血。用于跌打损伤，瘀血疼痛，外伤止血。

【注意】孕妇忌服，但可外用。

Major *Qi Li* Powder for Traumatic Injury

Name of Chinese Phonetic Alphabet Da Qi Li San

Formula Rhei Radix et Rhizoma (prepared with wine), Drynariae Rhizoma, Borax (calcined), Draconis Sanguis, Angelicae Sinensis Radix (tail part and prepared with wine), Olibanum (calcined), Myrrha (calcined), Notoginseng Radix et Rhizoma, Borneolum Syntheticum, Pyritum (calcined and quenched by vinegar) and Eupolyphaga seu Steleophaga (prepared with licorice root).

Actions and Indications Resolving stasis, reducing swelling, alleviating pain, relieving bleeding. It is used for traumatic injury with blood-stasis and pain and traumatic bleeding.

Warning It is contraindicated for pregnant women, but can be used externally.

大山楂冲剂

【处方】山楂、麦芽（炒）、六神曲（焦）。

【功能主治】开胃消食。用于食欲不振，消化不良，脘腹胀闷。

Chinese Hawthorn* Soluble Granules for Promoting Appetite

Name of Chinese Phonetic Alphabet Da Shan Zha Chong Ji

Formula Crataegi Fructus, Hordei Fructus Germinatus (fried) and Medicata Massa Fermentata (charred).

Actions and Indications Promoting digestion. It is used for poor appetite, dyspepsia and abdominal distention.

* 山楂

大川芎颗粒

【处方】川芎、天麻。

【功能主治】活血化瘀，平肝息风。主治头风及瘀血型头痛。症见头痛、脑胀、眩晕、颈项紧张不舒、上下肢及偏身麻木、舌部瘀斑。

【注意】重症患者请遵医嘱服用；外感头痛、孕妇、出血性脑血管急性期患者忌用。

Chuanxiong Ligusticum* and Gastrodia** Granules

Name of Chinese Phonetic Alphabet Da Chuan Xiong Ke Li

Formula Chuanxiong Rhizoma and Gastrodiae Rhizoma.

Actions and Indications Activating blood, resolving stasis, pacifying the liver and extinguishing wind. It is used for obstinate headache and blood-stasis type headache manifested as dizziness, rigidity of neck, numbness of limbs, hemilateral numbness and ecchymosis on the tongue.

Warning Severe cases should follow the physician's advice. It is contraindicated for pregnant women, headache due to external contraction and acute stage of hemorrhagic cerebrovascular disease.

* 川芎 ** 天麻

大补阴丸

【处方】熟地黄、知母（盐炒）、黄柏（盐炒）、龟甲（制）、猪脊髓。

【功能主治】滋阴降火。用于阴虚火旺，潮热盗汗，咳嗽咯血，耳鸣遗精。

Major Tonifying *Yin* Bolus

Name of Chinese Phonetic Alphabet Da Bu Yin Wan

Formula Rehmanniae Radix Praeparata, Anemarrhenae Rhizoma (fried with salt), Phellodendri Chinensis Cortex (fried with salt), Testudinis Carapax et Plastrum (prepared) and Suillus Spinalis Medulla.

Actions and Indications Enriching *yin*, downbearing fire. It is indicated for tidal fever, night sweating, cough, hemoptysis, tinnitus and nocturnal emission due to *yin*-deficiency with effulgent fire.

大枫子油

【处方】大枫子油、硼酸、冰片。

【功能主治】祛风除湿，润肤止痒。用于雀斑粉刺，酒渣鼻子，疥癣，鹅掌风。

【注意】外用药，切勿入口。

Chaulmoogra-tree* Oil

Name of Chinese Phonetic Alphabet Da Feng Zi You

Formula Hydnocarpi Anthelmintici Semen Oleum, Boric acid and Borneolum Syntheticum.

Actions and Indications Dispelling wind and dampness, moistening skin and relieving itching. It is used for freckle acne, rosacea, scabies, tinea and tinea manuum.

Warning It is for external use only.

* 大枫子

大活络丸

【处方】乌梢蛇、蕲蛇、麻黄、两头尖、威灵仙、绵马贯众、甘草、羌活、僵蚕（炒）、广藿香、乌药、黄连、没药（制）、大黄、木香、沉香、天南星（制）、赤芍、松香、丁香、乳香（制）、肉桂、细辛、青皮、白术（麸炒）、豆蔻、安息香、黄芩、香附（醋制）、玄参、何首乌、防风、龟甲（醋淬）、葛根、血竭、当归、虎骨（油酥）、地龙、犀角、麝香、熟地黄、牛黄、冰片、红参、制草乌、天麻、全蝎、骨碎补（烫、去毛）。

【功能主治】祛风止痛，除湿豁痰，舒筋活络。用于中风痰厥引起的瘫痪，足痿痹痛，筋脉拘急，腰腿疼痛及跌打损伤，行走不便，胸痹症。

【注意】孕妇忌服。

Major Collateral-activating Pill

Name of Chinese Phonetic Alphabet Da Huo Luo Wan

Formula Zaocys, Agkistrodon, Ephedrae Herba, Anemones Raddeanae Rhizoma, Clematidis Radix et Rhizoma, Dryopteridis Crassirhizomatis Rhizoma, Glycyrrhizae Radix et Rhizoma, Notopterygii Rhizoma et Radix, Bombyx Batryticatus (fried), Pogostemonis Herba, Linderae Radix, Coptidis Rhizoma, Myrrha (prepared), Rhei Radix et Rhizoma, Aucklandiae Radix, Aquilariae Lignum Resinatum, Arisaematis Rhizoma (prepared), Paeoniae Radix Rubra, Pini Resina, Caryophylli Flos, Olibanum (prepared), Cinnamomi Cortex, Asari Radix et Rhizoma, Citri Reticulatae Pericarpium Viride, Atractylodis Macrocephalae Rhizoma (fried with bran), Amomi Fructus Rotundus, Benzoinum, Scutellariae Radix, Cyperi Rhizoma (prepared with vinegar), Scrophularia Radix, Polygoni Multiflori Radix, Saposhnikoviae Radix, Testudinis Carapax et Plastrum (quenched by vinegar), Puerariae Lobatae Radix, Draconis Sanguis, Angelicae Sinensis Radix, Tigris Os (crisped by oil), Pheretima, Rhinocerotis Asiatici Cornu, Moschus, Rehmanniae Radix Praeparata, Bovis Calculus, Borneolum Syntheticum, Ginseng Radix et Rhizoma Rubra, Aconiti Kusnezoffii Radix Cocta, Gastrodiae Rhizoma, Scorpio and Psoraleae Fructus (scalded and removed hair).

Actions and Indications Dispelling wind, alleviating pain, eliminating dampness, expectorating phlegm, relaxing sinews, activating collaterals. It is indicated for paralysis due to apoplexy; leg wilting, muscular spasm, pain of waist and legs, injury due to fall and strike, difficult walking and chest impediment syndrome.

Warning It is contraindicated for pregnant women.

大黄䗪虫丸

【处方】熟大黄、土鳖虫（炒）、水蛭（制）、干漆（煅）、蛴螬（炒）、苦杏仁（炒）、地黄、白芍、黄芩、桃仁、甘草、虻虫（去翅足，炒）。

【功能主治】活血破瘀，通经消痞。用于淤血内停，腹部肿块，肌肤甲错，目眶黯黑，潮热羸瘦，闭经不行。

【注意】孕妇禁用；皮肤过敏者停服。

Rhubarb* and Ground Beetle** Bolus

Name of Chinese Phonetic Alphabet Da Huang Zhe Chong Wan

Formula Rehmanniae Radix Praeparata, Eupolyphaga seu Steleophaga (fried), Hirudo (prepared), Toxicodendri Resina (calcined), Holotrichiae Larva (fried), Armeniacae Semen Amarum (fried), Rehmanniae Radix, Paeoniae Radix Alba, Scutellariae Radix, Persicae Semen, Glycyrrhizae Radix et Rhizoma and Tabanus (removed wings and feet and fried).

Actions and Indications Activating blood, breaking stasis, regulating menstruation, dispersing stuffiness. It is used for abdominal mass, encrusted skin, dim orbit, tidal fever, emaciation and amenorrhea due to internal stagnation of blood-stasis.

Warning It is contraindicated for pregnant women and should be suspended in cases of skin allergy.

* 大黄 ** 土鳖虫

万氏牛黄清心浓缩丸

【处方】牛黄、朱砂、黄连、黄芩、栀子、郁金。

【功能主治】清热解毒，镇惊安神。用于邪热内闭，烦躁不安，神昏谵语，小儿高热惊厥。

【注意】孕妇慎用。

Wanshi Bezoar*Concentrative Pill

Name of Chinese Phonetic Alphabet Wan Shi Niu Huang Qing Xin Nong Suo Wan

Formula Bovis Calculus, Cinnabaris, Coptidis Rhizoma, Scutellariae Radix, Gardeniae Fructus and Curcumae Radix.

Actions and Indications Clearing heat and detoxifying, settling fright and tranquilizing the mind. It is used for vexation, coma, delirious speech and infantile high fever and convulsion due to internal block of heat pathogens.

Warning It should be used carefully for pregnant women.

* 牛黄

万应胶囊

【处方】胡黄连、黄连、儿茶、冰片、香墨、熊胆、麝香、牛黄、牛胆汁。

【功能主治】清热，镇惊，解毒。用于小儿高热，烦躁易惊，口舌生疮，牙龈、咽喉肿痛。

Heat-clearing Capsule for Children

Name of Chinese Phonetic Alphabet Wan Ying Jiao Nang

Formula Picrorhizae Rhizoma, Coptidis Rhizoma, Catechu, Borneolum Syntheticum, Chinese Ink, Ursi Fel, Moschus, Bovis Calculus and Bovis Bilis.

Actions and Indications Clearing heat, settling fright and detoxicating. It is indicated for children high fever, vexation and easiness to be frightened, aphthae, gingivitis and sore-throat.

万通炎康片

【处方】苦玄参、肿节风。

【功能主治】清热解毒，消肿止痛。用于咽喉肿痛，急、慢性咽喉炎，扁桃体炎，牙龈炎，疮疖。

Wan Tong Yan Kang Tablet for Relieving Laryngopharyngitis

Name of Chinese Phonetic Alphabet Wan Tong Yan Kang Pian

Formula Picriae Herba and Sarcandrae Herba.

Actions and Indications Clearing heat and detoxicating, dispersing swelling and relieving pain. It is indicated for sore-throat, acute and chronic laryngopharyngitis, tonsillitis, gingivitis, abscess and deep-rooted boil.

上清丸

【处方】菊花、薄荷、川芎、白芷、荆芥、防风、桔梗、连翘、栀子、黄芩（酒炒）、黄柏（酒炒）、大黄（酒炒）。

【功能主治】清热散风，解毒，通便。用于头晕耳鸣，目赤，鼻窦炎，口舌生疮，牙龈肿痛，大便秘结。

【注意】孕妇忌服。

Clearing Upper Energizer Heat Bolus

Name of Chinese Phonetic Alphabet Shang Qing Wan

Formula Chrysanthemi Flos, Menthae Haplocalycis Herba, Chuanxiong Rhizoma, Angelicae Dahuricae Radix, Schizonepetae Herba, Saposhnikoviae Radix, Platycodonis Radix, Forsythiae Fructus, Gardeniae Frucrus, Scutellariae Radix (fried with wine), Phellodendri Chinensis Cortex (fried with wine) and Rhei Radix et Rhizoma (fried with wine).

Actions and Indications Clearing heat and dispersing wind, detoxicating, relaxing the bowels. It is used for dizziness, tinnitus, conjunctive congestion, sinusitis, aphthae, gingivitis and constipation.

Warning It is contraindicated for pregnant women.

口炎清冲剂

【处方】天冬、麦冬、玄参、金银花、甘草。

【功能主治】滋阴清热，解毒消肿。用于阴虚火旺所致的口腔炎症。

Stomatitis-relieving Soluble Granules

Name of Chinese Phonetic Alphabet Kou Yan Qing Chong Ji

Formula Asparagi Radix, Ophiopogonis Radix, Scrophulariae Radix, Lonicerae Japonicae Flos and Glycyrrhizae Radix et Rhizoma.

Actions and Indications Nourishing *yin*, clearing heat, detoxifying, reducing swelling. It is used for stomatitis due to *yin*-deficiency with effulgent fire.

口腔溃疡散

【处方】青黛、白矾、冰片。

【功能主治】消溃止痛。用于复发性口腔溃疡，疱疹性口腔溃疡。

Relieving Ulcerative Stomatitis Powder

Name of Chinese Phonetic Alphabet Kou Qiang Kui Yang San

Formula Indigo Naturalis, Alumen and Borneolum Syntheticum.

Actions and Indications Promoting the healing

of stomatocace and relieving pain. It is indicated for recurrent ulcerative stomatitis, herpetic ulcerative stomatitis.

山东阿胶膏

【处方】阿胶、党参、黄芪、白术、枸杞子、甘草、白芍。

【功能主治】养血补血，补虚润燥。用于气血不足引起的虚劳咳嗽，肺萎吐血，妇女崩漏、胎动不安。

Soft Extract of Ass-hide Gelatin*

Name of Chinese Phonetic Alphabet Shan Dong E Jiao Gao

Formula Asini Corii Colla, Codonopsis Radix, Astragali Radix, Atractylodis Macrocephalae Rhizoma, Lycii Fructus, Glycyrrhizae Radix et Rhizoma and Paeoniae Radix Alba.

Actions and Indications Nourishing and tonifying blood, relieving deficiency syndrome and moistening dryness. It is indicated for cough due to consumptive disease and insufficiency of *qi* and blood; lung atrophy, hematemesis, metrorrhagia and threatened abortion.

* 阿胶

山玫胶囊

【处方】山楂、刺玫果。

【功能主治】益气化瘀。用于冠心病、脑动脉硬化、气滞血瘀证，症见胸痛，痛有定处，胸闷憋气；或眩晕、心悸、气短、乏力，舌质紫暗。

【注意】孕妇慎服。

Chinese Hawthorn* and Dahurian Rose** Capsule

Name of Chinese Phonetic Alphabet Shan Mei Jiao Nang

Formula Crataegi Fructus and Rosae Davuricae Fructus.

Actions and Indications Tonifying *qi*, resolving stasis. It is indicated for coronary heart disease and cerebeal arteriosclerosis due to *qi*-stagnation and blood-stasis and manifested as fixed pectoralgia, chest distress or vertigo, palpitation, shortness of breath, fatigue and purple tongue body.

Warning It should be used cautiously for pregnant women.

* 山楂 ** 山刺玫

山药丸

【处方】山药、杜仲（炭炒）、牛膝、甘草、木香、乳香（醋炙）、没药（醋炙）、千年健、羌活、地枫皮、红花、防风、续断、柴胡、狗脊（沙烫）、麻黄、马钱子粉、自然铜（煅醋淬）。

【功能主治】祛风通络，强筋壮骨。用于痹症，筋骨痿软，关节不利，跌打损伤。

【注意】孕妇忌服，久病体虚者勿服。

Chinese Yam* Pill for Relieving Impediment Syndrome

Name of Chinese Phonetic Alphabet Shan Yao Wan

Formula Dioscoreae Rhizoma, Eucommiae Cortex (carbonated), Achyranthis Bidentatae Radix, Glycyrrhizae Radix et Rhizoma, Aucklandiae Radix, Olibanum (prepared with vinegar), Myrrha (prepared with vinegar), Homalomenae Rhizoma, Notopterygii Rhizoma et Radix, Illicii Cortex, Carthami Flos, Saposhnikoviae Radix, Dipsaci Radix, Bupleuri Radix, Cibotii Rhizoma(scalded by sand), Ephedrae Herba, Strychni Semen Pulvis and Pyritum (calcined and quenched by vinegar).

Actions and Indications Dispelling wind and dredging collaterals, strengthening sinews and bone. It is used for impediment syndrome, marked by wilting of sinews and bone, immobility of joints and traumatic injury.

Warning It is contraindicated for pregnant women and cases with debility of constitution.

* 山药

山海丹胶囊

【处方】三七、人参、黄芪、红花、山羊血粉、决明子、葛根、佛手、海藻、何首乌、丹参、川芎等药加工制成的胶囊剂。

【功能主治】活血通络。用于心脉瘀阻，胸痹。

【注意】服药期间少数病人有口舌干燥感。

Shanhaidan Capsule for Chest Impediment

Name of Chinese Phonetic Alphabet Shan Hai Dan Jiao Nang

Formula Notoginseng Radix et Rhizoma, Ginseng Radix et Rhizoma, Astragali Radix, Carthami Flos, Caprinus Sanguis Pulvis, Cassiae Semen, Puerariae Lobatae Radix, Citri Sarcodactylis Fructus, Sargassum, Polygoni Multiflori Radix, Salviae Miltiorrhizae Radix et Rhizoma, Chuanxiong Rhizoma, etc.

Actions and Indications Activating blood, dredging collaterals. It is used for chest impediment disease due to obstruction of heart vessels.

Warning During administration, dry mouth and tongue occurs occasionally.

山绿茶降压片

【处方】山绿茶。

【功能主治】清热解毒，平肝潜阳。用于眩晕耳鸣，头痛头胀，心烦易怒，少寐多梦及高血压、高血脂见有上述证候者。

Green Tea* Tablet for Lowering Blood Pressure

Name of Chinese Phonetic Alphabet Shan Lü Cha Jiang Ya Pian

Formula Camelliae Sinensis Folium Gemmae (green tea).

Actions and Indications Clearing heat, detoxifying, pacifying the liver, subduing *yang*. It is used for vertigo, tinnitus, headache, distending pain in the head, vexation, profuse dreaming and also used for hypertension and hyperlipemia with the above mentioned symptoms.

* 绿茶

山楂降压片

【处方】山楂 、菊花、泽泻、夏枯草、小蓟、决明子。

【功能主治】平肝潜阳。用于阴虚阳亢型高血压病，症见头痛眩晕，耳鸣健忘，腰膝酸软，五心烦热，心悸失眠。

Chinese Hawthorn* Tablet for Lowering Blood Pressure

Name of Chinese Phonetic Alphabet Shan Zha Jiang Ya Pian

Formula Crataegi Fructus, Chrysanthemi Flos, Alismatis Rhizoma, Prunellae Spica, Cirsii Herba and Cassiae Semen.

Actions and Indications Pacifying the liver, subduing *yang*. It is used for hypertension of *yin* deficiency with *yang* hyperactivity type, and manifested as headache, vertigo, tinnitus, amnesia, soreness and weakness of waist and knees, vexing heat in the chest, palms and soles, palpitation, insomnia.

* 山楂

山楂精降脂片

【处方】本品为山楂提取物制成的片剂。

【功能主治】降血脂。用于治疗高脂血症，亦可作为冠心病和高血压的辅助治疗。

Chinese Hawthorn* Extract Tablet for Decreasing Blood-lipid

Name of Chinese Phonetic Alphabet Shan Zha Jing Jiang Zhi Pian

Formula Crataegi Fructus (extract).

Actions and Indications Decreasing blood-lipid. It is indicated for hyperlipemia and coronary heart disease, and as adjuvant treatment for coronary heart disease and hypertension.

*山楂

千金化痰丸

【处方】枳实、白术（麸炒）、陈皮、法半夏、茯苓、甘草、胆南星（酒炙）、白附子（矾炙）、浮海石（煅）、防风、当归、天麻、知母、天花粉、黄芩、黄柏、大黄。

【功能主治】清热化痰，行气。用于痰热互结，咳痰黄稠或眩晕，痰核流注，便秘。

【注意】孕妇忌服。

Qian Jin Pill for Resolving Phlegm

Name of Chinese Phonetic Alphabet Qian Jin Hua Tan Wan

Formula Aurantii Fructus Immaturus, Atractylodis Macrocephalae Rhizoma (fried with bran), Citri Reticulatae Pericarpium, Pinelliae Rhizoma Praeparatum, Poria, Glycyrrhizae Radix et Rhizoma, Arisaema cum Bile (prepared with wine), Typhonii Rhizoma (prepared with alum), Pumex (calcined), Saposhnikoviae Radix, Angelicae Sinensis Radix, Gastrodiae Rhizoma, Anemarrhenae Rhizoma, Trichosanthis Radix, Scutellariae Radix, Phellodendri Chinensis Cortex and Rhei Radix et Rhizoma.

Actions and Indications Clearing heat and resolving phlegm, moving *qi*. It is used for binding of phlegm and heat, marked by yellow and thick phlegm or vertigo, scrofula, metastatic abscess and constipation.

Warning It is contraindicated for pregnant women.

千柏鼻炎片

【处方】千里光、卷柏、羌活、决明子、麻黄、川芎、白芷。

【功能主治】清热解毒，活血祛风。用于急、慢性鼻炎，鼻窦炎，咽炎。

Ragwort* and Selaginella** Tablet for Rhinitis

Name of Chinese Phonetic Alphabet Qian Bai Bi Yan Pian

Formula Senecionis Scandentis Herba, Selaginellae Herba, Notopterygii Rhizoma et Radix, Cassiae Semen, Ephedrae Herba, Chuanxiong Rhizoma and Angelicae Dahuricae Radix.

Actions and Indications Clearing heat and detoxicating, activating blood and dispelling wind. It is indicated for acute and chronic rhinitis, nasal sinusitis, pharyngitis.

*千里光 **卷柏

千喜片

【处方】穿心莲、千里光。

【功能主治】清热解毒，消炎止痛，止泻止痢。用于肠炎，结肠炎，细菌性痢疾和鼻窦炎等。

Qian Xi Tablet for Relieving Enteritis

Name of Chinese Phonetic Alphabet Qian Xi Pian

Formula Andrographis Herba and Senecionis Scandentis Herba.

Actions and Indications Clearing heat and detoxicating, antiphlogistic and alleviating pain, relieving diarrhea and dysentery. It is indicated for enteritis, colitis, bacillary dysentery and nasosinusitis.

千金止带丸

【处方】党参、白术（炒）、当归、白芍、川芎、香附（醋制）、木香、砂仁、小茴香（盐炒）、延胡索（醋制）、杜仲（盐炒）、续断、补骨脂（盐炒）、鸡冠花、青黛、椿皮（炒）、牡蛎（煅）。

【功能主治】补虚止带，和血调经。用于赤白带下，月经不调，腰酸腹痛。

Leucorrhea-arresting Bolus

Name of Chinese Phonetic Alphabet Qian Jin

Zhi Dai Wan

Formula Codonopsis Radix, Atractylodis Macrocephalae Rhizoma (fried), Angelicae Sinensis Radix, Paeoniae Radix Alba, Chuanxiong Rhizoma, Cyperi Rhizoma (prepared with vinegar), Aucklandiae Radix, Amomi Fructus, Foeniculi Fructus (fried with salt), Corydalis Rhizoma (prepared with vinegar), Eucommiae Cortex (fried with salt), Dipsaci Radix, Psoraleae Fructus (fried with salt), Celosiae Cristatae Flos, Indigo Naturalis, Ailanthi Cortex (fried) and Ostreae Concha (calcined).

Actions and Indications Arresting leucorrhea, harmonizing blood and regulating menstruation. It is indicated for red and white vaginal discharge, irregular menstruation, soreness of waist and abdominal pain.

川贝枇杷糖浆

【处方】川贝母流浸膏、桔梗、枇杷叶、薄荷脑。

【功能主治】清热宣肺，化痰止咳。用于感冒咳嗽及支气管炎。

Syrup of Sichuan Fritillary* and Loquat Leaf**

Name of Chinese Phonetic Alphabet Chuan Bei Pi Pa Tang Jiang

Formula Fritillariae Cirrhosae Extractum, Platycodonis Radix, Eriobotryae Folium and Menthol.

Actions and Indications Clearing heat and diffusing the lung, resolving phlegm and relieving cough. It is indicated for cough due to common cold; and bronchitis.

*川贝母 **枇杷叶

川芎茶调口服液

【处方】川芎、白芷、羌活、细辛、防风、薄荷、荆芥、甘草。

【功能主治】疏风止痛。用于风邪头痛，或有恶寒、发热、鼻塞。

Chuanxiong Ligusticum* Oral Liquid

Name of Chinese Phonetic Alphabet Chuan Xiong Cha Tiao Kou Fu Ye

Formula Chuanxiong Rhizoma, Angelicae Dahuricae Radix, Notopterygii Rhizoma et Radix, Asari Radix et Rhizoma, Saposhnikoviae Radix, Menthae Haplocalycis Herba, Schizonepetae Herba and Glycyrrhizae Radix et Rhizoma.

Actions and Indications Dispersing wind to alleviate pain. It is used for headache due to pathogenic wind marked by aversion to cold, fever, nasal congestion.

*川芎

久芝清心丸

【处方】大黄、黄芩、桔梗、山药、丁香、牛黄、麝香、冰片、朱砂、雄黄、薄荷脑。

【功能主治】清热，泻火，通便。用于内热壅盛引起的头晕脑胀，口鼻生疮，咽喉肿痛，风火牙痛，大便秘结。

【注意】孕妇忌服。

Jiu Zhi Pill for Clearing Heat

Name of Chinese Phonetic Alphabet Jiu Zhi Qing Xin Wan

Formula Rhei Radix et Rhizoma, Scutellariae Radix, Platycodonis Radix, Dioscoreae Rhizoma, Caryophylli Flos, Bovis Calculus, Moschus, Borneolum Syntheticum, Cinnabaris, Realgar and Menthol.

Actions and Indications Clearing heat, purging fire, relaxing the bowels. It is used for dizziness, aphthae, sore-throat, toothache and constipation due to internal heat.

Warning It is contraindicated for pregnant women.

卫生宝丸

【处方】黄芩、玄参、天花粉、麦冬、竹茹、僵蚕（麸炒）、荆芥穗、薄荷、桔梗、柴胡、紫苏叶、苦杏仁（去皮炒）、六神曲（麸炒）、甘草、朱砂粉、羚羊角粉、水牛角浓缩粉、冰片、雄黄粉。

【功能主治】疏风解表，润肺化痰。用于外感风寒，内有蕴热而致的怕冷发热，四肢酸懒，头疼目眩，咳嗽痰多，口渴咽干。

Dispersing Exogenous Wind-cold Pill

Name of Chinese Phonetic Alphabet Wei Sheng Bao Wan

Formula Scutellariae Radix, Scorphulariae Radix, Trichosanthis Radix, Ophiopogonis Radix, Bambusae Caulis in Taenias, Bombyx Batryticatus (fried with bran), Schizonepetae Spica, Menthae Haplocalycis Herba, Platycodonis Radix, Bupleuri Radix, Perillae Folium, Armeniacae Semen Amarum (removed seed coat and fried), Medicata Massa Fermentata (fried with bran), Glycyrrhizae Radix et Rhizoma, Cinnabaris Pulvis, Saigae Tataricae Cornu Pulvis, Bubali Cornu Pulvis Concentratio, Borneolum Syntheticum and Realgar Pulvis.

Actions and Indications Dispersing wind, releasing the exterior, moistening the lung and resolving phlegm. It is indicated for cases with fear of cold, fever, soreness of limbs, headache, dizzy vision, productive cough, thirst and dry throat due to invasion of exogenous wind-cold and accumulation of heat in the interior.

女金丸

【处方】当归、白芍、川芎、熟地黄、党参、白术（炒）、茯苓、甘草、肉桂、益母草、牡丹皮、没药（制）、延胡索（醋制）、藁本、白芷、黄芩、白薇、香附（醋制）、砂仁、陈皮、赤石脂（煅）、鹿角霜、阿胶。

【功能主治】调经养血，理气止痛。用于月经不调，痛经，小腹胀痛，腰腿酸痛。

【注意】孕妇慎用。

Golden Bolus of Regulating Menstruation

Name of Chinese Phonetic Alphabet Nü Jin Wan

Formula Angelicae Sinensis Radix, Paeoniae Radix Alba, Chuanxiong Rhizoma, Rehmanniae Radix Praepatata, Codonopsis Radix, Atractylodis Macrocephalae Rhizoma (fried), Poria, Glycyrrhizae Radix et Rhizoma, Cinnamomi Cortex, Leonuri Herba, Moutan Cortex, Myrrha (prepared), Corydalis Rhizoma (prepared with vinegar), Ligustici Rhizoma et Radix, Angelicae Dahuricae Radix, Scutellariae Radix, Cynanchi Atrati Radix et Rhizoma, Cyperi Rhizoma (prepared with vinegar), Amomi Fructus, Citri Reticulatae Pericarpium, Halloysitum Rubrum (calcined), Cervi Cornu Degelatinatum and Asini Corii Colla.

Actions and Indications Regulating menstruation, nourishing *qi* and blood to alleviate pain. It is indicated for irregular menstruation, dysmemorrhea, distending pain in lower abdomen and soreness and pain of waist and legs.

Warning It should be used carefully for pregnant women.

小儿七珍丸

【处方】雄黄、天麻、天竺黄、全蝎、僵蚕（炒）、清半夏、钩藤、桔梗、黄芩、巴豆霜、胆南星、蝉蜕、蟾酥（制）、沉香、朱砂、羚羊角、人工牛黄、麝香、水牛角浓缩粉。

【功能主治】消积导滞，通便泻火，镇惊退热，化痰息风。用于小儿感冒发热，乳食停滞，大便不通，惊风抽搐，痰涎壅盛。

Children *Qizhen* Pill

Name of Chinese Phonetic Alphabet Xiao Er Qi Zhen Wan

Formula Realgar, Gastrodiae Rhizoma, Bambusae Concretio Silicea, Scorpio, Bombyx Batryticatus (fried), Pinelliae Rhizoma Praeparatum cum Alumine, Uncariae Ramulus cum Uncis, Platycodonis Radix, Scutellariae Radix, Crotonis Semen Pulveratum, Arisaema cum Bile, Cicadae Periostracum, Bufonis Venenum (prepared), Aquilariae Lignum Resinatum, Cinnabaris, Saigae Tataricae Cornu, Bovis Calculus Artifactus, Moschus and Bubali Cornu Pulvis Concentratio.

Actions and Indications Promoting digestion, relaxing the bowels and purging fire, settling fright and defervescing, resolving phlegm and extinguishing wind. It is indicated for children common cold, marked by fever, retention of food and milk, constipation, convulsion, spasm, dominance of phlegm.

小儿七星茶冲剂

【处方】薏苡仁、稻芽、山楂、淡竹叶、钩藤、蝉蜕、甘草。

【功能主治】定惊消滞。用于小儿消化不良，不思饮食，二便不畅，夜寐不安。

Qi Xing Cha Soluble Granules for Children Dyspepsia

Name of Chinese Phonetic Alphabet Xiao Er Qi Xing Cha Chong Ji

Formula Coicis Semen, Oryzae Fructue Germinatus, Crataegi Fructus, Lophatheri Herba, Uncariae Ramulus cum Uncis, Cicadae Periostracum and Glycyrrhizae Radix et Rhizoma.

Actions and Indications Tranquilizing the mind and removing food stagnation. It is used for children dyspepsia, anorexia, difficulty in urination and defecation, restless sleep.

小儿太极丸

【处方】胆南星、天竺黄、僵蚕（炒）、大黄、冰片、麝香、朱砂。

【功能主治】镇惊清热，涤痰消积。用于小儿急惊，手足抽搐，角弓反张，食积痞满，内热咳嗽。

【注意】泄泻者忌服。

Infantile *Tai Ji* Pill

Name of Chinese Phonetic Alphabet Xiao Er Tai Ji Wan

Formula Arisaema cum Bile, Bambusae Concretio Silicea, Bombyx Batryticatus (freid), Rhei Radix et Rhizoma, Borneolum Syntheticum, Moschus and Cinnabaris.

Actions and Indications Settling fright, clearing heat, removing phlegm, promoting digestion. It is used for acute infantile convulsion, tic, opisthotonos, indigestion, cough due to internal heat.

Warning It is contraindicated for cases with diarrhea.

小儿止泻安冲剂

【处方】赤石脂（煅）、肉豆蔻（煨）、伏龙肝、茯苓、陈皮、木香（煨）、砂仁。

【功能主治】健脾和胃，利湿止泻。用于小儿消化不良腹泻，脾虚腹泻。

Diarrhea-arresting Soluble Granules for Children

Name of Chinese Phonetic Alphabet Xiao Er Zhi Xie An Chong Ji

Formula Halloysitum Rubrum (calcined), Myristicae Semen (roasted),Terra Flava Usta, Poria, Citri Reticulatae Pericarpium, Aucklandiae Radix (roasted) and Amomi Fructus.

Actions and Indications Fortifying the spleen, harmonizing the stomach, draining dampness and arresting diarrhea. It is used for children dyspepsia and diarrhea due to deficiency of the spleen.

小儿止泻膏

【处方】本品由芋头干片等经加工制成的煎膏剂。

【功能主治】健脾止泻。用于小儿脾虚湿盛，伤乳伤食所致的腹泻及久泻。

Taro★ Extract for Children Diarrhea

Name of Chinese Phonetic Alphabet Xiao Er Zhi Xie Gao

Formula Colocasiae Esculentae Tuber.

Actions and Indications Fortifying the spleen and checking diarrhea. It is used for children diarrhea and chronic diarrhea due to spleen deficiency and abundant dampness, improper diet.

*芋

小儿止咳糖浆

【处方】甘草流浸膏、桔梗流浸膏、氯化铵、橙皮酊。

【功能主治】祛痰，镇咳。用于小儿感冒引起的咳嗽。

Syrup for Relieving Infantile Cough

Name of Chinese Phonetic Alphabet Xiao Er Zhi Ke Tang Jiang

Formula Glycyrrhizae Extractum, Platycodonis Extractum, Ammonium Chloride and Orange Tinctura.

Actions and Indications Dispelling phlegm and settling cough. It is indicated for cough due to infantile common cold.

小儿止嗽糖浆

【处方】玄参、麦冬、胆南星、杏仁水、槟榔（焦）、桔梗、竹茹、桑白皮、天花粉、川贝母、瓜蒌子、甘草、紫苏子（炒）、知母、紫苏叶油。

【功能主治】润肺清热，止嗽化痰。用于发热，咳嗽黄痰，口干舌燥，腹满便秘，久嗽痰盛。

Syrup for Relieving Children Cough

Name of Chinese Phonetic Alphabet Xiao Er Zhi Sou Tang Jiang

Formula Scrophulariae Radix, Ophiopogonis Radix, Arisaema cum Bile, Armeniacae Aqua Amarum, Arecae Semen (charred), Platycodonis Radix, Bambusae Caulis in Taenias, Mori Cortex, Trichosanthis Radix, Fritillariae Cirrhosae Bulbus, Trichosanthis Semen, Glycyrrhizae Radix et Rhizoma, Perillae Fructus (fried), Anemarrhenae Rhizoma and Perillae Folium Oleum.

Actions and Indications Moistening the lung and clearing heat, alleviating cough and resolving phlegm. It is indicated for fever, cough with yellow phlegm, dry mouth and tongue, abdominal fullness and constipation, chronic cough with profuse phlegm.

小儿化毒胶囊

【处方】牛黄、珍珠、雄黄、黄连、甘草、天花粉、川贝母、赤芍、乳香、没药、冰片、大黄。

【功能主治】清热解毒，活血消肿。用于小儿疹后余毒未尽，烦躁，口渴，口疮，便秘，疥肿溃烂。

Infantile Detoxicating Capsule

Name of Chinese Phonetic Alphabet Xiao Er Hua Du Jiao Nang

Formula Bovis Calculus, Margarita, Realgar, Coptidis Rhizoma, Glycyrrhizae Radix et Rhizoma, Trichosanthis Radix, Fritillariae Cirrhosae Bulbus, Paeoniae Radix Rubra, Olibanum, Myrrha, Borneolum Syntheticum and Rhei Radix et Rhizoma.

Actions and Indications Clearing heat and detoxicating, activating blood and dispersing swelling. It is used for residual toxin after measles, vexation, thirst, aphthae, constipation and scabies.

小儿化食丸

【处方】六神曲（炒焦）、山楂（炒焦）、麦芽（炒焦）、槟榔（炒焦）、莪术（醋制）、三棱（制）、牵牛子（炒焦）、大黄。

【功能主治】消食化滞，泻火通便。用于小儿胃热停食，肚腹胀满，恶心呕吐，烦躁口渴，大便干燥。

【注意】忌食辛辣油腻。

Promoting Children Digestion Pill

Name of Chinese Phonetic Alphabet Xiao Er Hua Shi Wan

Formula Medicata Massa Fermentata (charred), Crataegi Fructus (charred), Hordei Fructus Germinatus (charred), Arecae Semen (charred), Curcumae Rhizoma (prepared with vinegar), Sparganii Rhizoma (prepared),

Pharbitidis Semen (charred) and Rhei Radix et Rhizoma.

Actions and Indications Promoting digestion and removing food stagnation, purging fire and relaxing the bowels. It is used for children abdominal distention and fullness, nausea, vomiting, vexation, thirst and dry stool due to stomach heat.

Warning Pungent and oily foods should be avoided.

小儿牛黄散

【处方】钩藤、僵蚕（麸炒）、天麻、全蝎、黄连、胆南星（酒炙）、大黄、浙贝母、滑石、半夏（制）、橘红、天竺黄、朱砂、人工牛黄、麝香、冰片。

【功能主治】清热镇惊，散风化痰。用于小儿食滞内热引起的咳嗽身热，呕吐痰涎，烦躁起急，睡卧不安，惊风抽搐，神志昏迷，大便燥结。

Children Bezoar* Powder

Name of Chinese Phonetic Alphabet Xiao Er Niu Huang San

Formula Uncariae Ramulus cum Uncis, Bombyx Batryticatus (fried with bran), Gastrodiae Rhizoma, Scorpio, Coptidis Rhizoma, Arisaema cum Bile (prepared with wine), Rhei Radix et Rhizoma, Fritillariae Thunbergii Bulbus, Talcum, Pinellae Rhizoma Praeparata, Citri Exocarpium Rubrum, Bambusae Concretio Silicea, Cinnabaris, Bovis Calculus Artifactus, Moschus and Borneolum Syntheticum..

Actions and Indications Clearing heat, settling fright, dissipating wind, resolving phlegm. It is used for children cough, feverish sensation of body, phlegm vomitus, vexation, convulsive spasm, obnubilation and dry stool due to indigestion and internal heat.

* 牛黄

小儿百寿丸

【处方】钩藤、僵蚕（麸炒）、胆南星（酒炙）、天竺黄、桔梗、木香、砂仁、陈皮、苍术（制）、茯苓、山楂（炒）、六神曲（炒）、麦芽（炒）、薄荷、滑石、甘草、朱砂、牛黄。

【功能主治】清热散风，消食化滞，镇惊息风，化痰止咳。用于小儿外感风热，发热头痛，消化不良，停食停乳，厌食嗳气，咳嗽痰多，惊风。

Children Health Protection Pill

Name of Chinese Phonetic Alphabet Xiao Er Bai Shou Wan

Formula Uncariae Ramulus cum Uncis, Bombyx Batryticatus (fried with bran), Arisaema cum Bile (prepared with wine), Bambusae Concretio Silicea, Platycodonis Radix, Aucklandiae Radix, Amomi Fructus, Citri Reticulatae Pericarpium, Atractylodis Rhizoma (prepared), Poria, Crataegi Fructus (fried), Medicata Massa Fermentata (fried), Hordei Fructus Germinatus (fried), Menthae Haplocalycis Herba, Talcum, Glycyrrhizae Radix et Rhizoma, Cinnabaris and Bovis Calculus.

Actions and Indications Clearing heat and dissipating wind, promoting digestion and removing food stagnation, settling fright and extinguishing wind, resolving phlegm and suppressing cough. It is indicated for children external contraction of wind-heat, marked by fever, headache, dyspepsia, anorexia, belching, cough with profuse phlegm, convulsion.

小儿至宝丸

【处方】紫苏叶、广藿香、薄荷、羌活、陈皮、白附子（制）、胆南星、芥子（炒）、川贝母、槟榔、山楂（炒）、茯苓、六神曲（炒）、麦芽（炒）、琥珀、冰片、天麻、钩藤、僵蚕（炒）、蝉蜕、全蝎、牛黄、雄黄、滑石、朱砂。

【功能主治】疏风镇惊，化痰导滞。用于小儿风寒感冒，停食停乳，发热鼻塞，咳嗽痰多，呕吐泄泻，惊惕抽搐。

Children Precious Pill

Name of Chinese Phonetic Alphabet Xiao Er Zhi Bao Wan

Formula Perillae Folium, Pogostemonis Herba, Menthae Haplocalycis Herba, Notopterygii Rhizoma et Radix, Citri Reticulatae Pericarpium, Typhonii Rhizoma (prepared), Arisaema cum Bile, Sinapis Semen (fried), Fritillariae Cirrhosae Bulbus, Arecae Semen, Crataegi Fructus (fried), Poria, Medicata Massa Fermentata (fried), Hordei Fructus Germinatus (fried), Succinum, Borneolum Syntheticum, Gastrodiae Rhizoma, Uncariae Ramulus cum Uncis, Bombyx Batryticatus(fried), Cicadae Periostracum, Scorpio, Bovis Calculus, Realgar, Talcum and Cinnabaris.

Actions and Indications Dispersing wind and settling fright, resolving phlegm and removing food stagnation. It is indicated for commom cold in children, marked by retention of food and milk, fever, nasal congestion, productive cough and phlegm, vomiting, diarrhea, fright convulsion.

小儿回春丸

【处方】全蝎、朱砂、蛇含石（醋煅）、天竺黄、川贝母、胆南星、人工牛黄、白附子（制）、天麻、僵蚕（麸炒）、雄黄、防风、羌活、麝香、冰片、甘草、钩藤。

【功能主治】息风镇惊，化痰开窍。用于小儿急惊抽搐，痰涎壅盛，神昏气喘，烦躁发热。

Relieving Infantile Convulsion Pill

Name of Chinese Phonetic Alphabet Xiao Er Hui Chun Wan

Formula Scorpio, Cinnabaris, Limonitum (calcined by vinegar), Bambusae Concretio Silicea, Fritillariae Cirrhosae Bulbus, Arisaema cum Bile, Bovis Calculus Artifactus, Typhonii Rhizoma (prepared), Gastrodiae Rhizoma, Bombyx Batryticatus (fried with bran), Realgar, Saposhnikoviae Radix, Notopterygii Rhizoma et Radix, Moschus, Borneolum Syntheticum, Glycyrrhizae Radix et Rhizoma and Uncariae Ramulus cum Uncis.

Actions and Indications Extinguishing wind and settling fright, resolving phlegm and opening the orifices. It is indicated for infantile acute convulsion, excessive phlegm and saliva, loss of consciousness and dyspnea, vexation and fever.

小儿导赤片

【处方】大黄、滑石、地黄、栀子、甘草、关木通、茯苓。

【功能主治】清热利便。用于胃肠炽热，口舌生疮，咽喉肿痛，牙根出血，腮颊肿痛，暴发火眼，大便不利，小便赤黄。

Dao Chi Tablet for Children

Name of Chinese Phonetic Alphabet Xiao Er Dao Chi Pian

Formula Rhei Radix et Rhizoma, Talcum, Rehmanniae Radix, Gardeniae Fructus, Glycyrrhizae Radix et Rhizoma, Aristolochiae Manshuriensis Caulis and Poria.

Actions and Indications Clearing heat and promoting bowels movement. It is used for aphthae, sorethroat, bleeding of dental root, buccal swelling and pain, sudden conjunctivitis, constipation and dark yellow urine due to potent heat of the stomach and intestine.

小儿抗痫胶囊

【处方】太子参、茯苓、天麻、九节菖蒲、川芎、胆南星等。

【功能主治】豁痰息风，健脾理气。用于原发性全身性僵直发作型儿童癫痫风痰闭阻证，发作时症见四肢抽搐、口吐涎沫、二目上窜，甚至昏仆。

Children Epilepsy-relieving Capsule

Name of Chinese Phonetic Alphabet Xiao Er Kang Xian Jiao Nang

Formula Pseudostellariae Radix, Poria, Gastrodiae Rhizoma, Anemones Altaicae Rhizoma, Chuanxiong Rhizoma, Arisaema cum Bile, etc.

Actions and Indications Expelling phlegm, extinguishing wind, fortifying the spleen, regulating *qi*. It is used for children epilepsy marked by spasm of limbs, salivary vomitus and eyeballs-up or even coma.

小儿金丹片

【处方】朱砂、橘红、川贝母、胆南星、前胡、玄参、清半夏、大青叶、关木通、桔梗、荆芥穗、羌活、西河柳、地黄、枳壳（炒）、赤芍、钩藤、葛根、牛蒡子、天麻、甘草、防风、冰片、水牛角浓缩粉、羚羊角粉、薄荷脑 。

【功能主治】祛风化痰，清热解毒。用于感冒风热，痰火内盛，发热头痛，咳嗽气喘，咽喉肿痛，呕吐，高热惊风。

Children *Jin Dan* Tablet

Name of Chinese Phonetic Alphabet Xiao Er Jin Dan Pian

Formula Cinnabaris, Citri Exocarpium Rubrum, Fritillariae Cirrhosae Bulbus, Arisaema cum Bile, Peucedani Radix, Scrophulariae Radix, Pinelliae Rhizoma Praeparatum cum Alumine, Isatidis Folium, Aristolochiae Manshuriensis Caulis, Platycodonis Radix, Schizonepetae Spica, Notopterygii Rhizoma et Radix, Tamaricis Cacumen, Rehmanniae Radix, Aurantii Fructus (fried), Paeoniae Radix Rubra, Uncariae Ramulus cum Uncis, Puerariae Lobatae Radix, Arctii Fructus, Gastrodiae Rhizoma, Glycyrrhizae Radix et Rhizoma, Saposhnikoviae Radix, Borneolum Syntheticum, Bubali Cornu Pulvis Concentratio, Saigae Tataricae Cornu Pulvis and Menthol.

Actions and Indications Dispelling wind, resolving phlegm, clearing heat, detoxifying. It is used for children common cold of wind-heat type, fever, headache, cough and dyspnea due to phlegm-fire; sore-throat, vomiting, high fever, convulsion.

小儿肺热平胶囊

【处方】牛黄、地龙、珍珠（制）、拳参、牛胆粉、甘草、平贝母、麝香、射干、朱砂、黄连、黄芩、羚羊角、寒水石、冰片、紫草、柴胡。

【功能主治】清热化痰，止咳平喘，镇惊开窍。用于小儿肺热喘咳，吐痰黄稠，高热烦渴，神昏谵妄，抽搐，苔黄腻者。

Relieving Infantile Dyspnea and Cough Capsule

Name of Chinese Phonetic Alphabet Xiao Er Fei Re Ping Jiao Nang

Formula Bovis Calculus, Pheretima, Margarita (prepared), Bistortae Rhizoma, Bovis Fel Pulvis, Glycyrrhizae Radix et Rhizoma, Fritillariae Ussuriensis Bulbus, Moschus, Belamcandae Rhizoma, Cinnabaris, Coptidis Rhizoma, Scutellariae Radix, Saigae Tataricae Cornu, Gypsum Rubrum, Borneolum Syntheticum, Arnebiae Radix and Bupleuri Radix.

Actions and Indications Clearing heat and resolving phlegm, relieving cough and dyspnea, settling fright and opening the orifices. It is indicated for infantile dyspneic cough due to lung-heat; yellow and thick phlegm, high fever, excessive thirst, loss of consciousness, delirium, spasm, yellow and greasy tongue fur.

小儿肺热咳喘口服液

【处方】麻黄、杏仁、生石膏、甘草、金银花、连翘、板蓝根、麦冬等。

【功能主治】清热解毒，宣肺化痰。用于热邪犯于肺卫所致发热汗出，微恶风寒，咳嗽，痰黄，或兼喘息，口干而渴。

Clearing Heat Oral Liquid for Relieving Children Cough

Name of Chinese Phonetic Alphabet Xiao Er Fei Re Ke Chuan Kou Fu Ye

Formula Ephedrae Herba, Armeniacae Semen Amarum, Gypsum Fibrosum, Glycyrrhizae Radix et Rhizoma, Lonicerae Japonicae Flos, Forsythiae Fructus, Isatidis Radix, Ophiopogonis Radix, etc.

Actions and Indications Clearing heat and detoxicating, diffusing the lung and resolving phlegm. It is indicated for fever and sweating, slight aversion to cold, cough, yellow phlegm, or accompanied by dyspnea, dry mouth and thirst due to heat pathogen invading the lung.

小儿肺热咳喘颗粒

【处方】麻黄、苦杏仁、生石膏、甘草、金银花、连翘、知母、黄芩、板蓝根、麦冬、鱼腥草。

【功能主治】清热解毒，宣肺止咳，化痰平喘。用于感冒，支气管炎，肺炎属痰热壅肺证者。

Instant Granules for Children Common Cold

Name of Chinese Phonetic Alphabet Xiao Er Fei Re Ke Chuan Ke Li

Formula Ephedrae Herba, Armeniacae Semen Amarum, Gypsum Fibrosum, Glycyrrhizae Radix et Rhizoma, Lonicerae Japonicae Flos, Forsythiae Fructus, Anemarrhenae Rhizoma, Scutellariae Radix, Isatidis Radix, Ophiopogonis Radix and Houttuyniae Herba.

Actions and Indications Clearing heat and detoxicating, diffusing the lung and alleviating cough, resolving phlegm and relieving dyspnea. It is indicated for children common cold, bronchitis, pneumonia attributive to stagnation of phlegm-heat in the lung.

小儿泻速停冲剂

【处方】地锦草、儿茶、乌梅、山楂（炒焦）、茯苓、白芍、甘草等。

【功能主治】清热利湿，健脾止泻，解痉止痛。用于治疗小儿泄泻、腹痛，纳差（尤适用秋季腹泻及慢性腹泻）。

【注意】服药期间忌生冷、油腻。

Relieving Infantile Chronic Diarrhea Soluble Granules

Name of Chinese Phonetic Alphabet Xiao Er Xie Su Ting Chong Ji

Formula Euphorbiae Humifusae Herba, Catechu, Mume Fructus, Crataegi Fructus (charred), Poria, Paeoniae Radix Alba, Glycyrrhizae Radix et Rhizoma, etc.

Actions and Indications Clearing heat and draining dampness, fortifying the spleen and relieving diarrhea, releasing convulsion to alleviate pain. It is indicated for infantile diarrhea, abdominal pain, poor appetite, especially for diarrhea in autumn and chronic diarrhea.

Warning Uncooked, cold, and oily foods are prohibited during medication.

小儿泻痢片

【处方】葛根、黄芩、黄连、厚朴、白芍、茯苓、焦山楂、乌梅、甘草、滑石粉。

【功能主治】清热化湿，止泻止痢。用于湿热腹泻，红、白痢疾。

Infantile Dysentery-relieving Tablet

Name of Chinese Phonetic Alphabet Xiao Er Xie Li Pian

Formula Puerariae Lobatae Radix, Scutellariae Radix, Coptidis Rhizoma, Magnoliae Officinalis Cortex, Paeoniae Radix Alba, Poria, Crataegi Fructus (charred), Mume Fructus, Glycyrrhizae Radix et Rhizoma and Talci Pulvis.

Actions and Indications Clearing heat and resolving dampness, relieving diarrhea and dysentery. It is indicated for diarrhea or dysentery with mucous or with bloody stool.

小儿宝泰康冲剂

【处方】连翘、地黄、竹叶、柴胡、玄参、桑叶、浙贝母、马蓝、桔梗、紫草、莱菔子、甘草。

【功能主治】解表清热，止咳化痰。用于小儿风热外感，症见发热、流涕、咳嗽、脉浮。

Relieving Common Cold Soluble Granules for Children

Name of Chinese Phonetic Alphabet Xiao Er Bao Tai Kang Chong Ji

Formula Forsythiae Fructus, Rehmanniae Radix, Phyllostachydis Henonis Folium, Bupleuri Radix, Scrophulariae Radix, Mori Folium, Fritillariae

Thunbergii Bulbus, Baphicacanthi Cusiae Rhizoma et Radix, Platycodonis Radix, Arnebiae Radix, Raphani Semen and Glycyrrhizae Radix et Rhizoma.

Actions and Indications Releasing the exterior and clearing heat, relieving cough and resolving phlegm. It is indicated for external contraction of wind-heat in children, manifested as fever, rhinorrhea, cough, floating pulse.

小儿咽扁冲剂

【处方】金银花、射干、金果榄、桔梗、玄参、麦冬、牛黄、冰片。

【功能主治】清热利咽，解毒止痛。用于肺热引起的咽喉肿痛，口舌糜烂，咳嗽痰盛，咽炎喉炎，扁桃体炎。

Relieving Laryngitis and Tonsillitis Soluble Granules for Children

Name of Chinese Phonetic Alphabet Xiao Er Yan Bian Chong Ji

Formula Lonicerae Japonicae Flos, Belamcandae Rhizoma, Tinosporae Radix, Platycodonis Radix, Scrophulariae Radix, Ophiopogonis Radix, Bovis Calculus and Borneolum Syntheticum.

Actions and Indications Clearing heat and soothing the throat, detoxicating and relieving pain. It is used for sore-throat, aphthae, productive cough, pharyngitis laryngitis and tonsillitis due to lung-heat.

小儿咳喘冲剂

【处方】麻黄、川贝母、苦杏仁（炒）、黄芩、天竺黄、紫苏子（炒）、僵蚕（炒）、山楂（炒）、莱菔子（炒）、石膏、鱼腥草、细辛、茶叶、甘草、桔梗。

【功能主治】清热宣肺，化痰止咳，降逆平喘。用于小儿发热、咳嗽、气喘。

Infantile Cough-relieving Soluble Granules

Name of Chinese Phonetic Alphabet Xiao Er Ke Chuan Chong Ji

Formula Ephedrae Herba, Fritillariae Cirrhosae Bulbus, Armeniacae Semen Amarum (fried), Scutellariae Radix, Bambusae Concretio Silicea, Perillae Fructus (fried), Bombyx Batryticatus (fried), Crataegi Fructus (fried), Raphani Semen (fried), Gypsum Fibrosum, Houttuyniae Herba, Asari Radix et Rhizoma, Camelliae Sinensis Folium Gemmae, Glycyrrhizae Radix et Rhizoma and Platycodonis Radix.

Actions and Indications Clearing heat and diffusing the lung, resolving phlegm and relieving cough and dyspnea, directing *qi* downward. It is indicated for infantile fever, cough and dyspnea.

小儿咳喘灵冲剂

【处方】麻黄、金银花、苦杏仁、板蓝根、石膏、甘草、瓜蒌。

【功能主治】宣肺、清热，止咳、祛痰、平喘。用于上呼吸道感染，气管炎，肺炎，咳嗽。

Relieving Infantile Upper Respiratory Track Infection Soluble Granules

Name of Chinese Phonetic Alphabet Xiao Er Ke Chuan Ling Chong Ji

Formula Ephedrae Herba, Lonicerae Japonicae Flos, Armeniacae Semen Amarum, Isatidis Radix, Gypsum Fibrosum, Glycyrrhizae Radix et Rhizoma and Trichosanthis Fructus.

Actions and Indications Diffusing the lung, clearing heat, relieving cough and dyspnea, dispelling phlegm. It is indicated for upper respiratory tract infection, trachitis, pneumonia and cough.

小儿香橘丸

【处方】木香、陈皮、苍术（米泔炒）、白术（麸炒）、茯苓、甘草、白扁豆（去皮）、山药、莲子、薏苡仁（麸炒）、山楂（炒）、麦芽（炒）、六神曲（麸炒）、厚朴（姜炙）、枳实、香附（醋炙）、砂仁、半夏（制）、泽泻。

【功能主治】健脾和胃，消食止泻。用于小儿饮食不节引起的呕吐便泻，脾胃不和，身热腹胀，面黄肌瘦，不思饮食。

Common Aucklandia* and Mardarin Orange Peel** Pill for Children

Name of Chinese Phonetic Alphabet Xiao Er Xiang Ju Wan

Formula Aucklandiae Radix, Citri Reticulatae Pericarpium, Atractylodis Rhizoma (fried with rice swilled water), Atractylodis Macrocephalae Rhizoma (fried with bran), Poria, Glycyrrhizae Radix et Rhizoma, Lablab Semen Album (removed seed coat), Dioscoreae Rhizoma, Nelumbinis Semen, Coicis Semen (fried with bran), Crataegi Fructus (fried), Hordei Fructus Germinatus (fried), Medicata Massa Fermentata (fried with bran), Magnoliae Officinalis Cortex (prepared with ginger), Aurantii Fructus Immaturus, Cyperi Rhizoma (prepared with vinegar), Amomi Fructus, Pinelliae Rhizoma (prepared) and Alismatis Rhizoma.

Actions and Indications Fortifying the spleen and harmonizing the stomach, promoting digestion and relieving diarrhea. It is used for vomiting, diarrhea, disharmony of the spleen and stomach, abdominal distention with fever, sallow complexion, emaciation, and anorexia due to improper diet of children.

* 木香 ** 陈皮

小儿退热冲剂

【处方】大青叶、板蓝根、金银花、连翘、栀子、牡丹皮、淡竹叶、黄芩、地龙、重楼、柴胡、白薇。

【功能主治】疏风解表，解毒利咽。用于小儿风热感冒，发热恶风，头痛目赤，咽喉肿痛，痄腮。

Antipyretic Soluble Granules for Children

Name of Chinese Phonetic Alphabet Xiao Er Tui Re Chong Ji

Formula Isatidis Folium, Isatidis Radix, Lonicerae Japonicae Flos, Forsythiae Fructus, Gardeniae Fructus, Moutan Cortex, Lophatheri Herba, Scutellariae Radix, Pheretima, Paridis Rhizoma, Bupleuri Radix and Cynanchi Atrati Radix et Rhizoma.

Actions and Indications Dispersing wind and releasing the exterior, detoxicating and soothing the throat. It is indicated for common cold in children, marked by aversion to wind, fever, headache and conjunctival congestion, sore-throat and mumps due to attack of wind-heat.

小儿健脾贴膏

【处方】丁香、吴茱萸、五倍子、磁石、冰片、麝香。

【功能主治】疏通经络，温中健脾。用于小儿消化不良。

Fortifying Spleen Plaster for Children

Name of Chinese Phonetic Alphabet Xiao Er Jian Pi Tie Gao

Formula Caryophylli Flos, Euodiae Fructus, Galla Chinensis, Magnetitum, Borneolum Syntheticum and Moschus.

Actions and Indications Dredging the meridians and collaterals, warming the middle and fortifying the spleen. It is used for children dyspepsia.

小儿脐风散

【处方】全蝎、猪牙皂、大黄、当归、朱砂、巴豆霜、硇砂（炙）、牛黄。

【功能主治】清热驱风，镇惊祛痰。用于初生小儿胎火内热引起的睡卧易惊，啼哭不安，身热面赤，咳嗽痰多，大便不通，惊风抽搐。

【注意】不宜多服。

Infantile Umbilical Wind Relieving Powder

Name of Chinese Phonetic Alphabet Xiao Er Qi Feng San

Formula Scorpio, Gleditsiae Fructus Abnormalis, Rhei Radix et Rhizoma, Angelicae Sinensis Radix,

Cinnabaris, Crotonis Semen Pulveratum, Sal Ammoniacum (prepared) and Bovis Calculus.

Actions and Indications Clearing heat, expelling wind, settling fright, dispelling phlegm. It is used for neonatal frightened sleep, crying, feverish sensation of body, flushed complexion, productive cough, difficult bowels movement, convulsive spasm.

Warning Long-term medication is prohibited.

小儿疳积冲剂

【处方】稻芽（炒）、山楂、甘草、鸡内金、夜明砂、叶下珠、山药（炒）、茯苓、海螵蛸、党参、莲子、使君子。

【功能主治】利湿消积，驱虫助食，健脾益气。用于小儿疳积，暑热腹泻，纳呆自汗，烦躁失眠。

Relieving Children Malnutrition Soluble Granules

Name of Chinese Phonetic Alphabet Xiao Er Gan Ji Chong Ji

Formula Oryzae Fructus Germinatus (fried), Crataegi Fructus, Glycyrrhizae Radix et Rhizoma, Galli Gigerii Endothelium Corneum , Vespertilionis Faeces, Phyllanthi Urinariae Herba, Dioscoreae Rhizoma (fried), Poria, Sepiae Endoconcha, Codonopsis Radix, Nelumbinis Semen and Quisqualis Fructus.

Actions and Indications Draining dampness and resolving stagnation, expelling worms and promoting digestion, fortifying the spleen and replenishing *qi*. It is used for children malnutrition, diarrhea due to summer-heat; loss of appetite, spontaneous sweating, vexation and insomnia.

小儿消食片

【处方】鸡内金（炒）、山楂、六神曲（炒）、麦芽（炒）、槟榔、陈皮。

【功能主治】消食化滞，健脾和胃。用于脾胃不和，消化不良，食欲不振，便秘，疳积。

Digestion-promoting Tablet for Children

Name of Chinese Phonetic Alphabet Xiao Er Xiao Shi Pian

Formula Galli Gigerii Endothelium Corneum (fried), Crataegi Fructus, Medicata Massa Fermentata (fried), Hordei Fructus Germinatus (fried), Arecae Semen and Citri Reticulatae Pericarpium.

Actions and Indications Promoting digestion, fortifying the spleen and harmonizing the stomach. It is used for dyspepsia, poor appetite, constipation and malnutrition due to disharmony of the spleen and stomach.

小儿消积丸

【处方】枳壳（麸炒）、三棱（醋炒）、黄芩、莪术（醋煮）、厚朴（姜制）、槟榔、青皮（醋炒）、陈皮、大黄、牵牛子（炒）、香附（醋炒）、木香、巴豆霜、朱砂。

【功能主治】消食导滞，理气和胃，止痛。用于小儿各种停食积滞，脘腹胀痛，面色萎黄，身体瘦弱。

【注意】虚弱，滑泻，外感者均忌服，如服药后大便泄泻次数过多，食欲不振，应立即停药。

Improving Children Food Stagnation Pill

Name of Chinese Phonetic Alphabet Xiao Er Xiao Ji Wan

Formula Aurantii Fructus (fried with bran), Sparganii Rhizoma (prepared with vinegar), Scutellariae Radix, Curcumae Rhizoma (boiled with vinegar), Magnoliae Officinalis Cortex (prepared with ginger), Arecae Semen, Citri Reticulatae Pericarpium Viride (fried with vinegar), Citri Reticulatae Pericarpium, Rhei Radix et Rhizoma, Pharbitidis Semen (fried), Cyperi Rhizoma (fried with vinegar), Aucklandiae Radix, Crotonis Semen Pulveratum and Cinnabaris.

Actions and Indications Promoting digestion and removing food stagnation, regulating *qi* and harmonizing the stomach, relieving pain. It is used for various children food retention, abdominal distention and pain, sallow complexion, emaciation.

Warning It is contraindicated for cases with debility, frequent diarrhea, external contraction. In case with frequent diarrhea, poor appetite after medication, suspend the medicine immediately.

小儿消积止咳口服液

【处方】山楂、槟榔、枳实、瓜蒌等。

【功能主治】清热疏肺，消积止咳。用于小儿食积咳嗽属痰热证，症见咳嗽，喉间痰鸣，腹胀，口臭。

Children Cough-relieving Oral Liquid

Name of Chinese Phonetic Alphabet Xiao Er Xiao Ji Zhi Ke Kou Fu Ye

Formula Crataegi Fructus, Arecae Semen, Aurantii Fructus Immaturus, Trichosanthis Fructus, etc.

Actions and Indications Clearing heat and soothing the lung, removing food stagnation and alleviating cough. It is indicated for children cough due to dyspepsia attributive to phlegm-heat syndrome, manifested as cough, wheezing sound in the throat, abdominal distension and halitosis.

小儿麻甘冲剂

【处方】麻黄、黄芩、紫苏子、甘草、桑白皮、苦杏仁、地骨皮、石膏。

【功能主治】平喘止咳，利咽祛痰。用于小儿肺炎喘咳，咽喉炎。

Soluble Granules of Chinese Ephedra* and Licorice** for Relieving Children Cough

Name of Chinese Phonetic Alphabet Xiao Er Ma Gan Chong Ji

Formula Ephedrae Herba, Scutellariae Radix, Perillae Fructus, Glycyrrhizae Radix et Rhizoma, Mori Cortex, Armeniacae Semen Amarum, Lycii Cortex and Gypsum Fibrosum.

Actions and Indications Relieving dyspnea and cough, soothing the throat and dispelling phlegm. It is indicated for children pneumonia, cough, dyspnea and laryngopharyngitis.

* 麻黄 ** 甘草

小儿清肺止咳片

【处方】紫苏叶、菊花、葛根、川贝母、苦杏仁（去皮炒）、枇杷叶、紫苏子（炒）、桑白皮（蜜炙）、前胡、射干、栀子（姜炙）、黄芩、知母、板蓝根、牛黄、冰片。

【功能主治】清热解表，止咳化痰。用于内热肺火，外感风热引起的身热咳嗽，气促痰多，烦躁口渴，大便干燥。

Clearing Heat Tablet for Alleviating Children Cough

Name of Chinese Phonetic Alphabet Xiao Er Qing Fei Zhi Ke Pian

Formula Perillae Folium, Chrysanthemi Flos, Puerariae Lobatae Radix, Fritillariae Cirrhosae Bulbus, Armeniacae Semen Amarum (removed seed coat and fried), Eriobotryae Folium, Perillae Fructus (fried), Mori Cortex (prepared with honey), Peucedani Radix, Belamcandae Rhizoma, Gardeniae Fructus (prepared with ginger), Scutellariae Radix, Anemarrhenae Rhizoma, Isatidis Radix, Bovis Calculus and Borneolum Syntheticum.

Actions and Indications Clearing heat and releasing the exterior, alleviating cough and resolving phlegm. It is indicated for fever, cough, shortness of breath, profuse phlegm, vexation, thirst and dry stool due to internal heat and lung-fire, external contration of wind-heat.

小儿清肺化痰口服液

【处方】麻黄、前胡、黄芩、紫苏子（炒）、石膏、苦杏仁（去皮炒）、葶苈子、竹茹。

【功能主治】清热化痰，止咳平喘。用于小儿肺热感冒引起的呼吸气促，咳嗽痰喘，喉中作响。

【注意】脾虚泄泻者不宜服用。

Relieving Infantile Cough Oral Liquid

Name of Chinese Phonetic Alphabet Xiao Er Qing Fei Hua Tan Kou Fu Ye

Formula Ephedrae Herba, Peucedani Radix, Scutellariae Radix, Perillae Fructus (fried), Gypsum Fibrosum, Armeniacae Semen Amarum (removed seed coat and fried), Lepidii Semen and Bambusae Caulis in Taenias.

Actions and Indications Clearing heat and resolving phlegm, relieving cough and dyspnea. It is indicated for shortness of breath, cough, phlegm dyspnea and wheezy sound in the throat due to common cold of lung-heat.

Warning It is contraindicated for cases with diarrhea due to deficiency of the spleen.

小儿清肺散

【处方】黄芩、石膏、胆南星、清半夏、川贝母、百部、白前、冰片、茯苓、沉香。

【功能主治】清肺化痰，止咳平喘。用于咳嗽喘促，痰多色黄稠，咯吐不爽，面赤身热，气急鼻煽，胸闷胀满，舌红苔黄腻，脉滑数。又用于急性支气管炎，哮喘，肺炎等病属痰热壅肺证者。

【注意】本品对寒证、虚证之咳喘不宜。

Relieving Children Cough Powder

Name of Chinese Phonetic Alphabet Xiao Er Qing Fei San

Formula Scutellariae Radix, Gypsum Fibrosum, Arisaema cum Bile, Pinelliae Rhizoma Praeparatum cum Alumine, Fritillariae Cirrhosae Bulbus, Stemonae Radix, Cynanchi Stauntonii Rhizoma et Radix, Borneolum Syntheticum, Poria and Aquilariae Lignum Resinatum.

Actions and Indications Clearing lung-heat and resolving phlegm, alleviating cough and dyspnea. It is indicated for cough, dyspnea, profuse and yellow thick phlegm, difficult expectoration, red face and fever, shortness of breath, flapping of the nasal wings, chest distress and fullness, red tongue and yellow greasy fur, slippery and rapid pulse, also for acute bronchitis, asthma and pneumonia attributive to stagnation of phlegm-heat in the lung.

Warning It is not suitable for cases with cough and dyspnea due to cold and deficiency syndrome.

小儿清咽冲剂

【处方】玄参、蒲公英、薄荷、牛蒡子（炒）、蝉蜕、板蓝根、连翘、牡丹皮、青黛。

【功能主治】清热解表，解毒利咽。用于小儿外感风热引起的发热头痛，咳嗽音哑，咽喉肿痛。

Children Sore-throat-relieving Soluble Granules

Name of Chinese Phonetic Alphabet Xiao Er Qing Yan Chong Ji

Formula Scrophulariae Radix, Taraxaci Herba, Menthae Haplocalycis Herba, Arctii Fructus (fried) Cicadae Periostracum, Isatidis Radix, Forsythiae Fructus, Moutan Cortex and Indigo Naturalis.

Actions and Indications Clearing heat and releasing the exterior, detoxicating and soothing the throat. It is indicated for children fever, headache, cough, hoarseness and sore-throat due to exogenous wind-heat.

小儿清热止咳口服液

【处方】麻黄、苦杏仁（炒）、石膏、甘草、黄芩、板蓝根、北豆根。

【功能主治】清热，宣肺，平喘。用于小儿外感引起的发热恶寒，咳嗽痰黄，气促喘息，口干音哑，咽喉肿痛，乳蛾红肿。

Clearing Heat and Alleviating Children Cough Oral Liquid

Name of Chinese Phonetic Alphabet Xiao Er

Qing Re Zhi Ke Kou Fu Ye

Formula Ephedrae Herba, Armeniacae Semen Amarum (fried), Gypsum Fibrosum, Glycyrrhizae Radix et Rhizoma, Scutellariae Radix, Isatidis Radix and Menispermi Rhizoma.

Actions and Indications Clearing heat, diffusing the lung and relieving dyspnea. It is indicated for children fever, aversion to cold, cough with yellow phlegm, dyspnea, dry mouth, hoarseness, sore-throat, red and swelling tonsil due to external contraction.

小儿清热利肺口服液

【处方】金银花、连翘、石膏、麻黄、苦杏仁、牛蒡子、射干等。

【功能主治】清热宣肺，止咳平喘。用于小儿咳嗽属风热犯肺证。症见发热，咳嗽或咯痰，流涕或鼻塞，咽痛，口渴，舌红或苔黄。小儿急性支气管炎具有上述症候者。

【注意】脾胃虚弱者慎用。

Relieving Children Cough Oral Liquid

Name of Chinese Phonetic Alphabet Xiao Er Qing Re Li Fei Kou Fu Ye

Formula Lonicerae Japonicae Flos, Forsythiae Fructus, Gypsum Fibrosum, Ephedrae Herba, Armeniacae Semen Amarum, Arctii Fructus, Belamcandae Rhizoma, etc.

Actions and Indications Clearing heat and diffusing the lung, alleviating cough and dyspnea. It is indicated for children cough attributive to wind-heat invading the lung, masnifested as fever, cough or spitting phlegm, rhinorrhea or stuffy nose, sore-throat, thirst, red tongue or yellow tongue fur, etc. Also for children acute bronchitis with the above mentioned symptoms.

Warning It should be used carefully for cases with deficiency of the spleen and stomach.

小儿清感灵片

【处方】羌活、荆芥穗、防风、苍术（炒）、白芷、葛根、川芎、地黄、黄芩、甘草、牛黄、苦杏仁（炒）。

【功能主治】发汗解肌，清热透表。用于外感风寒引起的发热怕冷，肌表无汗，头痛口渴，咽痛鼻塞，咳嗽痰多，体倦。

Relieving Common Cold Tablet for Children

Name of Chinese Phonetic Alphabet Xiao Er Qing Gan Ling Pian

Formula Notopterygii Rhizoma et Radix, Schizonepetae Spica, Saposhnikoviae Radix, Atractylodis Rhizoma (fried), Angelicae Dahuricae Radix, Puerariae Lobatae Radix, Chuanxiong Rhizoma, Rehmanniae Radix, Scutellariae Radix, Glycyrrhizae Radix et Rhizoma, Bovis Calculus and Armeniacae Semen Amarum (fried).

Actions and Indications Promoting sweating, releasing the flesh, clearing heat and outthrusting through the exterior. It is indicated for fever, fear of cold, anhidrosis, headache, thirst, sore-throat, nasal congestion, cough with profuse phlegm and tiredness due to external contraction of wind-cold.

小儿智力糖浆

【处方】龟甲、龙骨、远志、石菖蒲、雄鸡。

【功能主治】调补阴阳，开窍益智。用于小儿脑功能轻微障碍综合征。

Children Intelligence-promoting Syrup

Name of Chinese Phonetic Alphabet Xiao Er Zhi Li Tang Jiang

Formula Testudinis Carapax et Plastrum, Draconis Os, Polygalae Radix, Acori Tatarinowii Rhizoma and Galli Caro Maris.

Actions and Indications Regulating and tonifying *yin* and *yang*, opening the orifices to promote intelligence. It is used for minimal brain disorder syndrome in children.

小儿感冒颗粒

【处方】广藿香、菊花、连翘、大青叶、板蓝根、地黄、地骨皮、白薇、薄荷、石膏。

【功能主治】疏风解表，清热解毒。用于小儿风热感冒，发热重，头胀痛，咳嗽痰黏，咽喉肿痛；流感见上述证候者。

Common Cold Relieving Soluble Granules for Children

Name of Chinese Phonetic Alphabet Xiao Er Gan Mao Ke Li

Formula Pogostemonis Herba, Chrysanthemi Flos, Forsythiae Fructus, Isatidis Folium, Isatidis Radix, Rehmanniae Radix, Lycii Cortex, Cynanchi Atrati Radix et Rhizoma, Menthae Haplocalycis Herba and Gypsum Fibrosum.

Actions and Indications Dispersing wind and releasing the exterior, clearing heat and detoxicating. It is indicated for common cold in children, marked by fever, distending pain over the head, cough with mucous phlegm, sore-throat, and is used for influenza with the above mentioned symptoms.

小儿腹泻宁糖浆

【处方】党参、白术、茯苓、葛根、甘草、广藿香、木香。

【功能主治】补气健脾，和胃生津。用于小儿腹泻呕吐，口渴，消化不良，消瘦倦怠，舌淡苔白。

【注意】呕吐腹泻后舌红口渴，小便短赤者慎用。

Relieving Children Diarrhea Syrup

Name of Chinese Phonetic Alphabet Xiao Er Fu Xie Ning Tang Jiang

Formula Codonopsis Radix, Atractylodis Macrocephalae Rhizoma, Poria, Puerariae Lobatae Radix, Glycyrrhizae Radix et Rhizoma, Pogostemonis Herba and Aucklandiae Radix.

Actions and Indications Tonifying *qi* and fortifying the spleen, harmonizing the stomach and engendering fluid. It is used for children diarrhea and vomiting, thirst, dyspepsia, emaciation and tiredness, pale tongue with white fur.

Warning It should be used carefully for cases with red tongue and thirst, scanty and dark urine after vomiting and diarrhea.

小儿解表冲剂

【处方】金银花、连翘、牛蒡子（炒）、蒲公英，黄芩、防风、紫苏叶、荆芥穗、葛根、牛黄。

【功能主治】宣肺解表，清热解毒。用于感冒初起引起的恶寒发热，头痛咳嗽，鼻塞流涕，咽喉痛痒。

Common-cold-relieving Soluble Granules for Children

Name of Chinese Phonetic Alphabet Xiao Er Jie Biao Chong Ji

Formula Lonicerae Japonicae Flos, Forsythiae Fructus, Arctii Fructus (fried), Taraxaci Herba, Scutellariae Radix, Saposhnikoviae Radix, Perillae Folium, Schizonepetae Spica, Puerariae Lobatae Radix and Bovis Calculus.

Actions and Indications Diffusing the lung and releasing the exterior, clearing heat and detoxicating. It is indicated for initial stage of common cold, marked by aversion to cold, fever, headache, cough, nasal congestion, rhinorrhea, pain and itch of throat.

小儿解热丸

【处方】胆南星、竹黄、青礞石（煅）、猪牙皂、陈皮、甘草、全蝎、僵蚕（炒）、蜈蚣、天麻、钩藤、羌活、麻黄、薄荷、防风、牛黄、琥珀、冰片、朱砂、珍珠、麝香等。

【功能主治】清热豁痰，息风定惊。治疗小儿急热惊风，痰热动风抽搐，舌绛脉数。

Children Heat-clearing Pill

Name of Chinese Phonetic Alphabet Xiao Er Jie Re Wan

Formula Arisaema cum Bile, Shiraiae Bambusicolae Stroma, Chloriti Lapis (calcined), Gleditsiae Fructus Abnomalis, Citri Reticulatae Pericarpium, Glycyrrhizae Radix et Rhizoma, Scorpio, Bombyx Batryticatus (fried), Scolopendra, Gastrodiae Rhizoma, Uncariae Ramulus cum Uncis, Notopterygii Rhizoma et Radix, Ephedrae Herba, Menthae Haplocalycis Herba, Saposhnikoviae Radix, Bovis Calculus, Succinum, Borneolum Syntheticum, Cinnabaris, Margarita, Moschus, etc.

Actions and Indications Clearing heat, expelling phlegm, extinguishing wind, settling fright. It is used for infantile acute convulsion, tic due to phlegm-heat, crimson tongue and rapid pulse.

小儿敷脐止泻散

【处方】黑胡椒。

【功能主治】温中散寒，止泻。主治小儿、腹泻，腹痛。

【注意】敷药期间忌食生冷油腻。只供外用。

Umbilical Compress Powder for Children Diarrhea

Name of Chinese Phonetic Alphabet Xiao Er Fu Qi Zhi Xie San

Formula Piperis Fructus Nigrum.

Actions and Indications Warming the middle and dissipating cold, relieving diarrhea. It is indicated for children diarrhea and abdominal pain.

Warning Uncooked, cold and oily foods should be avoided. It is for external use only.

小青龙颗粒

【处方】麻黄、桂枝、白芍、干姜、细辛、甘草（蜜制）、法半夏、五味子。

【功能主治】解表化饮，止咳平喘。用于风寒水饮，恶寒发热，无汗，喘咳痰稀。

【注意】凡风热咳喘及正气不足的虚喘不宜应用，阴虚干咳无痰者禁用。

Xiaoqinglong Granules

Name of Chinese Phonetic Alphabet Xiao Qing Long Ke Li

Formula Ephedrae Herba, Cinnamomi Ramulus, Paeoniae Radix Alba, Zingiberis Rhizoma, Asari Radix et Rhizoma, Glycyrrhizae Radix et Rhizoma (prepared with honey), Pinelliae Rhizoma Praeparatum and Schisandrae Chinensis Fructus.

Actions and Indications Releasing the exterior, resolving retained fluid, suppressing cough and calming panting. It is indicated for retained fluid, aversion to cold with fever, anhidrosis, dyspnea and cough with clear phlegm due to attack of wind-cold.

Warning It is contraindicated for cases with dyspnea, cough due to wind-heat and insufficiency of healthy *qi* and for cases with non-productive cough due to *yin*-deficiency.

小败毒膏

【处方】蒲公英、金银花、天花粉、黄柏、大黄、白芷、陈皮、乳香（醋炙）、当归、赤芍、木鳖子（打碎）、甘草。

【功能主治】清热解毒，消肿止痛。用于湿热蕴结、热毒壅盛引起的疮疡初起，红肿硬痛，周身刺痒，乳痈胀痛，大便燥结。

【注意】孕妇忌服，忌食辛辣鱼腥食物。

Relieving Sore Soft Extract

Name of Chinese Phonetic Alphabet Xiao Bai Du Gao

Formula Taraxaci Herba, Lonicerae Japonicae Flos, Trichosanthis Radix, Phellodendri Chinensis Cortex, Rhei Radix et Rhizoma, Angelicae Dahuricae Radix, Citri Reticulatae Pericarpium, Olibanum (prepared with vinegar), Angelicae Sinensis Radix, Paeoniae Radix Rubra, Momordicae Semen (crushed) and Glycyrrhizae Radix et Rhizoma.

Actions and Indications Clearing heat and detoxicating, dispersing swelling and relieving pain. It is used for initial stage of sore and ulcer with red, swelling and pain, itching of the whole body, acute mastitis and dry stool due to damp-heat accumulation and excessive heat-toxin.

Warning It is contraindicated for pregnant women. Pungent and fish foods should be avoided.

小金丸

【处方】麝香、没药（制）、乳香（制）、枫香脂、制草乌、当归（酒炒）、地龙、香墨、五灵脂（醋炒）、木鳖子（去壳去油）。

【功能主治】散结消肿，化瘀止痛。用于阴疽初起，皮色不变，肿硬作痛，多发性脓肿，瘿瘤，瘰疬，乳岩，乳癖。

【注意】孕妇禁用。

Xiao Jin Pill

Name of Chinese Phonetic Alphabet Xiao Jin Wan

Formula Moschus, Myrrha (prepared), Olibanum (prepared), Liquidambaris Resina, Aconiti Kusnezoffii Radix Cocta, Angelicae Sinensis Radix (fried with wine), Pheretima, Chinese Ink, Trogopterori Faeces (fried with vinegar) and Momordicae Semen (removed seed coat and oil).

Actions and Indications Dissipating mass, reducing swelling, resolving stasis, alleviating pain. It is used for initial stage of deep-rooted carbuncle with swelling, hard and painful, multiple abscesses, goiter, scrofula, mammary rocky mass, hyperplasia of mammary gland.

Warning It is contraindicated for pregnant women.

小建中冲剂

【处方】桂枝、白芍、甘草（蜜炙）、生姜、大枣。

【功能主治】温中补虚，止痛。用于脾胃虚寒，脘腹疼痛，喜温喜按，嘈杂吞酸，食少，心悸，胃及十二指肠溃疡。

Middle-energizer-warming Soluble Granules

Name of Chinese Phonetic Alphabet Xiao Jian Zhong Chong Ji

Formula Cinnamomi Ramulus, Paeoniae Radix Alba, Glycyrrhizae Radix et Rhizoma (prepared with honey), Zingiberis Rhizoma Recens and Jujubae Fructus.

Actions and Indications Warming the middle energizer and replenishing deficiency, alleviating pain. It is indicated for abdominal pain, like warmth and pressing, gastric upset, acid regurgitation, anorexia, palpitation and gastroduodenal ulcer due to deficiency-cold of the spleen and stomach.

小活络丸

【处方】胆南星、制川乌、制草乌、地龙、乳香（制）、没药（制）。

【功能主治】祛风除湿，活血通痹。用于风寒湿痹，肢体疼痛，麻木拘挛。

【注意】孕妇禁用。

Arthralgia-relieving Pill

Name of Chinese Phonetic Alphabet Xiao Huo Luo Wan

Formula Arisaema cum Bile, Aconiti Radix Cocta, Aconiti Kusnezoffii Radix Cocta, Pheretima, Olibanum (prepared) and Myrrha (prepared).

Actions and Indications Dispelling wind and dampness, activating blood and freeing impediment. It is indicated for wind-cold-dampness impediment syndrome (arthralgia), general pain, numbness and spasm of the body.

Warning It is contraindicated for pregnant women.

小柴胡冲剂

【处方】柴胡、姜半夏、黄芩、党参、甘草、生姜、大枣。

【功能主治】解表散热，疏肝和胃。用于寒热往来，胸胁苦满，心烦喜吐，口苦咽干。

Soluble Granules of Minor Chinese Hare's Ear★

Name of Chinese Phonetic Alphabet Xiao Chai Hu Chong Ji

Formula Bupleuri Radix, Pinelliae Rhizoma Praeparatum cum Zingibere et Alumine, Scutellariae Radix, Codonopsis Radix, Glycyrrhizae Radix et Rhizoma, Zingiberis Rhizoma Recens and Jujubae Fructus.

Actions and Indications Releasing the exterior and dissipating heat, soothing the liver and harmonizing the stomach. It is indicated for alternate attacks of chill and fever, fullness and oppression in the hypochondrium, dysphoria, vomiting, bitter mouth and dry throat.

* 柴胡

子龙丸

【处方】甘遂、京大戟、芥子。

【功能主治】逐饮祛痰。用于痰涎伏饮停伏于胸膈上下之忽然胸背、颈项、腰胯隐痛不可忍，筋骨牵引灼痛，走窜不定，或手足冷痹，或头痛，或神志昏倦，以及痰迷癫痫。

Zi Long Pill

Name of Chinese Phonetic Alphabet Zi Long Wan

Formula Kansui Radix, Euphorbiae Pekinensis Radix and Sinapis Semen.

Actions and Indications Expelling retained fluid and dispelling phlegm. It is indicated for sudden and wandering pain in the chest, nape, neck, waist and hip, scorching pain in the sinew and bone, or cold and numbness of limbs, or headache, loss of consciousness, and epilepsy due to retention of phlegm in the thorax.

四画

开光复明丸

【处方】栀子（姜炙）、黄芩、黄连、黄柏、大黄、龙胆、蒺藜（去刺盐炒）、菊花、防风、石决明、玄参、红花、当归尾、赤芍、地黄、泽泻、羚羊角粉、冰片。

【功能主治】清热散风，退翳明目。用于肝胆热盛引起的暴发火眼，红肿痛痒，眼睑赤烂，羞明。

【注意】孕妇及脾胃虚寒者忌服。忌食辛辣食物。

Improving Vision Bolus

Name of Chinese Phonetic Alphabet Kai Guang Fu Ming Wan

Formula Gardeniae Fructus (prepared with ginger), Scutellariae Radix, Coptidis Rhizoma, Phellodendri Chinensis Cortex, Rhei Radix et Rhizoma, Gentianae Radix et Rhizoma, Tribuli Fructus (removed thorn and fried with salt), Chrysanthemi Flos, Saposhnikoviae Radix, Haliotidis Concha, Scrophulariae Radix, Carthami Flos, Angelicae Sinensis Radix (tail part), Paeoniae Radix Rubra, Rehmanniae Radix, Alismatis Rhizoma, Saigae Tataricae Cornu Pulvis and Borneolum Syntheticum.

Actions and Indications Clearing heat and dissipating wind, removing nebula to improve vision. It is used for sudden conjunctivitis, pain, swelling and itching of the eyes, blepharitis marginalis and photophobia due to exuberant heat of the liver and gall.

Warning It is contraindicated for pregnant women and cases with deficiency-cold of the spleen and stomach. Pungent foods should be avoided.

开胃山楂丸

【处方】山楂、六神曲（炒）、槟榔、山药、白扁豆（炒）、鸡内金（炒）、枳壳（麸炒）、麦芽（炒）、砂仁。

【功能主治】健脾胃，助消化。用于饮食积滞，脘腹胀满，食后疼痛，消化不良。

Chinese Hawthorn* Bolus for Promoting Digestion

Name of Chinese Phonetic Alphabet Kai Wei Shan Zha Wan

Formula Crataegi Fructus, Medicata Massa Fermentata (fried), Arecea Semen, Dioscoreae Rhizoma, Lablab Semen Album (fried), Galli Gigerii Endothelium Corneum (fried), Aurantii Fructus (fried with bran), Hordei Fructus Germinatus (fried) and Amomi Fructus.

Actions and Indications Fortifying the spleen and stomach, promoting digestion. It is used for food stagnation, abdominal distention and fullness with pain after meal, dyspepsia.

* 山楂

开胃健脾丸

【处方】白术、党参、茯苓、木香、黄连、六神曲（炒）、陈皮、砂仁、麦芽（炒）、山楂、山药、肉豆蔻（煨）、甘草（蜜炙）。

【功能主治】开胃健脾。用于脾胃不和，消化不良，食欲不振，嗳气吞酸。

Appetite-improving Pill

Name of Chinese Phonetic Alphabet Kai Wei Jian Pi Wan

Formula Atractylodis Macrocephalae Rhizoma, Codonopsis Radix, Poria, Aucklandiae Radix, Coptidis Rhizoma, Medicata Massa Fermentata (fried), Citri Reticulatae Pericarpium, Amomi Fructus, Hordei Fructus Germinatus (fried), Crataegi Fructus, Dioscoreae Rhizoma, Myristicae Semen (roasted) and Glycyrrhizae Radix et Rhizoma (prepared with honey).

Actions and Indications Promoting appetite and fortifying the spleen. It is used for dyspepsia, poor appetite, eructation and acid regurgitation due to disharmony of the spleen and stomach.

开胸顺气丸

【处方】槟榔、牵牛子（炒）、陈皮、木香、厚朴（姜制）、三棱（醋制）、莪术（醋制）、猪牙皂。

【功能主治】消积化滞，行气止痛。用于停食停水，气郁不舒，胸胁胀满，胃脘胀痛。

【注意】孕妇禁用，年老体弱者慎用。

Qi-fluency Pill

Name of Chinese Phonetic Alphabet Kai Xiong Shun Qi Wan

Formula Arecae Semen, Pharbitidis Semen (fried), Citri Reticulatae Pericarpium, Aucklandiae Radix, Magnoliae Officinalis Cortex (prepared with ginger), Sparganii Rhizoma (prepared with vinegar), Curcumae Rhizoma (prepared with vinegar) and Gleditsiae Fructus Abnormalis.

Actions and Indications Dispersing accumulation and food retention, moving *qi* to alleviate pain. It is used for hypochondriac fullness and stomach duct pain due to food and *qi* stagnation.

Warning It is contraindicated for pregnant women and should be used carefully for senile debility.

天一止咳糖浆

【处方】百部流浸膏、桔梗流浸膏、远志流浸膏、盐酸麻黄碱、氯化铵、薄荷脑。

【功能主治】用于感冒、咳嗽、多痰、支气管性气喘。

Tian Yi Syrup for Alleviating Cough

Name of Chinese Phonetic Alphabet Tian Yi Zhi Ke Tang Jiang

Formula Stemonae Extractum, Platycodonis Extractum, Polygalae Extractum, Ephedrine Hydrochloride, Ammonium Chloride and Menthol.

Actions and Indications It is indicated for common cold, cough, profuse phlegm, bronchial dyspnea.

天王补心浓缩丸

【处方】丹参、当归、石菖蒲、党参、茯苓、五味子、麦冬、天冬、地黄、玄参、远志（制）、酸枣仁、柏子仁、桔梗、甘草、朱砂。

【功能主治】滋阴，养血，补心安神。用于心阴不足，心悸健忘，失眠多梦，大便干燥。

Cardiotonic Concentrative Bolus

Name of Chinese Phonetic Alphabet Tian Wang Bu Xin Nong Suo Wan

Formula Salviae Miltiorrhizae Radix et Rhizoma, Angelicae Sinensis Radix, Acori Tatarinowii Rhizoma, Codonopsis Radix, Poria, Schisandrae Chinensis Fructus, Ophiopogonis Radix, Asparagi Radix, Rehmanniae Radix, Scrophulariae Radix, Polygalae Radix (prepared), Ziziphi Spinosae Semen, Platycladi Semen, Platycodonis Radix, Glycyrrhizae Radix et Rhizoma and Cinnabaris.

Actions and Indications Enriching *yin*, nourishing blood, tonifying the heart, tranquilizing the mind. It is used for palpitation, amnesia, insomnia, profuse dreaming, and dry stool due to insufficiency of heart-*yin*.

天和追风膏

【处方】生草乌、麻黄、细辛、羌活、乌药、白芷、高良姜、独活、威灵仙、生川乌、肉桂、红花、桃仁、苏木、赤芍、乳香、没药、当归、蜈蚣、蛇蜕、海风藤、牛膝、续断、香加皮、红大戟、麝香酮、血竭、肉桂油、冰片、薄荷脑、辣椒流浸膏、丁香罗勒油、月桂氮卓酮、樟脑、水杨酸甲酯。

【功能主治】温经通络，祛风除湿，活血止痛。用于风湿痹痛，腰背酸痛，四肢麻木，经脉拘挛。

【注意】孕妇禁用。

Tian He Plaster for Relieving Rheumalgia

Name of Chinese Phonetic Alphabet Tian He Zhui Feng Gao

Formula Aconiti Kusnezoffii Radix, Ephedrae Herba, Asari Radix et Rhizoma, Notopterygii Rhizoma et Radix, Linderae Radix, Angelicae Dahuricae Radix, Alpiniae Officinarum Rhizoma, Angelicae Pubescentis Radix, Clematidis Radix et Rhizoma, Aconiti Radix, Cinnamomi Cortex, Carthami Flos, Persicae Semen, Sappan Lignum, Paeoniae Radix Rubra, Olibanum, Myrrha, Angelicae Sinensis Radix, Scolopendra, Serpentis Periostracum, Piperis Kadsurae Caulis, Achyranthis Bidentatae Radix, Dipsaci Radix, Periplocae Cortex, Knoxiae Radix, Musk Ketone, Draconis Sanguis, Cinnamomi Oleum, Borneolum Syntheticum, Menthol, Capsici Extractum, Ocimi Basilici Oleum, Laurocapram, Camphora and Methylsalicylate.

Actions and Indications Warming the meridians and activating collaterals, dispelling wind and dampness, activating blood and alleviating pain. It is indicated for rheumalgia , aching pain of the waist and back, numbness and spasm of the limbs.

Warning It is contraindicated for pregnant women.

天麻丸

【处方】天麻、羌活、独活、杜仲（盐炒）、牛膝、粉萆薢、附子（制）、当归、地黄、玄参。

【功能主治】祛风除湿，舒筋通络，活血止痛。用于肢体拘挛，手足麻木，腰腿酸痛。

【注意】孕妇慎服。

Gastrodia* Honey Bolus for Relieving Numbness of Limbs

Name of Chinese Phonetic Alphabet Tian Ma Wan

Formula Gastrodiae Rhizoma, Notopterygii Rhizoma et Radix, Angelicae Pubescentis Radix, Eucommiae Cortex (fried with salt), Achyranthis Bidentatae Radix, Dioscoreae Hypoglaucae Rhizoma, Aconiti Lateralis Radix Praeparata,, Angelicae Sinensis Radix, Rehmanniae Radix and Scrophulariae Radix.

Actions and Indications Dispelling wind and dampness, relaxing sinews and dredging collaterals, activating blood and relieving pain. It is used for spasm and numbness of limbs, soreness and pain of waist and legs.

Warning It should be used carefully for pregnant women.

* 天麻

天麻头痛片

【处方】天麻、白芷、川芎、荆芥、当归、乳香(醋制)。

【功能主治】养血祛风，散寒止痛。用于风寒头痛、血虚头痛、血瘀头痛。

Gastrodia* Headache-relieving Tablet

Name of Chinese Phonetic Alphabet Tian Ma Tou Tong Pian

Formula Gastrodiae Rhizoma, Angelicae Dahuricae Radix, Chuanxiong Rhizoma, Schizonepetae Herba, Angelicae Sinensis Radix and Olibanum (prepared with vinegar).

Actions and Indications Nourishing blood and dispelling wind, dissipating cold and relieving pain. It is indicated for headache due to wind-cold, blood-deficiency and blood-stasis respectively.

* 天麻

天麻钩藤颗粒

【处方】天麻、钩藤、石决明、栀子、黄芩、牛膝、杜仲(盐制)、益母草、茯苓、桑寄生、首乌藤。

【功能主治】平肝息风，清热安神。用于肝阳上亢，高血压等所引起的头痛、眩晕、耳鸣、眼花、震颤、失眠。

Gastrodia* and Gambir Vine** Granules

Name of Chinese Phonetic Alphabet Tian Ma Gou Teng Ke Li

Formula Gastrodiae Rhizoma, Uncariae Ramulus cum Uncis, Haliotidis Concha, Gardeniae Fructus, Scutellariae Radix, Achyranthis Bidentatae Radix, Eucommiae Cortex (prepared with salt), Leonuri Herba, Poria, Taxilli Herba and Polygoni Multiflori Caulis.

Actions and Indications Pacifying the liver, extinguishing wind, clearing heat, tranquilizing the mind. It is used for headache, vertigo, tinnitus, blurred vision, tremor and insomnia due to ascendant hyperactivity of liver-*yang* and hypertension.

* 天麻 ** 钩藤

天麻首乌片

【处方】天麻、白芷、何首乌、熟地黄、丹参、川芎、当归、蒺藜、桑叶、墨旱莲、白芍、女贞子、黄精、甘草。

【功能主治】滋补肝肾，养血息风，定眩止痛，乌须黑发。用于肝肾不足所致的眩晕头痛，口苦咽干，耳鸣耳聋，视物昏花，神疲健忘，须发早白，舌红少苔，脉象弦细；脑动脉硬化，早期高血压，血管性头痛，脂溢性皮炎属上述证候者。

Gastrodia* and Chinese Knotweed** Tablet

Name of Chinese Phonetic Alphabet Tian Ma Shou Wu Pian

Formula Gastrodiae Rhizoma, Angelicae Dahuricae Radix, Polygoni Multiflori Radix, Rehmanniae Radix Praeparata, Salviae Miltiorrhizae Radix et Rhizoma, Chuanxiong Rhizoma, Angelicae Sinensis Radix, Tribuli Fructus, Mori Folium, Ecliptae Herba, Paeoniae Radix Alba, Ligustri Lucidi Fructus, Polygonati Rhizoma and Glycyrrhizae Radix et Rhizoma.

Actions and Indications Enriching the liver and kidney, nourishing blood, extinguishing wind, relieving vertigo, alleviating pain, blackening hair and beard. It is used for vertigo, headache, bitter taste in the mouth, dry throat, tinnitus, deafness, blurred vision, lassitude of spirit, amnesia, premature graying of hair, red tongue with few coating, string-like and fine pulse due to insufficiency of the liver and kidney; and also for cerebral arteriosclerosis, early stage of hypertension, vascular headache, seborrheic dermatitis.

* 天麻 ** 何首乌

天麻祛风补片

【处方】天麻（姜汁制）、当归、附片（砂炒）、杜仲（盐炙）、独活、茯苓、川牛膝（酒炙）、地黄、肉桂、羌活、玄参。

【功能主治】温肾养肝，除湿止痛。用于肝肾亏损引起的头昏、头晕、耳鸣，畏寒肢冷，四肢关节疼痛，腰酸膝软，手足麻木等症。

【注意】感冒忌用。

Gastrodia* Tablet for Dispelling Wind

Name of Chinese Phonetic Alphabet Tian Ma Qu Feng Bu Pian

Formula Gastrodiae Rhizoma (prepared with ginger juice), Angelicae Sinensis Radix, Aconiti Lateralis Radix Praeparata (sliced and fried with sand), Eucommiae Cortex (prepared with salt), Angelicae Pubescentis Radix, Poria, Cyathulae Radix (prepared with wine), Rehmanniae Radix, Cinnamomi Cortex, Notopterygii Rhizoma et Radix and Scrophulariae Radix.

Actions and Indications Warming the kidney and tonifying the liver, eliminating dampness and alleviating pain. It is indicated for dizziness, tinnitus, fear of cold, cold limbs, arthralgia, soreness of waist and weakness of knees, and numbness of limbs due to dual depletion of the liver and kidney.

Warning It is contraindicated for cases with common cold.

* 天麻

元胡止痛滴丸

【处方】延胡索（醋制）、白芷。

【功能主治】理气，活血，止痛。用于气滞血瘀的胃痛，胁痛头痛及月经痛等。

*Yanhusuo** Drop Pill for Alleviating Pain

Name of Chinese Phonetic Alphabet Yuan Hu Zhi Tong Di Wan

Formula Corydalis Rhizoma (prepared with vinegar) and Angelicae Dahuricae Radix.

Actions and Indications Regulating *qi*, activating blood, alleviating pain. It is indicated for stomachache, hypochondriac pain, headache and dysmenorrhea due to *qi*-stagnation and blood-stasis.

* 延胡索

无极丸

【处方】甘草、石膏、滑石粉、糯米（蒸熟）、薄荷脑、冰片、丁香、砂仁、豆蔻、肉桂、牛黄等。

【功能主治】清热祛暑，止呕。用于中暑，呕吐恶心，烦倦，头目晕眩，伤酒伤食，消化不良，水土不服，晕车晕船。

Wu Ji Pill for Summer-heat Stroke

Name of Chinese Phonetic Alphabet Wu Ji Wan

Formula Glycyrrhizae Radix et Rhizoma, Gypsum Fibrosum, Talci Pulvis, Oryzae Glutinosae Fructus (steamed), Menthol, Borneolum Syntheticum, Caryophylli Flos, Amomi Fructus, Amomi Fructus Rotundus, Cinnamomi Cortex, Bovis Calculus, etc.

Actions and Indications Clearing heat and dispelling summer-heat, relieving vomiting. It is indicated for summer-heat stroke, vomiting, nausea, tiredness, dizziness, dizzy vision, excessive drinking and improper diet, indigestion, unaccustomedness to the climate of a new place, car sickness and naupathia.

无烟灸条

【处方】羌活、细辛、白芷、甘松、木香、艾叶炭。

【功能主治】行气血，逐寒湿。用于风寒湿痹，肌肉酸麻，关节四肢疼痛，脘腹冷痛。

Smokeless Moxa-roll

Name of Chinese Phonetic Alphabet Wu Yan

Jiu Tiao

Formula Notopterygii Rhizoma et Radix, Asari Radix et Rhizoma, Angelicae Dahuricae Radix, Nardostachyos Radix et Rhizoma, Aucklandiae Radix and Artemisiae Argyi Folium Carbonisatus.

Actions and Indications Moving *qi* and blood, eliminating cold-dampness. It is used for wind-cold-dampness impediment syndrome marked by aching and numbness of muscles, pain of the joints and limbs, abdominal cold and pain.

云香精

【处方】白芷、朱砂根、鸡骨香、莪术、五味藤、白木香、千斤拔、皂角、羊耳菊、枫荷桂、虎杖、桂枝、过江龙、穿壁风、风藤、木香、了刁竹、山豆根、细辛、樟脑、薄荷脑等。

【功能主治】祛风除湿，活血止痛。用于风湿骨痛，伤风感冒，头痛，肚痛，心胃气痛，冻疮。

【注意】孕妇与未满3岁儿童忌内服。

Yun Xiang Essence

Name of Chinese Phonetic Alphabet Yun Xiang Jing

Formula Angelicae Dahuricae Radix, Ardisiae Crenatae Radix, Crotonis Crassifolii Radix, Curcumae Rhizoma, Securidacae Inappendiculatae Radix, Stephaniae Tetrandrae Radix, Flemingiae Philippinensis Radix, Gleditsiae Fructus, Inulae Cappae Herba, Sassafratis Tzumu Radix, Polygoni Cuspidati Rhizoma et Radix , Cinnamomi Ramulus, Lycopodii Complanati Herba, Piperis Hancei Caulis et Folium, Fici Martini Radix et Caulis, Aucklandiae Radix, Cynanchi Paniculati Radix et Rhizoma, Sophorae Tonkinensis Radix et Rhizoma, Asari Radix et Rhizoma, Camphora, Menthol, etc.

Actions and Indications Dispelling wind and dampness, activating blood and relieving pain. It is indicated for rheumatic ostealgia, common cold, headache, abdominal pain, precordial pain, chilblain.

Warning It is contraindicated for pregnant women and children under 3 years of age.

木瓜丸

【处方】木瓜、当归、川芎、白芷、威灵仙、狗脊（制）、牛膝、鸡血藤、海风藤、人参、制川乌、制草乌。

【功能主治】祛风散寒，活络止痛。用于风寒湿痹，四肢麻木，周身疼痛，腰膝无力，步履艰难。

【注意】孕妇禁用。

Chinese-quince* Pill for Relieving Impediment Syndrome

Name of Chinese Phonetic Alphabet Mu Gua Wan

Formula Chaenomelis Fructus, Angelicae Sinensis Radix, Chuanxiong Rhizoma, Angelicae Dahuricae Radix, Clematidis Radix et Rhizoma, Cibotii Rhizoma(prepared), Achyranthis Bidentatae Radix, Spatholobi Caulis, Piperis Kadsurae Caulis, Ginseng Radix et Rhizoma, Aconiti Radix Cocta and Aconiti Kusnezoffii Radix Cocta.

Actions and Indications Dispelling wind and dissipating cold, activating collaterals and alleviating pain. It is indicated for wind-cold-dampness impediment syndrome, marked by numbness of the limbs, general pain, weakness of the waist and knees, difficulty for walk.

Warning It is contraindicated for pregnant women.

* 木瓜

木香分气丸

【处方】木香、砂仁、丁香、檀香、香附（醋炙）、广藿香、陈皮、厚朴（姜炙）、枳实、豆蔻、莪术（醋炙）、山楂（炒）、白术（麸炒）、甘松、槟榔、甘草。

【功能主治】宽胸消胀，止呕。用于肝郁气滞，脾胃不和，胸膈痞闷，两胁胀满，胃脘疼痛，倒饱嘈杂，呕吐恶心，嗳气吞酸。

【注意】孕妇慎用。

Common Aucklandia* Pill

Name of Chinese Phonetic Alphabet Mu Xiang

Fen Qi Wan

Formula Aucklandiae Radix, Amomi Fructus, Caryophylli Flos, Santali Albi Lignum, Cyperi Rhizoma (prepared with vinegar), Pogostemonis Herba, Citri Reticulatae Pericarpium, Magnoliae Officinalis Cortex (prepared with vinegar), Aurantii Fructus Immaturus, Amomi Fructus Rotundus, Curcumae Rhizoma (prepared with vinegar), Crataegi Fructus (fried), Atractylodis Macrocephalae Rhizoma (fried with bran), Nardostachyos Radix et Rhizoma, Arecae Semen and Glycyrrhizae Radix et Rhizoma.

Actions and Indications Soothing the chest, dispersing fullness, relieving vomiting. It is used for chest stuffiness and depression, hypochondriac fullness, pain in stomach duct, gastric upset, vomiting, nausea, eructation and acid regurgitation due to stagnation of liver-*qi* and disharmony of the spleen and stomach.

Warning It should be used cautiously for pregnant women.

* 木香

木香顺气丸

【处方】木香、砂仁、香附（醋制）、槟榔、甘草、陈皮、厚朴（制）、枳壳（炒）、苍术（炒）、青皮（炒）。

【功能主治】行气化湿，健脾和胃。用于湿浊阻滞气机，胸膈痞闷，脘腹胀痛，呕吐恶心，嗳气纳呆。

Qi-moving Pill of Common Aucklandia*

Name of Chinese Phonetic Alphabet Mu Xiang Shun Qi Wan

Formula Aucklandiae Radix, Amomi Fructus, Cyperi Rhizoma (prepared with vinegar), Arecae Semen, Glycyrrhizae Radix et Rhizoma, Citri Reticulatae Pericarpium, Magnoliae Officinalis Cortex (prepared), Aurantii Fructus (fried), Atractylodis Rhizoma (fried) and Citri Reticulatae Pericarpium Viride (fried).

Actions and Indications Moving *qi*, resolving dampness, fortifying the spleen and harmonizing the stomach. It is used for stuffiness and depression of hypochondrium, abdominal fullness and pain, vomiting, nausea, eructation and loss of appetite caused by stagnation of *qi* movement and dampness-turbidity.

* 木香

木香槟榔丸

【处方】木香、槟榔、枳壳（炒）、陈皮、青皮（醋炒）、香附（醋制）、三棱（醋制）、莪术（醋制）、黄连、黄柏（酒炒）、大黄、牵牛子（炒）、芒硝。

【功能主治】行气导滞，泻热通便。用于赤白痢疾，里急后重，胃肠积滞，脘腹胀痛，大便不通。

【注意】孕妇禁用。

Common Aucklandia* and Betel Nut** Pill for Dysentery-relieving

Name of Chinese Phonetic Alphabet Mu Xiang Bing Lang Wan

Formula Aucklandiae Radix, Arecae Semen, Aurantii Fructus (fried), Citri Reticulatae Pericarpium, Citri Reticulatae Pericarpium Viride (fried with vinegar), Cyperi Rhizoma (prepared with vinegar), Sparganii Rhizoma (prepared with vinegar), Curcumae Rhizoma (prepared with vinegar), Coptidis Rhizoma, Phellodendri Chinensis Cortex (fried with wine), Rhei Radix et Rhizoma, Pharbitidis Semen (fried) and Natrii Sulfas.

Actions and Indications Moving *qi* and removing food stagnation, purging fire and relaxing the bowels. It is used for dysentery with purulent and bloody stools, tenesmus, food stagnation, abdominal distention and pain, constipation.

Warning It is contraindicated for pregnant women.

* 木香 ** 槟榔

五子衍宗丸

【处方】枸杞子、菟丝子（炒）、覆盆子、五味子（醋蒸）、车前子（盐炒）。

【功能主治】补肾益精。用于肾虚腰痛，尿后余沥，遗精早泄，阳痿不育。

Five Seeds Bolus for Tonifying Kidney

Name of Chinese Phonetic Alphabet Wu Zi Yan Zong Wan

Formula Lycii Fructus, Cuscutae Semen (fried), Rubi Fructus, Schisandrae Chinensis Fructus (steamed by wine) and Plantaginis Semen (fried with salt).

Actions and Indications Tonifying the kidney and essence. It is used for lumbago, dripping urination, nocturnal emission, ejaculatio praecox, impotence and sterility due to deficiency of the kidney.

五灵丸

【处方】柴胡、灵芝、丹参、五味子。

【功能主治】疏肝健脾活血。用于肝郁脾虚夹瘀，症见纳呆，腹胀嗳气，胁肋胀痛，疲乏无力。

【注意】孕妇慎用。有溃疡病史者，请在医生指导下用。

Wu Ling Bolus

Name of Chinese Phonetic Alphabet Wu Ling Wan

Formula Bupleuri Radix, Ganoderma, Salviae Miltiorrhizae Radix et Rhizoma and Schisandrae Chinensis Fructus.

Actions and Indications Soothing the liver , tonifying the spleen and activating blood. It is indicated for anorexia, abdominal distention, eructation, hypochondriac distention and pain, tiredness and fatigue due to liver depression, spleen deficiency with blood stasis.

Warning It should be used carefully for pregnant women. Cases with a ulcerous history should follow the physician's advice.

五苓片

【处方】茯苓、泽泻、猪苓、桂枝、白术。

【功能主治】温阳化气，利湿行水。用于小便不利，水肿腹胀，呕逆泄泻，口不思饮。

Wu Ling Tablet for Inducing Diuresis

Name of Chinese Phonetic Alphabet Wu Ling Pian

Formula Poria, Alismatis Rhizoma, Polyporus, Cinnamomi Ramulus and Atractylodis Macrocephalae Rhizoma.

Actions and Indications Warming *yang* and transforming *qi*, inducing diuresis. It is indicated for difficult urination, edema, vomiting, diarrhea and undesiredness to drink.

五味子糖浆

【处方】本品为五味子制成的糖浆。

【功能主治】益气补肾，镇静安神。用于神经衰弱、头晕、失眠。

Five-flavor-fruit* Syrup

Name of Chinese Phonetic Alphabet Wu Wei Zi Tang Jiang

Formula Schisandrae Chinensis Fructus.

Actions and Indications Tonifying *qi* and the kidney, tranquilizing the mind. It is indicated for neurasthenia, dizziness and insomnia.

* 五味子

五味黄连丸

【处方】黄连、红花、诃子等。

【功能主治】消炎，止泻，止痛。用于胃肠炎，久泻腹痛，胆热偏盛引起的厌食。

Golden Thread* Pill for Relieving Gastroenteritis

Name of Chinese Phonetic Alphabet Wu Wei Huang Lian Wan

Formula Coptidis Rhizoma, Carthami Flos, Chebulae Fructus, etc.

Actions and Indications Antiphlogistic, relieving diarrhea and pain. It is indicated for gastroenteritis, abdominal pain, chronic diarrhea, anorexia due to exuberance of gallbladder-heat.

＊黄连

五味麝香丸

【处方】麝香、诃子（去核）、草乌、木香、藏菖蒲。

【功能主治】消炎，止痛，祛风。用于扁桃体炎，咽峡炎，流行性感冒，炭疽病，风湿性关节炎，神经痛，胃痛，牙痛。

【注意】本品有毒，慎用；孕妇忌服。

Musk★ Pill

Name of Chinese Phonetic Alphabet Wu Wei She Xiang Wan

Formula Moschus, Chebulae Fructus (removed nucleus), Aconiti Kusnezoffii Radix, Aucklandiae Radix and Acori Calami Rhizoma.

Actions and Indications Counteracting inflammation, relieving pain, dispelling wind. It is indicated for tonsillitis, angina, influenza, anthrax, rheumatic arthritis, neuralgia, stomachache and toothache.

Warning The preparation is toxic and should be used cautiously. It is contraindicated for pregnant women.

＊麝香

五香丸

【处方】香附（醋炙）、丁香、木香、五灵脂（醋炙）、牵牛子（炒）。

【功能主治】消积化痞，宽胸止痛。用于气郁结滞，宿食停水引起的胸胁胀满，胃寒腹痛，嗳气嘈杂，积聚痞块，大便不畅。

【注意】孕妇忌服。

Wu Xiang Pill

Name of Chinese Phonetic Alphabet Wu Xiang Wan

Formula Cyperi Rhizoma (prepared with vinegar), Caryophylli Flos, Aucklandiae Radix, Trogopterori Faeces (prepared with vinegar) and Pharbitidis Semen (fried).

Actions and Indications Relieving distention and resolving mass, soothing the chest and relieving pain. It is used for hypochondriac distention and fullness, abdominal pain, belching, gastric upset, abdominal mass and difficulty in defecation due to *qi* stagnation, foods retention.

Warning It is contraindicated for pregnant women.

五淋丸

【处方】海金沙、关木通、栀子（姜制）、黄连、石韦（去毛）、茯苓皮、琥珀、地黄、白芍、川芎、当归、甘草。

【功能主治】清热利湿，分清止淋。用于下焦湿热引起的尿频尿急，小便涩痛，浑浊不清。

【注意】孕妇慎服。

Relieving Strangury Pill

Name of Chinese Phonetic Alphabet Wu Lin Wan

Formula Lygodii Spora, Aristolochiae Manshuriensis Caulis, Gardeniae Fructus (prepared with ginger), Coptidis Rhizoma, Pyrrosiae Folium (removed hair), Poriae Cutis, Succinum, Rehmanniae Radix, Paeoniae Radix Alba, Chuanxiong Rhizoma, Angelicae Sinensis Radix and Glycyrrhizae Radix et Rhizoma.

Actions and Indications Clearing heat and draining dampness, separating the pure substance from the turbid, relieving strangury. It is indicated for frequent urination and urgent urination, drippling, painful and turbid urination due to damp-heat of lower energizer.

Warning It should be used carefully for pregnant women.

五羚丹胶囊

【处方】五味子（醋制）、丹参、羚羊角。

【功能主治】益气活血，解毒。用于气阴不足，邪毒蕴结，瘀血阻滞所致的胸胁疼痛，口苦咽干，倦怠纳差，以及慢性、迁延性肝炎长期谷丙转氨酶单项不降见上述证候者。

Five-flavor-fruit* Antelope Horn** and Redroot Sage*** Capsule

Name of Chinese Phonetic Alphabet Wu Ling Dan Jiao Nang

Formula Schisandrae Chinensis Fructus (prepared with vinegar), Salviae Miltiorrhizae Radix et Rhizoma and Saigae Tataricae Cornu.

Actions and Indications Tonifying *qi*, activating blood, detoxifying. It is used for hypochondriac pain due to dual insufficiency of *qi* and *yin*; bitter mouth, dry throat, tiredness, poor appetite due to accumulation of pathogens and also used for chronic, persistent hepatitis with high glutamic pyruvic transaminase.

* 五味子 ** 羚羊角 *** 丹参

五粒回春丸

【处方】黄连、黄芩、关木通、大青叶、地黄、葛根、玄参、赤芍、前胡、柴胡、淡豆豉、天花粉、桔梗、浙贝母、荆芥穗、西河柳、羚羊角、牛蒡子（炒）、水牛角浓缩粉。

【功能主治】解肌透疹，清热化痰。用于感冒发热，鼻流清涕，隐疹不出，咳嗽。

【注意】服药避风。发疹、有便泻者忌服。

Wu Li Hui Chun Pill

Name of Chinese Phonetic Alphabet Wu Li Hui Chun Wan

Formula Coptidis Rhizoma, Scutellariae Radix, Aristolochiae Manshuriensis Caulis, Isatidis Folium, Rehmanniae Radix, Puerariae Lobatae Radix, Scrophulariae Radix, Paeoniae Radix Rubra, Peucedani Radix, Bupleuri Radix, Sojae Semen Praeparatum, Trichosanthis Radix, Platycodonis Radix, Fritillariae Thunbergii Bulbus, Schizonepetae Spica, Tamaricis Cacumen, Saigae Tataricae Cornu, Arctii Fructus (fried) and Bubali Cornu Pulvis Concentratio.

Actions and Indicationss Releasing the flesh and outthrusting the rashes, clearing heat and resolving phlegm. It is indicated for common cold, marked by fever, clear nasal discharge, latent urticaria and cough.

Warning During administration, draught should be avoided. It is contraindicated for cases with rashes and diarrhea.

五福化毒丸

【处方】连翘、青黛、黄连、桔梗、玄参、地黄、芒硝、赤芍、甘草、牛蒡子（炒）、水牛角浓缩粉。

【功能主治】清热解毒，凉血消肿。用于小儿疮疖，痱毒，咽喉肿痛，口舌生疮，牙龈出血，痄腮。

Wu Fu Detoxifying Pill for Relieving Infantile Miliaria

Name of Chinese Phonetic Alphabet Wu Fu Hua Du Wan

Formula Forsythiae Fructus, Indigo Naturalis, Coptidis Rhizoma, Platycodonis Radix, Scrophulariae Radix, Rehmanniae Radix, Natrii Sulfas, Paeoniae Radix Rubra, Glycyrrhizae Radix et Rhizoma, Arctii Fructus (fried) and Bubali Cornu Pulvis Concentratio.

Actions and Indications Clearing heat and detoxicating, cooling blood and dispersing swelling. It is used for infantile sores and furuncle, miliaria, sore-throat, aphthae, gingival bleeding and mumps.

太和妙灵丸

【处方】钩藤、僵蚕（麸炒）、天竺黄、天麻、羌活、荆芥穗、法半夏、柴胡、薄荷、蓼大青叶、金银花、防风、全蝎、天南星（制）、化橘红、赤芍、黄芩、栀子（姜炙）、关木通、麦冬、玄参、羚羊角粉、琥珀粉、甘草、朱砂、冰片。

【功能主治】散寒解表，清热镇惊，化痰止咳。用于小儿肺胃痰热，外感风寒引起的发热恶寒，头痛鼻塞，咳嗽气促，烦躁不安，内热惊风，四肢抽搐。

Tai He Miraculous Effectiveness Pill

Name of Chinese Phonetic Alphabet Tai He Miao Ling Wan

Formula Uncariae Ramulus cum Uncis, Bombyx Batryticatus (fried with bran), Bambusae Concretio Silicea, Gastrodiae Rhizoma, Notopterygii Rhizoma et Radix, Schizonepetae Spica, Pinelliae Rhizoma Praeparatum, Bupleuri Radix, Menthae Haplocalycis Herba, Polygoni Tinctorii Folium, Lonicerae Japonicae Flos, Saposhnikoviae Radix, Scorpio, Arisaematis Rhizoma (prepared), Citri Grandis Exocarpium, Paeoniae Radix Rubra, Scutellariae Radix, Gardeniae Fructus (prepared with ginger), Aristolochiae Manshuriensis Caulis, Ophiopogonis Radix, Scrophulariae Radix, Saigae Tataricae Cornu Pulvis, Succini Pulvis, Glycyrrhizae Radix et Rhizoma, Cinnabaris and Borneolum Syntheticum.

Actions and Indications Dispersing cold and releasing the exterior, clearing heat and settling fright, resolving phlegm and relieving cough. It is indicated for children with manifestations as fever, aversion to cold, headache, nasal congestion, cough and shortness of breath, vexation, convulsion and spasm of limbs due to phlegm-heat of the lung and stomach and exogenous wind-cold.

止血片

【处方】拳参、墨旱莲、地锦草、土大黄、珍珠母（煅）。

【功能主治】清热凉血，止血。用于因血热引起的月经过多，鼻衄，咳血，吐血。

Bleeding-relieving Tablet

Name of Chinese Phonetic Alphabet Zhi Xue Pian

Formula Bistortae Rhizoma, Ecliptae Herba, Euphorbiae Humifusae Herba, Rumicis Nepalensis Radix and Margaritifera Concha (calcined).

Actions and Indications Clearing heat, cooling blood, relieving bleeding. It is used for hypermenorrhea, epistaxis, hemoptysis and hematemesis due to blood-heat.

止血灵胶囊

【处方】扶芳藤、蒲公英、黄芪、地榆。

【功能主治】清热，解毒，止血。用于子宫肌瘤出血，恶露不净，经间出血，放环出血，痔疮出血，鼻衄。

Miraculous Bleeding-relieving Capsule

Name of Chinese Phonetic Alphabet Zhi Xue Ling Jiao Nang

Formula Euonymi Fortunei Caulis seu Folium, Taraxaci Herba, Astragali Radix and Sanguisorbae Radix.

Actions and Indications Clearing heat, detoxifying, relieving bleeding. It is used for bleeding of hysteromyoma, profuse discharge of lochia, intermenstrual bleeding, bleeding due to setting of contraceptive ring, hemorrhoidal bleeding, epistaxis.

止血宝胶囊

【处方】小蓟。

【功能主治】凉血止血，祛瘀消肿。用于鼻出血、吐血、尿血、便血、崩漏下血。

Field Thistle* Capsule

Name of Chinese Phonetic Alphabet Zhi Xue Bao Jiao Nang

Formula Cirsii Herba.

Actions and Indications Cooling blood, relieving bleeding, dispelling stasis, reducing swelling. It is used for epistaxis, hematemesis, hematuria, hematochezia, metrorrhagia.

* 小蓟

止血定痛片

【处方】三七、甘草、花蕊石（煅）、海螵蛸。

【功能主治】散瘀，止血，止痛。用于十二指肠溃疡疼痛，出血，胃酸过多。

Duodenal Ulcer Bleeding and Pain Relieving Tablet

Name of Chinese Phonetic Alphabet Zhi Xue Ding Tong Pian

Formula Notoginseng Radix et Rhizoma, Glycyrrhizae Radix et Rhizoma, Ophicalcitum (calcined) and Sepiae Endoconcha.

Actions and Indications Dissipating stasis, relieving bleeding, alleviating pain. It is used for pain and bleeding due to duodenal ulcer and gastroxia.

止血复脉合剂

【处方】阿胶、附子、川芎、大黄。

【功能主治】止血祛痰，滋阴复脉。用于上消化道出血量多，症见烦躁，肢冷，汗出，脉弱无力。可作为失血性休克的辅助治疗药物。

Relieving Bleeding and Restoring Normal Pulse Beating Mixture

Name of Chinese Phonetic Alphabet Zhi Xue Fu Mai He Ji

Formula Asini Corii Colla, Aconiti Lateralis Radix Praeparata, Chuanxiong Rhizoma and Rhei Radix et Rhizoma.

Actions and Indications Relieving bleeding and dispelling phlegm, nourishing *yin* and restoring normal pulse beating. It is used for hemorrhage of the upper digestive tract, manifested as vexation, cold limbs, sweating, weak pulse, also used as adjuvant medicine for hemorrhagic shock.

止红肠澼丸

【处方】当归、黄芩、栀子、荆芥穗、槐花、阿胶、白芍、地榆（炭）、黄连、乌梅、升麻、地黄（炭）、侧柏叶（炭）。

【功能主治】清热，凉血，止血，养血。用于肠风便血，痔疮下血。

Relieving Hemorrhoidal Bleeding Bolus

Name of Chinese Phonetic Alphabet Zhi Hong Chang Pi Wan

Formula Angelicae Sinensis Radix, Scutellariae Radix, Gandeniae Fructus, Schizonepetae Spica, Sophorae Flos, Asini Corii Colla, Paeoniae Radix Alba, Sanguisorbae Radix (carbonated), Coptidis Rhizoma, Mume Fructus, Cimicifugae Rhizoma, Rehmanniae Radix (carbonated) and Platycladi Cacumen (carbonated).

Actions and Indications Clearing heat, cooling blood, relieving bleeding and nourishing blood. It is used for fresh blood in stool, hemorrhoidal bleeding.

止泻利颗粒

【处方】杨梅根、钻地风、山楂、金银花。

【功能主治】收敛止泻，解毒消食。用于湿热泄泻，痢疾，久泻，久痢，伤食泄泻。

Diarrhea-arresting Granules

Name of Chinese Phonetic Alphabet Zhi Xie Li Ke Li

Formula Myricae Rubrae Radix, Schizophragmatis Integrifolii Cortex, Grataegi Fructus and Lonicerae Japonicae Flos.

Actions and Indications Arresting diarrhea, promoting digestion and detoxifying. It is used for diarrhea of damp-heat type, dysentery, chonic diarrhea, chronic dysentery and diarrhea due to improper diet.

止咳川贝枇杷露

【处方】枇杷叶、桔梗、水半夏、平贝母流浸膏、薄荷脑。

【功能主治】镇咳祛痰。用于感冒及支气管炎引起的咳嗽。

Sichuan Fritillary* and Loquat Leaf** Distillate for Relieving Cough

Name of Chinese Phonetic Alphabet Zhi Ke Chuan Bei Pi Pa Lu

Formula Eriobotryae Folium, Platycodonis Radix, Pinelliae Cordatae Tuber, Fritillariae Ussuriensis Extractum and Menthol.

Actions and Indications Relieving cough and dispelling phlegm. It is indicated for cough due to common cold and bronchitis.

*川贝母 **枇杷叶

止咳丸

【处方】川贝母、罂粟壳、防风、桔梗、葶苈子、紫苏子、法半夏（砂炒）、麻黄、白前、前胡、紫苏叶、厚朴（姜炙）、白果、桑叶、黄芩（酒炙）、硼砂、南沙参、薄荷、陈皮、枳壳（麸炒）、茯苓、甘草。

【功能主治】降气化痰，止咳定喘。用于风寒入肺引起的咳嗽痰多，喘促胸闷，周身酸痛或久咳不止，以及老年急、慢性支气管炎。

Alleviating Cough Pill

Name of Chinese Phonetic Alphabet Zhi Ke Wan

Formula Fritillariae Cirrhosae Bulbus, Papaveris Pericarpium, Saposhnikoviae Radix, Platycodonis Radix, Lepidii Semen, Perillae Fructus, Pinelliae Rhizoma Praeparatum (sliced and fried with sand), Ephedrae Herba, Cynanchi Stauntonii Rhizoma et Radix, Peucedani Radix, Perillae Folium, Magnoliae Officinalis Cortex (prepared with ginger), Ginkgo Semen, Mori Folium, Scutellariae Radix (prepared with wine), Borax, Adenophorae Radix, Menthae Haplocalycis Herba, Citri Reticulatae Pericarpium, Aurantii Fructus (fried with bran), Poria and Glycyrrhizae Radix et Rhizoma.

Actions and Indications Downbearing *qi* and resolving phlegm, alleviating cough and calming dyspnea. It is indicated for cough with profuse phlegm, dyspnea, chest distress, general aching pain and chronic cough due to wind-cold invading the lung; and also for acute, chronic bronchitis in the aged.

止咳平喘糖浆

【处方】麻黄、苦杏仁、石膏、水半夏（制）、陈皮、茯苓、桑白皮、罗汉果、鱼腥草、甘草、薄荷油。

【功能主治】清热宣肺，止咳平喘。用于风热感冒，急性支气管炎等引起的咳喘，气粗痰多，咽痛。

【注意】高血压患者慎用。

Alleviating Cough and Dyspnea Syrup

Name of Chinese Phonetic Alphabet Zhi Ke Ping Chuan Tang Jiang

Formula Ephedrae Herba, Armeniacae Semen Amarum, Gypsum Fibrosum, Pinelliae Cordatae Tuber(prepared), Citri Reticulatae Pericarpium, Poria, Mori Cortex, Siraitiae Fructus, Houttuyniae Herba, Glycyrrhizae Radix et Rhizoma and Menthae Haplocalycis Oleum.

Actions and Indications Clearing heat and diffusing the lung, alleviating cough and calming dyspnea. It is indicated for cough, shortness of breath, profuse phlegm and sore-throat due to common cold of wind-heat type and acute bronchitis.

Warning It should be used carefully for cases with hypertension.

止咳宁嗽胶囊

【处方】桔梗、荆芥、百部、紫菀（制）、白前（制）、前胡、款冬花（蜜炙）、麻黄（蜜炙）、陈皮、苦杏仁（炒）、防风。

【功能主治】疏风散寒，宣肺解表，镇咳祛痰。用于风寒咳嗽，呕吐，咽喉肿痛。

Cough-alleviating Capsule

Name of Chinese Phonetic Alphabet Zhi Ke

Ning Sou Jiao Nang

Formula Platycodonis Radix, Schizonepetae Herba, Stemonae Radix, Asteris Radix et Rhizoma (prepared), Cynanchi Stauntonii Rhizoma et Radix (prepared), Peucedani Radix, Farfarae Flos (prepared with honey), Ephedrae Herba (prepared with honey), Citri Reticulatae Pericarpium, Armeniacae Semen Amarum (fried) and Saposhnikoviae Radix.

Actions and Indications Dispersing wind and dissipating cold, diffusing the lung and releasing the exterior, alleviating cough and dispelling phlegm. It is indicated for cough due to wind-cold; vomiting, sore-throat.

止咳枇杷糖浆

【处方】枇杷叶、白前、桔梗、桑白皮、百部、薄荷脑。

【功能主治】清肺、止咳、化痰。用于咳嗽多痰，支气管炎。

Syrup of Loquat Leaf* for Relieving Cough

Name of Chinese Phonetic Alphabet Zhi Ke Pi Pa Tang Jiang

Formula Eriobotryae Folium, Cynanchi Stauntonii Rhizoma et Radix, Platycodonis Radix, Mori Cortex, Stemonae Radix and Menthol.

Actions and Indications Clearing lung-heat, relieving cough and resolving phlegm. It is indicated for cough with profuse phlegm, bronchitis.

* 枇杷叶

止咳宝片

【处方】本品为紫菀、橘红、桔梗、枳壳、百部、五味子、陈皮、干姜、荆芥、罂粟壳浸膏、甘草等药经加工制成的片剂。

【功能主治】理肺祛痰，止咳平喘。用于外感咳嗽，痰多清稀，色白而黏，痰多不易咯出以及慢性支气管炎与上呼吸道感染所致的久咳。

【注意】孕妇、婴儿及哺乳期妇女忌服。

Cough-alleviating Tablet

Name of Chinese Phonetic Alphabet Zhi Ke Bao Pian

Formula Asteris Radix et Rhizoma, Citri Exocarpium Rubrum, Platycodonis Radix, Aurantii Fructus, Stemonae Radix, Schisandrae Chinensis Fructus, Citri Reticulatae Pericarpium, Zingiberis Rhizoma, Schizonepetae Herba, Papaveris Pericarpium Extractum, Glycyrrhizae Radix et Rhizoma, etc.

Actions and Indications Regulating the lung and dispelling phlegm, alleviating cough and calming dyspnea. It is indicated for cough due to external contraction, marked by profuse and thin, white and sticky phlegm, difficult expectoration and chronic cough due to chronic bronchitis and upper respiratory tract infection.

Warning It is contraindicated for pregnant women, infants and women in breast feeding period.

止咳定喘片

【处方】香白芷、虎刺、矮地茶、罗汉果、水田七。

【功能主治】止咳祛痰，消炎定喘。用于支气管哮喘，哮喘性支气管炎。

Relieving Cough and Dyspnea Tablet

Name of Chinese Phonetic Alphabet Zhi Ke Ding Chuan Pian

Formula Angelicae Dahuricae Radix, Damnacanthi Indici Herba seu Radix, Ardisiae Japonicae Herba, Siraitiae Fructus and Taccae Tuber.

Actions and Indications Relieving cough and dyspnea, dispelling phlegm and antiphlogistic. It is indicated for bronchial asthma, asthmatic bronchitis.

止咳橘红口服液

【处方】化橘红、陈皮、法半夏、茯苓、甘草、紫苏子（炒）、苦杏仁（去皮炒）、紫菀、款冬花、麦冬、瓜蒌皮、知母、桔梗、地黄、石膏。

【功能主治】清肺润燥，止嗽化痰。用于肺热燥咳，痰多气促，口苦咽干。

【注意】忌食辛辣油腻物。

Huazhou Pummelo Oral Liquid for Relieving Cough

Name of Chinese Phonetic Alphabet Zhi Ke Ju Hong Kou Fu Ye

Formula Citri Grandis Exocarpium, Citri Reticulatae Pericarpium, Pinelliae Rhizoma Praeparatum, Poria, Glycyrrhizae Radix et Rhizoma, Perillae Fructus (fried), Armeniacae Semen Amarum (removed seed coat and fried), Asteris Radix et Rhizoma, Farfarae Flos, Ophiopogonis Radix, Trichosanthis Pericarpium, Anemarrhenae Rhizoma, Platycodonis Radix, Rehmanniae Radix and Gypsum Fibrosum.

Actions and Indications Clearing lung-heat and moistening dryness, relieving cough and resolving phlegm. It is indicated for dry cough due to lung-heat; marked by profuse phlegm and shortness of breath, bitter mouth and dry throat.

Warning Pungent and oily foods are prohibited.

*化橘红

止喘灵气雾剂

【处方】洋金花总生物碱等。

【功能主治】本品为抗胆碱药和选择性β-受体兴奋剂的中西药复方制剂，有舒张支气管作用。

Dyspnea-relieving Aerosol

Name of Chinese Phonetic Alphabet Zhi Chuan Ling Qi Wu Ji

Formula Datura Total Alkaloids, etc.

Actions and Indications Compound preparation containing anticholinergic and selective β-receptor stimulant, and possessing an effect of dilating bronchus.

止喘灵注射液

【处方】本品为麻黄、杏仁等药经加工制成的注射液。

【功能主治】平喘，止咳，祛痰。用于哮喘，咳嗽，胸闷痰多；支气管哮喘、喘息性气管炎。

Asthma-relieving Injection

Name of Chinese Phonetic Alphabet Zhi Chuan Ling Zhu She Ye

Formula Ephedrae Herba, Armeniacae Semen Amarum, etc.

Actions and Indications Calming dyspnea, relieving cough and dispelling phlegm. It is indicated for asthma, cough, chest distress, profuse phlegm; and bronchial asthma, asthmatic trachitis.

止痛化癥胶囊

【处方】党参、黄芪（蜜炙）、白术（炒）、丹参、当归、鸡血藤、三棱、莪术、芡实、山药、延胡索、川楝子、鱼腥草、败酱草、蜈蚣、全蝎、土鳖虫、炮姜、肉桂。

【功能主治】活血调经，化癥止痛。用于癥瘕积聚，痛经闭经，赤白带下及慢性盆腔炎。

Pain-alleviating and Mass-dispersing Capsule

Name of Chinese Phonetic Alphabet Zhi Tong Hua Zheng Jiao Nang

Formula Codonopsis Radix, Astragali Radix (prepared with honey), Atractylodis Rhizoma Macrocphalae (fried), Salviae Miltiorrhizae Radix et Rhizoma, Angelicae Sinensis Radix, Spatholobi Caulis, Sparganii Rhizoma, Curcumae Rhizoma, Euryales Semen, Dioscoreae Rhizoma, Corydalis Rhizoma, Toosendan Fructus, Houttuyniae Herba, Patriniae Herba, Scolopendra, Scorpio, Eupolyphaga seu Steleophaga, Zingiberis Rhizoma Praeparatum and Cinnamomi Cortex.

Actions and Indications Activating blood, regulating menstruation, resolving mass, alleviating pain. It is used for abdominal mass, dysmenorrhea, amenorrhea, red-white vaginal discharge and chronic pelvic inflammation.

止痛透骨膏

【处方】急性子、白芷等。

【功能主治】祛风散寒，活血行滞，通络止痛。用于膝、腰椎部骨性关节炎属血瘀、风寒阻络证者。症见关节疼痛、肿胀、压痛或功能障碍、舌质暗或有瘀斑。

Arthritis-relieving Plaster

Name of Chinese Phonetic Alphabet Zhi Tong Tou Gu Gao

Formula Impatientis Semen, Angelicae Dahuricae Radix, etc.

Actions and Indications Dispelling wind, dissipating cold, activating blood, dredging collaterals, alleviating pain. It is used for osteoarthritis of knees and lumbar vertebrae marked by arthralgia, swelling, tenderness or dysfunction, purple tongue with ecchymosis due to blood-stasis and wind-cold obstructing the collaterals.

止嗽化痰颗粒

【处方】桔梗、知母、前胡、罂粟壳、半夏、川贝母、苦杏仁、百部等。

【功能主治】清肺止咳，化痰定喘。用于久嗽、痰喘气逆、喘息不眠。

Relieving Cough Soluble Granules

Name of Chinese Phonetic Alphabet Zhi Sou Hua Tan Ke Li

Formula Platycodonis Radix, Anemarrhenae Rhizoma, Peucedani Radix, Papaveris Pericarpium, Pinelliae Rhizoma, Fritillariae Cirrhosae Bulbus, Armeniacae Semen Amarum, Stemonae Radix, etc.

Actions and Indications Clearing lung-heat and relieving cough, resolving phlegm and calming dyspnea. It is indicated for chronic cough, phlegm dyspnea, *qi* counterflow, dyspnea with sleeplessness.

止嗽青果合剂

【处方】西青果、麻黄、苦杏仁（去皮炒）、石膏、甘草、紫苏子（炒）、紫苏叶、半夏（制）、浙贝母、桑白皮（蜜炙）、白果、黄芩、款冬花、冰片。

【功能主治】宣肺化痰，止咳定喘。用于风寒束肺引起的咳嗽痰盛，胸膈满闷，气促作喘，口燥咽干。

【注意】肺痨，气促痰喘者忌服。

Mixture of Myrobalan* for Alleviating Cough

Name of Chinese Phonetic Alphabet Zhi Sou Qing Guo He Ji

Formula Chebulae Fructus, Ephedrae Herba, Armeniacae Semen Amarum (removed seed coat and fried), Gypsum Fibrosum, Glycyrrhizae Radix et Rhizoma, Perillae Fructus (fried), Perillae Folium, Pinelliae Rhizoma (prepared), Fritillariae Thunbergii Bulbus, Mori Cortex (prepared with honey), Ginkgo Semen, Scutellariae Radix, Farfarae Flos and Borneolum Syntheticum.

Actions and Indications Diffusing the lung and resolving phlegm, alleviating cough and dyspnea. It is indicated for cough with profuse phlegm, chest distress, shortness of breath, dry mouth and throat due to wind-cold residing in the lung.

Warning It is contraindicated for cases with pulmonary tuberculosis and shortness of breath.

* 西青果

少阳感冒冲剂

【处方】柴胡、黄芩、生晒参、甘草、半夏、干姜、大枣、青蒿。

【功能主治】扶正解表，清热和中。用于寒热往来，口苦咽干，头晕目眩，不思饮食，心烦恶心。

Soluble Granules for Lesser *Yang* Common Cold

Name of Chinese Phonetic Alphabet Shao Yang Gan Mao Chong Ji

Formula Bupleuri Radix, Scutellariae Radix, Ginseng Radix et Rhizoma Exsiccatus, Glycyrrhizae Radix et Rhizoma, Pinelliae Rhizoma, Zingiberis Rhizoma, Jujubae Fructus and Artemisiae Annuae Herba.

Actions and Indications Reinforcing the healthy *qi* and releasing the exterior, clearing heat and harmonizing the middle. It is indicated for alternating chills and fever, bitter taste in the mouth, dry throat, dizziness, dizzy vision, anorexia, vexation and nausea.

少腹逐瘀丸

【处方】当归、蒲黄、五灵脂（醋炒）、赤芍、小茴香（盐炒）、延胡索（醋制）、没药（炒）、川芎、肉桂、炮姜。

【功能主治】活血化瘀，祛寒止痛。用于血瘀有寒引起的月经不调，小腹胀痛，腰痛，白带。

Relieving Irregular Menstruation Bolus

Name of Chinese Phonetic Alphabet Shao Fu Zhu Yu Wan

Formula Angelicae Sinensis Radix, Typhae Pollen, Trogopterori Faeces (prepared with vinegar), Paeoniae Radix Rubra, Foeniculi Fructus (fried with salt), Corydalis Rhizoma (prepared with vinegar), Myrrha (fried), Chuanxiong Rhizoma, Cinnamomi Cortex and Zingiberis Rhizoma Praeparatum.

Actions and Indications Activating blood, resolving stasis, dispelling cold, alleviating pain. It is used for irregular menstruation, distending pain in the lower abdomen, lumbago and leucorrhea due to blood-stasis and cold.

中风回春片

【处方】当归（酒制）、川芎（酒制）、红花、桃仁、丹参、鸡血藤、忍冬藤、络石藤、地龙（炒）、土鳖虫（炒）、伸筋草、川牛膝、蜈蚣、茺蔚子（炒）、全蝎、威灵仙（酒制）、僵蚕（麸炒）、木瓜、金钱白花蛇。

【功能主治】活血化瘀，舒筋通络。用于中风偏瘫，肢体麻木。

【注意】脑出血急性期忌服。

Miraculous Tablet for Apoplexy

Name of Chinese Phonetic Alphabet Zhong Feng Hui Chun Pian

Formula Angelicae Sinensis Radix (prepared with wine), Chuanxiong Rhizoma (prepared with wine), Carthami Flos, Persicae Semen, Salviae Miltiorrhizae Radix et Rhizoma, Spatholobi Caulis, Lonicerae Japonicae Caulis, Trachelospermi Caulis et Folium, Pheretima (fried), Eupolyhaga seu Steleophaga (fried), Lycopodii Herba, Cyathulae Radix, Scolopendra, Leonuri Fructus (fried), Scorpio, Clematidis Radix et Rhizoma (prepared with wine), Bombyx Batryticatus (fried with bran), Chaenomelis Fructus and Bangarus Parvus.

Actions and Indications Activating blood, resolving stasis, relaxing sinews and dredging collaterals. It is indicated for hemiparalysis, and numbness of extremities due to apoplexy.

Warning It is contraindicated for acute stage of cerebral hemorrhage.

中华跌打丸

【处方】栀子、苍术、假蒟叶、地耳草、红杜仲、鬼画符、乌药、金不换、牛马蕨、丁茄根、急性子、木鳖子、山橘叶、大力王、刘寄奴、鹅不食草、牛膝、鸡血藤、毛老虎、穿破石、两面针、丢了棒、岗梅、过江龙、香附、桂枝、樟脑、半边莲、独活、制川乌、丁香等。

【功能主治】消肿止痛，舒筋活络，止血生肌，活血祛瘀。用于挫伤筋骨，创伤出血，风湿瘀痛。

【注意】孕妇忌服。

Zhong Hua Traumatic Injury Bolus

Name of Chinese Phonetic Alphabet Zhong Hua Die Da Wan

Formula Gardeniae Fructus, Atractylodis Rhizoma, Piperis Sarmentosi Folium, Hyperici Japonici Herba, Parabarii Micranthi Caulis seu Radix, Breyniae Fruticosae Folium, Linderae Radix, Stephaniae Sinicae Radix, Smilacis Nipponicae Rhizoma et Radix, Solani Surattensis Radix, Impatientis Semen, Momordicae Semen, Fortunellae Hindsii Folium, Cardui Crispi Herba, Artemisiae Anomalae Herba, Centipedae Herba, Achyranthis Bidentatae Radix, Spatholobi Caulis, Inulae Cappae Herba, Cudraniae Radix, Zanthoxyli Radix, Claoxyli Polot Radix et Folium, Ilicis Asprellae Folium seu Radix, Lycopodii Complanati Herba, Cyperi Rhizoma, Cinnamomi Ramulus, Camphora, Lobeliae Chinensis Herba, Angelicae Pubescentis Radix, Aconiti Radix Cocta, Caryophylli Flos, etc.

Actions and Indications Reducing swelling, alleviating pain, relaxing sinews, activating collaterals, relieving bleeding, promoting tissue regeneration, activating blood, dispelling stasis. It is used for contusion of sinews, traumatic bleeding, rheumatalgia.

Warning It is contraindicated for pregnant women.

中满分消丸

【处方】党参、白术（麸炒）、茯苓、甘草、陈皮、半夏（制）、砂仁、枳实、厚朴（姜炙）、猪苓、泽泻、黄芩、黄连、知母、姜黄。

【功能主治】健脾行气，利湿清热。用于脾虚气滞，湿热郁结引起的宿食蓄水，脘腹胀痛，烦热口苦，倒饱嘈杂，二便不利。

Dyspepsia-promoting Pill

Name of Chinese Phonetic Alphabet Zhong Man Fen Xiao Wan

Formula Codonopsis Radix, Atractylodis Macrocephalae Rhizoma (fried with bran), Poria, Glycyrrhizae Radix et Rhizoma, Citri Reticulatae Pericarpium, Pinelliae Rhizoma (prepared), Amomi Fructus, Aurantii Fructus Immaturus, Magnoliae Officinalis Cortex (prepared with ginger), Polyporus, Alismatis Rhizoma, Scutellariae Radix, Coptidis Rhizoma, Anemarrhenae Rhizoma and Curcumae Longae Rhizoma.

Actions and Indications Fortifying the spleen and moving *qi*, draining dampness and clearing heat. It is indicated for dyspepsia, water retention syndrome, abdominal distention and pain, heat vexation, bitter taste in the mouth, gastric discomfort, difficulty in urination and defecation due to *qi*-stagnation, spleen deficiency and retention of dampness-heat.

内消瘰疬丸

【处方】夏枯草、玄参、大青盐、海藻、浙贝母、薄荷、天花粉、蛤壳（煅）、白蔹、连翘、熟大黄、甘草、地黄、桔梗、枳壳、当归、玄明粉。

【功能主治】软坚散结。用于瘰疬痰核或肿或痛。

Relieving Scrofula Pill

Name of Chinese Phonetic Alphabet Nei Xiao Luo Li Wan

Formula Prunellae Spica, Scrophulariae Radix, Halitum, Sargassum, Fritillariae Thunbergii Bulbus, Menthae Haplocalycis Herba, Trichosanthis Radix, Meretricis Concha (calcined), Ampelopsis Radix, Forsythiae Fructus, Rhei Radix et Rhizoma, Glycyrrhizae Radix et Rhizoma, Rehmanniae Radix, Platycodonis Radix, Aurantii Fructus, Angelicae Sinensis Radix and Natrii Sulfas Exsiccatus.

Actions and Indications Softening mass. It is indicated for scrofula with swelling or pain.

贝母梨膏

【处方】川贝母、梨膏。

【功能主治】润肺，止咳，化痰。用于咳嗽痰多，咯痰不爽，咽喉干痛。

Sichuan Fritillary* and Pear Soft Extract

Name of Chinese Phonetic Alphabet Bei Mu Li Gao

Formula Fritillariae Cirrhosae Bulbus and Pyri Fructus (extract).

Actions and Indications Moistening the lung, relieving cough, resolving phlegm. It is used for productive cough, difficult expectoration, sore-throat.

*川贝母

贝羚胶囊

【处方】本品为川贝母、羚羊角、麝香等药味经加工制成的胶囊剂。

【功能主治】清热化痰。用于小儿肺炎咳喘，喘息性支气管炎引起的痰壅气急；也可用于成人慢性支气管炎引起的痰壅气急。

【注意】大便溏薄者不宜使用。

Sichuan Fritillary* and Antelope Horn** Capsule for Relieving Children Pneumonia

Name of Chinese Phonetic Alphabet Bei Ling Jiao Nang

Formula Fritillariae Cirrhosae Bulbus, Saigae Tataricae Cornu, Moschus, etc.

Actions and Indications Clearing heat and resolving phlegm. It is indicated for children shortness of breath due to cough and asthma of pneumonia and asthmatic bronchitis; also for shortness of breath due to chronic bronchitis in adult.

Warning It is contraindicated for cases with sloppy stool.

*川贝母 **羚羊角

仁丹

【处方】陈皮、檀香、砂仁、豆蔻（去果皮）、甘草、木香、丁香、广藿香叶、儿茶、肉桂、薄荷脑、冰片、朱砂。

【功能主治】清暑开窍。用于中暑呕吐，烦躁恶心，胸中满闷，头目晕眩，晕车晕船，水土不服。

Ren Dan Pill

Name of Chinese Phonetic Alphabet Ren Dan

Formula Citri Reticulatae Pericarpium, Santali Albi Lignum, Amomi Fructus, Amomi Fructus Rotundus (removed peel), Glycyrrhizae Radix et Rhizoma, Aucklandiae Radix, Caryophylli Flos, Pogostemonis Folium, Catechu, Cinnamomi Cortex, Menthol, Borneolum Syntheticum and Cinnabaris.

Actions and Indications Clearing summer-heat and opening the orifices. It is indicated for summer-heat stroke, vomiting, vexation, nausea, chest distress, dizziness and dizzy vision, car-sickness and naupathia, unaccustomedness to the climate of a new place.

仁青芒觉

【处方】毛诃子、蒲桃、西红花、牛黄、麝香、朱砂等。

【功能主治】清热解毒，益肝养胃，愈疮醒神，滋补强身。用于各种中毒症，急、慢性胃溃疡，腹水，麻风病。

【注意】服药期间，禁用酸腐、生冷及油腻食物。

Renqing Mangjue Pill (A Tibetan Formula)

Name of Chinese Phonetic Alphabet Ren Qing Mang Jue

Formula Terminaliae Belliricae Fructus, Syzygii Jambos Pericarpium, Croci Stigma, Bovis Calculus, Moschus, Cinnabaris, etc.

Actions and Indications Clearing heat and detoxicating, tonifying the liver and nourishing the stomach, healing sore. It is used for various toxic disorders, acute or chronic gastric ulcer, ascites and leprosy.

Warning During medication, sour, rotten, uncooked and oily foods are prohibited.

仁青常觉

【处方】珍珠、朱砂、檀香、降香、沉香、诃子、牛黄、麝香、西红花等。

【功能主治】清热，解毒，滋补。用于陈旧性胃肠炎、溃疡，萎缩性胃炎，各种中毒症，陈旧热病。

【注意】服药期间，禁用酸、腐、生冷食物。

Renqing Changjue Pill (A Tibetan Formula)

Name of Chinese Phonetic Alphabet Ren Qing Chang Jue

Formula Margarita, Cinnabaris, Santali Albi Lignum, Dalbergiae Odoriferae Lignum, Aquilariae Lignum Resinatum, Chebulae Fructus, Bovis Calculus, Moschus, Croci Stigma, etc.

Actions and Indications Clearing heat, detoxicating and tonifying. It is used for remote gastroenteritis, ulcer, atrophic gastritis, various toxic disorders and remote heat disease.

Warning During medication, sour, rotton, uncooked and cold foods are prohibited.

化积口服液

【处方】本品为茯苓（去皮）、莪术（醋制）、雷丸、海螵蛸、三棱、红花、鸡内金（炒）等药经加工制成的口服液。

【功能主治】消积治疳。用于小儿疳气型疳积，腹胀腹痛；面黄肌瘦，消化不良。

Relieving Children Malnutrition Oral Liquid

Name of Chinese Phonetic Alphabet Hua Ji Kou Fu Ye

Formula Poria (removed exoperidium), Curcumae Rhizoma (prepared with vinegar), Omphalia, Sepiae Endoconcha, Sparganii Rhizoma, Carthami Flos, Galli Gigerii Endothelium Corneum (fried), etc.

Actions and Indications Relieving malnutrition. It is used for children malnutrition marked by abdominal fullness and pain, sallow complexion, emaciation and dyspepsia.

化瘀祛斑胶囊

【处方】柴胡、薄荷、黄芩、赤芍、当归、红花。

【功能主治】疏风清热，活血化瘀。用于黄褐斑、酒渣鼻、粉刺。

【注意】宜持续服用 1~2 个月。

Freckle-eliminating Capsule

Name of Chinese Phonetic Alphabet Hua Yu Qu Ban Jiao Nang

Formula Bupleuri Radix, Menthae Haplocalycis Herba, Scutellariae Radix, Paeoniae Radix Rubra, Angelicae Sinensis Radix and Carthami Flos.

Actions and Indications Dispersing wind, clearing heat, activating blood, resolving stasis. It is used for chloasma, rosacea and acne.

Warning Apply the medicine for 1 ~ 2 months continuously.

化癥回生片

【处方】益母草、红花、花椒（炭）、水蛭（制）、当归、苏木、三棱（醋炙）、两头尖、川芎、降香、香附（醋炙）、人参、高良姜、姜黄、没药（醋制）、苦杏仁（炒）、大黄、麝香、小茴香（盐炒）、桃仁、虻虫、鳖甲胶、五灵脂（醋炙）、丁香、白芍、蒲黄（炭）、延胡索（醋炙）、艾叶（炙）、阿魏、肉桂、干漆（煅）、乳香（醋炙）、熟地黄、紫苏子、吴茱萸（甘草水炙）。

【功能主治】消癥化瘀。用于癥积血痹，妇女干血痨，产后瘀血，少腹疼痛拒按。

【注意】孕妇禁用。

Dispersing Abdominal Mass Tablet

Name of Chinese Phonetic Alphabet Hua Zheng

Hui Sheng Pian

Formula Leonuri Herba, Carthami Flos, Zanthoxyli Pericarpium (carbonated), Hirudo (prepared), Angelicae Sinensis Radix, Sappan Lignum, Sparganii Rhizoma (prepared with vinegar), Anemones Raddeanae Rhizoma, Chuanxiong Rhizoma, Dalbergiae Odoriferae Lignum, Cyperi Rhizoma (prepared with vinegar), Ginseng Radix et Rhizoma, Alpiniae Officinarum Rhizoma, Curcumae Longae Rhizoma, Myrrha (prepared with vinegar), Armeniacae Semen Amarum (fried), Rhei Radix et Rhizoma, Moschus, Foeniculi Fructus (fried with salt), Persicae Semen, Tabanus, Trionycis Carapacis Colla, Trogopterori Faeces (prepared with vinegar), Caryophylli Flos, Paeoniae Radix Alba, Typhae Pollen (carbonated), Corydalis Rhizoma (prepared with vinegar), Artemisiae Argyi Folium (prepared), Ferulae Resina, Cinnamomi Cortex, Toxicodendri Resina (calcined), Olibanum (prepared with vinegar), Rehmanniae Radix Praeparata, Perillae Fructus and Euodiae Fructus (prepared with licorice water).

Actions and Indications Dispersing mass, resolving stasis. It is used for consumptive disease due to blood-stasis in women; puerperal blood-stasis, tenderness and pain of lower abdomen due to abdominal mass.

Warning It is contraindicated for pregnant women.

气管炎橡胶膏

【处方】赤芍、乌药、白芷、桂枝、生草乌、紫苏子、白附子、荜澄茄、生天南星、罂粟壳、芥子、皂荚、冰片、樟脑、薄荷脑、松节油、水杨酸甲酯。

【功能主治】温肺化痰、平喘止咳。用于受寒引起的气管炎，并有预防气管炎的作用。

【注意】有咳血史和高血压患者忌用。

Relieving Trachitis Adhesive Plaster

Name of Chinese Phonetic Alphabet Qi Guan Yan Xiang Jiao Gao

Formula Paeoniae Radix Rubra, Linderae Radix, Angelicae Dahuricae Radix, Cinnamomi Ramulus, Aconiti Kusnezoffii Radix, Perillae Fructus, Typhonii Rhizoma, Fructus Litseae, Arisaematis Rhizoma, Papaveris Pericarpium, Sinapis Semen, Gleditsiae Fructus, Borneolum Syntheticum, Camphora, Menthol, Terebinthinae Oleum and Methylsalicylate.

Actions and Indications Warming the lung and resolving phlegm, calming dyspnea and relieving cough. It is indicated for trachitis due to cold and it has effect of preventing trachitis.

Warning It is contraindicated for cases with history of hematemesis and hypertension.

气滞胃痛片

【处方】柴胡、延胡索（炙）、枳壳、香附（炙）、白芍、甘草（炙）。

【功能主治】舒肝理气，和胃止痛。用于肝郁气滞，胸痞胀满，胃脘疼痛。

【注意】孕妇慎用。

Stomachache-relieving Tablet

Name of Chinese Phonetic Alphabet Qi Zhi Wei Tong Pian

Formula Bupleuri Radix, Corydalis Rhizoma (prepared), Aurantii Fructus, Cyperi Rhizoma (prepared), Paeoniae Radix Alba and Glycyrrhizae Radix et Rhizoma (prepared).

Actions and Indications Soothing the liver, regulating *qi*, harmonizing the stomach, alleviating pain. It is used for stuffiness and fullness in chest and stomach duct pain due to stagnation of liver-*qi*.

Warning It should be used carefully for pregnant women.

毛鸡药酒

【处方】当归、茯苓、千年健、桃仁、川芎、白芷、红花、赤芍、干毛鸡（或鲜毛鸡，均除去毛、内脏）。

【功能主治】温经祛风，活血化瘀。用于产后眩晕，四肢酸痛无力，痛经。

【注意】感冒发热，喉痛，眼赤等忌服。

Crow Pheasant* Medicated Wine

Name of Chinese Phonetic Alphabet Mao Ji Yao Jiu

Formula Angelicae Sinensis Radix, Poria, Homalomenae Rhizoma, Persicae Semen, Chuanxiong Rhizoma, Angelicae Dahuricae Radix, Carthami Flos, Paeoniae Radix Rubra, Centropodis Sinensis Caro (removed feather and internal organs).

Actions and Indications Warming meridians, dispelling wind, activating blood, resolving stasis. It is indicated for puerperal vertigo, soreness, pain and weakness of limbs, dysmenorrhea.

Warning It is contraindicated for cases with common cold, fever, sore-throat, conjunctivitis.

* 毛鸡

午时茶颗粒

【处方】苍术、柴胡、羌活、防风、白芷、川芎、广藿香、前胡、连翘、陈皮、山楂、枳实、麦芽（炒）、甘草、桔梗、六神曲（炒）、紫苏叶、厚朴、红茶。

【功能主治】解表和中。用于感受风寒，内伤食积，寒热吐泻。

Wu Shi Cha Granules for Improving Dyspepsia

Name of Chinese Phonetic Alphabet Wu Shi Cha Ke Li

Formula Atractylodis Rhizoma, Bupleuri Radix, Notopterygii Rhizoma et Radix, Saposhnikoviae Radix, Angelicae Dahuricae Radix, Chuanxiong Rhizoma, Pogostemonis Herba, Peucedani Radix, Forsythiae Fructus, Citri Reticulatae Pericarpium, Crataegi Fructus, Aurantii Fructus Immaturus, Hordei Fructus Germinatus (fried), Glycyrrhizae Radix et Rhizoma, Platycodonis Radix, Medicata Massa Fermentata (fried), Perillae Folium, Magnoliae Officinalis Cortex and Camelliae Sinensis Folium Gemmae Fermentatio.

Actions and Indications Releasing the exterior and harmonizing the middle energizer. It is used for dyspepsia, vomiting and diarrhea.

牛黄上清丸

【处方】牛黄、石膏、薄荷、菊花等。

【功能主治】清热泻火，散风止痛。用于头痛眩晕，目赤耳鸣，咽喉肿痛，口舌生疮，牙龈肿痛，大便燥结。

【注意】孕妇慎用。

Bezoar* Bolus for Purging Heat

Name of Chinese Phonetic Alphabet Niu Huang Shang Qing Wan

Formula Bovis Calculus, Gypsum Fibrosum, Menthae Haplocalycis Herba, Chrysanthemi Flos, etc.

Actions and Indications Clearing heat and purging fire, dissipating wind and relieving pain. It is used for headache, vertigo, conjunctival congestion, tinnitus, sore-throat, aphthae, gingivitis and dry stool.

Warning It should be used cautiously for pregnant women.

* 牛黄

牛黄千金散

【处方】全蝎、僵蚕（制）、牛黄、朱砂、冰片、胆南星、黄连、天麻、甘草。

【功能主治】清热解毒，镇痉定惊。用于小儿惊风高热，手足抽搐，痰涎壅盛，神昏谵语。

【注意】忌辛辣饮食（乳母同忌），慢惊风忌用。

Qian Jin Bezoar* Powder

Name of Chinese Phonetic Alphabet Niu Huang Qian Jin San

Formula Scorpio, Bombyx Batryticatus (prepared), Bovis Calculus, Cinnabaris, Boneolum Syntheticum, Arisaema cum Bile, Coptidis Rhizoma, Gastrodiae Rhizoma and Glycyrrhizae Radix et Rhizoma.

Actions and Indications Clearing heat, detoxifying, settling fright and spasm. It is indicated for infantile convulsion marked by high fever, spasm of limbs, excessive phlegm, loss of consciousness, delirium.

Warning It is contraindicated for cases with chronic convulsion and pungent foods should be avoided in foster-nurse.

*牛黄

牛黄化毒片

【处方】天南星（制）、连翘、金银花、白芷、甘草、乳香、没药、牛黄。

【功能主治】解毒消肿，散结止痛。用于疮疡、乳痛、红肿。

Bezoar* Tablet for Detoxifying

Name of Chinese Phonetic Alphabet Niu Huang Hua Du Pian

Formula Arisaematis Rhizoma (prepared), Forsythiae Fructus, Lonicerae Japonicae Flos, Angelicae Dahuricae Radix, Glycyrrhizae Radix et Rhizoma, Olibanum, Myrrha and Bovis Calculus.

Actions and Indications Detoxifying and dispersing swelling, dissipating mass, relieving pain. It is used for sore, mastalgia with red and swelling.

*牛黄

牛黄至宝丸

【处方】连翘、栀子、大黄、芒硝、石膏、青蒿、 陈皮、木香、广藿香、牛黄、冰片、雄黄。

【功能主治】清热解毒，泻火通便。用于胃肠积热引起的头痛眩晕，目赤耳鸣，口燥咽干，大便燥结。

【注意】孕妇忌服。

Treasure Bolus of Bezoar*

Name of Chinese Phonetic Alphabet Niu Huang Zhi Bao Wan

Formula Forsythiae Fructus, Gardeniae Fructus, Rhei Radix et Rhizoma, Natrii Sulfas, Gypsum Fibrosum, Artemisiae Annuae Herba, Citri Reticulatae Pericarpium, Aucklandiae Radix, Pogostemonis Herba, Bovis Calculus, Borneolum Syntheticum and Realgar.

Actions and Indications Clearing heat and detoxifying, purging fire, relaxing the bowels. It is used for headache, vertigo, conjunctival congestion, tinnitus, dry mouth and throat and dry stool due to accumulation of heat in the stomach and intestines.

Warning It is contraindicated for pregnant women.

*牛黄

牛黄抱龙丸

【处方】牛黄、胆南星、天竺黄、茯苓、琥珀、僵蚕（炒）、全蝎、麝香、雄黄、朱砂。

【功能主治】清热镇惊，祛风化痰。用于小儿风痰壅盛，高热神昏，惊风抽搐。

Bao Long Bezoar* Pill

Name of Chinese Phonetic Alphabet Niu Huang Bao Long Wan

Formula Bovis Calculus, Arisaema cum Bile, Bambusae Concretio Silicea, Poria, Succinum, Bombyx Batryticatus (fried), Scorpio, Moschus, Realgar and Cinnabaris.

Actions and Indications Clearing heat, settling fright, dispelling wind, resolving phlegm. It is used for infantile excessive wind-phlegm, high fever, obnubilation, convulsive spasm.

*牛黄

牛黄降压胶囊

【处方】牛黄、羚羊角、珍珠、冰片、黄芪、郁金、白芍等。

【功能主治】清心化痰，镇静降压。用于肝火旺盛，头晕目眩，烦躁不安，痰火壅盛，高血压症。

【注意】腹泻者忌服。

Bezoar* Capsule for Hypertension-

relieving

Name of Chinese Phonetic Alphabet Niu Huang Jiang Ya Jiao Nang

Formula Bovis Calculus, Saigae Tataricae Cornu, Margarita, Borneolum Syntheticum, Astragali Radix, Curcumae Radix, Paeoniae Radix Alba, etc.

Actions and Indications Clearing heart-fire, resolving phlegm, tranquilizing the mind and lowering blood pressure. It is used for dizziness, dizzy vision and vexation due to intense liver-fire; hypertension due to intense phlegm-fire.

Warning It is contraindicated for cases with diarrhea.

* 牛黄

牛黄益金片

【处方】黄柏、硼砂、玄明粉、牛黄、薄荷脑、薄荷油。

【功能主治】清热利咽，消肿止痛。用于急、慢性咽炎。

Bezoar* Tablet for Throat Trouble

Name of Chinese Phonetic Alphabet Niu Huang Yi Jin Pian

Formula Phellodendri Chinensis Cortex, Borax, Natrii Sulfas Exsiccatus, Bovis Calculus, Menthol and Menthae Haplocalycis Oleum.

Actions and Indications Clearing heat and soothing the throat, dispersing swelling and relieving pain. It is indicated for acute and chronic pharyngitis.

* 牛黄

牛黄消炎灵胶囊

【处方】牛黄、黄芩、栀子、朱砂、珍珠母、郁金、雄黄、冰片、石膏、盐酸小檗碱、水牛角浓缩粉。

【功能主治】消炎退热，通窍，镇静，降压安神。用于病毒性感冒，上呼吸道感染，肺炎，气管炎及其他细菌性感染引起的高热不退等症。

Bezoar* Capsule for Anti-inflammation

Name of Chinese Phonetic Alphabet Niu Huang Xiao Yan Ling Jiao Nang

Formula Bovis Calculus, Scutellariae Radix, Gardeniae Fructus, Cinnabaris, Margaritifera Concha, Curcumae Radix, Realgar, Borneolum Syntheticum, Gypsum Fibrosum, Berberine Hydrochloride and Bubali Cornu Pulvis Concentratio.

Actions and Indications Anti-inflammation, abating fever, inducing resuscitation, depressurization and tranquilization. It is indicted for viral common cold, upper respiratory infection, pneumonia, trachitis and unmitigated hyperpyrexia due to bacterial infection.

* 牛黄

牛黄蛇胆川贝散

【处方】牛黄、蛇胆汁、川贝母。

【功能主治】清热，化痰，止咳。用于外感咳嗽中的热痰咳嗽，燥痰咳嗽。

Powder of Bezoar* Forest Cobra Bile** and Sichuan Fritillary***

Name of Chinese Phonetic Alphabet Niu Huang She Dan Chuan Bei San

Formula Bovis Calculus, Naja Bilis and Fritillariae Cirrhosae Bulbus.

Actions and Indications Clearing heat, resolving phlegm and relieving cough. It is indicated for cough due to heat-phlegm; cough due to dryness-phlegm.

* 牛黄 ** 蛇胆汁 *** 川贝母

牛黄清火丸

【处方】大黄、黄芩、桔梗、山药、丁香、牛黄、冰片、雄黄、薄荷脑。

【功能主治】清热，散风，解毒。用于肝胃肺蕴热引起的头晕目眩，口鼻生疮，风火牙疼，咽喉肿痛，痄腮红肿，耳鸣。

【注意】孕妇忌服。

Bezoar* Pill for Clearing Fire

Name of Chinese Phonetic Alphabet Niu Huang Qing Huo Wan

Formula Rhei Radix et Rhizoma, Scutellariae Radix, Platycodonis Radix, Dioscoreae Rhizoma, Caryophylli Flos, Bovis Calculus, Borneolum Syntheticum, Realgar and Menthol.

Actions and Indications Clearing heat, dissipating wind, detoxicating. It is indicated for dizziness, dizzy vision, aphthae, toothache, sore-throat, mumps and tinnitus due to accumulation of heat in the liver, stomach and lung.

Warning It is contraindicated for pregnant women.

*牛黄

牛黄清心丸

【处方】牛黄、当归、白术（炒）、阿胶、山药、黄芩、苦杏仁（炒）、茯苓、甘草、川芎、大豆黄卷、桔梗、防风、柴胡、大枣（去核）、干姜、麝香、人参、六神曲（炒）、肉桂、白蔹、麦冬、蒲黄（炒）、白芍、冰片、羚羊角、朱砂、雄黄、水牛角浓缩粉。

【功能主治】清心化痰，镇惊祛风。用于神志混乱，言语不清，痰涎壅盛，头晕目眩，癫痫惊风，痰迷心窍，痰火痰厥。

【注意】孕妇慎用。

Bezoar* Pill for Clearing Heart-fire

Name of Chinese Phonetic Alphabet Niu Huang Qing Xin Wan

Formula Bovis Calculus, Angelicae Sinensis Radix, Atractylodis Macrocephalae Rhizoma (fried), Asini Corii Colla, Dioscoreae Rhizoma, Scutellariae Radix, Armeniacae Semen Amarum (fried), Poria, Glycyrrhizae Radix et Rhizoma, Chuanxiong Rhizoma, Sojae Semen Germinatum, Platycodonis Radix, Saposhnikoviae Radix, Bupleuri Radix, Jujubae Fructus (removed nucleus), Zingiberis Rhizoma, Moschus, Ginseng Radix et Rhizoma, Medicata Massa Fermentata (fried), Cinnamomi Cortex, Ampelopsis Radix, Ophiopogonis Radix, Typhae Pollen (fried), Paeoniae Radix Alba, Borneolum Syntheticum, Saigae Tataricae Cornu, Cinnabaris, Realgar and Bubali Cornu Pulvis Concentratio.

Actions and Indications Clearing heart-fire, resolving phlegm, settling fright, dispelling wind. It is used for unconsciousness, alalia, dizziness, dizzy vision, epilepsy, convulsion, phlegm syncope.

Warning It should be used cautiously for pregnant women.

*牛黄

牛黄清肺散

【处方】牛黄、茯苓、川贝母、白前、沉香、黄芩、胆南星、水牛角浓缩粉、百部（制）、清半夏、石膏、冰片。

【功能主治】清肺化痰，消炎止咳。用于肺热咳嗽，痰涎壅盛，胸满喘促。

Bezoar* Powder for Relieving Cough

Name of Chinese Phonetic Alphabet Niu Huang Qing Fei San

Formula Bovis Calculus, Poria, Fritillariae Cirrhosae Bulbus, Cynanchi Stauntonii Rhizoma et Radix, Aquilariae Lignum Resinatum, Scutellariae Radix, Arisaema cum Bile, Bubali Cornu Pulvis Concentratio, Stemonae Radix (prepared), Pinelliae Rhizoma Praeparatum cum Alumine, Gypsum Fibrosum and Borneolum Syntheticum.

Actions and Indications Clearing lung-heat and resolving phlegm, antiphlogistic and alleviating cough. It is indicated for cough due to lung-heat, marked by profuse phlegm, chest distress and dyspnea.

*牛黄

牛黄清胃丸

【处方】牛黄、大黄、菊花、麦冬、薄荷、石膏、栀子、玄参、番泻叶、黄芩、甘草、桔梗、黄柏、连翘、牵牛子（炒）、枳实（沙烫）、冰片。

【功能主治】清胃泻火，润燥通便。用于心胃火盛，头晕目眩，口舌生疮，牙龈肿痛，乳蛾咽痛，便秘尿赤。

【注意】孕妇忌服。

Bezoar* Bolus for Clearing Stomach-fire

Name of Chinese Phonetic Alphabet Niu Huang Qing Wei Wan

Formula Bovis Calculus, Rhei Radix et Rhizoma, Chrysanthemi Flos, Ophiopogonis Radix, Menthae Haplocalycis Herba, Gypsum Fibrosum, Gardeniae Fructus, Scrophulariae Radix, Sennae Folium, Scutellariae Radix, Glycyrrhizae Radix et Rhizoma, Platycodonis Radix, Phellodendri Chinensis Cortex, Forsythiae Fructus, Pharbitidis Semen (fried), Aurantii Fructus Immaturus (scalded by heated soil) and Borneolum Syntheticum.

Actions and Indications Clearing stomach-fire, moistening dryness and relaxing the bowels. It is used for dizziness, dizzy vision, aphthae, gingivitis, tonsillitis, sore-throat, constipation and dark urine due to intense stomach-fire.

Warning It is contraindicated for pregnant women.

*牛黄

牛黄清宫丸

【处方】牛黄、麦冬、黄芩、莲子心、天花粉、甘草、大黄、栀子、地黄、连翘、郁金、玄参、雄黄、犀角、朱砂、冰片、金银花、麝香。

【功能主治】清热解毒，镇惊安神，止渴除烦。用于身热烦躁，昏迷不醒，舌赤唇干，谵语狂躁，头痛眩晕，惊悸不安，小儿急热惊风。

【注意】孕妇忌服。

Qinggong Pill of Bezoar*

Name of Chinese Phonetic Alphabet Niu Huang Qing Gong Wan

Formula Bovis Calculus, Ophiopogonis Radix, Scutellariae Radix, Nelumbinis Plumula, Trichosanthis Radix, Glycyrrhizae Radix et Rhizoma, Rhei Radix et Rhizoma, Gardeniae Fructus, Rehmanniae Radix, Forsythiae Fructus, Curcumae Radix, Scrophulariae Radix, Realgar, Rhinocerotis Cornu, Cinnabaris, Borneolum Syntheticum, Lonicerae Japonicae Flos and Moschus.

Actions and Indications Clearing heat and detoxifying, settling fright, tranquilizing the mind, quenching thirst and relieving vexation. It is used for generalized fever, vexation, coma, red tongue, dry lips, delirious speech, mania, headache, vertigo, fright and infantile acute convulsion of heat type.

Warning It is contraindicated for pregnant women.

*牛黄

牛黄清热胶囊

【处方】黄连、黄芩、栀子、郁金、寒水石、牛黄、水牛角浓缩粉、琥珀粉、玳瑁粉、朱砂、冰片。

【功能主治】清热镇惊。用于温邪入里引起的高热痉厥，四肢抽动，烦躁不安，痰浊壅塞。

Heat-clearing Capsule of Bezoar*

Name of Chinese Phonetic Alphabet Niu Huang Qing Re Jiao Nang

Formula Coptidis Rhizoma, Scutellariae Radix, Gardeniae Fructus, Curcumae Radix, Gypsum Rubrum, Bovis Calculus, Bubali Cornu Pulvis Concentratio, Succini Pulvis, Eretmochelydis Carapax Pulvis, Cannabaris and Borneolum Syntheticum.

Actions and Indications Clearing heat and settling fright. It is used for hight fever, convulsive spasm, spasm of limbs, vexation, restlessness and stagnation of phlegm-turbidity due to warm pathogens entering the interior.

*牛黄

牛黄解毒片

【处方】牛黄、雄黄、石膏、大黄、黄芩、桔梗、冰片、甘草。

【功能主治】清热解毒。用于火热内盛，咽喉肿痛，牙龈肿痛，口舌生疮，目赤肿痛。

【注意】孕妇禁用。

Bezoar* Tablet for Detoxicating

Name of Chinese Phonetic Alphabet Niu Huang Jie Du Pian

Formula Bovis Calculus, Realgar, Gypsum Fibrosum, Rhei Radix et Rhizoma, Scutellariae Radix, Platycodonis Radix, Borneolum Syntheticum and Glycyrrhizae Radix et Rhizoma.

Actions and Indications Clearing heat and detoxicating. It is used for sore-throat, gingivitis, aphthae and conjunctival congestion due to internal prevailing heat.

Warning It is contraindicated for pregnant women.

* 牛黄

牛黄镇惊丸

【处方】牛黄、全蝎、僵蚕（炒）、白附子（制）、麝香、朱砂、雄黄、半夏（制）、钩藤、防风、琥珀、胆南星、珍珠、天麻、天竺黄、冰片、薄荷、甘草。

【功能主治】镇惊安神，祛风豁痰。用于小儿惊风，高热抽搐，牙关紧闭，烦躁不安。

【注意】风寒表证不宜用；慢惊风禁用；忌食辛辣肥甘厚味（乳母同忌）。

Bezoar* Pill for Convulsion-settling

Name of Chinese Phonetic Alphabet Niu Huang Zhen Jing Wan

Formula Bovis Calculus, Scorpio, Bombyx Batryticatus (fried) Typhonii Rhizoma (prepared), Moschus, Cinnabaris, Realgar, Pinellae Rhizoma Praeparata, Uncariae Ramulus cum Uncis, Saposhnikoviae Radix, Succinum, Arisaema cum Bile, Margarita, Gastrodiae Rhizoma, Bambusae Concretio Silicea, Borneolum Syntheticum, Menthae Haplocalycis Herba and Glycyrrhizae Radix et Rhizoma.

Actions and Indications Settling fright, tranquilizing the mind, dispelling wind, expelling phlegm. It is used for infantile convulsion marked by high fever, spasm, lockjaw, vexation.

Warning It is contraindicated for cases with exterior syndrome of wind-cold type and chronic convulsion. Pungent and fatty foods should be avoided in lactating mother.

* 牛黄

牛黄醒脑丸

【处方】黄连、水牛角浓缩粉、黄芩、冰片、栀子、麝香、郁金、朱砂、雄黄、牛黄、珍珠、玳瑁。

【功能主治】清热解毒，镇惊，开窍。用于热病高热，昏迷惊厥，烦躁不安，小儿惊风抽搐，失眠。

【注意】孕妇慎用。

Heat-clearing Pill of Bezoar*

Name of Chinese Phonetic Alphabet Niu Huang Xing Nao Wan

Formula Coptidis Rhizoma, Bubali Cornu Pulvis Concentratio, Sculellariae Radix, Borneolum Syntheticum, Gardeniae Fructus, Moschus, Curcumae Radix, Cinnabaris, Realgar, Bovis Calculus, Margarita and Eretmochelydis Carapax.

Actions and Indications Clearing heat and detoxifying, settling fright and inducing resuscitation. It is used for heat disease marked by high fever, coma, convulsion, vexation, restlessness, and also used for infantile convulsion, spasm, and insomnia.

Warning It should be used carefully for pregnant women.

* 牛黄

牛黄醒消丸

【处方】牛黄、麝香、乳香（制）、没药（制）、雄黄。

【功能主治】清热解毒，消肿止痛。用于痈疽发背，瘰疬流注，乳痈乳岩，无名肿毒。

【注意】孕妇忌服。

Bezoar* Pill for Dispersing Swelling

Name of Chinese Phonetic Alphabet Niu Huang Xing Xiao Wan

Formula Bovis Calculus, Moschus, Olibanum (prepared), Myrrha (prepared) and Realgar.

Actions and Indications Clearing heat and detoxicating, dispersing swelling, relieving pain. It is used for abscess and deep-rooted carbucle, scrofula, deep multiple abscess, acute mastitis, rocky mass in the breast, inflammatory swelling of unknown origin.

Warning It is contraindicated for pregnant women.

* 牛黄

升血灵冲剂

【处方】皂矾、黄芪、山楂、阿胶、大枣。

【功能主治】补气养血，消积理脾。用于治疗缺铁性贫血。

【注意】禁用茶水冲服。

Relieving Iron-deficiency Anemia Soluble Granules

Name of Chinese Phonetic Alphabet Sheng Xue Ling Chong Ji

Formula Malanteritum, Astragali Radix, Crataegi Fructus, Asini Corii Colla and Jujubae Fructus.

Actions and Indications Tonifying *qi*, nourishing blood and regulating the spleen. It is used for iron-deficiency anemia.

Warning The soluble granules cannot be mixed with tea for oral use.

升血调元汤

【处方】鸡血藤、骨碎补、何首乌、黄芪、麦芽、女贞子、党参、佛手。

【功能主治】益气养血，补肾健脾。用于提升外周血白细胞和其他原因引起的白细胞减少症及病后虚弱。

Tonifying Blood Decoction

Name of Chinese Phonetic Alphabet Sheng Xue Tiao Yuan Tang

Formula Spatholobi Caulis, Drynariae Rhizoma, Polygoni Multiflori Radix, Astragali Radix, Hordei Fructus Germinatus, Ligustri Lucidi Fructus, Codonopsis Radix and Citri Sarcodactylis Fructus.

Actions and Indications Tonifying *qi* and blood, fortifying the kidney and spleen. It is indicated for rising peripheral leukocytes, leukopenia due to various causes, and debility after illness.

片仔癀

【处方】本品为牛黄、麝香、三七、蛇胆等药经加工制成的锭剂。

【功能主治】清热解毒，凉血化瘀，消肿止痛。用于热毒血瘀所致的急、慢性病毒性肝炎，痈疽疔疮，无名肿毒，跌打损伤及各种炎症。

【注意】孕妇忌服。

Pien Tze Huang Troche

Name of Chinese Phonetic Alphabet Pian Zai Huang

Formula Bovis Calculus, Moschus, Notoginseng Radix et Rhizoma, Naja Fel, etc.

Actions and Indications Clearing heat and detoxicating, cooling the blood and resolving stasis, dispersing swelling and relieving pain. It is indicated for acute and chronic viral hepatitis, abscess and deep-rooted boil, swelling and pain of unknown origin, traumatic injury and inflammation due to heat-toxin and blood-stasis.

Warning It is contraindicated for pregnant women.

乌贝颗粒

【处方】海螵蛸（去壳）、浙贝母。

【功能主治】制酸止痛，收敛止血。用于胃痛反酸，胃及十二指肠溃疡。

Cuttle Bone* and Thunberg Fritillary** Granules

Name of Chinese Phonetic Alphabet Wu Bei Ke Li

Formula Sepiae Endoconcha (removed coat) and Fritillariae Thunbergii Bulbus.

Actions and Indications Inhibiting acidity, alleviating pain, relieving bleeding. It is indicated for stomachache, acid regurgitation, gastric and duodenal ulcer.

* 海螵蛸 ** 浙贝母

乌军治胆片

【处方】乌梅、大黄、佛手、枳实、牛至、栀子、甘草、槟榔、威灵仙、姜黄。

【功能主治】疏肝解郁，利胆排石，清里泄热，理气止痛。用于胆囊炎，胆道感染，胆道手术后综合征属肝胆湿热证者。

Japanese Apricot* and Rhubarb** Tablet for Infection of Biliary Tract

Name of Chinese Phonetic Alphabet Wu Jun Zhi Dan Pian

Formula Mume Fructus, Rhei Radix et Rhizoma, Citri Sarcodactylis Fructus, Aurantii Fructus Immaturus, Origani Vulgaris Herba, Gandeniae Fructus, Glycyrrhizae Radix et Rhizoma, Arecae Semen, Clematidis Radix et Rhizoma and Curcumae Rhizoma Longae.

Actions and Indications Soothing the liver, relieving depression, draining the biliary tract to eliminate stone, clearing heat, regulating *qi* to alleviate pain. It is indicated for cholecystitis, infection of biliary tract, post-operation syndrome of biliary tract attributed to dampness-heat syndrome of the liver and gallbladder.

* 乌梅 ** 大黄

乌鸡白凤口服液

【处方】乌鸡（去毛爪肠）、人参、白芍、丹参、香附（醋炙）、当归、牡蛎（煅）、鹿角、桑螵蛸、甘草、青蒿、天冬、熟地黄、地黄、川芎、黄芪、银柴胡、芡实（炒）、山药。

【功能主治】补气养血，调经止带。用于气血两亏引起的月经不调，行经腹痛，崩漏带下，小腹冷痛，体弱乏力，腰酸腿软，产后虚弱，阴虚盗汗。

Silky Chicken* Oral Liquid

Name of Chinese Phonetic Alphabet Wu Ji Bai Feng Kou Fu Ye

Formula Galli Caro cum Osse Nigro (removed claws and intestines), Ginseng Radix et Rhizoma, Paeoniae Radix Alba, Salviae Miltiorrhizae Radix et Rhizoma, Cyperi Rhizoma (prepared with vinegar), Angelicae Sinensis Radix, Ostreae Concha (calcined), Cervi Cornu, Mantidis Ootheca, Glycyrrhizae Radix et Rhizoma, Artemisiae Annuae Herba, Asparagi Radix, Rehmanniae Radix Praeparata, Rehmanniae Radix, Chuanxiong Rhizoma, Astragali Radix, Stellariae Radix, Euryales Semen (fried) and Dioscoreae Rhizoma.

Actions and Indications Tonifying *qi* and blood, regulating menstruation and relieving white vaginal discharge. It is indicated for irregular menstruation, abdominal pain during menstruation, metrorrhagia, white vaginal discharge, cold-pain in the lower abdomen, general debility, soreness of waist and weakness of legs, puerperal debility and night sweating due to dual deficiency of *qi* and blood.

* 乌鸡

乌鸡白凤丸

【处方】乌鸡（去毛爪肠）、鹿角胶、鳖甲（制）、牡蛎（煅）、桑螵蛸、人参、黄芪、当归、白芍、香附（醋制）、天冬、甘草、地黄、熟地黄、川芎、银柴胡、丹参、山药、芡实（炒）、鹿角霜。

【功能主治】补气养血，调经止带。用于气血两虚，身体瘦弱，腰膝酸软，月经不调，崩漏带下。

Silky Chicken* Bolus

Name of Chinese Phonetic Alphabet Wu Ji Bai

Feng Wan

Formula Galli Caro cum Osse Nigro (removed claws and intestines), Cervi Corus Colla, Trionycis Carapax (prepared), Ostreae Concha (calcined), Mantidis Ootheca, Ginseng Radix et Rhizoma, Astragali Radix, Angelicae Sinensis Radix, Paeoniae Radix Alba, Cyperi Rhizoma (prepared with vinegar), Asparagi Radix, Glycyrrhizae Radix et Rhizoma, Rehmanniae Radix, Rehmanniae Radix Praeparata, Chuanxiong Rhizoma, Stellariae Radix, Salviae Miltiorrhizae Radix et Rhizoma, Dioscoreae Rhizoma, Euryales Semen (fried) and Cervi Cornu Degelatinatum.

Actions and Indications Tonifying *qi* and blood, regulating menstruation and relieving white vaginal discharge. It is indicated for emaciation of women, soreness of waist and weakness of legs, irregular menstruation, metrorrhagia and white vaginal discharge due to dual deficiency of *qi* and blood.

* 乌鸡

乌梅丸

【处方】乌梅、干姜、附子、细辛、花椒、桂枝、人参、当归、黄连、黄柏。

【功能主治】温脏安蛔。用于蛔厥、久痢、厥阴头痛症见腹痛，胸闷，呕吐，四肢冰冷，脉沉细或弦紧。

【注意】孕妇慎用。

Japanese Apricot★ Bolus

Name of Chinese Phonetic Alphabet Wu Mei Wan

Formula Mume Fructus, Zingiberis Rhizoma, Aconiti Lateralis Radix Praeparata, Asari Radix et Rhizoma, Zanthoxyli Pericarpium, Cinnamomi Ramulus, Ginseng Radix et Rhizoma, Angelicae Sinensis Radix, Coptidis Rhizoma and Phellodendri Chinensis Cortex.

Actions and Indications Warming the viscera and expelling ascaris. It is used for ascariasis, chronic dysentery and *jueyin* headache, manifested as abdominal pain, chest distress, vomiting, cold limbs, sunken and fine pulse or string-like and tight pulse.

Warning It should be used cautiously for pregnant women.

* 乌梅

乌蛇止痒丸

【处方】乌梢蛇、防风、蛇床子、黄柏、人参须、苍术、牡丹皮、当归、苦参、人工牛黄、蛇胆汁。

【功能主治】养血祛风，燥湿止痒。用于皮肤瘙痒，荨麻疹等属血虚郁热。

Garter Snake★ Pill for Relieving Itching

Name of Chinese Phonetic Alphabet Wu She Zhi Yang Wan

Formula Zaocys, Saposhnikoviae Radix, Cnidii Fructus, Phellodendri Chinensis Cortex, Ginseng Radix Fibrosa, Atractylodis Rhizoma, Moutan Cortex, Angelicae Sinensis Radix, Sophorae Flavescentis Radix, Bovis Calculus Artifactus and Naja Bilis.

Actions and Indications Nourishing blood, dispelling wind, drying dampness, relieving itching. It is used for cutaneous pruritus and urticaria attributed to blood deficiency and stagnation of heat.

* 乌梢蛇

丹七片

【处方】丹参、三七。

【功能主治】活血化瘀。用于血瘀气滞，心胸痹痛，眩晕头痛，经期腹痛。

Redroot Sage★ and *Sanchi*★★ Tablet

Name of Chinese Phonetic Alphabet Dan Qi Pian

Formula Salviae Miltiorrhizae Radix et Rhizoma and Notoginseng Radix et Rhizoma.

Actions and Indications Activating blood and resolving stasis. It is used for impediment and pain of the heart and chest, vertigo, headache and dysmenorrhea due to blood-stasis and *qi*-stagnation.

* 丹参 ** 三七

丹红化瘀口服液

【处方】丹参、当归、川芎、桃仁、红花、柴胡枳壳。

【功能主治】活血化瘀，行气通络。用于视网膜中央静脉阻塞吸收期的气滞血瘀证。

【注意】用药期间定期检查凝血时间。有出血倾向者，视网膜中央阻塞出血期患者以及孕妇禁用。

Redroot Sage★ and Safflower★★ Oral Liquid for Resolving Stasis

Name of Chinese Phonetic Alphabet Dan Hong Hua Yu Kou Fu Ye

Formula Salviae Miltiorrhizae Radix et Rhizoma, Angelicae Sinensis Radix, Chuanxiong Rhizoma, Persicae Semen, Carthami Flos, Bupleuri Radix and Aurantii Fructus.

Actions and Indications Activating blood, resolving stasis, moving *qi*, activating collaterals. It is used for obstructive absorption period of central vein of retina attributed to *qi*-stagnation and blood-stasis syndrome.

Warning During medication, periodic examination of the clotting time is needed. This oral liquid is contraindicated for cases with bleeding tendency, obstructive bleeding period of central vein of retina, and pregnant women.

* 丹参 ** 红花

丹参片

【处方】本品为丹参制成的片剂。

【功能主治】活血化瘀，清心除烦。用于冠心病引起的心绞痛及心神不宁。

Redroot Sage★ Tablet

Name of Chinese Phonetic Alphabet Dan Shen Pian

Formula Salviae Miltiorrhizae Radix et Rhizoma.

Actions and Indications Activating blood and resolving stasis, clearing heart-fire, relieving vexation. It is indicated for angina pectoris and irritability due to coronary heart disease.

* 丹参

丹参酮胶囊

【处方】本品为丹参经适宜加工制成的胶囊。

【功能主治】抗菌消炎。用于骨髓炎，痤疮，扁桃体炎，外耳道炎，疖，痈，外伤感染，烧伤感染，乳腺炎，蜂窝织炎。

Tanshinone★ Capsule

Name of Chinese Phonetic Alphabet Dan Shen Tong Jiao Nang

Formula Salviae Miltiorrhizae Radix et Rhizoma.

Actions and Indications Antisepsis, anti-inflammation. It is indicated for osteomyelitis, acne, tonsillitis, otitis externa, furuncle, abscess, traumatic infection, burn, mastitis, cellulitis.

* 丹参酮

丹羚心舒胶囊

【处方】丹参提取物、羚羊角粉、人参、当归、三七、蟾酥、麝香、冰片、猪胆膏。

【功能主治】益气活血，芳香开窍，化瘀止痛。用于气血淤滞，心窍闭阻之胸中憋闷、心悸、心痛、抽搐惊厥。

Redroot Sage★ and Antelope Horn★★ Capsule

Name of Chinese Phonetic Alphabet Dan Ling Xin Shu Jiao Nang

Formula Salviae Miltiorrhizae Radix et Rhizoma

(extract), Saigae Tataricae Cornu Pulvis, Ginseng Radix et Rhizoma, Angelicae Sinensis Radix, Notoginseng Radix et Rhizoma, Bufonis Venenum, Moschus, Borneolum Syntheticum and Suillus Fel Extractum.

Actions and Indications Tonifying *qi*, activating blood, opening orifices, resolving stasis, alleviating pain. It is used for chest distress, palpitation, cardialgia, spasm and faint from fright due to stagnation of *qi*, blood and heart orifice.

*丹参 **羚羊角

风热咳嗽软胶囊

【处方】桑叶、菊花、黄芩、薄荷、桔梗等。

【功能主治】祛风解热，止咳化痰。用于风热咳嗽，鼻流稠涕，发热头昏，咽干舌燥。

Relieving Cough Soft Capsule

Name of Chinese Phonetic Alphabet Feng Re Ke Sou Ruan Jiao Nang

Formula Mori Folium, Chrysanthemi Flos, Scutellariae Radix, Menthae Haplocalycis Herba, Platycodonis Radix, etc.

Actions and Indications Dispelling wind and clearing heat, relieving cough and resolving phlegm. It is indicated for cough due to wind-heat; marked by thick nasal discharge, fever dizziness, dry throat and tongue.

风热清口服液

【处方】金银花、熊胆粉、青黛、桔梗、瓜蒌皮、甘草。

【功能主治】清热解毒，宣肺透表，利咽化痰。用于外感风热所致的发热、微恶风寒、头痛、咳嗽、流涕、口渴、咽痛，以及急性上呼吸道感染见上述症状者。

Heat-clearing Oral Liquid for Relieving Common Cold

Name of Chinese Phonetic Alphabet Feng Re Qing Kou Fu Ye

Formula Lonicerae Japonicae Flos, Ursi Fel Pulvis, Indigo Naturalis, Platycodonis Radix, Trichosanthis Pericarpium and Glycyrrhizae Radix et Rhizoma.

Actions and Indications Clearing heat and detoxicating, diffusing the lung and outthrusting through the exterior, soothing the throat and resolving phlegm. It is indicated for fever, mild aversion to wind-cold, headache, cough, rhinorrhea, thirst, sore-throat due to external contraction of wind-heat, and acute upper respiratory tract infection with the above mentioned symptoms.

风热感冒冲剂

【处方】板蓝根、连翘、薄荷、荆芥穗、桑叶、芦根、牛蒡子、菊花、苦杏仁、桑枝、六神曲。

【功能主治】清热解毒，宣肺利咽。用于感冒身热，鼻塞，头痛，咳嗽，痰多。

Common Cold Relieving Soluble Granules

Name of Chinese Phonetic Alphabet Feng Re Gan Mao Chong Ji

Formula Isatidis Radix, Forsythiae Fructus, Menthae Haplocalycis Herba, Schizonepetae Spica, Mori Folium, Phragmitis Rhizoma, Arctii Fructus, Chrysanthemi Flos, Armeniacae Semen Amarum, Mori Ramulus and Medicata Massa Fermentata.

Actions and Indications Clearing heat and detoxicating, diffusing the lung and soothing the throat. It is indicated for common cold marked by fever, nasal congestion, headache, cough, profuse phlegm.

风痛安胶囊

【处方】防己、通草、桂枝、姜黄、石膏、薏苡仁、木瓜、海桐皮、忍冬藤、黄柏、滑石粉、连翘。

【功能主治】清热利湿，活血通络。用于急、慢性风湿性关节炎，慢性风湿性关节炎活动期。

Relieving Chronic Rheumatic Arthritis Capsule

Name of Chinese Phonetic Alphabet Feng Tong An Jiao Nang

Formula Stephaniae Tetrandrae Radix, Tetrapanacis Medulla, Cinnamomi Ramulus, Curcumae Longae Rhizoma, Gypsum Fibrosum, Coicis Semen, Chaenomelis Fructus, Erythrinae Orientalis Cortex, Lonicerae Japonicae Caulis, Phellodendri Chinensis Cortex, Talci Pulvis and Forsythiae Fructus.

Actions and Indications Clearing heat and draining dampness, activating blood and dredging collaterals. It is indicated for acute, chronic rheumatic arthritis or active stage of chronic rheumatic arthritis.

风湿马钱片

【处方】马钱子（制）、僵蚕（炒）、没药（炒）、苍术、全蝎、牛膝、乳香（炒）、麻黄、甘草。

【功能主治】祛风，除湿，镇痛。用于风湿性关节炎，类风湿，坐骨神经痛。

【注意】孕妇，高血压患者，心、肝、肾疾患者忌服；儿童、老弱者慎服，不宜久服多服。

Strychnine Seed* Tablet for Relieving Rheumatic Arthritis

Name of Chinese Phonetic Alphabet Feng Shi Ma Qian Pian

Formula Strychni Semen (prepared), Bombyx Batryticatus (fried), Myrrha (fried), Atractylodis Rhizoma, Scorpio, Achyranthis Bidentatae Radix, Olibanum (fried), Ephedrae Herba and Glycyrrhizae Radix et Rhizoma.

Actions and Indications Dispelling wind and dampness, settling pain. It is indicated for rheumatic arthritis, rheumatoid arthritis and sciatica.

Warning It is contraindicated for pregnant women and cases with hypertension, and should be used carefully for children and the aged, and long-term use is prohibited.

* 马钱子

风湿圣药胶囊

【处方】土茯苓、桃仁、玉竹、五味子、黄柏、防风、羌活、独活、防己、威灵仙、蚕砂、绵萆薢、桂枝、当归、红花、人参、青风藤、穿山龙。

【功能主治】祛风除湿，舒筋通络止痛。用于风湿性关节炎及类风湿性关节炎（关节未变形者）。

【注意】孕妇忌服。

Miraculous Capsule for Relieving Rheumatic Arthritis

Name of Chinese Phonetic Alphabet Feng Shi Sheng Yao Jiao Nang

Formula Smilacis Glabrae Rhizoma, Persicae Semen, Polygonati Odorati Rhizoma, Schisandrae Chinensis Fructus, Phellodendri Chinensis Cortex, Saposhnikoviae Radix, Notopterygii Rhizoma et Radix, Angelicae Pubescentis Radix, Stephaniae Tetrandrae Radix, Clematidis Radix et Rhizoma, Bombycis Feculae, Dioscoreae Spongiosae Rhizoma, Cinnamomi Ramulus, Angelicae Sinensis Radix, Carthami Flos, Ginseng Radix et Rhizoma, Sinomenii Caulis and Dioscoreae Nipponicae Rhizoma.

Actions and Indications Dispelling wind and dampness, relaxing sinews and dredging collaterals, alleviating pain. It is indicated for rheumatic and rheumatoid arthritis without deformation of the joints.

Warning It is contraindicated for pregnant women.

风湿灵仙液

【处方】土茯苓、蚕砂、地龙、当归、桃仁（炒）、红花、威灵仙、广防己、青风藤、独活、人参、黄柏（盐制）、粉萆薢、玉竹、防风、羌活、桂枝、五味子。

【功能主治】祛风除湿，通经活络，止痛。用于类风湿性关节炎，风湿性关节炎，坐骨神经痛，骨质增生。

【注意】孕妇忌服。

Chinese Clematis* Oral Liquid for Relieving Rheumatoid Arthritis

Name of Chinese Phonetic Alphabet Feng Shi Ling Xian Ye

Formula Smilacis Glabrae Rhizoma, Bombycis Feculae, Pheretima, Angelicae Sinensis Radix, Persicae Semen (fried), Carthami Flos, Clematidis Radix et Rhizoma, Aristolochiae Fangchi Radix, Sinomenii Caulis, Angelicae Pubescentis Radix, Ginseng Radix et Rhizoma, Phellodendri Chinensis Cortex (prepared with salt), Dioscoreae Hypoglaucae Rhizoma, Polygonati Odorati Rhizoma, Saposhnikoviae Radix, Notopterygii Rhizoma et Radix, Cinnamomi Ramulus and Schisandrae Chinensis Fructus.

Actions and Indications Dispelling wind and dampness, dredging the meridians and activating collaterals, alleviating pain. It is indicated for rheumatoid and rheumatic arthritis, sciatica and hyperosteogeny.

Warning It is contraindicated for pregnant women.

*威灵仙

风湿定片

【处方】八角枫根、白芷、徐长卿、甘草。

【功能主治】活血通络，除痹止痛。用于风湿性关节炎，类风湿关节炎，颈肋神经痛，坐骨神经痛。

【注意】儿童、孕妇、心脏病患者、过度衰弱有并发症者禁服。

Tablet for Dispelling Wind-dampness

Name of Chinese Phonetic Alphabet Feng Shi Ding Pian

Formula Alangii Radix, Angelicae Dahuricae Radix, Cynanchi Paniculati Radix et Rhizoma and Glycyrrhizae Radix et Rhizoma.

Actions and Indications Activating blood and dredging collaterals, relieving impediment syndrome and alleviating pain. It is indicated for rheumatic and rheumatoid arthritis, cervical rib neuralgia and sciatica.

Warning It is contraindicated for children, pregnant women and cases with heart diseases or complicatd severe debility.

风湿骨痛丸

【处方】制川乌、制草乌、红花、甘草、木瓜、乌梅、麻黄。

【功能主治】温经散寒，通络止痛。用于风寒湿痹所致的风湿性关节炎。

【注意】本品含毒性药，不可多服，孕妇忌服。

Relieving Rheumatic Arthritis Pill

Name of Chinese Phonetic Alphabet Feng Shi Gu Tong Wan

Formula Aconiti Radix Cocta, Aconiti Kusnezoffii Radix Cocta, Carthami Flos, Glycyrrhizae Radix et Rhizoma, Chaenomelis Fructus, Mume Fructus and Ephedrae Herba.

Actions and Indications Warming the meridians and dissipating cold, activating collaterals and alleviating pain. It is indicated for rheumatic arthritis due to wind-cold-damp impediment.

Warning The preparation contains toxic drugs, overdosage is prohibited and it is contraindicated for pregnant women.

风湿液

【处方】独活、桑寄生、羌活、防风、秦艽、木瓜、鹿角胶、鳖甲胶、牛膝、当归、白芍、川芎、红花、白术、甘草、红曲。

【功能主治】补养肝肾，养血通络，祛风除湿。用于肝肾血亏、风寒湿痹引起的骨节疼痛，四肢麻木，以及风湿性、类风湿性疾病。

【注意】孕妇忌服。

Relieving Rheumatic Disease Oral Liquid

Name of Chinese Phonetic Alphabet Feng Shi Ye

Formula Angelicae Pubescentis Radix, Taxilli

Herba, Notopterygii Rhizoma et Radix, Saposhnikoviae Radix, Gentianae Macrophyllae Radix, Chaenomelis Fructus, Cervi Cornus Colla, Trionycis Carapacis Colla, Achyranthis Bidentatae Radix, Angelicae Sinensis Radix, Paeoniae Radix Alba, Chuanxiong Rhizoma, Carthami Flos, Atractylodis Macrocephalae Rhizoma, Glycyrrhizae Radix et Rhizoma and Oryzae Fructus Monascus.

Actions and Indications Tonifying the liver, kidney and blood, activating collaterals, dispelling wind-dampness. It is indicated for arthralgia, numbness of extremities, rheumatic or rheumatoid diseases due to depletion of the liver, kidney and blood, and stagnation of wind-cold-damp.

Warning It is contraindicated for pregnant women.

风湿痛药酒

【处方】石南藤、麻黄、枳壳、桂枝、蚕砂、黄精、陈皮、厚朴、苦杏仁、泽泻、山药、苍术、牡丹皮、川芎、白术、白芷、木香、石耳、羌活、小茴香、猪牙皂、补骨脂、香附、菟丝子、没药、当归、乳香。

【功能主治】祛风除湿，活络止痛。用于风湿骨痛，手足麻木，腰痛腿痛，跌打损伤。

【注意】孕妇忌服。

Medicated Wine for Relieving Rheumatalgia

Name of Chinese Phonetic Alphabet Feng Shi Tong Yao Jiu

Formula Photiniae Serrulatae Herba, Ephedrae Herba, Aurantii Fructus, Cinnamomi Ramulus, Bombycis Feculae, Polygonati Rhizoma, Citri Reticulatae Pericarpium, Magnoliae Officinalis Cortex, Armeniacae Semen Amarum, Alismatis Rhizoma, Dioscoreae Rhizoma, Atractylodis Rhizoma, Moutan Cortex, Chuanxiong Rhizoma, Atractylodis Macrocephalae Rhizoma, Angelicae Dahuricae Radix, Aucklandiae Radix, Umbilicariae Esculentae Carpophorum, Notopterygii Rhizoma et Radix, Foeniculi Fructus, Gleditsiae Fructus Abnormalis, Psoraleae Fructus, Cyperi Rhizoma, Cuscutae Semen, Myrrha, Angelicae Sinensis Radix and Olibanum.

Actions and Indications Dispelling wind and dampness, activating collaterals and alleviating pain. It is indicated for rheumatalgia, numbness of the hands and feet, pain of the waist and legs and traumatic injury.

Warning It is contraindicated for pregnant women.

风寒咳嗽丸

【处方】陈皮、法半夏、青皮、苦杏仁、麻黄、紫苏叶、五味子、桑白皮、甘草（蜜炙）。

【功能主治】温肺散寒，祛痰止咳。用于外感风寒，头痛鼻塞，痰多咳嗽，胸闷气喘。

Cough-relieving Pill

Name of Chinese Phonetic Alphabet Feng Han Ke Sou Wan

Formula Citri Reticulatae Pericarpium, Pinelliae Rhizoma Praeparatum, Citri Reticulatae Pericarpium Viride, Armeniacae Semen Amarum, Ephedrae Herba, Perillae Folium, Schisandrae Chinensis Fructus, Mori Cortex and Glycyrrhizae Radix et Rhizoma (prepared with honey).

Actions and Indications Warming the lung and dissipating cold, dispelling phlegm and relieving cough. It is indicated for headache, nasal congestion, cough with profuse phlegm, chest distress and panting due to external contraction of wind-cold.

风寒感冒冲剂

【处方】麻黄、葛根、紫苏叶、防风、桂枝、白芷、陈皮、苦杏仁、桔梗、甘草、干姜。

【功能主治】解表发汗，疏风散寒。用于感冒身热，头痛，咳嗽，鼻塞，流涕。

Relieving Common Cold Soluble Granules

Name of Chinese Phonetic Alphabet Feng Han

Gan Mao Chong Ji

Formula Ephedrae Herba, Puerariae Lobatae Radix, Perillae Folium, Saposhnikoviae Radix, Cinnamomi Ramulus, Angelicae Dahuricae Radix, Citri Reticulatae Pericarpium, Armeniacae Semen Amarum, Platycodonis Radix, Glycyrrhizae Radix et Rhizome and Zingiberis Rhizoma.

Actions and Indications Releasing the exterior, promoting sweating, dispersing wind and dissipating cold. It is indicated for common cold of wind-cold type, marked by generalized fever, headache, cough, stuffy nose and rhinorrhea.

六一散

【处方】滑石粉、甘草。

【功能主治】清暑利湿。内服用于暑热身倦，口渴泄泻，小便黄少；外治痱子刺痒。

Six to One Powder for Relieving Summer-heat

Name of Chinese Phonetic Alphabet Liu Yi San

Formula Talci Pulvis (weight 6) and Glycyrrhizae Pulvis (weight 1).

Actions and Indications Clearing summer-heat, draining dampness. For internal use: it is used for lassitude, thirst, diarrhea and scanty yellow urine due to summer-heat. For external use: it is used for miliaria.

六合定中丸

【处方】广藿香、紫苏叶、香薷、木香、檀香、厚朴（姜制）、枳壳（炒）、陈皮、桔梗、甘草、茯苓、木瓜、白扁豆（炒）、山楂（炒）、六神曲（炒）、麦芽（炒）、稻芽（炒）。

【功能主治】祛暑除湿，和中消食。用于宿食停滞，头痛，胸闷恶心，吐泻腹痛。

Harmonizing the Middle Energizer Bolus

Name of Chinese Phonetic Alphabet Liu He Ding Zhong Wan

Formula Pogostemonis Herba, Perillae Folium, Moslae Herba, Aucklandiae Radix, Santali Albi Lignum, Magnoliae Officinalis Cortex (prepared with ginger), Aurantii Fructus (fried), Citri Reticulatae Pericarpium, Platycodonis Radix, Glycyrrhizae Radix et Rhizoma, Poria, Chaenomelis Fructus, Lablab Semen Album (fried), Crataegi Fructus (fried), Medicate Massa Fermentata (fried), Hordei Fructus Germinatus (fried) and Oryzae Fructus Germinatus (fried).

Actions and Indications Dispelling summer-heat and eliminating dampness, harmonizing the middle energizer and promoting digestion. It is indicated for headache, chest distress, nausea, vomiting, diarrhea and abdominal pain due to foods stagnation.

六君子丸

【处方】党参、白术（麸炒）、茯苓、半夏（制）、陈皮、甘草（蜜炙）。

【功能主治】补脾益气，燥湿化痰。用于脾胃虚弱，食量不多，气虚痰多，腹胀便溏。

Six Mild-medicinal Pill

Name of Chinese Phonetic Alphabet Liu Jun Zi Wan

Formula Codonopsis Radix, Atractylodis Macrocephalae Rhizoma(fried with bran), Poria, Pinelliae Rhizoma (prepared), Citri Reticulatae Pericarpium and Glycyrrhizae Radix et Rhizoma (prepared with honey).

Actions and Indications Tonifying the spleen, replenishing *qi*, drying dampness and resolving phlegm. It is used for poor appetite due to hypofunction of the spleen and stomach; profuse phlegm due to *qi*-deficiency; abdominal distension and sloppy stool.

六味木香胶囊

【处方】木香、栀子、石榴皮、闹羊花、豆蔻、荜茇。

【功能主治】开郁行气，止痛。用于胃痛，腹痛，嗳气呕吐。

Common Aucklandia* Capsule

Name of Chinese Phonetic Alphabet Liu Wei Mu Xiang Jiao Nang

Formula Aucklandiae Radix, Gardeniae Fructus, Granati Pericarpium, Rhododendri Mollis Flos, Amomi Fructus Rotundus and Piperis Longi Fructus.

Actions and Indications moving *qi* and alleviating pain. It is indicated for stomachache, abdominal pain, eructation and vomiting.

* 木香

六味地黄丸

【处方】熟地黄、山茱萸（制）、牡丹皮、山药、茯苓、泽泻。

【功能主治】滋阴补肾。用于肾阴亏损，头晕耳鸣，腰膝酸软，骨蒸潮热，盗汗遗精，消渴。

Pill of Six Ingredients Containing Chinese Fox-glove*

Name of Chinese Phonetic Alphabet Liu Wei Di Huang Wan

Formula Rehmanniae Radix Praeparata, Corni Fructus (prepared), Moutan Cortex, Dioscoreae Rhizoma, Poria and Alismatis Rhizoma.

Actions and Indications Enriching *yin* and tonifying the kidney. It is indicated for dizziness, tinnitus, soreness of waist and weakness of knees, tidal fever, night sweating, nocturnal emission and wasting-thirst due to depletion of kidney-*yin*.

* 地黄

六味安消胶囊

【处方】土木香、大黄、山柰、寒水石（煅）、诃子等。

【功能主治】和胃健脾，导滞消积，行血止痛。用于胃痛胀满，消化不良，便秘，痛经。

【注意】孕妇忌服。

Regulating Digestion Capsule

Name of Chinese Phonetic Alphabet Liu Wei An Xiao Jiao Nang

Formula Inulae Radix, Rhei Radix et Rhizoma, Kaempferiae Rhizoma, Gypsum Rubrum (calcined), Chebulae Fructus, etc.

Actions and Indications Harmonizing the stomach and fortifying the spleen, removing food stagnation, moving blood to relieve pain. It is used for stomachache with distention and fullness, dyspepsia, constipation and dysmenorrhea.

Warning It is contraindicated for pregnant women.

六味能消胶囊

【处方】大黄、藏木香、诃子等。

【功能主治】宽中理气，润肠通便，调节血脂。用于胃脘胀痛，厌食纳差，大便秘结；还适用于高脂血症及肥胖症。

【注意】妊娠及哺乳期妇女忌用。

Regulating Blood-lipid Capsule

Name of Chinese Phonetic Alphabet Liu Wei Neng Xiao Jiao Nang

Formula Rhei Radix et Rhizoma, Inulae Radix, Chebulae Fructus, etc.

Actions and Indications Regulating *qi* to soothe the middle, moistening the intestines to relax the bowels, regulating blood-lipid. It is used for stomachache with distention and fullness, anorexia, constipation, also used for hyperlipoidemia and adiposity.

Warning It is contraindicated for pregnant and breast feeding women.

六神丸

【处方】本品由麝香等药经加工制成的小丸剂。

【功能主治】清凉解毒，消炎止痛。用于烂喉丹痧，咽喉肿痛，单双乳蛾，小儿热疖，痈疡疔疮，乳痈发背，无名肿毒。

Miraculous Pill of Six Ingredients

Name of Chinese Phonetic Alphabet Liu Shen Wan

Formula Moschus, etc.

Actions and Indications Refreshing and detoxicating, antiphlogistic and relieving pain. It is used for sore-throat, unilateral or bilateral tonsillitis, infantile furuncle, abscess and deep-rooted boil, suppurative mastitis, swelling and pain of unknown origin.

心力丸

【处方】人参、附片、蟾酥、麝香、红花、冰片、灵芝、珍珠、人工牛黄。

【功能主治】温阳益气，活血化瘀。用于心阳不振、气滞血瘀所致的胸痹心痛，胸闷气短，心悸怔忡，冠心病，心绞痛等。

【注意】孕妇慎用。

Tonifying Heart-*yang* Pill

Name of Chinese Phonetic Alphabet Xin Li Wan

Formula Ginseng Radix et Rhizoma, Aconiti Lateralis Radix Praeparata (sliced), Bufonis Venenum, Moschus, Carthami Flos, Borneolum Syntheticum, Ganoderma, Margarita and Bovis Calculus Artifactus.

Actions and Indications Warming *yang*, tonifying *qi*, activating blood and resolving stasis. It is used for cardialgia, chest distress, shortness of breath, palpitation, fearful throbbing, coronary heart disease and angina pectoris due to declination of heart-*yang*, *qi*-stagnation and blood-stasis.

Warning It should be used carefully for pregnant women.

心元胶囊

【处方】制何首乌、灵芝、丹参、地黄、麦冬等。

【功能主治】滋肾养心，活血化瘀。用于胸痹心肾阴虚、心血瘀阻引起的胸闷不适，胸部刺痛或绞痛，或胸痛彻背，固定不移，入夜更甚，心悸盗汗，心烦不寐，腰酸膝软，耳鸣头晕等冠心病稳定性劳累性心绞痛、高脂血症见上述证候者。

Relieving Heart Trouble Capsule

Name of Chinese Phonetic Alphabet Xin Yuan Jiao Nang

Formula Polygoni Multiflori Radix Praeparata, Ganoderma, Salviae Miltiorrhizae Radix et Rhizoma, Rehmanniae Radix, Ophiopogonis Radix, etc.

Actions and Indications Enriching the kidney and heart, activating blood and resolving stasis. It is indicated for chest distress, stabbing or colicky pain, or fixative pain in the chest referring to the back which is even more severe at night, palpitation, night sweating, vexation, insomnia, soreness of waist and weakness of knees, tinnitus, dizziness, and exertional angina pectoris and hyperlipemia with the above mentioned symptoms.

心可宁胶囊

【处方】丹参、三七、冰片、水牛角浓缩粉、蟾酥、红花、牛黄、人参须。

【功能主治】活血散瘀，开窍止痛。用于冠心病、心绞痛，胸闷，心悸，眩晕。

Relieving Coronary Heart Disease Capsule

Name of Chinese Phonetic Alphabet Xin Ke Ning Jiao Nang

Formula Salviae Miltiorrhizae Radix et Rhizoma, Notoginseng Radix et Rhizoma, Borneolum Symtheticum, Bubali Cornu Pulvis Concentratio, Bufonis Venenum, Carthami Flos, Bovis Calculus and Ginseng Radix Fibrosa.

Actions and Indications Activating blood, dissipating stasis, inducing resuscitation, alleviating pain. It is indicated for coronary heart disease, angina pectoris, chest distress, palpitation and vertigo.

心可舒片

【处方】山楂、丹参、葛根、三七、木香。

【功能主治】活血化瘀，行气止痛。用于冠心病，心绞痛。

Coronary Heart Disease Relieving Tablet

Name of Chinese Phonetic Alphabet Xin Ke Shu Pian

Formula Crataegi Fructus, Salviae Miltiorrhizae Radix et Rhizoma, Puerariae Lobatae Radix, Notoginseng Radix et Rhizoma and Aucklandiae Radix.

Actions and Indications Activating blood, resolving stasis, moving *qi* to alleviate pain. It is indicated for coronary heart disease and angina pectoris.

心达康片

【处方】本品为沙棘经提取加工制成的片剂。

【功能主治】补益心气，化瘀通脉，消痰运脾。用于心气虚弱，心脉瘀阻，痰湿困脾所致的心慌、心悸、心痛，气短胸闷，血脉不畅等症。

Sand Thorn* Tablet

Name of Chinese Phonetic Alphabet Xin Da Kang Pian

Formula Hippophae Fructus (extract).

Actions and Indications Tonifying heart-*qi*, resolving stasis, dredging vessels, resolving phlegm, invigorating the spleen. It is used for fluster, palpitation, cardialgia, shortness of breath and chest distress due to weakness of heart-*qi*, stagnation of vessels and stagnation of phlegm-dampness in the spleen.

*沙棘

心血宁片

【处方】葛根提取物、山楂提取物。

【功能主治】活血化瘀，通络止痛。用于心血瘀阻、瘀阻脑络引起的胸痹，眩晕，以及冠心病、高血压、心绞痛、高脂血症等见上述证候者。

Heart-blood-soothing Tablet

Name of Chinese Phonetic Alphabet Xin Xue Ning Pian

Formula Puerariae Lobatae Radix (extract) and Crataegi Fructus (extract).

Actions and Indications Activating blood, resolving stasis, dredging collaterals, alleviating pain. It is used for chest distress, vertigo due to stagnation of heart-blood and stagnation of collaterals; and also used for coronary heart disease, hypertension, angina pectoris and hyperlipemia with the above mentioned symptoms.

心肝宝胶囊

【处方】本品为人工虫草菌丝粉制成的胶囊。

【功能主治】补虚损，益精气，保肺益肾，扶正固本。用于乙型慢性活动性肝炎，肝硬化；房性、室性早搏，心动过速、心动过缓；顽固性失眠症及肾病综合征，癌症辅助治疗。

Hypha Cordyceps* Capsule

Name of Chinese Phonetic Alphabet Xin Gan Bao Jiao Nang

Formula Cordyceps (fungus) Hypha Pulvis.

Actions and Indications Tonifying essential *qi*, lung and kidney, reinforcing the healthy *qi* and strengthening the body resistance. It is indicated for chronic active hepatitis B, cirrhosis; atrial, ventricular premature beating, tachycardia, bradycardia; intractable insomnia, nephrotic syndrome and supplementary treament of tumor.

*虫草菌丝

心宝丸

【处方】洋金花、人参、肉桂、附子、鹿茸、冰片、麝香、三七。

【功能主治】温补心气，益气助阳，活血通脉。用于治疗心肾阳虚，心脉瘀阻引起的慢性心功能不全；窦房结功能不全引起的心动过缓、病窦综合征以及缺血心脏病引起的心绞痛及心电图缺血性改变。

【注意】孕妇、青光眼患者忌服。

Xinbao Bolus for Cardiac Insufficiency

Name of Chinese Phonetic Alphabet Xin Bao Wan

Formula Daturae Flos, Ginseng Radix et Rhizoma, Cinnamomi Cortex, Aconiti Lateralis Radix Praeparata, Cervi Cornu Pantotrichum, Borneolum Syntheticum, Moschus and Notoginseng Radix et Rhizoma.

Actions and Indications Warming and tonifying heart-*qi* and assisting *yang*, activating blood to drain the vessels. It is indicated for chronic cardiac insufficiency due to dual deficiency of heart-kidney *yang* and heart vessel obstruction; bradycardia and sick sinus syndrome due to sinus node insufficiency, angina pectoris and ischemic change of electrocardiogram due to ischemic heart disease.

Warning It is contraindicated for pregnant women and glaucoma patients.

心荣口服液

【处方】黄芪、地黄、赤芍、麦冬、五味子、桂枝。

【功能主治】助阳，益气，养阴。用于心阳不振，气阴两虚型冠心病。症见胸闷隐痛，心悸气短，头晕目眩，倦怠懒言，面色少华等。

Tonifying Heart-*yang* Oral Liquid

Name of Chinese Phonetic Alphabet Xin Rong Kou Fu Ye

Formula Astragali Radix, Rehmanniae Radix, Paeoniae Radix Rubra, Ophiopogonis Radix, Schisandrae Chinensis Fructus and Cinnamomi Ramulus.

Actions and Indications Assisting *yang*, tonifying *qi* and nourishing *yin*. It is used for coronary heart disease due to declination of heart-*yang* and dual deficiency of *qi* and *yin*, and manifested as chest distress with dull pain, palpitation, shortness of breath, dizziness, dizzy vision, tiredness, indolent speaking and pale complexion.

心脉通片

【处方】当归、决明子、钩藤、丹参、牛膝、夏枯草、三七、葛根、槐花、毛冬青。

【功能主治】活血化瘀，通脉养心，降压降脂。用于高血压、高脂血症等。

Relieving Hypertension and Hyperlipemia Tablet

Name of Chinese Phonetic Alphabet Xin Mai Tong Pian

Formula Angelicae Sinensis Radix, Cassiae Semen, Uncariae Ramulus cum Uncis, Salviae Miltiorrhizae Radix et Rhizoma, Achyranthis Bidentatae Radix, Prunellae Spica, Notoginseng Radix et Rhizoma, Puerariae Lobatae Radix, Sophorae Flos and Ilecis Pubescentis Radix.

Actions and Indications Activating blood, resolving stasis, dredging vessels, nourishing the heart, lowering blood pressure and blood-lipid. It is indicated for hypertension and hyperlipemia.

心脑健片

【处方】本品为茶叶提取物制成的胶囊剂。

【功能主治】清利头目，醒神健脑，化浊降脂。用于头晕目眩，胸闷气短，倦怠乏力，精神不振，记忆力减退等症。对心血管病伴高纤维蛋白原症及动脉粥样硬化，肿瘤放疗、化疗所致的白细胞减少症有防治作用。

Tea Extract Tablet

Name of Chinese Phonetic Alphabet Xin Nao

Jian Pian

Formula Camelliae Sinensis Folium Gemmae Extractum.

Actions and Indications Soothing the mind, fortifying the brain, resolving turbidity, decreasing lipid. It is used for dizziness, dizzy vision, chest distress, shortness of breath, tiredness, fatigue, lassitude of spirit and hypomnesis. It also acts for preventing angiocardiopathy accompanied with hyperfibrinogensis, atherosclerosis and leukopenia due to chemotherapy and radiotherapy in the treatment of tumor.

心脑康软胶囊

【处方】赤芍、川芎、丹参、地龙、甘草、葛根、枸杞子、红花、九节、菖蒲、鹿心粉、牛膝、酸枣仁、郁金、远志、泽泻、制首乌。

【功能主治】活血化瘀，通窍止痛，扩张血管，增加冠状动脉血流量。用于冠心病，心绞痛及脑动脉硬化症。

Relieving Coronary Heart Disease Soft Capsule

Name of Chinese Phonetic Alphabet Xin Nao Kang Ruan Jiao Nang

Formula Paeoniae Radix Rubra, Chuanxiong Rhizoma, Salviae Miltiorrhizae Radix et Rhizoma, Pheretima, Glycyrrhizae Radix et Rhizoma, Puerariae Lobatae Radix, Lycii Fructus, Carthami Flos, Anemones Altaicae Rhizoma, Cervi Cor Pulvis, Achyranthis Bidentatae Radix, Ziziphi Spinosae Semen, Curcumae Radix, Polygalae Radix, Alismatis Rhizoma and Polygoni Multiflori Radix Praeparata.

Actions and Indications Activating blood and resolving stasis, dredging the orifices and relieving pain, dilating blood vessels and increasing blood flow volume of coronary artery. It is indicated for coronary heart disease, angina pectoris and cerebral arteriosclerosis.

心脑舒通胶囊

【处方】本品为蒺藜经提取加工制成的胶囊。

【功能主治】活血化瘀，舒利血脉。用于胸痹心痛，中风恢复期的半身不遂、语言障碍和动脉硬化等心脑血管缺血性疾患，以及各种血液高黏症。

【注意】颅内出血后尚未完全止血者忌用；有出血史或血液低黏症患者慎用。

Caltrop* Capsule for Soothing Heart and Brain

Name of Chinese Phonetic Alphabet Xin Nao Shu Tong Jiao Nang

Formula Tribuli Fructus (extract).

Actions and Indications Activating blood, resolving stasis, soothing blood vessels. It is used for chest impediment syndrome, cardialgia, hemiparalysis in convelescent period of apoplexy, lalopathy and arteriosclerosis, and various blood hyperviscosity.

Warning It is contraindicated for intracranial hemorrhage and should be used cautiousley for patients with a hemorrhagic history or blood hypoviscosity.

*蒺藜

心脑静片

【处方】莲子心、珍珠母、槐角、黄柏、木香、黄芩、夏枯草、钩藤、龙胆、淡竹叶、威灵仙、天南星（制）、甘草、牛黄、朱砂、冰片。

【功能主治】清心清脑，镇惊安神，降低血压，疏通经络，防治中风。用于头晕目眩，烦躁不宁，言语不清，手足不遂。

【注意】孕妇忌服。

Mind-tranquilizing Tablet

Name of Chinese Phonetic Alphabet Xin Nao Jing Pian

Formula Nelumbinis Plumula, Margaritifera Concha, Sophorae Fructus, Phellodendri Chinensis Cortex, Aucklandiae Radix, Scutellariae Radix, Prunellae Spica, Uncariae Ramulus cum Uncis,

Gentianae Radix et Rhizoma, Lophatheri Herba, Clematidis Radix et Rhizoma, Arisaematis Rhizoma (prepared), Glycyrrhizae Radix et Rhizoma, Bovis Calculus, Cinnabaris and Borneolum Syntheticum.

Actions and Indications Clearing heart-fire, tranquilizing the mind, lowering blood pressure, dredging meridians and collaterals, preventing apoplexy. It is used for dizziness, dizzy vision, vexation, alalia, numbness of limbs.

Warning It is contraindicated for pregnant women.

心通口服液

【处方】黄芪、党参、麦冬、何首乌、淫羊藿、葛根、当归、丹参、皂角刺、海藻、昆布、牡蛎、枳实。

【功能主治】益气养阴，软坚化痰。用于气阴两虚、痰瘀交阻型胸痹，症见心痛，心悸，胸闷气短，心烦乏力，脉沉细、弦滑、结代及冠心病心绞痛见上述证候者。

【注意】孕妇禁用。如服后反酸，可于饭后服用。

Relieving Chest Distress Oral Liquid

Name of Chinese Phonetic Alphabet Xin Tong Kou Fu Ye

Formula Astragali Radix, Codonopsis Radix, Ophiopogonis Radix, Polygoni Multiflori Radix, Epimedii Folium, Puerariae Lobatae Radix, Angelicae Sinensis Radix, Salviae Miltiorrhizae Radix et Rhizoma, Gleditsiae Spina, Sargassum, Laminariae et Eckloniae Thallus, Ostreae Concha and Aurantii Fructus Immaturus.

Actions and Indications Tonifying *qi* and nourishing *yin*, softening hardness and resolving phlegm. It is indicated for chest impediment syndrome due to stagnation of phlegm and stasis, and manifested as heart pain, palpitation, chest distress, shortness of breath, vexation, fatigue, sunken, fine, string-like and slippery pulse or bound and intermittent pulse, and for coronary heart disease and angina pectoris with the above mentioned symptoms.

Warning It is contraindicated for pregnant women. In case with acid regurgitation after administration, it should be administrated after meal.

心痛康胶囊

【处方】本品为白芍、红参、淫羊藿、山楂等药材经加工制成的胶囊。

【功能主治】益气活血，温阳养阴，散结止痛。用于气滞血瘀所致的心胸刺痛或闷痛，痛有定处，心悸气短或兼有神疲自汗，咽干心烦，冠心病，心绞痛。

【注意】凡肝火亢盛或虚阳上亢而头目眩晕胀痛者慎用；服药期间不宜饮酒和食用辛辣之品。

Chest-pain-relieving Capsule

Name of Chinese Phonetic Alphabet Xin Tong Kang Jiao Nang

Formula Paeoniae Radix Alba, Ginseng Radix et Rhizoma Rubra, Epimedii Folium, Crataegi Fructus, etc.

Actions and Indications Tonifying *qi*, activating blood, warming *yang* and nourishing *yin*, dissipating stagnation to alleviate pain. It is used for fixed stabbing pain in chest or distress, palpitation, shortness of breath or complicated with lassitude of spirit, spontaneous sweating, dry throat and vexation due to stagnation of *qi* and blood-stasis; and also used for coronary heart disease, angina pectoris.

Warning It should be used cautiously for cases with intense liver-fire or deficiency-*yang* floating upward marked by dizziness and dizzy vision; during medication, wine and pungent foods are prohibited.

心痛舒喷雾剂

【处方】牡丹皮、川芎、冰片。

【功能主治】活血化瘀，凉血止痛。用于缓解或改善心血瘀阻所致冠心病，心绞痛急性发作时的临床症状和心电图异常。

【注意】用药后病情不能缓解者，应加用其他综合措施。

Relieving Coronary Heart Disease Spray

Name of Chinese Phonetic Alphabet Xin Tong Shu Pen Wu Ji

Formula Moutan Cortex, Chuanxiong Rhizoma and Borneolum Syntheticum.

Actions and Indications Activating blood, resolving stasis, cooling blood, alleviating pain. It is used for relieving or improving the clinical symptoms and electrocardiographic abnormality of acute attack in coronary heart disease and angina pectoris.

Warning In case the state of illness is not relieved yet after spray, the comprehensive treatment should be applied .

双虎肿痛宁

【处方】搜山虎、黄杜鹃根、生川乌、生草乌、生天南星、生半夏、樟脑、薄荷脑。

【功能主治】化瘀行气，消肿止痛，舒筋活络，驱风除湿。用于跌打损伤，扭伤，摔伤，风湿关节痛，并可作骨折及脱臼复位等手术局部麻醉止痛用。

【注意】严禁内服。

Shuang Hu Oils for Relaxing Sinews

Name of Chinese Phonetic Alphabet Shuang Hu Zhong Tong Ning

Formula Atropanthes Sinensis Radix, Rhododendri Mollis Radix, Aconiti Radix (fresh), Aconiti Kusnezoffii Radix (fresh), Arisaematis Rhizoma (fresh), Pinelliae Rhizoma (fresh), Camphora and Menthol.

Actions and Indications Resolving stasis, moving *qi*, reducing swelling, alleviating pain, relaxing sinews, dredging collaterals, expelling wind and damp. It is used for traumatic injury, sprain injury due to fall, rheumatic arthralgia, and also used for topical analgesic during operations of fracture and reposition for dislocation.

Warning It is for external use only.

双黄连片

【处方】金银花、黄芩、连翘。

【功能主治】辛凉解表，清热解毒。主治外感风热引起的发热、咳嗽、咽痛。

Shuang Huang Lian Tablet

Name of Chinese Phonetic Alphabet Shuang Huang Lian Pian

Formula Lonicerae Japonicae Flos, Scutellariae Radix and Forsythiae Fructus.

Actions and Indications Releasing the exterior, clearing heat and detoxicating. It is indicated for fever, cough, sore-throat due to external contraction of wind-heat.

双清口服液

【处方】温郁金、金银花、连翘、广藿香、知母、大青叶、生地黄、桔梗、甘草、石膏、蜂蜜、山梨酸钾。

【功能主治】清解表邪，清热解毒。适用于风温肺热，卫气同病，症见发热兼恶风寒，口渴，咳嗽，痰黄，头痛，舌红苔黄或兼白，脉滑数或浮数，以及急性气管炎见上述证候者。

【注意】孕妇及肝、肾功能不良者慎用。

Shuang Qing Oral Liquid for Clearing Heat

Name of Chinese Phonetic Alphabet Shuang Qing Kou Fu Ye

Formula Curcumae Radix，Lonicerae Japonicae Flos, Forsythiae Fructus, Pogostemonis Herba, Anemarrhenae Rhizoma, Isatidis Folium, Rehmanniae Radix, Platycodonis Radix, Glycyrrhizae Radix et Rhizoma, Gypsum Fibrosum, Mel and Potassium Sorbate.

Actions and Indications Relieving the exterior, clearing heat and detoxicating. It is used for cases attacked by wind-heat in the lung, or disease of both defense and *qi* aspects, manifested as fever, aversion to wind and cold, thirst, cough, yellow phlegm, headache, red tongue with yellow or white fur, slippery and rapid pulse or floating and rapid pulse. And it is also used for acute trachitis with the above mentioned symptoms.

Warning It should be used cautiously for pregnant women and cases with hepatic and renal insufficiency.

五画

功劳去火片

【处方】功劳木、黄柏、黄芩、栀子。

【功能主治】清热解毒。用于实热火毒型急性咽喉炎、急性胆囊炎、急性肠炎。

Leatherleaf Mahonia* Tablet for Clearing Heat

Name of Chinese Phonetic Alphabet Gong Lao Qu Huo Pian

Formula Mahoniae Caulis, Phellodendri Chinensis Cortex, Scutellariae Radix and Gardeniae Fructus.

Actions and Indications Clearing heat and detoxicating. It is used for acute laryngopharyngitis, acute cholecystitis and acute enteritis due to excess heat toxin.

* 功劳木

艾附暖宫丸

【处方】艾叶(炭)、香附(醋制)、吴茱萸(制)、肉桂、当归、川芎、白芍(酒炒)、地黄、黄芪(蜜炙)、续断。

【功能主治】理气补血，暖宫调经。用于子宫虚寒，月经不调，经来腹痛，腰酸带下。

Argy Wormwood* and Nut-grass** Bolus for Warming Uterus

Name of Chinese Phonetic Alphabet Ai Fu Nuan Gong Wan

Formula Artemisiae Argyi Folium (carbonated), Cyperi Rhizoma (prepared with vinegar), Euodiae Fructus (prepared), Cinnamomi Cortex, Angelicae Sinensis Radix, Chuanxiong Rhizoma, Paeoniae Radix Alba (fried with wine), Rehmanniae Radix, Astragali Radix (prepared with honey) and Dipsaci Radix.

Actions and Indications Regulating *qi* and tonifying blood, warming the uterus and regulating menstruation. It is used for irregular menstruation, dysmenorrhea, soreness of the waist and vaginal discharge due to deficiency-cold of the uterus.

* 艾叶 ** 香附

艾迪注射液

【处方】斑蝥、人参、黄芪、刺五加。

【功能主治】清热解毒，消瘀散结。用于原发性肝癌，肺癌，直肠癌，恶性淋巴瘤，妇科恶性肿瘤等。

Large Blister Beetle* Injection

Name of Chinese Phonetic Alphabet Ai Di Zhu She Ye

Formula Mylabris, Ginseng Radix et Rhizoma, Astragali Radix and Acanthopanacis Senticosi Radix et Rhizoma seu Caulis.

Actions and Indications Clearing heat, detoxifying, dispersing mass. It is used for primary liver cancer, lung cancer, rectal cancer, malignant lymphoma and gynecological malignant tumor.

* 斑蝥

平安丸

【处方】木香、丁香、母丁香、沉香、香附(醋炙)、砂仁、青皮(醋炙)、陈皮、枳实、延胡索(醋炙)、茯苓、草果、肉豆蔻(煨)、豆蔻、山楂(炒)、六神曲(麸炒)、麦芽(炒)、槟榔、白术(麸炒)。

【功能主治】舒肝理气，和胃止痛。用于肝气犯胃引起的胃痛，胁痛，吞酸倒饱，呃逆，脘腹胀满等症。

【注意】孕妇忌服。

Stomachache-relieving Bolus

Name of Chinese Phonetic Alphabet Ping An Wan

Formula Aucklandiae Radix, Caryophylli Flos, Caryophylli Fructus, Aquilariae Lignum Resinatum, Cyperi Rhizoma (prepared with vinegar), Amomi Fructus, Citri Reticulatae Pericarpium Viride (prepared with vinegar), Citri Reticulatae Pericarpium, Aurantii Fructus Immaturus, Corydalis Rhizoma (prepared with vinegar), Poria, Tsaoko Fructus, Myristicae Semen (roasted), Amomi Fructus Rotundus, Crataegi Fructus (fried), Medicata Massa Fenmentata (fried with bran), Hordei Fructus Germinatus (fried), Arecae Semen and Atractylodis Macrocephalae Rhizoma (fried with bran).

Actions and Indications Soothing the liver, regulating *qi*, harmonizing the stomach, alleviating pain. It is indicated for stomachache, hypochondriac pain, acid regurgitation, hiccup and abdominal fullness due to liver-*qi* invading the stomach.

Warning It is contraindicated for pregnant women.

平肝舒络丸

【处方】柴胡、青皮（醋炙）、陈皮、佛手、乌药、香附（醋炙）、木香、檀香、丁香、沉香、广藿香、砂仁、豆蔻、厚朴（姜炙）、枳壳（去瓤麸炒）、羌活、白芷、威灵仙（酒炙）、细辛、木瓜、防风、钩藤、僵蚕（麸炒）、胆南星（酒炙）、天竺黄、桑寄生、何首乌（黑豆酒炙）、牛膝、川芎、熟地黄、龟甲（砂烫醋淬）、延胡索（醋炙）、乳香（醋炙）、没药（醋炙）、白及、人参、白术（麸炒）、茯苓、肉桂、黄连、冰片、朱砂、羚羊角粉。

【功能主治】平肝疏络，活血祛风。用于肝气郁结，经络不疏引起的胸胁胀满，肩背窜痛，手足麻木，筋脉拘挛。

Liver-pacifying Bolus

Name of Chinese Phonetic Alphabet Ping Gan Shu Luo Wan

Formula Bupleuri Radix, Citri Reticulatae Pericarpium Viride (prepared with vinegar), Citri Reticulatae Pericarpium, Citri Sarcodactylis Fructus, Linderae Radix, Cyperi Rhizoma (prepared with vinegar), Aucklandiae Radix, Santali Albi Lignum, Caryophylli Flos, Aquilariae Lignum Resinatum, Pogostemonis Herba, Amomi Fructus, Amomi Fructus Rotundis, Magnoliae Officinalis Cortex (prepared with ginger), Aurantii Fructus (removed pulp and fried with bran), Notopterygii Rhizoma et Radix, Angelicae Dahuricae Radix, Clematidis Radix et Rhizoma (prepared with wine), Asari Radix et Rhizoma, Chaenomelis Fructus, Saposhnikoviae Radix, Uncariae Ramulus cum Uncis, Bombyx Batryticatus(fried with bran), Arisaema cum Bile (prepared with wine), Bambusae Concretio Silicea, Taxilli Herba, Polygoni Multiflori Radix (prepared with wine), Achyranthis Bidentatae Radix, Chuanxiong Rhizoma, Rehmanniae Radix Praeparata, Testudinis Carapax et Plastrum (scalded by sand and quenched by vinegar), Corydalis Rhizoma (prepared with vinegar), Olibanum (prepared with vinegar), Myrrha (prepared with vinegar), Bletillae Rhizoma, Ginseng Radix et Rhizoma, Atractylodis Macrocephalae Rhizoma (fried with bran), Poria, Cinnamomi Cortex, Coptidis Rhizoma, Borneolum Syntheticum, Cinnabaris and Saigae Tataricae Cornu Pulvis.

Actions and Indications Pacifying the liver, draining collaterals, activating blood and dispelling wind. It is used for fullness and pain of hypochondrium, pain in shoulder and back, numbness of extremities and muscular spasm due to stagnation of liver-*qi* and collaterals.

平消胶囊

【处方】郁金、仙鹤草、五灵脂、白矾、硝石、干漆（制）、枳壳（麸炒）、马钱子粉。

【功能主治】活血化瘀，止痛散结，清热解毒，扶正祛邪。对肿瘤具有一定的缓解症状、缩小瘤体、抑制肿瘤生长、提高人体免疫力。

【注意】可与手术治疗、放疗、化疗同时进行。

Tumor-relieving Capsule

Name of Chinese Phonetic Alphabet Ping Xiao Jiao Nang

Formula Curcumae Radix, Agrimoniae Herba, Trogopterori Faeces, Alumen, Nitrum, Toxicodendri Resina (prepared), Aurantii Fructus (fried with bran) and Strychni Semen Pulvis.

Actions and Indications Activating blood, redsolving stasis, alleviating pain, dispersing mass, clearing heat, detoxifying, supporting healthy *qi*, dispelling pathogen. The preparation possesses remittent action for tumor, reducing the size of tumor, inhibiting the growth of tumor, increasing the immunologic function of human body.

Warning The preparation can be applied with the treatment of operation, radiotherapy and chemotherapy simultaneously.

正天丸

【处方】钩藤、白芍、川芎、当归、地黄、白芷、防风、羌活、桃仁、红花、细辛、独活、麻黄、附片、鸡血藤。

【功能主治】疏风活血，养血平肝，通络止痛。用于外感风邪、瘀血阻络、血虚失养、肝阳上亢引起的多种头痛，神经性头痛，颈椎病型头痛，经前头痛。

Headache-relieving Pill

Name of Chinese Phonetic Alphabet Zheng Tian Wan

Formula Uncariae Ramulus cum Uncis, Paeoniae Radix Alba, Chuanxiong Rhizoma, Angelicae Sinensis Radix, Rehmanniae Radix, Angelicae Dahuricae Radix, Saposhnikoviae Radix, Notopterygii Rhizoma et Radix, Persicae Semen, Carthami Flos, Asari Radix et Rhizoma, Angelicae Pubescentis Radix, Ephedrae Herba, Aconiti Lateralis Radix Praeparata (sliced) and Spatholobi Caulis.

Actions and Indications Dispersing wind, activating and nourishing blood, pacifying the liver, dredging collaterals, alleviating pain. It is indicated for many types of headache, nervous headache, cervical type headache and premenstrual headache due to exogenous wind pathogen, blood-stasis, blood deficiency and ascendant hyperactivity of liver-*yang*.

正心泰胶囊

【处方】黄芪、葛根、槲寄生、丹参、山楂、川芎。

【功能主治】补气活血，通络止痛。适用于冠心病，心绞痛表现为气瘀或肾虚证候者，症见胸痛、胸闷、心悸、乏力、眩晕、腰膝酸软。

Relieving Coronary Heart Disease Capsule

Name of Chinese Phonetic Alphabet Zheng Xin Tai Jiao Nang

Formula Astragali Radix, Puerariae Lobatae Radix, Visci Herba, Salviae Miltiorrhizae Radix et Rhizoma, Crataegi Fructus and Chuanxiong Rhizoma.

Actions and Indications Tonifying *qi*, activating blood, dredging collaterals, alleviating pain. It is indicated for coronary heart disease and angina pectoris manifested as chest pain and distress, palpitation, fatigue, vertigo, soreness and weakness of waist and knees attributed to *qi*-stagnation or deficiency of the kidney.

正骨水

【处方】土鳖虫、过江龙、薄荷脑、降香、两面针、樟脑、虎杖、五味藤、横经席、穿壁风、鹰不扑、草乌、碎骨木、羊耳菊、木香、风藤、鸡骨香、了刁竹、千斤拔、朱砂根、皂荚、五加皮、莪术等。

【功能主治】舒筋活络，散瘀镇痛，祛风除湿。用于跌打扭伤，各种骨折。

【注意】忌内服；不能搽入伤口。

Bone-knitting Aqua

Name of Chinese Phonetic Alphabet Zheng Gu

Shui

Formula Eupolyphaga seu Steleophaga, Lycopodii Complanati Herba, Menthol, Dalbergiae Odoriferae Lignum, Zanhtoxyli Radix, Camphora, Polygoni Cuspidati Rhizoma et Radix , Securidacae Inappendiculatae Radix, Calophylli Membranacei Radix, Piperis Hancei Caulis et Folium, Araliae Armatae Radix et Folium, Aconiti Kusnezoffii Radix, Ilicis Rotundae Cortex, Inulae Cappae Herba, Aucklandiae Radix, Fici Martini Radix et Caulis, Crotonis Crassifolii Radix, Cynanchi Paniculati Radix et Rhizoma, Flemingiae Philippinensis Radix, Ardisiae Crenatae Radix, Gleditsiae Fructus, Acanthopanacis Cortex, Curcumae Rhizoma, etc.

Actions and Indications Relaxing sinews, activating collaterals, dissipating stasis, alleviating pain, dispelling wind and dampness. It is used for traumatic sprain and various fractures.

Warning It is for external use only and is contraindicated for cases with wound of skin.

正柴胡饮颗粒

【处方】柴胡、陈皮、防风、甘草、赤芍、生姜。

【功能主治】表散风寒，解热止痛。用于外感风寒初起：发热恶寒、无汗、头痛、鼻塞、喷嚏、咽痒咳嗽、四肢酸痛。适用于流行性感冒初起、轻度上呼吸道感染。

Chinese Hare's Ear★ Soluble Granules

Name of Chinese Phonetic Alphabet Zheng Chai Hu Yin Ke Li

Formula Bupleuri Radix, Citri Reticulatae Pericarpium, Saposhnikoviae Radix, Glycyrrhizae Radix et Rhizoma, Paeoniae Radix Rubra and Zingiberis Recens Rhizoma.

Actions and Indications Dispersing wind-cold, releasing heat and relieving pain. It is used for initial stage of external contraction of wind-cold manifested as aversion to cold with fever, anhidrosis, headache, stuffy nose, sneezing, itching throat and cough, aching pain of the limbs. It is suitable for initial stage of influenza, mild upper respiratory infection.

＊柴胡

正清风痛宁

【处方】本品为青风藤经加工制成的片剂。

【功能主治】祛风除湿，活血通络，消肿止痛。用于风寒寒痹症。症见肌肉酸痛，关节肿胀、疼痛，屈伸不利，麻木僵硬等及风湿与类风湿性关节炎具有上述证候者。

Orientvine★ Tablet for Relieving Impediment Syndrome

Name of Chinese Phonetic Alphabet Zheng Qing Feng Tong Ning

Formula Sinomenii Caulis.

Actions and Indications Dispelling wind and dampness, activating blood and dredging collatrals, reducing swelling and relieving pain. It is used for impediment syndrome, manifested as muscular soreness and pain, swelling and pain of joint, immobility and numbness of limbs, and is also for rheumatism and rheumatoid arthritis with the above mentioned symptoms.

＊青风藤

玉丹荣心丸

【处方】玉竹、丹参等。

【功能主治】益气养阴，活血化瘀，清热解毒，强心复脉。可用于病毒性心肌炎，心脏病。症见胸闷心慌，气短乏力，头晕，多汗，心前区不适或疼痛等。

Solomon's Seal★ and Redroot Sage★★ Pill for Myocarditis

Name of Chinese Phonetic Alphabet Yu Dan Rong Xin Wan

Formula Polygonati Odorati Rhizoma, Salviae Miltiorrhizae Radix et Rhizoma, etc.

Actions and Indications Tonifying *qi* and nourishing *yin*, activating blood, resolving stasis, clearing heat and detoxifying, strengthening the heart to restore normal pulse beat. It is indicated for viral myocarditis and cardiac disease manifested as chest distress, fluster, shortness of breath, fatigue, dizziness, hyperhidrosis and precordial pain.

* 玉竹 ** 丹参

玉叶解毒冲剂

【处方】玉叶金花、金银花、菊花、野菊花、岗梅、山芝麻、积雪草。

【功能主治】清热解毒，辛凉解表，清暑利湿，生津利咽。用于防治外感风热引起的感冒，咳嗽，咽喉炎，尿路感染及预防中暑。

Erose Mussaenda* Detoxicating Soluble Granules

Name of Chinese Phonetic Alphabet Yu Ye Jie Du Chong Ji

Formula Mussaendae Erosae Folium, Lonicerae Japonicae Flos, Chrysanthemi Flos, Chrysanthemi Indici Flos, Ilicis Asprellae Folium seu Radix, Helicteris Angustifoliae Radix and Centellae Herba.

Actions and Indications Clearing heat and detoxicating, releasing the exterior, clearing summer-heat and draining dampness, engendering fluid, soothing the throat. It is used for preventing and treating external contraction of wind-heat, marked by common cold, cough, laryngopharyngitis, urinary tract infection and heat stroke prevention.

* 玉叶金花

玉泉丸

【处方】葛根、天花粉、地黄、麦冬、五味子、甘草。

【功能主治】生津止渴，清热除烦，养阴滋肾，益气和中。用于糖尿病。

Promoting Fluid-engendering Pill

Name of Chinese Phonetic Alphabet Yu Quan Wan

Formula Puerariae Lobatae Radix, Trichosanthis Radix, Rehmanniae Radix, Ophiopoganis Radix, Schisandrae Chinensis Fructus and Glycyrrhizae Radix et Rhizoma.

Actions and Indications Promoting fluid-engendering to quench thirst, clearing heat, relieving vexation, nourishing *qi* and kidney-*yin*, harmonizing the middle energizer. It is indicated for diabetes.

玉屏风胶囊

【处方】黄芪、防风、白术（炒）。

【功能主治】益气，固表，止汗。用于表虚不固，自汗恶风，面色㿠白，或体虚易感风邪者。

Qi-Tonifying and Exterior-securing Capsule

Name of Chinese Phonetic Alphabet Yu Ping Feng Jiao Nang

Formula Astragali Radix, Saposhnikoviae Radix and Atractylodis Macrocephalae Rhizoma (fried).

Actions and Indications Tonifying *qi*, securing the exterior, relieving sweating. It is used for spontaneous sweating, aversion to cold, bright pale complexion, or susceptibleness of wind pathogen due to physical debility.

玉真散

【处方】生白附子、防风、白芷、生天南星、天麻、羌活。

【功能主治】祛风，解痉，止痛。用于破伤风；外治跌扑损伤。

【注意】孕妇禁用。

Yu Zhen Powder

Name of Chinese Phonetic Alphabet Yu Zhen San

Formula Typhonii Rhizoma (fresh), Saposhnikoviae Radix, Angelicae Dahuricae Radix, Arisaematis Rhizoma (fresh), Gastrodiae Rhizoma and

Notopterygii Rhizoma et Radix.

Actions and Indications Dispelling wind, relieving spasm, alleviating pain. It is used for tetanus, externally used for traumatic injury.

Warning It is contraindicated for pregnant women.

古汉养生精片

【处方】人参、黄芪（蜜炙）、枸杞子、女贞子（制）、黄精等。

【功能主治】滋肾益精，补脑安神。用于头昏心悸，目眩耳鸣，健忘无力。亦可用于脑动脉硬化，冠心病，前列腺增生，更年期综合征，病后虚弱。

Preserving Healthy Essence Tablet

Name of Chinese Phonetic Alphabet Gu Han Yang Sheng Jing Pian

Formula Ginseng Radix et Rhizoma, Astragali Radix (prepared with honey), Lycii Fructus, Ligustri Lucidi Fructus (prepared), Polygonati Rhizoma, etc.

Actions and Indications Enriching the kidney and essence, tonifying the brain to tranquilize the mind. It is used for dizziness, palpitation, dizzy vision, tinnitus, amnesia. It is also used for cerebral arteriosclerosis, coronary heart disease, hyperplasia of prostate, menopausal syndrome, and debility after illness.

甘霖洗剂

【处方】甘草、苦参、白鲜皮、土荆皮等。

【功能主治】清热除湿，祛风止痒。用于风湿热蕴于肌肤所致皮肤瘙痒和下焦湿热所致外阴瘙痒。

【注意】本品为外用药；对酒精过敏者忌用。

Gan Lin Washings

Name of Chinese Phonetic Alphabet Gan Lin Xi Ji

Formula Glycyrrhizae Radix et Rhizoma, Sophorae Flavescentis Radix, Dictamni Cortex, Pseudolaricis Cortex, etc.

Actions and Indications Clearing heat and dispelling dampness, dispelling wind and relieving itching. It is indicated for cutaneous pruritus due to wind-damp-heat in the skin; and vulva itching duc to lower energizer dampness-heat.

Warning The preparation is for external use only and is contraindicated for allergic cases to alcohol.

甘露膏

【处方】当归、益母草、川芎、丹参、白芍、香附、泽兰、附子、小茴香、红花、吴茱萸、延胡索、艾叶、乌药、莪术、三棱、牛膝、木香、胡椒、肉桂、没药、甘草。

【功能主治】温经止带，暖子宫，调经血。用于妇女经期不准，行经腹痛，血寒白带。

【注意】孕妇忌用。

Sweet Dew Plaster

Name of Chinese Phonetic Alphabet Gan Lu Gao

Formula Angelicae Sinensis Radix, Leonuri Herba, Chuanxiong Rhizoma, Salviae Miltiorrhizae Radix et Rhizoma, Paeoniae Radix Alba, Cyperi Rhizoma, Lycopi Herba, Aconiti Lateralis Radix Praeparata, Foeniculi Fructus, Carthami Flos, Euodiae Fructus, Corydalis Rhizoma, Artemisiae Argyi Folium, Linderae Radix, Curcumae Rhizoma, Sparganii Rhizoma, Achyranthis Bidentatae Radix, Aucklandiae Radix, Piperis Fructus, Cinnamomi Cortex, Myrrha and Glycyrrhizae Radix et Rhizoma.

Actions and Indications Warming the meridians, relieving leukorrhea, warming the uterus, regulating menstruation. It is used for irregular menstruation, dysmenorrhea, leukorrhagia.

Warning It is contraindicated for pregnant women.

东方活血膏

【处方】生川乌、生草乌、红花、川芎、乳香（制）、没药（制）、羌活、独活、穿山甲（制）、当归、血竭、全蝎、自然铜、天麻、狗骨、木鳖子、黑木耳、雄黄、白矾、檀香、冰片、金银花、石膏、蘑菇、金针菇、儿茶、细辛。

【功能主治】祛风散寒，活血化瘀，舒筋活络。用于风寒湿痹所致的肩臂腰腿疼痛、肢体麻木。

【注意】孕妇、丹毒患者禁用。

Blood-activating Plaster

Name of Chinese Phonetic Alphabet Dong Fang Huo Xue Gao

Formula Aconiti Radix (raw), Aconiti Kusnezoffii Radix (raw), Carthami Flos, Chuanxiong Rhizoma, Olibanum (prepared), Myrrha (prepared), Notopterygii Rhizoma et Radix, Angelicae Pubescentis Radix, Manis Squama (prepared), Angelicae Sinensis Radix, Draconis Sanguis, Scorpio, Pyritum, Gastrodiae Rhizoma, Canis Os, Momordicae Semen, Auriculariae Sporocarpium, Realgar, Alumen, Santali Albi Lignum, Borneolum Syntheticum, Lonicerae Japonicae Flos, Gypsum Fibrosum, Agarici Campestris Sporocarpium, Collybiae Sporocarpium, Catechu and Asari Radix et Rhizoma.

Actions and Indications Expelling wind, dissipating cold, activating blood, resolving stasis, relaxing sinews and activating collaterals. It is used for pain of shoulder, waist and legs and numbness of extremities due to impediment syndrome of wind-cold-damp.

Warning It is contraindicated for pregnant women and cases with erysipelas.

石斛明目丸

【处方】石斛、青葙子、决明子（炒）、蒺藜（去刺盐炙）、地黄、熟地黄、枸杞子、菟丝子、肉苁蓉（酒炙）、人参、山药、茯苓、天冬、麦冬、五味子（醋炙）、甘草、枳壳（麸炒）、菊花、防风、黄连、牛膝、川芎、苦杏仁（去皮炒）、石膏、磁石（煅醋淬）、水牛角浓缩粉。

【功能主治】平肝清热，滋肾明目。用于肝肾两亏，虚火上升引起的瞳孔散大，夜盲昏花，视物不清，内障抽痛，头目眩晕，精神疲倦。

【注意】忌食辛辣食物。

Noble Dendrobium* Pill for Improving Vision

Name of Chinese Phonetic Alphabet Shi Hu Ming Mu Wan

Formula Dendrobii Caulis, Celosiae Semen, Cassiae Semen (fried), Tribuli Fructus (removed the thorn and prepared with salt), Rehmanniae Radix, Rehmanniae Radix Praepatata, Lycii Fructus, Cuscutae Semen, Cistanches Caulis Carnosus (prepared with wine), Ginseng Radix et Rhizoma, Dioscoreae Rhizoma, Poria, Asparagi Radix, Ophiopogonis Radix, Schisandrae Chinensis Fructus (prepared with vinegar), Glycyrrhizae Radix et Rhizoma, Aurantii Fructus (fried with bran), Chrysanthemi Flos, Saposhnikoviae Radix, Coptidis Rhizoma, Achyranthis Bidentatae Radix, Chuanxiong Rhizoma, Armeniacae Semen Amarum (removed the seed coat and fried), Gypsum Fibrosum, Magnetitum (calcined and quenched by vinegar), and Bubali Cornu Pulvis Concentratio.

Actions and Indications Pacifying the liver, clearing heat, enriching the kidney to improve vision. It is indicated for platycoria, nyctalopia, blurred vision, cataract, vertigo and lassitude of spirit due to dual deficiency of liver and kidney, and deficiency-fire flaming upward.

Warning The pungent food is prohibited.

* 石斛

石斛夜光丸

【处方】石斛、人参、山药、茯苓、甘草、肉苁蓉、枸杞子、菟丝子、地黄、熟地黄、五味子、天冬、麦冬、苦杏仁、防风、川芎、枳壳、黄连、牛膝、菊花、蒺藜、青葙子、决明子、水牛角浓缩粉、羚羊角。

【功能主治】滋阴补肾，清肝明目。用于肝肾两亏，阴虚火旺，内障目暗，视物昏花。

Night Clear Vision Bolus of Noble Dendrobium*

Name of Chinese Phonetic Alphabet Shi Hu Ye Guang Wan

Formula Dendrobii Caulis, Ginseng Radix et Rhizoma, Dioscoreae Rhizoma, Poria, Glycyrrhizae Radix et Rhizoma, Cistanches Caulis Carnosus, Lycii Fructus, Cuscutae Semen, Rehmanniae Radix, Rehmanniae Radix Praeparata, Schisandrae Chinensis Fructus, Asparagi Radix, Ophiopogonis Radix, Armeniacae Semen Amarum, Saposhnikoviae Radix, Chuanxiong Rhizoma, Aurantii Fructus, Coptidis Rhizoma, Achyranthis Bidentatae Radix, Chrysanthemi Flos, Tribuli Fructus, Celosiae Semen, Cassiae Semen, Bubali Cornu Pulvis Concentratio and Saigae Tartaricae Cornu.

Actions and Indications Enriching *yin*, tonifying the kidney, clearing liver-fire to improve vision. It is indicated for cataract and blurred vision due to dual deficiency of the liver and kidney, and *yin*-deficiency with effulgent fire.

*石斛

石淋通片

【处方】广金钱草浸膏。

【功能主治】清湿热，利尿，排石。用于尿路结石，肾盂肾炎，胆囊炎。

Snowbellleaf Tickclover* Tablet for Relieving Strangury

Name of Chinese Phonetic Alphabet Shi Lin Tong Pian

Formula Desmodii Styracifolii Extractum.

Actions and Indications Clearing dampness-heat, inducing diuresis and removing stone. It is indicated for lithangiuria, pyelonephritis and cholecystitis.

*广金钱草

石榴健胃散

【处方】石榴子、肉桂、荜茇、红花、豆蔻。

【功能主治】温胃益火，化滞除湿。用于消化不良，食欲不振，寒性腹泻。

Pomegranate Fruit* Powder for Warming Stomach

Name of Chinese Phonetic Alphabet Shi Liu Jian Wei San

Formula Granati Fructus, Cinnamomi Cortex, Piperis Longi Fructus, Carthami Flos and Amomi Fructus Rotundus.

Actions and Indications Warming the stomach and enriching fire, resolving stagnation and eliminating dampness. It is indicated for indigestion, poor appetite and diarrhea.

*石榴子

石膏散

【处方】石膏、冰片。

【功能主治】清热祛火，消肿止痛。用于胃火上升引起的牙齿疼痛；口舌糜烂，牙龈出血。

【注意】忌食辛辣食物。阴虚火旺者忌用。

Gypsum* Powder

Name of Chinese Phonetic Alphabet Shi Gao San

Formula Gypsum Fibrosum and Borneolum Syntheticum.

Actions and Indications Clearing heat and dispelling fire, dispersing swelling and relieving pain. It is used for toothache, aphthae, gingival bleeding due to upward attacking of stomach-fire.

Warning Pungent foods should be avoided. It should be used carefully for cases with *yin*-deficiency and effulgent fire.

*石膏

右归丸

【处方】熟地黄、附子（炮附片）、肉桂、山药、山茱萸（酒炙）、菟丝子、鹿角胶、枸杞子、当归、杜仲（盐炒）。

【功能主治】温补肾阳，填精止遗。用于肾阳不足，命门火衰，腰膝酸冷，精神不振，怯寒畏冷，阳痿遗精，大便溏薄，尿频而清。

Warming Kidney-*yang* Bolus

Name of Chinese Phonetic Alphabet You Gui Wan

Formula Rehmanniae Radix Praeparata, Aconiti Lateralis Radix Praeparata (sliced), Cinnamomi Cortex, Dioscoreae Rhizoma, Corni Fructus (prepared with wine), Cuscutae Semen, Cervi Cornus Colla, Lycii Fructus, Angelicae Sinensis Radix and Eucommiae Cortex (fried with salt).

Actions and Indications Warming and tonifying kidney-*yang*, relieving spermatorrhea. It is used for soreness and cold of waist and knees, lassitude fo spirit, fear of cold, impotence, nocturnal emission, sloppy stool, freguent and clear urine due to insufficiency of kidney-*yang* and debilitation of the life gate fire.

左归丸

【处方】熟地黄、菟丝子、牛膝、龟甲胶、鹿角胶、山药、山茱萸、枸杞子。

【功能主治】滋阴补肾。用于真阴不足，腰酸膝软，盗汗遗精，神疲口燥。

Tonifying Kidney-*yin* Pill

Name of Chinese Phonetic Alphabet Zuo Gui Wan

Formula Rehmanniae Radix Praeparata, Cuscutae Semen, Achyranthis Bidentatae Radix, Testudinis Carapacis et Plastri Colla, Cervi Cornus Colla, Dioscoreae Rhizoma, Corni Fructus and Lycii Fructus.

Actions and Indications Enriching kidney-*yin*. It is indicated for soreness of waist and weakness of knees, night sweating, nocturnal emission, lassitude of spirit and dry mouth due to insufficiency of genuine *yin*.

左金胶囊

【处方】黄连、吴茱萸。

【功能主治】泻火，疏肝，和胃，止痛。用于肝火犯胃，脘胁胀痛。口苦嘈杂，呕吐酸水。

Zuo Jin Capsule

Name of Chinese Phonetic Alphabet Zuo Jin Jiao Nang

Formula Coptidis Rhizoma and Euodiae Fructus.

Actions and Indications Purging fire, soothing the liver, harmonizing the stomach, relieving pain. It is used for liver-fire invading the stomach, marked by hypochondriac distention and pain, bitter taste in the mouth, gastric upset, acid vomiting.

龙凤宝胶囊

【处方】淫羊藿、山楂、党参、白附片、玉竹、肉苁蓉、黄芪、牡丹皮、冰片。

【功能主治】补肾壮阳，健脾益气，宁神益智。用于更年期综合征及神经衰弱。

Relieving Menopausal Syndrome Capsule

Name of Chinese Phonetic Alphabet Long Feng Bao Jiao Nang

Formula Epimedii Folium, Crataegi Fructus, Codonopsis Radix, Typhonii Rhizoma (sliced), Polygonati Odorati Rhizoma, Cistanches Caulis Carnosus, Astragali Radix, Moutan Cortex and Borneolum Syntheticum.

Actions and Indications Tonifying kidney-*yang*, fortifying the spleen and tonifying *qi*, tranquilizing the mind. It is indicated for menopausal syndrome, neurasthenia.

龙牡壮骨冲剂

【处方】本品为黄芪、麦冬、龟甲、白术、山药、龙骨、牡蛎、鸡内金、维生素D_2等加工制成的颗粒。

【功能主治】强筋壮骨，和胃健脾。用于治疗和预防小儿佝偻病、软骨病，对小儿多汗，夜惊，食欲不振，消化不良，发育迟缓等症也有治疗作用。

Strengthening Bone Soluble Granules for Children

Name of Chinese Phonetic Alphabet Long Mu Zhuang Gu Chong Ji

Formula Astragali Radix, Ophiopogonis Radix, Testudinis Carapax et Plastrum, Atractylodis Macrocephalae Rhizoma, Dioscoreae Rhizoma, Draconis Os, Ostreae Concha, Galli Gigerii Endothelium Corneum and Vitamin D_2, etc.

Actions and Indications Strengthening the tendon and bone, harmonizing the stomach and fortifying the spleen. It is indicated for the prevention and treatment of children rickets, osteomalacia, and also effective for hyperhidrosis, poor appetite, indigestion and developmental retardation in children.

龙胆泻肝片

【处方】龙胆、柴胡、黄芩、栀子（炒）、泽泻、关木通、车前子（盐炒）、当归（酒炒）、地黄、甘草（蜜炙）。

【功能主治】清肝胆，利湿热。用于肝胆湿热，头晕目赤，耳鸣耳聋，耳痛，胁痛口苦，尿赤涩痛，湿热带下。

【注意】孕妇慎用。

Scabrous Gentian* Tablet for Purging Liver-fire

Name of Chinese Phonetic Alphabet Long Dan Xie Gan Pian

Formula Gentianae Radix et Rhizoma, Bupleuri Radix, Scutellariae Radix, Gardeniae Fructus (fried), Alismatis Rhizoma, Aristolochiae Manshuriensis Caulis, Plantaginis Semen (fried with salt), Angelicae Sinensis Radix (fried with wine), Rehmanniae Radix and Glycyrrhizae Radix et Rhizoma (prepared with honey).

Actions and Indications Clearing the liver-fire and gallbladder-fire, draining dampness and heat. It is indicated for damp-heat of the liver and gallbladder, dizziness, conjunctival congestion, tinnitus, deafness, otalgia, hypochondriac pain, bitter taste in the mouth, dark and scanty urine and vaginal discharge due to damp-heat of the liver and gallbladder.

Warning It should be used cautiously for pregnant women.

*龙胆

龙珠软膏

【处方】硼砂、炉甘石、冰片、人工牛黄、珍珠等。

【功能主治】清热解毒、消肿止痛、祛腐生肌；用于热毒蕴结的疖、痈。

【注意】孕妇禁用。

Long Zhu Soft Ointment

Name of Chinese Phonetic Alphabet Long Zhu Ruan Gao

Formula Borax, Calamina, Borneolum Syntheticum, Bovis Calculus Artifactus, Margarita, etc.

Actions and Indications Clearing heat and detoxicating, dispersing swelling and relieving pain, removing necrosis and promoting tissue regeneration. It is used for furuncle and abscess due to accumulation of heat-toxin.

Warning It is contraindicated for pregnant women.

可达灵片

【处方】本品为延胡索经加工制成的浸膏片。

【功能主治】活血化瘀，行利气止痛。用于冠心病，心绞痛，急性心肌梗死，陈旧性心肌梗死之胸闷憋气、心悸眩晕。

*Yanhusuo** Tablet

Name of Chinese Phonetic Alphabet Ke Da Ling Pian

Formula Corydalis Extractum.

Actions and Indications Activating blood, resolving stasis, moving *qi* to alleviate pain. It is indicated for coronary heart disease, angina pectoris, acute myocardial infarction, remote myocardial infarction marked by chest distress, palpitation and vertigo.

* 延胡索

归芍地黄丸

【处方】当归、白芍（酒炒）、熟地黄、山茱萸（制）、牡丹皮、山药、茯苓、泽泻。

【功能主治】滋肝肾，补阴血，清虚热。用于肝肾两亏，阴虚血少，头晕目眩，耳鸣咽干，午后潮热，腰腿酸痛，脚跟疼痛。

Bolus of Chinese Angelica* White Peony** and Chinese Fox-glove***

Name of Chinese Phonetic Alphabet Gui Shao Di Huang Wan

Formula Angelicae Sinensis Radix, Paeoniae Radix Alba (fried with wine), Rehmanniae Radix Praeparata, Corni Fructus (prepared), Moutan Cortex, Dioscoreae Rhizoma, Poria and Alismatis Rhizoma.

Actions and Indications Enriching the liver and kidney, tonifying *yin*-blood, clearing deficiency-heat. It is used for dizziness, dizzy vision, tinnitus, dry throat, afternoon tidal fever, soreness and pain of waist and legs, and painful heels due to dual depletion of the liver and kidney, *yin*-deficiency and insufficiency of blood.

* 当归 ** 白芍 *** 地黄

归脾丸

【处方】党参、白术（炒）、黄芪（蜜炙）、甘草（蜜炙）、茯苓、远志（制）、酸枣仁、龙眼肉、当归、木香、大枣（去核）、生姜。

【功能主治】益气健脾，养血安神。用于心脾两虚，气短心悸，失眠多梦，头昏头晕，肢倦乏力，食欲不振，崩漏便血。

Fortifying Spleen and Nourishing Blood Bolus

Name of Chinese Phonetic Alphabet Gui Pi Wan

Formula Codonopsis Radix, Atractylodis Macrocephalae Rhizoma (fried), Astragali Radix (prepared with honey), Glycyrrhizae Radix et Rhizoma (prepared with honey), Poria, Polygalae Radix (prepared), Ziziphi Spinosae Semen, Longan Arillus, Angelicae Sinensis Radix, Aucklandiae Radix, Jujubae Fructus (removed nucleus) and Zingiberis Rhizoma Recens.

Actions and Indications Tonifying *qi*, fortifying the spleen, nourishing blood and tranquilizing the mind. It is indicated for dual deficiency of the heart and spleen marked by shortness of breath, palpitation, insomnia, profuse dreaming, dizziness, tiredness, fatigue, poor appetite, metrorrhagia and hematochezia.

北豆根片

【处方】本品为北豆根中提取的总生物碱片。

【功能主治】清热解毒，止咳，祛痰。用于咽喉肿痛，扁桃体炎，慢性支气管炎。

Siberian Moonseed* Tablet for Relieving Sore-throat

Name of Chinese Phonetic Alphabet Bei Dou Gen Pian

Formula Menispermi Rhizoma (total alkaloids).

Actions and Indications Clearing heat and detoxicating, relieving cough and dispelling phlegm. It is used for sore-throat, tonsillitis, chronic bronchitis.

* 北豆根

北芪五加片

【处方】黄芪干浸膏、刺五加浸膏。

【功能主治】益气，健脾，安神。用于体虚乏力，腰膝酸软，失眠多梦，食欲不振。

Milkveteh* and Manyprickle Acanthopanax** Tablet

Name of Chinese Phonetic Alphabet Bei Qi Wu Jia Pian

Formula Astragali Extractum and Acanthopanacis

Senticosi Extractum.

Actions and Indications Tonifying *qi* and fortifying the spleen, tranquilizing. It is used for physical debility, fatigue, soreness and weakness of the waist and knees, insomnia and profuse dreaming, poor appetite.

* 黄芪 ** 刺五加

田七补丸

【处方】乌鸡（去毛爪肠）、熟地黄、当归、三七（香油炸黄）、党参、女贞子（酒炙）、香附（醋炙）、白术（麸炒）、山药、墨旱莲。

【功能主治】补肝益肾，益气养血。用于气血不足引起的面色苍白，心悸气短，精神疲倦，体虚潮热，腰酸腿软，妇女产后失血过多。

【注意】血热引起的失血禁用。

*Sanchi** Tonic Bolus

Name of Chinese Phonetic Alphabet Tian Qi Bu Wan

Formula Galli Caro cum Osse Nigro (removed the claws and intestines), Rehmanniae Radix Praeparata, Angelicae Sinensis Radix, Notoginseng Radix et Rhizoma (fried with vegetable oil), Codonopsis Radix, Ligustri Lucidi Fructus (prepared with wine), Cyperi Rhizoma (prepared with vinegar), Atractylodis Macrocephalae Rhizoma (fried with bran), Dioscoreae Rhizoma and Ecliptae Herba.

Actions and Indications Tonifying the liver, kidney, *qi* and blood. It is indicated for pale complexion, palpitation, shortness of breath, lassitude of spirit, general debility, tidal fever, soreness of waist and weakness of legs and puerperal massive hemorrhage due to insufficiency of *qi* and blood.

Warning It is contraindicated for cases with loss of blood due to blood-heat.

* 三七

田七痛经胶囊

【处方】三七、五灵脂、蒲黄、木香、延胡索、川芎、小茴香、冰片。

【功能主治】通调气血，止痛调经。用于经期腹痛及因寒所致的月经失调。

*Sanchi** Capsule for Dysmenorrhea-relieving

Name of Chinese Phonetic Alphabet Tian Qi Tong Jing Jiao Nang

Formula Notoginseng Radix et Rizoma, Trogopterori Faeces, Typhae Pollen, Aucklandiae Radix, Corydalis Rhizoma, Chuanxiong Rhizoma, Foeniculi Fructus and Borneolum Syntheticum.

Actions and Indications Regulating *qi* and blood, alleviating pain, regulating menstruation. It is used for abdominal pain during menstrual period or irregular menstruation due to cold pathogen.

* 三七

甲亢灵片

【处方】墨旱莲、丹参、牡蛎（煅）、龙骨（煅）、夏枯草、山药。

【功能主治】平肝潜阳，软坚散结。用于具有心悸、汗多、烦躁易怒、咽干、脉数等症状的甲状腺功能亢进症。

【注意】腹胀食少者慎用。

Relieving Hyperthyroidism Tablet

Name of Chinese Phonetic Alphabet Jia Kang Ling Pian

Formula Ecliptae Herba, Salviae Miltiorrhizae Radix et Rhizoma, Ostreae Concha (calcined), Draconis Os (calcined), Prunellae Spica and Dioscoreae Rhizoma.

Actions and Indications Pacifying the liver to subdue *yang*, softening hardness and mass. It is indicated for hyperthyroidism, manifested as palpitation, profuse sweating, vexation, easiness to be angry, dry throat, rapid pulse.

Warning It should be used carefully for cases with abdominal distention and anorexia.

四方胃片

【处方】海螵蛸、浙贝母、沉香、黄连、川楝子（去皮酒炒）、柿霜、苦杏仁、延胡索（醋制）、吴茱萸（盐水制）。

【功能主治】舒肝和胃，制酸止痛。用于肝胃不和所致胃痛，胃酸过多，消化不良，以及胃、十二指肠溃疡见上述症状者。

Stomachache and Dyspepsia Relieving Tablet

Name of Chinese Phonetic Alphabet Si Fang Wei Pian

Formula Sepiae Endoconcha, Fritillariae Thunbergii Bulbus, Aquilariae Lignum Resinatum, Coptidis Rhizoma, Toosendan Fructus (removed pericarp and fried with wine), Kaki Fructus Pulveratum, Armeniacae Semen Amarum, Corydalis Rhizoma (prepared with vinegar) and Euodiae Fructus (prepared with salt water).

Actions and Indications Soothing the liver, harmonizing the stomach, inhibiting acidity and alleviating pain. It is indicated for stomachache, gastroxia and dyspepsia, due to disharmony of the liver and stomach, and also used for gastroduodenal ulcer with the above mentioned symptoms.

四正丸

【处方】广藿香、香薷、紫苏叶、白芷、檀香、木瓜、法半夏、厚朴（姜制）、大腹皮、陈皮、白术（麸炒）、桔梗、茯苓、槟榔、枳壳（麸炒）、山楂（炒）、六神曲（麸炒）、麦芽（炒）、白扁豆（去皮）、甘草。

【功能主治】祛暑解表，化湿止泻。用于内伤湿滞，外感风寒，头晕身重，恶寒发热，恶心呕吐，饮食无味，腹胀泄泻。

Si Zheng Bolus

Name of Chinese Phonetic Alphabet Si Zheng Wan

Formula Pogostemonis Herba, Moslae Herba, Perillae Folium, Angelicae Dahuricae Radix, Santali Albi Lignum, Chaenomelis Fructus, Pinelliae Rhizoma Praeparatum, Magnoliae Officinalis Cortex (prepared with ginger), Arecae Pericarpium, Citri Reticulatae Pericarpium, Atractylodis Macrocephalae Rhizoma (fried with bran), Platycodonis Radix, Poria, Arecae Semen, Aurantii Fructus (fried with bran), Crataegi Fructus (fried), Medicate Massa Fermentata (fried with bran), Hordei Fructus Germinatus (fried), Lablab Semen Album (removed seed coat) and Glycyrrhizae Radix et Rhizoma.

Actions and Indications Dispelling summer-heat and releasing the exterior, resolving dampness and relieving diarrhea. It is indicated for dizziness and heavy sensation of the body, aversion to cold, fever, nausea, vomiting, anorexia, abdominal distention and diarrhea due to internal dampness stagnation and exogenous wind-cold.

四红丹

【处方】当归、地榆（炭）、大黄（炭）、当归（炭）、大黄、槐花（炭）。

【功能主治】清热止血。用于吐血、衄血、便血、妇女崩漏下血。

Si Hong Bolus

Name of Chinese Phonetic Alphabet Si Hong Dan

Formula Angelicae Sinensis Radix, Sanguisorbae Radix (carbonated), Rhei Radix et Rhizoma (carbonated), Angelicae Sinensis Radix (carbonated), Rhei Radix et Rhizoma and Sophorae Flos (carbonated).

Actions and Indications Clearing heat, relieving bleeding. It is used for hematemesis, epistaxis, hematochezia, metrorrhagia.

四物合剂

【处方】当归、川芎、白芍、熟地黄。

【功能主治】调经养血。用于营血虚弱，月经不调。

Four Medicinals Mixture

Name of Chinese Phonetic Alphabet Si Wu He Ji

Formula Angelicae Sinensis Radix, Chuanxiong Rhizoma, Paeoniae Radix Alba and Rehmanniae Radix Praeparata.

Actions and Indications Regulating menstruation and nourishing blood. It is used for irregular menstruation due to deficiency of nutrient and blood.

四逆汤

【处方】附子（制）、干姜、甘草（蜜炙）。

【功能主治】温中祛寒，回阳救逆。用于阳虚欲脱，冷汗自出，四肢厥逆，下利清谷，脉微欲绝。

Saving from Collapse Decoction

Name of Chinese Phonetic Alphabet Si Ni Tang

Formula Aconiti Lateralis Radix (prepared), Zingiberis Rhizoma and Glycyrrhizae Radix et Rhizoma (prepared with honey).

Actions and Indications Warming the middle and dissipating cold, restoring *yang* to save from collapse. It is used for *yang*-deficiency collapse, cold sweating, cold extremities , clear food diarrhea and fainting pulse.

代温灸膏

【处方】本品为肉桂、辣椒等药经加工制成的橡胶膏剂。

【功能主治】温通经脉，散寒镇痛。用于脘腹冷痛，虚寒泄泻，腰背、四肢关节冷痛；慢性虚寒型胃肠炎、慢性风湿性关节炎。

Analgesic Adhesive Plaster

Name of Chinese Phonetic Alphabet Dai Wen Jiu Gao

Formula Cinnamomi Cortex, Capsici Fructus. etc.

Actions and Indications Warming and dredging meridians and collaterals, dissipating cold, alleviating pain. It is used for abdominal cold-pain, diarrhea, cold-pain in back and joints of limbs, chronic gastroenteritis, chronic rheumatic arthritis.

仙乐雄胶囊

【处方】人参、鹿茸、狗鞭、牛鞭、淫羊藿、熟地黄。

【功能主治】温肾补气，益精助阳。用于肾阳不足，精气亏损所致的头昏耳鸣，腰膝酸软，惊悸健忘，阳痿不举。

Celestial Capsule

Name of Chinese Phonetic Alphabet Xian Le Xiong Jiao Nang

Formula Ginseng Radix et Rhizoma, Cervi Cornu Pantotrichum, Canis Testis et Penis, Bovis Testis et Penis, Epimedii Folium and Rehmanniae Radix Praeparata.

Actions and Indications Warming the kidney, tonifying *qi*, essence and *yang*. It is used for dizziness, tinnitus, soreness and weakness of waist and knees, palpitation, amnesia, impotence and erect disorder due to insufficiency of kidney-*yang*.

外用应急软膏

【处方】本品为黄芩、白芍、丹参、补骨脂、人参、党参、金银花、茯苓、益母草、鱼腥草、鸭跖草、辛夷、甘草、青蒿、樟脑等药经加工制成的软膏。

【功能主治】消肿，止痛，抗感染，促进伤口愈合。用于冻疮，I~II 度烫伤，手足皲裂及小面积轻度擦挫伤。

【注意】只供外用，涂药后不可用塑料薄膜覆盖。

Emergency Ointment for External Application

Name of Chinese Phonetic Alphabet Wai Yong Ying Ji Ruan Gao

Formula Scutellariae Radix, Paeoniae Radix Alba, Salviae Miltiorrhizae Radix et Rhizoma, Psoraleae Fructus, Ginseng Radix et Rhizoma, Codonopsis Radix, Lonicerae Japonicae Flos, Poria, Leonuri Herba, Houttuyniae Herba, Commelinae Herba, Magnoliae Flos, Glycyrrhizae Radix et Rhizoma, Artemisiae Annuae Herba, Camphora, etc.

Actions and Indications Dispersing swelling and relieving pain, anti-infectious, promoting wound healing. It is used for pernio, wound healing, I~II degree burn, rhagades of the hand and foot, mild sprain.

Warning It is for external use only; and plastic membrance is prohibited from covering the wound after medication.

外搽白灵酊

【**处方**】当归尾、红花、红花夹竹桃（叶）、苏木、没药、白芷、白矾、马齿苋。

【**功能主治**】活血化瘀，增加光敏作用，用于白癜风。

【**注意**】本品为外用药，严禁口服。

Vitiligo-relieving Tincture

Name of Chinese Phonetic Alphabet Wai Cha Bai Ling Ding

Formula Angelicae Sinensis Radix (tail part), Carthami Flos, Nerii Indici Folium, Sappan Lignum, Myrrha, Angelicae Dahuricae Radix, Alumen and Portulacae Herba.

Actions and Indications Activating blood, resolving stasis, increasing photosensitivity. It is indicated for vitiligo.

Warning The tincture is applied for external use only.

孕妇金花丸

【**处方**】栀子（姜制）、当归、白芍、川芎、金银花、地黄、黄芩、黄柏、黄连。

【**功能主治**】清热，安胎。用于孕妇头痛，眩晕，口鼻生疮，咽喉肿痛，双目赤肿，牙龈疼痛，或胎动下坠，小腹作痛，心烦不安，口干咽燥，渴喜冷饮，小便短黄。

【**注意**】忌食辛辣食物。

Honeysuckle Flower* Pill for Pregnant Women

Name of Chinese Phonetic Alphabet Yun Fu Jin Hua Wan

Formula Gardeniae Fructus (prepared with ginger), Angelicae Sinensis Radix, Paeoniae Radix Alba, Chuanxiong Rhizoma, Lonicerae Japonicae Flos, Rehmanniae Radix, Scutellariae Radix, Phellodendri Chinensis Cortex and Coptidis Rhizoma.

Actions and Indications Clearing heat, preventing abortion. It is used for headache, vertigo, aphthae, sore-throat, conjunctivitis and gingival pain in pregnant women or threatened abortion, lower abdominal pain, restlessness, dry mouth and throat, desired cold drink and scanty dark urine.

Warning Pungent foods should be avoided.

* 金银花

孕妇清火丸

【**处方**】黄芩、知母、石斛、柴胡、地黄、薄荷、白芍、白术（麸炒）、甘草。

【**功能主治**】清火安胎。用于孕妇胎热口干，胸腹灼热，或口舌生疮，咽喉燥痛，或大便秘结，小便黄赤。

Gravida-soothing Pill

Name of Chinese Phonetic Alphabet Yun Fu Qing Huo Wan

Formula Scutellariae Radix, Anemarrhenae Rhizoma, Dendrobii Caulis, Bupleuri Radix, Rehmanniae Radix, Menthae Haplocalycis Herba, Paeoniae Radix Alba, Atractylodis Macrocephalae Rhizoma (fried with bran) and Glycyrrhizae Radix et Rhizoma.

Actions and Indications Clearing fire, preventing abortion. It is used for fetal heat in pregnant women marked by dry mouth, chest and abdominal heat sensation, aphthae, sore-throat or constipation, dark yellow urine.

孕康口服液

【处方】本品为山药、续断、黄芪、当归、白芍、补骨脂等经加工制成的口服液。

【功能主治】健脾固肾，养血安胎。用于肾虚型和气血虚弱型先兆性流产和习惯性流产。

【注意】服药期间，忌食辛辣刺激性食物，避免剧烈运动以及重体力劳动；凡难产、异位妊娠、葡萄胎等非本品适用范围。

Abortion-preventing Oral Liquid

Name of Chinese Phonetic Alphabet Yun Kang Kou Fu Ye

Formula Dioscoreae Rhizoma, Dipsaci Radix, Astragali Radix, Angelicae Sinensis Radix, Paeoniae Radix Alba, Psoraleae Fructus, etc.

Actions and Indications Fortifying the spleen and kidney, nourishing blood and preventing abortion. It is indicated for threatened abortion and habitual abortion due to kidney-deficiency and deficiency of *qi* and blood.

Warning Pungent and irritant foods, strenuous exercise and heavy physical labour should be avoided. It is contraindicated for difficult labour, heterotopic pregnancy and grape mole.

冬凌草片

【处方】本品为冬凌草制成的片剂。

【功能主治】清热解毒。用于慢性扁桃体炎、咽炎、喉炎、口腔炎。

Blushed Rabdosia* Tablet for Relieving Tonsillitis

Name of Chinese Phonetic Alphabet Dong Ling Cao Pian

Formula Rabdosiae Rubescentis Folium.

Actions and Indications Clearing heat and detoxicating. It is indicated for chronic tonsillitis, pharyngitis, laryngitis, stomatitis .

*冬凌草

生力雄丸

【处方】人参、鹿茸、淫羊藿、韭菜子、蛇床子、蜻蜓、蚕蛾、咖啡因、马钱子、蟾酥。

【功能主治】补肾壮阳，益髓填精，用于肾精亏损，性欲减退，阳痿早泄，夜尿频多，腰膝酸冷，白发脱发。

【注意】感冒者忌服。

Furious Energy Pill

Name of Chinese Phonetic Alphabet Sheng Li Xiong Wan

Formula Ginseng Radix et Rhizoma, Cervi Cornu Pantotrichum, Epimedii Folium, Allii Tuberosi Semen, Cnidii Fructus, Acestra, Bombycis Imagine Masculi, Caffeine, Strychni Semen and Bufonis Venenum.

Actions and Indications Tonifying kidney-*yang*, marrow and essence. It is used for sexual hypoesthesia, impotence, ejaculatio praecox, frequent urination at night, soreness and cold of waist and knees, gray hair and alopecia due to depletion of kidney-essence.

Warning It is contraindicated for cases with common cold.

生化丸

【处方】当归、川芎、桃仁、甘草、干姜（炒炭）。

【功能主治】养血祛瘀。用于产后受寒恶露不行或行而不畅，夹有血块，小腹冷痛。

Lochiostasis-relieving Bolus

Name of Chinese Phonetic Alphabet Sheng Hua Wan

Formula Angelicae Sinensis Radix, Chuanxiong Rhizoma, Persicae Semen, Glycyrrhizae Radix et

Rhizoma and Zingiberis Rhizoma (carbonated).

Actions and Indications Nourishing blood, dispelling stasis. It is used for puerperal lochiostasis complicated by blood clot and cold-pain of lower abdomen.

生尔发糖浆

【处方】熟地黄、制何首乌、菟丝子、赤芍、当归、黄芪、桑椹、女贞子、墨旱莲、五味子(醋制)。

【功能主治】滋补肝肾，补气养血。用于肝肾不足，气血亏虚所引起的各种脱发。

【注意】忌食辛辣食物。

Engendering Hair Syrup

Name of Chinese Phonetic Alphabet Sheng Er Fa Tang Jiang

Formula Rehmanniae Radix Praeparata, Polygoni Multiflori Radix Praeparata, Cuscutae Semen, Paeoniae Radix Rubra, Angelicae Sinensis Radix, Astragali Radix, Mori Fructus, Ligustri Lucidi Fructus, Ecliptae Herba and Schisandrae Chinensis Fructus (prepared with vinegar).

Actions and Indications Enriching the liver and kidney, tonifying *qi* and blood. It is used for various alopecia due to deficiency of *qi* and blood.

Warning Pungent foods are prohibited.

生发丸

【处方】制何首乌、补骨脂(盐制)、牛膝、当归、茯苓、枸杞子、菟丝子(盐制)、女贞子、墨旱莲、桑椹、黑芝麻、熟地黄、桑寄生、核桃仁、沙苑子、蛇床子、紫河车、骨碎补、黄芪、黄精(制)、五味子、灵芝、地黄、侧柏叶、苦参、山楂。

【功能主治】填精补血，补肝滋肾，乌须黑发。用于肝肾不足、精血气衰所致的须发早白，头发稀疏、干枯，斑秃脱发。

Engendering Hair Bolus

Name of Chinese Phonetic Alphabet Sheng Fa Wan

Formula Polygoni Multiflori Radix Praeparata, Psoraleae Fructus (prepared with salt), Achyranthis Bidentatae Radix, Angelicae Sinensis Radix, Poria, Lycii Fructus, Cuscutae Semen (prepared with salt), Ligustri Lucidi Fructus, Ecliptae Herba, Mori Fructus, Sesami Semen Nigrum, Rehmanniae Radix Praeparata, Taxilli Herba, Juglandis Semen, Astragali Complanati Semen, Cnidii Fructus, Hominis Placenta, Drynariae Rhizoma, Astragali Radix, Polygonati Rhizoma (prepared), Schisandrae Chinensis Fructus, Ganoderma, Rehmanniae Radix, Platycladi Cacumen, Sophorae Flavescentis Radix and Crataegi Fructus.

Actions and Indications Tonifying the essence and blood, enriching the liver and kidney, and blackening the beard and hair. It is indicated for premature graying of beard and hair, thin and dry hair and alopecia due to declination of essence, *qi* and blood.

生发酊

【处方】闹金花、补骨脂、生姜。

【功能主治】温经通脉。用于斑秃脱发症。

【注意】外用药。本品有毒，切勿入口。

Engendering Hair Tincture

Name of Chinese Phonetic Alphabet Sheng Fa Ding

Formula Rhododendri Mollis Flos, Psoraleae Fructus and Zingiberis Rhizoma Recens.

Actions and Indications Warming the meridians and draining the vessels. It is used for alopecia areata.

Warning It is for external use only. This preparation is toxic and should not be touched by the mouth.

生血丸

【处方】鹿茸、黄柏、白术、山药、紫河车等。

【功能主治】补肾健脾，填精补髓。用于失血血亏，放、化疗后全血细胞减少及再生障碍性贫血。

Honeyed Pill for Tonifying Blood

Name of Chinese Phonetic Alphabet Sheng Xue Wan

Formula Cervi Cornu Pantotrichum, Phellodendri Chinensis Cortex, Atractylodis Macrocephalae Rhizoma, Dioscoreae Rhizoma, Hominis Placenta, etc.

Actions and Indications Tonifying the kidney and fortifying the spleen, tonifying the vital essence and blood. It is used for pancytopenia due to radiotherapy and chemotherapy, and also used for aplastic anemia.

生血宝

【处方】制何首乌、女贞子、桑椹、墨旱莲、白芍、黄芪、狗脊。

【功能主治】养肝肾，益精血。用于恶性肿瘤、放化疗所致的白细胞减少及神疲乏力，腰膝疲软，头晕耳鸣，心悸，气短，失眠，咽干，纳差食少。

Engendering Blood Soluble Granules

Name of Chinese Phonetic Alphabet Sheng Xue Bao

Formula Polygoni Multiflori Radix Praeparata, Ligustri Lucidi Fructus, Mori Fructus, Ecliptae Herba, Paeoniae Radix Alba, Astragali Radix and Cibotii Rhizoma.

Actions and Indications Tonifying the liver and kidney, essence and blood. It is used for leukopenia caused by radiotherapy and chemotherapy in the treatment of malignant tumor, and manifested as lassitude of spirit, fatigue weakness of waist and knees, dizziness, tinnitus, palpitation, shortness of breath, insomnia, dry throat and poor appetite.

生肌散

【处方】象皮（滑石烫）、儿茶、赤石脂、龙骨（煅）、血竭、乳香（醋炙）、没药（醋炙）、冰片。

【功能主治】解毒，生肌。用于疮疖久溃。

【注意】外用药，溃烂初期禁用。

Promoting Tissue Regeneration Powder

Name of Chinese Phonetic Alphabet Sheng Ji San

Formula Elephantis Corium (scalded by talc), Catechu, Halloysitum Rubrum, Draconis Os (calcined), Draconis Sanguis, Olibanum (prepared with vinegar), Myrrha (prepared with vinegar) and Borneolum Syntheticum.

Actions and Indications Detoxicating and promoting tissue regeneration. It is used for prolonged diabrosis of sore and furuncle.

Warning It is for external use only and is contraindicated for initial ulceration.

生乳灵

【处方】当归、地黄、黄芪（蜜炙）、党参、玄参、麦冬、穿山甲（沙烫醋淬）、知母。

【功能主治】滋补气血，通络下乳。用于气血不足，乳络阻滞引起的乳汁少，稀薄灰黄。

Improving Puerperal Oligogalactia Oral Liquid

Name of Chinese Phonetic Alphabet Sheng Ru Ling

Formula Angelicae Sinensis Radix, Rehmanniae Radix, Astragali Radix (prepared with honey), Codonopsis Radix, Scrophulariae Radix, Ophiopogonis Radix, Manis Squma (scalded by heated soil and quenched by vinegar) and Anemarrhenae Rhizoma.

Actions and Indications Tonifying *qi* and blood, dredging the collaterals. It is indicated for oligogalactia due to dual insufficiency of *qi* and blood.

生脉饮注射液

【处方】人参、麦冬、五味子。

【功能主治】益气复脉，养阴生津。用于气阴两亏，心悸气短，脉微自汗。

Injection of Restoring Normal Pulse Beat

Name of Chinese Phonetic Alphabet Sheng Mai Yin Zhu She Ye

Formula Ginseng Radix et Rhizoma, Ophiopogonis Radix and Schisandrae Chinensis Fructus.

Actions and Indications Tonifying *qi*, restoring normal pulse beat, nourishing *yin* and engendering fluid. It is indicated for palpitation, shortness of breath, faint pulse and spontaneous sweating due to dual depletion of qi and *yin*.

白石清热冲剂

【处方】葛根、薄荷、生石膏、板蓝根、白花蛇舌草。

【功能主治】疏风清热，解毒利咽。用于外感风热，或风寒热化，症见发热、微恶风，头痛鼻塞，咳嗽痰黄，咽红肿痛，口干而渴，舌苔薄白或薄黄，脉浮数。还可用于呼吸道感染，急性扁桃体炎见上述证候者。

Soluble Granules of Spreading Hedyotis* Gypsum** for Clearing Heat

Name of Chinese Phonetic Alphabet Bai Shi Qing Re Chong Ji

Formula Puerariae Lobatae Radix, Menthae Haplocalycis Herba, Gypsum Fibrosum, Isatidis Radix and Hedyotis Diffusae Herba.

Actions and Indications Dispersing wind and clearing heat, detoxicating and soothing the throat. It is used for cases attacked by exogenous wind-heat, or wind-cold transforming into heat, manifested as fever, slight aversion to cold, headache, nasal congestion, cough with yellow phlegm, sore-throat, dry mouth, thirst, thin and white or thin and yellow tongue fur, floating and rapid pulse. It is also used for respiratory tract infection and acute tonsillitis with the above mentioned symptoms.

* 白花蛇舌草 ** 石膏

白花蛇舌草注射液

【处方】本品为白花蛇草经提取制成的灭菌水溶液。

【功能主治】清热解毒，利湿消肿。用于湿热蕴毒所致的呼吸道感染，扁桃体炎，肺炎，胆囊炎，阑尾炎，痈疖脓肿及手术后感染，亦可用于癌症辅助治疗。

Injection of Spreading Hedyotis*

Name of Chinese Phonetic Alphabet Bai Hua She She Cao Zhu She Ye

Formula Hedyotis Diffusae Herba (extract).

Actions and Indications Clearing heat and detoxicating, draining dampness and dispersing swelling. It is indicated for respiratory tract infection, tonsillitis, pneumonia, cholecystitis, appendicitis, abscess and deep-rooted boil due to damp-heat accumulation, and also used for postoperative infection, adjuvant treatment of cancer.

* 白花蛇舌草

白灵片

【处方】当归、三七、红花、牡丹皮、桃仁、防风、黄芪、马齿苋、苍术、白芷、赤芍。

【功能主治】活血化瘀，增加光敏作用。用于白癜风。

Vitiligo-relieving Tablet

Name of Chinese Phonetic Alphabet Bai Ling Pian

Formula Angelicae Sinensis Radix, Notoginseng Radix et Rhizoma, Carthami Flos, Moutan Cortex, Persicae Semen, Saposhnikoviae Radix, Astragali Radix, Portulacae Herba, Atractylodis Rhizoma, Angelicae Dahuricae Radix and Paeoniae Radix Rubra.

Actions and Indications Activating blood, resolving stasis, increasing photosensitivity. It is indicated for vitiligo.

白带丸

【处方】黄柏（酒炒）、椿皮、白芍、当归、香附（醋制）。

【功能主治】清湿热，止带下。用于湿热下注，赤白带下。

Relieving Leucorrhea Pill

Name of Chinese Phonetic Alphabet Bai Dai Wan

Formula Phellodendri Chinensis Cortex (fried with wine), Ailanthi Cortex, Paeoniae Radix Alba, Angelicae Sinensis Radix and Cyperi Rhizoma (prepared with vinegar).

Actions and Indications Clearing damp-heat, relieving vaginal discharge. It is indicated for red and white vaginal discharge due to downward attack of damp-heat.

白蚀丸

【处方】紫草、灵芝、降香、牡丹皮、补骨脂、丹参、红花、苍术、何首乌、海螵蛸、龙胆、蒺藜、黄药子、甘草。

【功能主治】补益肝肾，活血祛瘀，养血祛风。用于治疗白癜风。

【注意】孕妇禁用。服药过程患部宜常日晒。

Vitiligo-relieving Pill

Name of Chinese Phonetic Alphabet Bai Shi Wan

Formula Arnebiae Radix, Ganoderma, Dalbergiae Odoriferae Lignum, Moutan Cortex, Psoraleae Fructus, Salviae Miltiorrhizae Radix et Rhizoma, Carthami Flos, Atractylodis Rhizoma, Polygoni Multiflori Radix, Sepiae Endoconcha, Gentianae Radix et Rhizoma, Tribuli Fructus, Dioscoreae Bulbiferae Tuber and Glycyrrhizae Radix et Rhizoma.

Actions and Indications Tonifying the liver and kidney, activating and nourishing blood, dispelling stasis and wind. It is indicated for vitiligo.

Warning It is contraindicated for pregnant women. During medication, the affected part should be exposed to the sun frequently.

白清胃散

【处方】石膏、玄明粉、硼砂、冰片。

【功能主治】清热、消肿、止痛。用于胃火上升引起的牙龈疼痛，口舌生疮。

【注意】不可内服。忌食辛辣食物。

Clearing Stomach-fire Powder

Name of Chinese Phonetic Alphabet Bai Qing Wei San

Formula Gypsum Fibrosum, Natrii Sulfas Exsiccatus, Borax and Borneolum Syntheticum.

Actions and Indications Clearing heat, dispersing swelling, relieving pain. It is indicated for gingivitis, aphthae due to ascendent stomach-fire.

Warning Oral use is prohibited. Pungent foods should be avoided.

白癜风胶囊

【处方】补骨脂、黄芪、红花、川芎、当归、香附、桃仁、丹参、乌梢蛇、紫草、白鲜皮、山药、干姜、龙胆、蒺藜。

【功能主治】益气行滞，活血解毒，利湿消斑，驱风止痒。用于白癜风。

Vitiligo-relieving Capsule

Name of Chinese Phonetic Alphabet Bai Dian Feng Jiao Nang

Formula Psoraleae Fructus, Astragali Radix, Carthami Flos, Chuanxiong Rhizoma, Angelicae Sinensis Radix, Cyperi Rhizoma, Persicae Semen, Salviae Miltiorrhizae Radix et Rhizoma, Zaocys, Arnebiae Radix, Dictamni Cortex, Dioscoreae

Rhizoma, Zingiberis Rhizoma, Gentianae Radix et Rhizoma and Tribuli Fructus.

Actions and Indications Tonifying *qi*, activating blood, detoxifying, draining dampness, eliminating leukoplakia, dispelling wind to relieve itching. It is indicated for vitiligo.

瓜霜退热灵胶囊

【处方】西瓜霜、麝香、冰片、羚羊角、石膏、丁香、沉香、甘草等。

【功能主治】清热解毒，开窍，镇静。用于热病高热，惊厥抽搐，咽喉肿痛。

Capsule of Watermelon Mirabilite* for Heat Disease

Name of Chinese Phonetic Alphabet Gua Shuang Tui Re Ling Jiao Nang

Formula Mirabilitum Praeparatum, Moschus, Borneolum Syntheticum, Saigae Tataricae Cornu, Gypsum Fibrosum, Caryophylli Flos, Aquilariae Lignum Resinatum, Glycyrrhizae Radix et Rhizoma, etc.

Actions and Indications Clearing heat and detoxicating, opening the orifices, tranquilizing. It is used for heat disease marked by high fever, convulsion, syncope, spasm and sore-throat.

* 西瓜霜

乐儿康糖浆

【处方】党参、太子参、黄芪、茯苓、山药、薏苡仁、麦冬、制何首乌、大枣、山楂（焦）、麦芽（炒）、陈皮、桑枝。

【功能主治】益气健脾，和中开胃。用于小儿食欲不振，营养不良。

Harmonizing Stomach Syrup for Children

Name of Chinese Phonetic Alphabet Le Er Kang Tang Jiang

Formula Codonopsis Radix, Pseudostellariae Radix, Astragali Radix, Poria, Dioscoreae Rhizoma, Coicis Semen, Ophiopogonis Radix, Polygoni Multiflori Radix Praeparata, Jujubae Fructus, Grataegi Fructus (charred), Hordei Fructus Germinatus (fried), Citri Reticulatae Pericarpium and Cinnamomi Ramulus.

Actions and Indications Tonifying *qi* and fortifying the spleen, harmonizing the middle and increasing the appetite. It is used for poor appetite and malnutrition of children.

乐脉颗粒

【处方】丹参、川芎、赤芍、山楂、红花、香附、木香。

【功能主治】行气活血，解郁化瘀，养血通脉。用于冠心病、动脉硬化、肺心病、多发性梗死性痴呆等心脑血管疾病属气滞血瘀所致的头痛、眩晕、胸痛、心悸。

Relieving Coronary Heart Disease and Arteriosclerosis Granules

Name of Chinese Phonetic Alphabet Le Mai Ke Li

Formula Salviae Miltiorrhizae Radix et Rhizoma, Chuanxiong Rhizoma, Paeoniae Radix Rubra, Crataegi Fructus, Carthami Flos, Cyperi Rhizoma and Aucklandiae Radix.

Actions and Indications Moving *qi*, activating blood, relieving depression, resolving stasis, nourishing blood, dredging the vessels. It is indicated for coronary heart disease, arteriosclerosis, pulmonary heart disease, multiple infarctional dementia attributed to *qi*-stagnation and blood-stasis, and manifested as headache, vertigo, chest pain and palpitation.

冯了性风湿跌打药酒

【处方】丁公藤、桂枝、麻黄、羌活、当归、川芎、白芷、补骨脂、乳香、猪牙皂、陈皮、苍术、厚朴、香附、木香、枳壳、白术、山药、黄精、菟丝子、小茴香、苦杏仁、泽泻、五灵脂、蚕砂、牡丹皮、没药。

【功能主治】祛风除湿，活血止痛。用于风寒湿痹，手足麻木，腰腿酸痛，跌打损伤。

【注意】孕妇禁内服。

Fengliaoxing Medicated Wine for Traumatic Injury

Name of Chinese Phonetic Alphabet Feng Liao Xing Feng Shi Die Da Yao Jiu

Formula Erycibes Caulis, Cinnamomi Ramulus, Ephedrae Herba, Notopterygii Rhizoma et Radix, Angelicae Sinensis Radix, Chuanxiong Rhizoma, Angelicae Dahuricae Radix, Psoraleae Fructus, Olibanum, Gleditsiae Fructus Abnormalis, Citri Reticulatae Pericarpium, Atractylodis Rhizoma, Magnoliae Officinalis Cortex, Cyperi Rhizoma, Aucklandiae Radix, Aurantii Fructus, Atractylodis Macrocephalae Rhizoma, Dioscoreae Rhizoma, Polygonati Rhizoma, Cuscutae Semen, Foeniculi Fructus, Armeniacae Semen Amarum, Alismatis Rhizoma, Trogopterori Faeces, Bombycis Feculae, Moutan Cortex and Myrrha.

Actions and Indications Dispelling wind and dampness, activating blood and alleviating pain. It is indicated for wind-cold-damp impediment syndrome, numbness of the limbs, aching pain of the waist and legs, and is for traumatic injury.

Warning It is contraindicated for pregnant women.

玄麦甘桔颗粒

【处方】玄参、麦冬、甘草、桔梗。

【功能主治】滋阴清热，祛痰利咽。用于虚火上炎，口鼻干燥，咽喉肿痛。

Figwort* and Lily-turf** Soluble Granules

Name of Chinese Phonetic Alphabet Xuan Mai Gan Jie Ke Li

Formula Scrophulariae Radix, Ophiopogonis Radix, Glycyrrhizae Radix et Rhizoma and Platycodonis Radix.

Actions and Indications Nourishing *yin*, clearing heat, dispelling phlegm, soothing the throat. It is used for dry nose and mouth, sore-throat due to deficiency fire flaming upward.

* 玄参 ** 麦冬

汉桃叶片

【处方】本品为汉桃叶浸膏片。

【功能主治】祛风止痛，舒筋活络。用于三叉神经痛，坐骨神经痛，风湿关节痛。

Scandent Schefflera* Tablet for Relieving Sciatica

Name of Chinese Phonetic Alphabet Han Tao Ye Pian

Formula Schefflerae Arboricolae Extractum.

Actions and Indications Dispelling wind and relieving pain, relaxing sinews and activating collaterals. It is indicated for prosopalgia, sciatica and rheumatic arthralgia.

* 汉桃叶

宁坤养血丸

【处方】人参、茯苓、白术（麸炒）、甘草、当归、白芍、地黄、川芎、丹参、红花、柴胡、香附（醋炙）、厚朴（姜炙）、陈皮、肉桂。

【功能主治】补气和营，养血调经。用于气虚血少，月经不调，经期后延，行经小腹冷痛或经后小腹痛。

【注意】孕妇忌服。

Ning Kun Bolus for Nourishing Blood

Name of Chinese Phonetic Alphabet Ning Kun Yang Xue Wan

Formula Ginseng Radix et Rhizoma, Poria, Atractylodis Macrocephalae Rhizoma (fried with bran), Glycyrrhizae Radix et Rhizoma, Angelicae Sinensis Radix, Paeoniae Radix Alba, Rehmanniae Radix, Chuanxiong Rhizoma, Salviae Miltiorrhizae Radix et Rhizoma, Carthami Flos, Bupleuri Radix, Cyperi

Rhizoma (prepared with vinegar), Magnoliae Officinalis Cortex (prepared with ginger), Citri Reticulatae Pericarpium and Cinnamomi Cortex.

Actions and Indications Tonifying *qi* and harmonizing nutrient, nourishing blood to regulate menstruation. It is indicated for irregular menstruation, delayed menstrual period, cold-pain in the lower abdomen during menstrual period or after menstruation due to dual deficiency of *qi* and blood.

Warning It is contraindicated for pregnant women.

宁嗽糖浆剂

【处方】麻黄、紫菀、百部（蒸）、甘草、苦杏仁。

【功能主治】止咳化痰。用于伤风咳嗽，急、慢性支气管炎。

Calming Cough Syrup

Name of Chinese Phonetic Alphabet Ning Sou Tang Jiang Ji

Formula Ephedrae Herba, Asteris Radix et Rhizoma, Stemonae Radix (steamed), Glycyrrhizae Radix et Rhizoma and Armeniacae Semen Amarum.

Actions and Indications Relieving cough and resolving phlegm. It is indicated for cough due to common cold; acute or chronic bronchitis.

半夏天麻丸

【处方】法半夏、天麻、黄芪（蜜炙）、人参、苍术（米泔水炙）、白术（麸炒）、茯苓、陈皮、泽泻、六神曲（麸炒）、麦芽（炒）、黄柏。

【功能主治】健脾祛湿，化痰息风。用于脾虚聚湿生痰；眩晕，头痛，胸脘满闷。

【注意】忌食生冷油腻。

Ternate Pinellia* and Gastrodia** Pill

Name of Chinese Phonetic Alphabet Ban Xia Tian Ma Wan

Formula Pinelliae Rhizoma Praeparatum, Gastrodiae Rhizoma, Astragali Radix (preppared with honey), Ginseng Radix et Rhizoma, Atractylodis Rhizoma (prepared with rice swilled water), Atractylodis Macrocephalae Rhizoma (fried with bran), Poria, Citri Reticulatae Pericarpium, Alismatis Rhizoma, Medicata Massa Fermentata (fried with bran), Hordei Fructus Germinatus (fried) and Phellodendri Chinensis Cortex.

Actions and Indications Fortifying the spleen and dispelling dampness, resolving phlegm and extinguishing wind. It is indicated for accumulation of phlegm-dampness due to spleen-deficiency; vertigo, headache and chest upset.

Warning Uncooked, cold, oily foods are prohibited.

* 半夏 ** 天麻

半夏糖浆

【处方】生半夏、麻黄、紫菀、桔梗、枇杷叶、远志（制）、陈皮、甘草、薄荷油。

【功能主治】止咳化痰。用于咳嗽痰多，支气管炎。

Syrup of Ternate Pinellia* for Relieving Cough

Name of Chinese Phonetic Alphabet Ban Xia Tang Jiang

Formula Pinelliae Rhizoma, Ephedrae Herba, Asteris Radix et Rhizoma, Platycodonis Radix, Eriobotryae Folium, Polygalae Radix (prepared), Citri Reticulatae Pericarpium, Glycyrrhizae Radix et Rhizoma and Menthae Haplocalycis Oleum.

Actions and Indications Relieving cough and resolving phlegm. It is indicated for cough with profuse phlegm, bronchitis.

* 半夏

加味八珍益母膏

【处方】益母草、甘草、茯苓、人参、泽兰、桃仁（制）、红花、当归、熟地黄、川芎、赤芍、丹参、炮姜、香附（制）、白术（炒）。

【功能主治】补气养血，祛瘀调经。用于妇女气血不足，月经不调（经期后移或经行不畅，量少，闭经），产后恶露不尽，腹痛。

【注意】月经过多，月经提前者慎用，孕妇忌用。

Additional Chinese Motherwort* Extract

Name of Chinese Phonetic Alphabet Jia Wei Ba Zhen Yi Mu Gao

Formula Leonuri Herba, Glycyrrhizae Radix et Rhizoma, Poria, Ginseng Radix et Rhizoma, Lycopi Herba, Persicae Semen (prepared), Carthami Flos, Angelicae Sinensis Radix, Rehmanniae Radix Praeparata, Chuanxiong Rhizoma, Paeoniae Radix Rubra, Salviae Miltiorrhizae Radix et Rhizoma, Zingiberis Rhizoma Praeparatum, Cyperi Rhizoma (prepared) and Atractylodis Macrocephalae Rhizoma (fried).

Actions and Indications Tonifying *qi* and blood, dispelling stasis and regulating menstruation. It is indicated for irregular menstruation, delayed menstruation, scanty menstruation, amenorrhea, puerperal lochiorrhea and abdominal pain due to insufficiency of *qi* and blood.

Warning It should be used carefully for hypermenorrhea and preceded menstrual periods, and is contraindicated for pregnant women.

*益母草

加味左金丸

【处方】黄连（姜炙）、吴茱萸（甘草炙）、黄芩、柴胡、木香、香附（醋炙）、郁金、白芍、青皮（醋炙）、枳壳（去瓤麸炒）、陈皮、延胡索（醋炙）、当归、甘草。

【功能主治】平肝降逆，疏郁止痛。用于肝胃不和引起：胸脘痞闷，急躁易怒，嗳气吞酸，胃痛少食。

Additional *Zuojin* Pill

Name of Chinese Phonetic Alphabet Jia Wei Zuo Jin Wan

Formula Coptidis Rhizoma (prepared with ginger), Fructus Euodiae (prepared with licorice root), Scutellariae Radix, Bupleuri Radix, Aucklandiae Radix, Cyperi Rhizoma (prepared with vinegar), Curcumae Radix, Paeoniae Radix Alba, Citri Reticulatae Pericarpium Viride (prepared with vinegar), Aurantii Fructus (removed pulp and fried with bran), Citri Reticulatae Pericarpium, Corydalis Rhizoma (prepared with vinegar), Angelicae Sinensis Radix and Glycyrrhizae Radix et Rhizoma.

Actions and Indications Pacifying the liver, directing *qi* downward, relieving depression and alleviating pain. It is used for stuffiness and depression of hypochondrium, impatience, eructation, acid regurgitation, stomachache and poor appetite due to disharmony of the liver and stomach.

加味生化颗粒

【处方】当归、桃仁、益母草、赤芍、艾叶、川芎、炙甘草、炮姜、荆芥、阿胶。

【功能主治】活血化瘀，温经止痛。用于产后恶露不净，小腹疼痛，胎盘残留及功能性子宫出血。

Additional Granules for Lochiorrhagia

Name of Chinese Phonetic Alphabet Jia Wei Sheng Hua Ke Li

Formula Angelicae Sinensis Radix, Persicae Semen, Leonuri Herba, Paeoniae Radix Rubra, Artemisiae Argyi Folium, Chuanxiong Rhizoma, Glycyrrhizae Radix et Rhizoma Praeparata cum Melle, Zingiberis Rhizoma Praeparatum, Schizonepetae Herba and Asini Corii Colla.

Actions and Indications Activating blood, resolving stasis, warming the meridians, alleviating pain. It is indicated for puerperal lochiorrhea, pain of lower abdomen, remanent placenta, dysfunctional uterine bleeding.

加味保和丸

【处方】白术（麸炒）、茯苓、陈皮、厚朴（姜炙)、枳实、枳壳(麸炒)、香附(醋炙)、山楂(炒)、六神曲(麸炒)、麦芽(炒)、法半夏。

【功能主治】健胃理气，利湿和中。用于饮食不消，胸膈闷满，嗳气呕恶。

Bao He Additional Pill

Name of Chinese Phonetic Alphabet Jia Wei Bao He Wan

Formula Atractylodis Macrocephalae Rhizoma (fried with bran), Poria, Citri Reticulatae Pericarpium, Magnoliae Officinalis Cortex (prepared with ginger), Aurantii Fructus Immaturus, Aurantii Fructus (fried with bran), Cyperi Rhizoma (prepared with vinegar), Crataegi Fructus (fried), Medicata Massa Fermentata (fried with bran), Hordei Fructus Germinatus (fried) and Pinelliae Rhizoma Praeparatum.

Actions and Indications Fortifying the stomach and regulating *qi*, draining dampness and harmonizing the middle. It is used for dyspepsia, chest distress, eructation, vomiting and nausea.

加味逍遥丸

【处方】柴胡、当归、白芍、白术(麸炒)、茯苓、甘草、牡丹皮、栀子(姜炙)、薄荷。

【功能主治】舒肝清热，健脾养血。用于肝郁血虚，肝脾不和，两胁胀痛，头晕目眩，倦怠食少，月经不调，脐腹胀痛。

【注意】忌劳碌，忌食生冷油腻。

Additional *Xiao Yao* Pill

Name of Chinese Phonetic Alphabet Jia Wei Xiao Yao Wan

Formula Bupleuri Radix, Angelicae Sinensis Radix, Paeoniae Radix Alba, Atractylodis Macrocephalae Rhizoma (fried with bran), Poria, Glycyrrhizae Radix et Rhizoma, Moutan Cortex, Gardeniae Fructus (prepared with ginger) and Menthae Haplocalycis Herba.

Actions and Indications Soothing the liver and clearing heat, tonifying the spleen and nourishing blood. It is indicated for liver depression and blood deficiency, disharmony of the liver and spleen, hypochondriac pain, dizziness, dizzy vision, tiredness, poor appetite, irregular menstruation, distention and pain of umbilicus and abdomen.

Warning Overexertion, uncooked and oily foods are prohibited.

幼泻宁冲剂

【处方】白术(焦)、炮姜、车前草。

【功能主治】健脾利湿，温中止泻。用于小儿脾失健运、消化不良引起的腹泻。

Relieving Infantile Diarrhea Soluble Granules

Name of Chinese Phonetic Alphabet You Xie Ning Chong Ji

Formula Atractylodis Macrocephalae Rhizoma (charred), Zingiberis Rhizoma Praeparatum and Plantaginis Herba.

Actions and Indications Fortifying the spleen and draining dampness, warming the middle and relieving diarrhea. It is indicated for diarrhea due to spleen failing in transportion and dyspepsia of infant.

皮肤病血毒丸

【处方】茜草、桃仁、荆芥穗(炭)、蛇蜕(酒炙)、赤芍、当归、白茅根、地肤子、地黄、连翘、苍耳子(炒)、金银花、苦地丁、土茯苓、黄柏、皂角刺、桔梗、益母草、防风、赤茯苓、白芍、蝉蜕、牛蒡子(炒)、牡丹皮、白鲜皮、熟地黄、大黄(酒炒)、忍冬藤、紫草、土贝母、川芎(酒炙)、甘草、白芷、天葵子、紫荆皮、鸡血藤、浮萍、红花、苦杏仁(去皮炒)。

【功能主治】清热解毒，消肿止痒。用于经络不和，湿热血燥引起的风疹，湿疹，皮肤刺痒，雀斑粉刺，面赤鼻皶，疮疡肿毒，脚气疥癣，头目眩晕，大便燥结。

【注意】感冒期间停服，孕妇忌服。

Blood-toxin Dermatosis Relieving Pill

Name of Chinese Phonetic Alphabet Pi Fu Bing

Xue Du Wan

Formula Rubiae Radix, Persicae Semen, Schizonepetae Spica (carbonated), Serpentis Periostracum (prepared with wine), Paeoniae Radix Rubra, Angelicae Sinensis Radix, Imperatae Rhizoma, Kochiae Fructus, Rehmanniae Radix, Forsythiae Fructus, Xanthii Fructus (fried), Lonicerae Japonicae Flos, Corydalis Bungeanae Herba, Smilacis Glabrae Rhizoma, Phellodendri Chinensis Cortex, Gleditsiae Spina, Platycodonis Radix, Leonuri Herba, Saposhnikoviae Radix, Poria Rubra, Paeoniae Radix Alba, Cicadae Periostracum, Arctii Fructus (fried), Moutan Cortex, Dictamni Cortex, Rehmanniae Radix Praeparata, Rhei Radix et Rhizoma (fried with wine), Lonicerae Japonicae Caulis, Arnebiae Radix, Bolbostemmae Rhizoma, Chuanxiong Rhizoma (prepared with wine), Glycyrrhizae Radix et Rhizoma, Angelicae Dahuricae Radix, Semiaquilegiae Radix, Cercis Chinensis Cortex, Spatholobi Caulis, Spirodelae Herba, Carthami Flos and Armeniacae Semen Amarum (removed seed coat and fried).

Actions and Indications Clearing heat, detoxifying. Dispersing swelling, relieving itching. It is used for rubella, eczema, itching of skin, freckle, acne, reddish complexion, epistaxis, sore and ulcer of skin, scabies, tinea, vertigo and dry stools due to disharmony of meridians and collaterals and blood-dryness.

Warning It is contraindicated for pregnant women and should be suspended during common cold.

皮肤康洗液

【处方】金银花、蒲公英、马齿苋等。

【功能主治】清热解毒，凉血除湿，杀虫止痒。主治湿疮，见瘙痒、红斑、丘疹、水泡、糜烂等或湿热下注所致阴痒、白带量多等症。急性湿疹或阴道炎见有上述证候者。

【注意】本品为外用药；若有皮肤过敏反应者立即停用。

Medicated Skin Washing Liquid

Name of Chinese Phonetic Alphabet Pi Fu Kang Xi Ye

Formula Lonicerae Japonicae Flos, Taraxaci Herba, Portulacae Herba, etc.

Actions and Indications Clearing heat and detoxicating, cooling blood and eliminating dampness, killing worms and relieving itching. It is indicated for eczema, manifested as itching, rashes, pimple, blister, erosion, or pruritus vulvae, profuse vaginal discharge due to downward attack of dampness-heat, or for acute eczema or vaginitis with the above mentioned symptoms.

Warning Only for external use; for cases with allergic reaction, suspend the preparation immediately.

六画

地榆槐角丸

【处方】大黄、黄芩、地黄、槐角（蜜炙）、当归、赤芍、荆芥穗、枳壳（麸炒）、防风、红花、槐花（炒）、地榆（炭）。

【功能主治】疏风凉血，解热润燥。用于脏腑实热，大肠火盛，肠风便血，痔疮漏疮，湿热便秘，肛门肿痛。

【注意】忌食辛辣。孕妇忌服。

Burnet Bloodwort★ and Japanese Pagodatree★★ Bolus

Name of Chinese Phonetic Alphabet Di Yu Huai Jiao Wan

Formula Rhei Radix et Rhizoma, Scutellariae Radix, Rehmanniae Radix, Sophorae Fructus (preapared with honey), Angelicae Sinensis Radix, Paeoniae Radix Rubra, Schizonepetae Spica, Aurantii Fructus (fried with bran), Saposhnikoviae Radix, Carthami Flos, Sophorae Flos (fried) and Sanguisorbae Radix (carbonated).

Actions and Indications Dispersing wind, cooling blood, releasing heat, moistening dryness. It is used for fresh blood in stool, hemorrhoid and anal fistula due to excessive heat of large intestine; constipation of damp-heat type, swelling and pain of anus.

Warning It is contraindicated for pregnant women. Pungent foods should be avoided.

* 地榆 ** 槐

朴沉化郁丸

【处方】香附（醋制）、延胡索（醋制）、枳壳（麸炒）、檀香、木香、片姜黄、柴胡、厚朴（姜制）、丁香、沉香、高良姜、青皮（醋制）、陈皮、甘草、豆蔻、莪术（醋制）、砂仁、肉桂。

【功能主治】舒肝化瘀，开胃消食。用于胸腹胀满，消化不良，呕吐恶心，气滞闷郁，胃脘刺痛。

【注意】孕妇遵医嘱服用。

Magnolia Bark* and Chinese Eaglewood** Bolus for Relieving Dyspepsia

Name of Chinese Phonetic Alphabet Po Chen Hua Yu Wan

Formula Cyperi Rhizoma (prepared with vinegar), Corydalis Rhizoma (prepared with vinegar), Aurantii Fructus (fried with bran), Santali Albi Lignum, Aucklandiae Radix, Wenyujin Rhizoma Concisum, Bupleuri Radix, Magnoliae Officinalis Cortex (prepared with ginger), Caryophylli Flos, Aquilariae Lignum Resinatum, Alpiniae Officinarum Rhizoma, Citri Reticulatae Pericarpium Viride (prepared with vinegar), Citri Reticulatae Pericarpium, Glycyrrhizae Radix et Rhizoma, Amomi Fructus Rotundus, Curcumae Rhizoma (prepared with vinegar), Amomi Fructus and Cinnamomi Cortex

Actions and Indications Soothing the liver, resolving stasis, promoting appetite and digestion. It is used for fullness of chest and abdomen, dyspepsia, vomiting, nausea, depression due to stagnation of *qi*; stabbing pain in stomach duct.

Warning The pregnant women should follow the physician's advice.

* 厚朴 ** 沉香

芒果止咳片

【处方】芒果叶干浸膏、合成鱼腥草素、扑尔敏。

【功能主治】宣肺化痰，止咳平喘。用于咳嗽，气喘，多痰。

Tablet of Mango* for Relieving Cough

Name of Chinese Phonetic Alphabet Mang Guo Zhi Ke Pian

Formula Mangiferae Indicae Folium Extractum, Synthetic Houttuynine and Chlorpheniramine.

Actions and Indications Diffusing the lung and resolving phlegm, relieving cough and calming dyspnea. It is indicated for cough, dyspnea and profuse phlegm.

* 芒果

芎菊上清丸

【处方】川芎、菊花、黄芩、栀子、蔓荆子（炒）、黄连、薄荷、连翘、荆芥穗、羌活、藁本、桔梗、防风、甘草、白芷。

【功能主治】清热解表，散风止痛。用于外感风邪引起的恶风身热，偏正头痛，鼻流清涕，牙疼，喉痛。

【注意】体虚者慎用。

Chuanxiong Ligusticum* and Chrysanthemum** Pill

Name of Chinese Phonetic Alphabet Xiong Ju Shang Qing Wan

Formula Chuanxiong Rhizoma, Chrysanthemi Flos, Scutellariae Radix, Gardeniae Fructus, Viticis Fructus (fried), Coptidis Rhizoma, Menthae Haplocalycis Herba, Forsythiae Fructus, Schizonepetae Spica, Notopterygii Rhizoma et Radix, Ligustici Rhizoma et Radix, Platycodonis Radix, Saposhnikoviae Radix, Glycyrrhizae Radix et Rhizoma and Angelicae Dahuricae Radix.

Actions and Indications Clearing heat and releasing the exterior, dispersing wind and relieving pain. It is indicated for aversion to wind with fever, migraine headache, clear nasal discharge, toothache and sore-throat due to exogenous wind.

Warning It should be used carefully for cases with physical debility.

* 川芎 ** 菊花

吉如心片

【处方】广枣提取物。

【功能主治】行气活血，养心安神。主治心血瘀阻型胸痹，症见胸部刺痛、绞痛或胸部闷痛、胸闷弊气，心悸。用于治疗冠心病心绞痛及预防心绞痛发作。

Axillary Choerospondias* Tablet

Name of Chinese Phonetic Alphabet Ji Ru Xin Pian

Formula Choerospondiatis Fructus (extract).

Actions and Indications Moving *qi*, activating blood, nourishing the heart, tranquilizing the mind. It is used for chest impediment syndrome due to stagnation of heart-blood manifested as stabbing pain in chest, colicky pain, chest distress and palpitation. The preparation is suitable for coronary heart disease, angina pectoris and also used for preventing the paroxysm of angina pectoris.

* 广枣

老蔻丸

【处方】豆蔻、砂仁、肉桂、丁香、当归、川芎、山楂（炒）、六神曲（炒）、白术（麸炒）、甘草、青皮（醋制）、陈皮、乌药、莱菔子（炒）、大黄（酒蒸）、牵牛子（炒）、木香、枳壳（麸炒）、厚朴（姜制）、三棱（醋制）、莪术（醋制）、清半夏、草果、槟榔（炒）。

【功能主治】开郁舒气，温胃消食。用于肝郁气滞，饮食不消，腹闷胀饱，胃脘疼痛偏胃寒型。

【注意】孕妇忌服，忌食生冷食物油腻。

Krervanh* Bolus

Name of Chinese Phonetic Alphabet Lao Kou Wan

Formula Amomi Fructus Rotundus, Amomi Fructus, Cinnamomi Cortex, Caryophylli Flos, Angelicae Sinensis Radix, Chuanxiong Rhizoma, Crataegi Fructus (fried), Medicata Massa Fermentata (fried), Atractylodis Macrocephalae Rhizoma (fried with bran), Glycyrrhizae Radix et Rhizoma, Citri Reticulatae Pericarpium Viride (prepared with vinegar), Citri Reticulate Pericarpium, Linderae Radix, Raphani Semen (fried), Rhei Radix et Rhizoma (steamed by wine), Pharbitidis Semen (fried), Aucklandiae Radix, Aurantii Fructus (fried with bran), Magnoliae Officinalis Cortex (prepared with ginger), Sparganii Rhizoma (prepared with ginger), Curcumae Rhizoma (prepared with vinegar), Pinelliae Rhizoma Praeparatum cum Alumine, Tsaoko Fructus and Arecae Semen (fried).

Actions and Indications Relieving depression, soothing *qi*, warming the stomach to promote digestion. It is used for dyspepsia, abdominal fullness and pain in stomach duct due to stagnation of liver-*qi*.

Warning It is contraindicated for pregnant women; uncooked, cold and oily foods should be avoided.

* 豆蔻

西瓜霜润喉片

【处方】西瓜霜、冰片、薄荷油、薄荷脑。

【功能主治】清音利咽，消肿止痛。用于咽喉肿痛，声音嘶哑，喉痹，喉痈，口舌生疮，牙痈，急、慢性咽喉炎，扁桃体炎，口腔溃疡，口腔炎，牙龈肿痛等上呼吸道及口腔疾病。

Watermelon Mirabilite* Tablet for Throat-soothing

Name of Chinese Phonetic Alphabet Xi Gua Shuang Run Hou Pian

Formula Marabilitum Praeparatum, Borneolum Syntheticum, Menthae Haplocalycis Oleum and Menthol.

Actions and Indications Soothing the throat, dispersing swelling and relieving pain. It is indicated for sore-throat, hoarseness, throat abscess, aphthae, gingival abscess, acute and chronic laryngopharyngitis, tonsillitis, oral ulcer, stomatitis, gingivitis, upper respiratory tract and oral diseases.

* 西瓜霜

西红多苷片

【处方】西红花提取物。

【功能主治】活血化瘀，通脉止痛。用于胸痹心痛，症见胸痛，胸闷，憋气，舌紫或有瘀点、瘀斑。

Saffron* Tablet

Name of Chinese Phonetic Alphabet Xi Hong Duo Gan Pian

Formula Croci Stigma (extract).

Actions and Indications Activating blood, resolving stasis, dredging vessels, alleviating pain. It is indicated for cardialgia manifested as chest pain, depression of chest, suffocated feeling, purple tongue body or spots or patches on the tongue.

* 西红花

西黄丸

【处方】牛黄、麝香、乳香（醋制）、没药（醋制）。

【功能主治】清热解毒，和营消肿。用于痈疽疔毒，瘰疬，流注，癌肿。

【注意】孕妇忌服。

Xi Huang Pill

Name of Chinese Phonetic Alphabet Xi Huang Wan

Formula Bovis Calculus, Moschus, Olibanum (prepared with vinegar) and Myrrha (prepared with vinegar).

Actions and Indications Clearing heat and detoxicating, harmonizing the nutrient and dispersing swelling. It is used for deep-rooted boil, scrofula, deep multiple abscess, cancer.

Warning It is contraindicated for pregnant women.

西黄清醒丸

【处方】藏青果、黄芩、金果榄、栀子、防己、槟榔、木香、甘草、薄荷、冰片。

【功能主治】清利咽喉，解热除烦。用于肺胃蕴热引起的口苦舌燥，咽喉肿痛，烦躁不安，气滞胸满，头晕耳鸣。

【注意】忌食辛辣厚味。

Myrobalan* and Baical Skullcap** Bolus

Name of Chinese Phonetic Alphabet Xi Huang Qing Xing Wan

Formula Chebulae Fructus, Scutellariae Radix, Tinosporae Radix, Gardeniae Fructus, Stephaniae Tetrandrae Radix, Arecae Semen, Aucklandiae Radix, Glycyrrhizae Radix et Rhizoma, Menthae Haplocalycis Herba and Borneolum Syntheticum.

Actions and Indications Soothing the throat, clearing heat, relieving vexation. It is used for bitter taste in the mouth, dry tongue, sore-throat, vexation, restlessness, chest distress, dizziness and tinnitus due to heat accumulation in the lung and stomach.

Warning Pungent and fat foods are prohibited.

* 藏青果 ** 黄芩

再造丸

【处方】蕲蛇肉、全蝎、地龙、穿山甲（制）、豹骨（制）、牛黄、麝香、水牛角浓缩粉、僵蚕（炒）、防风、朱砂、天麻、龟甲（制）、羌活、白芷、川芎、附子（制）、葛根、麻黄、桑寄生、油松节、细辛、肉桂、粉萆薢、威灵仙（酒炒）、当归、赤芍、片姜黄、乳香（制）、血竭、三七、天竺黄、没药（制）、人参、黄芪、白术（炒）、骨碎补（炒）、茯苓、甘草、何首乌（制）、熟地黄、玄参、黄连、草豆蔻、化橘红、沉香、檀香、两头尖（醋制）、广藿香、冰片、乌药、母丁香、青皮（醋炒）、豆蔻、大黄、香附（醋制）、六神曲、红曲。

【功能主治】祛风化痰，活血通络。用于中风，口眼歪斜，半身不遂，手足麻木，疼痛拘挛，语言謇涩。

【注意】孕妇禁用。

Zai Zao Bolus for Apoplexy

Name of Chinese Phonetic Alphabet Zai Zao Wan

Formula Agkistrodon Caro, Scorpio, Pheretima, Manis Squma (prepared), Pardi Os (prepaned), Bovis Calculus, Moschus, Bubali Cornu Pulvis Concentratio, Bombyx Batryticatus (fried), Saposhnikoviae Radix, Cinnabaris, Gastrodiae Rhizoma, Testudinis Carapax et Plastrum (prepared), Notopterygii Rhizoma et Radix, Angelicae Dahuricae Radix, Chuanxiong Rhizoma, Aconiti Lateralis Radix Praeparata, Puerariae Lobatae Radix, Ephedrae Herba, Taxilli Herba, Pini Lignum Nodi , Asari Radix et Rhizoma, Cinnamomi Cortex, Dioscoreae Hypoglaucae Rhizoma, Clematidis Radix et Rhizoma (fried with wine), Angelicae Sinensis Radix, Paeoniae Radix Rubra, Wenyujin Rhizoma Concisum, Olibanum (prepared), Draconis Sanguis, Notoginseng Radix et Rhizoma, Bambusae Concretio Silicea, Myrrha (prepared), Ginseng Radix et Rhizoma, Astragali Radix, Atractylodis Macrocephalae Rhizoma (fried), Drynariae Rhizoma (fried), Poria, Glycyrrhizae Radix et Rhizoma, Polygoni Multiflori Radix (prepared), Rehmanniae Radix Praeparata, Scrophulariae Radix, Coptidis Rhizoma, Alpiniae Katsumadai Semen, Citri Grandis Exocarpium, Aquilariae Lignum Resinatum, Santali Albi Lignum, Anemones Raddeanae Rhizoma (prepared with vinegar), Pogostemonis Herba, Borneolum Syntheticum, Linderae Radix, Caryophylli Fructus, Citri Reticulatae Pericarpium Viride (prepared with vinegar), Amomi Fructus Rotundus, Rhei Radix et Rhizoma, Cyperi Rhizoma (prepared with vinegar), Medicata Massa Fermentata and Oryzae Fructus Monascus.

Actions and Indications Dispelling wind, resolving phlegm, activating blood, dredging collaterals. It is used for apoplexy, deviated mouth and eyes, hemiparalysis, numbness, pain and spasm of limbs, dysphasia.

Warning It is contraindicated for pregnant women.

再障生血片

【处方】菟丝子（酒制）、红参、鸡血藤、阿胶、当归、女贞子、黄芪。

【功能主治】补肝健脾，益气养血。用于肝肾不足，气血亏虚所致的再生障碍性贫血。

Relieving Aplastic Anemia Tablet

Name of Chinese Phonetic Alphabet Zai Zhang Sheng Xue Pian

Formula Cuscutae Semen (prepared with wine), Ginseng Radix et Rhizoma Rubra, Spatholobi Caulis, Asini Corii Colla, Angelicae Sinensis Radix, Ligustri Lucidi Fructus and Astragali Radix.

Actions and Indications Tonifying the liver, fortifying the spleen, tonifying *qi* and nourishing blood. It is indicated for aplastic anemia due to dual insufficiency of the liver and kidney and dual depletion of *qi* and blood.

耳聋丸

【处方】龙胆、黄芩、地黄、泽泻、关木通、栀子、当归、九节菖蒲、甘草、羚羊角。

【功能主治】清肝泻火，利湿通窍。用于上焦湿热，头晕头痛，耳聋耳鸣，耳内流脓。

Improving Audition Bolus

Name of Chinese Phonetic Alphabet Er Long Wan

Formula Gentianae Radix et Rhizoma, Scutellariae Radix, Rehmanniae Radix, Alismatis Rhizoma, Aristochiae Manshuriensis Caulis, Gardeniae Fructus, Angelicae Sinensis Radix, Anemones Altaicae Rhizoma, Glycyrrhizae Radix et Rhizoma and Saigae Tataricae Cornu.

Actions and Indications Clearing liver-fire,

draining dampness and dredging the orifices. It is used for dizziness, headache, dysaudia, tinnitus and otopyosis due to damp-heat of upper energizer.

耳聋左慈丸

【处方】磁石（煅）、熟地黄、山茱萸（制）、牡丹皮、山药、茯苓、泽泻、竹叶、柴胡。

【功能主治】滋肾平肝。用于肝肾阴虚，耳鸣耳聋，头晕目眩。

Magnetite* Bolus for Dysaudia

Name of Chinese Phonetic Alphabet Er Long Zuo Ci Wan

Formula Magnetitum (calcined), Rehmanniae Radix Pracparata, Corni Fructus (prepared), Moutan Cortex, Dioscoreae Rhizoma, Poria, Alismatis Rhizoma and Bupleuri Radix.

Actions and Indications Enriching the kidney, pacifying the liver. It is indicated for tinnitus, dysaudia, dizziness and dizzy vision due to dual *yin*-deficiency of the liver and kidney.

*磁石

百令胶囊

【处方】本品为发酵虫草菌粉制成的胶囊。

【功能主治】补肺肾，益精气。用于肺肾两虚引起的咳嗽、气喘、咯血、腰背酸痛及慢性支气管炎的辅助治疗。

Bailing Capsule

Name of Chinese Phonetic Alphabet Bai Ling Jiao Nang

Formula Cordyceps Fungus Pulvis.

Actions and Indications Tonifying the lung and kidney and replenishing essence and *qi*. It is indicated for cough, dyspnea, hemoptysis, aching pain of the waist and back due to dual deficiency of the lung and kidney; and also used for chronic bronchitis.

百合固金口服液

【处方】百合、熟地黄、麦冬、川贝母、玄参、地黄、当归、白芍、桔梗、甘草。

【功能主治】养阴润肺，祛痰止咳。治疗肺肾阴虚、虚火上炎、热伤肺络出现的咳嗽气喘，呛咳少痰，咳痰带血，咽喉干痛，音哑，潮热盗汗，五心烦热，胸闷气短，便干尿赤，舌红苔少，脉弦细数。

Lily Bulb* Oral Liquid

Name of Chinese Phonetic Alphabet Bai He Gu Jin Kou Fu Ye

Formula Lilii Bulbus, Rehmanniae Radix Praeparata, Ophiopogonis Radix, Fritillariae Cirrhosae Bulbus, Scrophulariae Radix, Rehmanniae Radix, Angelicae Sinensis Radix, Paeoniae Radix Alba, Platycodonis Radix and Glycyrrhizae Radix et Rhizoma.

Actions and Indications Nourishing *yin*, moistening the lung, dispelling phlegm, relieving cough. It is used for cough and dyspnea with few productive and blood-stained phlegm, sore-throat, dysphasia, tidal fever, night sweating, vexing heat in the chest, palms and soles, chest distress, shortness of breath, dry stool, brown urine, red tongue with few fur, string-like, fine and rapid pulse.

*百合

百补增力丸

【处方】六神曲（麸炒）、陈皮、白芍、麦芽、苍术（米泔水炒）、谷芽（炒）、山楂、枳壳、法半夏、川芎、厚朴（姜制）、香附（醋炒）、茯苓、甘草、鹿角霜、泽泻、人参、大黄（炭）、棕榈（炭）、山药、附子、荷叶、栀子（姜制）、侧柏叶（炭）、山茱萸（酒制）、当归、大蓟、小蓟、白茅根、牡丹皮、白术（麸炒）、肉桂、茜草、紫河车、黄芪（蜜炙）、黄芩、党参。

【功能主治】开胃健脾，益气养血。用于肾水不足，脾胃失和引起的自汗盗汗，腰腿疼痛，精神疲倦，劳伤过度，咳嗽咯血，食欲不振，消化不良。

Spleen-fortifying and Stomach-harmonizing Pill

Name of Chinese Phonetic Alphabet Bai Bu Zeng Li Wan

Formula Medicata Massa Fermentata (fried with bran), Citri Reticulatae Pericarpium, Paeoniae Radix Alba, Hordei Fructus Germinatus, Atractylodis Rhizoma (fried with rice swilled water), Setariae Fructus Germinatus (fried), Crataegi Fructus, Aurantii Fructus, Pinelliae Rhizoma Praeparatum, Chuanxiong Rhizoma, Magnoliae Officinallis Cortex (prepared with ginger), Cyperi Rhizoma (fried with vinegar), Poria, Glycyrrhizae Radix et Rhizoma, Cervi Cornu Degelatinatum, Alismatis Rhizoma, Ginseng Radix et Rhizoma, Rhei Radix et Rhizoma (carbonated), Trachycarpi Petiolus Carbonisatus, Dioscoreae Rhizoma, Aconiti Lateralis Radix Praeparata, Nelumbinis Folium, Gardeniae Fructus (prepared with ginger), Platycladi Cacumen (carbonated), Corni Fructus (prepared with wine), Angelicae Sinensis Radix, Cirsii Japonici Herba, Cirsii Herba, Imperatae Rhizoma, Moutan Cortex, Atractylodis Macrocephalae Rhizoma (fried with bran), Cinnamomi Cortex, Rubiae Radix, Hominis Placenta, Astragali Radix (prepared with honey), Scutellariae Radix and Codonopsis Radix.

Actions and Indications Increasing appetite, fortifying the spleen, tonifying *qi* and nourishing blood. It is used for spontaneous sweating, night sweating, pain of waist and legs, lassitude of spirit, overexertion, cough, hemoptysis, poor appetite and dyspepsia due to insufficiency of kidney-fluid and disharmony of the spleen and stomach.

百咳静糖浆

【处方】陈皮、麦冬、前胡、苦杏仁（炒）、清半夏、黄芩、百部（蜜炙）、黄柏、桑白皮、甘草、麻黄（蜜炙）、葶苈子（炒）、紫苏子（炒）、天南星（炒）、桔梗、瓜蒌子（炒）。

【功能主治】清热化痰、平喘止咳。用于百日咳，感冒及急、慢性气管炎引起的咳嗽。

Syrup for Relieving Cough

Name of Chinese Phonetic Alphabet Bai Ke Jing Tang Jiang

Formula Citri Reticulatae Pericarpium, Ophiopogonis Radix, Peucedani Radix, Armeniacae Semen Amarum (fried), Pinelliae Rhizoma Praeparatum cum Alumine, Scutellariae Radix, Stemonae Radix (prepared with honey), Phellodendri Chinensis Cortex, Mori Cortex, Glycyrrhizae Radix et Rhizoma, Ephedrae Herba (prepared with honey), Lepidii Semen (fried), Perillae Fructus (fried), Arisaematis Rhizoma (fried), Platycodonis Radix and Trichosanthis Semen (fried).

Actions and Indications Clearing heat and resolving phlegm, calming dyspnea and relieving cough. It is indicated for cough due to pertussis, common cold, and acute, chronic bronchitis.

至圣保元丸

【处方】胆南星（酒炙）、僵蚕（麸炒）、全蝎、蜈蚣、猪牙皂、天麻、天竺黄、青礞石（煅）、钩藤、羌活、防风、麻黄、薄荷、陈皮、茯苓、甘草、琥珀粉、牛黄、冰片、珍珠、朱砂。

【功能主治】祛风化痰，解热镇惊。用于小儿痰热内闭，外感风寒，身热面赤，咳嗽痰盛，气粗喘促以及风热急惊。

Holy Pill for Chidren

Name of Chinese Phonetic Alphabet Zhi Sheng Bao Yuan Wan

Formula Arisaema cum Bile (prepared with wine), Bombyx Batryticatus (fried with bran), Scorpio, Scolopendra, Fructus Gleditsiae Abnormalis, Gastrodiae Rhizoma, Bambusae Concretio Silicea, Chloriti Lapis (calcined), Uncariae Ramulus cum Uncis, Notopterygii Rhizoma et Radix, Saposhnikoviae Radix, Ephedrae Herba, Menthae Haplocalycis Herba, Citri Reticulatae Pericarpium, Poria, Glycyrrhizae Radix et Rhizoma, Succini Pulvis, Bovis Calculus, Borneolum Syntheticum, Margarita and Cinnabaris.

Actions and Indications Dispelling wind and resolving phlegm, releasing heat and settling fright. It is indicated for infant with manifestations as generalized fever, flushed complexion, productive cough, and acute convulsion due to internal blockage of phlegm-heat and exogenous wind-heat.

至灵胶囊

【处方】本品为由冬虫夏草幼虫分离的孢霉属真菌经人工培养发酵的菌丝体加工制成的胶囊。

【功能主治】补肺益肾。用于肺肾两虚所致咳喘、浮肿，亦可用于各类肾病、慢性支气管哮喘、慢性肝炎及肿瘤的辅助治疗。

Mycelium Mortierellae Capsule

Name of Chinese Phonetic Alphabet Zhi Ling Jiao Nang

Formula Mortierellae (fungus) Mycelium.

Actions and Indications Tonifying the lung and kidney. It is indicated for cough, dyspnea and edema due to dual deficiency of the lung and kidney, also applied for various nephroses, chronic bronchial asthma, chronic hepatitis and supplementary treatment of tumor.

贞芪扶正胶囊

【处方】女贞子、黄芪等。

【功能主治】补气养阴。用于久病虚损，气阴不足。配合手术、放疗、化疗，促进正常功能的恢复。

Chinese Privet* and Milkvetch** Capsule

Name of Chinese Phonetic Alphabet Zhen Qi Fu Zheng Jiao Nang

Formula Ligustri Lucidi Fructus, Astragali Radix, etc.

Actions and Indications Tonifying *qi* and nourishing *yin*. It is used for consumptive disease due to dual insufficiency of *qi* and *yin*. Also used for promoting the recovery of normal function of patients from operation, radiotherapy and chemotherapy.

* 女贞 ** 黄芪

当飞利肝宁胶囊

【处方】水飞蓟、当药。

【功能主治】清利湿热，益肝退黄。用于黄疸，急性黄疸型肝炎，传染性肝炎，慢性肝炎。

Diluted Swertia* and Blessed Thistle** Capsule for Relieving Hepatitis

Name of Chinese Phonetic Alphabet Dang Fei Li Gan Ning Jiao Nang

Formula Silybi Fructus and Swertiae Herba.

Actions and Indications Clearing and draining dampness and heat, nourishing the liver and relieving jaundice. It is indicated for jaundice, acute icteric hepatitis, infective hepatitis and chronic hepatitis.

* 当药 ** 水飞蓟

当归龙荟丸

【处方】当归（酒炒）、龙胆（酒炒）、芦荟、青黛、栀子、黄连（酒炒）、黄芩（酒炒）、黄柏（盐炒）、大黄（酒炒）、木香、麝香。

【功能主治】泻火通便。用于肝胆火旺，心烦不宁，头晕目眩，耳鸣耳聋，胁肋疼痛，大便秘结。

【注意】孕妇禁用。

Chinese Angelica* Scabrous Gentian** and Cape Aloe*** Bolus

Name of Chinese Phonetic Alphabet Dang Gui Long Hui Wan

Formula Angelicae Sinensis Radix (prepared with wine), Gentianae Radix et Rhizoma (prepared with wine), Aloe, Indigo Naturalis, Gardeniae Fructus, Coptidis Rhizoma (prepared with wine), Scutellariae Radix (prepared with wine), Phellodendri Chinensis Cortex (fried with salt), Rhei Radix et Rhizoma (prepared with wine), Aucklandiae Radix and Moschus.

Actions and Indications Purging fire and relaxing the bowels. It is indicated for vexation, dizziness, dizzy vision, tinnitus, deafness, hypochondriac pain and constipation due to effulgent fire of the liver and gallbladder.

Warning It is contraindicated for pregnant women.

* 当归 ** 龙胆 *** 芦荟

当归补血胶囊

【处方】当归、黄芪。

【功能主治】补养气血。用于身体虚弱，气血两亏者。

Chinese Angelica* Capsule for Tonifying Blood

Name of Chinese Phonetic Alphabet Dang Gui Bu Xue Jiao Nang

Formula Angelicae Sinensis Radix and Astragali Radix.

Actions and Indications Tonifying *qi* and blood. It is indicated for general debility due to dual depletion of *qi* and blood.

* 当归

当归苦参丸

【处方】当归、苦参。

【功能主治】凉血、祛湿。用于血燥湿热引起的粉刺疙瘩，湿疹刺痒，酒渣鼻等。

【注意】忌烟、酒及辛辣物。

Chinese Angelica* and Shrubby Sophora** Bolus

Name of Chinese Phonetic Alphabet Dang Gui Ku Shen Wan

Formula Angelicae Sinensis Radix and Sophorae Flavescentis Radix.

Actions and Indications Cooling blood and dispelling dampness. It is indicated for comedo, eczema, itching, brandy nose due to blood-dryness and damp-heat.

Warning Cigarette, wine and pungent foods are prohibited.

* 当归 ** 苦参

当归拈痛丸

【处方】当归、葛根、党参、苍术（炒）、升麻、苦参、泽泻、白术（炒）、知母、防风、羌活、黄芩、猪苓、茵陈、甘草。

【功能主治】清热利湿，祛风止痛。用于风湿阻络，骨节疼痛，湿热下注，足胫红肿热痛，或溃破流脓水者。

Chinese Angelica* Pill for Relieving Pain

Name of Chinese Phonetic Alphabet Dang Gui Nian Tong Wan

Formula Angelicae Sinensis Radix, Puerariae Lobatae Radix, Codonopsis Radix, Atractylodis Rhizoma (fried), Cimicifugae Rhizoma, Sophorae Flavescentis Radix, Alismatis Rhizoma, Atractylodis Macrocephalae Rhizoma (fried), Anemarrhenae Rhizoma, Saposhnikoviae Radix, Notopterygii Rhizoma et Radix, Scutellariae Radix, Polyporus, Artemisiae Scopariae Herba and Glycyrrhizae Radix et Rhizoma.

Actions and Indications Clearing heat and draining dampness, dispelling wind and alleviating pain. It is indicated for ostealgia, red, swelling and pain of the feet and diabrotic sore with pus due to wind-damp obstructing collaterals or downward attack of damp-heat.

* 当归

当归养血丸

【处方】当归、白芍（炒）、地黄、黄芪（蜜炙）、阿胶、牡丹皮、香附（制）、茯苓、杜仲（炒）、白术（炒）。

【功能主治】养血调经。用于气血两虚，月经不调。

Chinese Angelica★ Bolus for Tonifying Blood

Name of Chinese Phonetic Alphabet Dang Gui Yang Xue Wan

Formula Angelicae Sinensis Radix, Paeoniae Radix Alba (fried), Rehmanniae Radix, Astragali Radix (prepared with honey), Asini Corii Colla, Moutan Cortex, Cyperi Rhizoma (prepared), Poria, Eucommiae Cortex (fried) and Atractylodis Macrocephalae Rhizoma (fried).

Actions and Indications Tonifying blood to regulate menstruation. It is indicated for irregular menstruation due to dual deficiency of *qi* and blood.

* 当归

同仁大活络丸

【处方】蕲蛇（酒制）、乌梢蛇（酒制）、豹骨（制）、威灵仙（酒制）、全蝎、僵蚕（麸炒）、附子（制）、两头尖（醋制）、草乌（炙）、天麻、麻黄、何首乌（黑豆酒制）、羌活、细辛、防风、水牛角浓缩粉、官桂、丁香、赤芍、血竭、甘草、乳香（醋制）、地龙、龟甲（醋淬）、当归、熟地黄、白术（炒）、没药（醋制）、骨碎补、茯苓、玄参、青皮（醋制）、人参、绵马贯众、广藿香、香附（醋制）、沉香、熟大黄、豆蔻、天南星（制）、黄芩、葛根、松香（制）、黄连、乌药、木香、牛黄、安息香、冰片、麝香。

【功能主治】祛风，舒筋，活络，除湿。用于风寒湿痹引起的肢体疼痛，手足麻木，筋脉拘挛，中风瘫痪，口眼歪斜，半身不遂，语言不清。

【注意】孕妇忌服。

Tongren Bolus for Activating Collaterals

Name of Chinese Phonetic Alphabet Tong Ren Da Huo Luo Wan

Formula Agkistrodon (prepared with wine), Zaocys (prepared with wine), Pardi Os (prepared), Clematidis Radix et Rhizoma (prepared with wine), Scorpio, Bombyx Batryticatus (fried with bran), Aconiti Lateralis Radix Praeparata, Anemones Raddeanae Rhizoma (prepared with vinegar), Aconiti Kusnezoffii Radix (prepared), Gastrodiae Rhizoma, Ephedrae Herba, Polygoni Multiflori Radix (prepared with wine), Notopterygii Rhizoma et Radix, Asari Radix et Rhizoma, Saposhnikoviae Radix, Bubali Cornu Pulvis Concentratio, Cinnamomi Cortex, Caryophylli Flos, Paeoniae Radix Rubra, Draconis Sanguis, Glycyrrhizae Radix et Rhizoma, Olibanum (prepared with vinegar), Pheretima, Testudinis Carapax et Plastrum (quenched by vinegar), Angelicae Sinensis Radix, Rehmanniae Radix Praeparata, Atractylodis Macrocephalae Rhizoma (fried), Myrrha (prepared with vinegar), Drynariae Rhizoma, Poria, Scrophulariae Radix, Citri Reticulatae Pericarpium Viride (prepared with vinegar), Ginseng Radix et Rhizoma, Dryopteridis Crassirhizomatis Rhizoma, Pogostemonis Herba, Cyperi Rhizoma (prepared with vinegar), Aquilariae Lignum Resinatum, Rhei Radix et Rhizoma, Amomi Fructus Rotundus, Arisaematis Rhizoma (prepared), Scutellariae Radix, Puerariae Lobatae Radix, Pini Resina (prepared), Coptidis Rhizoma, Linderae Radix, Aucklandiae Radix, Bovis Calculus, Benzoinum, Borneolum Syntheticum and Moschus.

Actions and Indications Dispelling wind, relaxing sinews, activating collaterals, eliminating dampness. It is used for pain and numbness of limbs, mascular spasm, apoplexy, paralysis, deviated eyes and mouth, hemiparalysis and alalia due to wind-cold-damp impediment.

Warning It is contraindicated for pregnant women.

同仁牛黄清心丸

【处方】当归、川芎、甘草、山药、黄芩、白芍、麦冬、白术（麸炒）、六神曲（麸炒）、蒲黄（炒）、大枣（去核）、阿胶、茯苓、人参、防风、干姜、柴胡、肉桂、白蔹、桔梗、大豆黄卷、苦杏仁（炒）、牛黄、麝香、水牛角浓缩粉、羚羊角、冰片。

【功能主治】益气养血，镇惊安神，化痰息风。用于气血不足，痰热上扰引起的胸中郁热，惊悸虚烦，头目眩晕，中风不语，口眼歪斜，半身不遂，言语不清，神志昏迷，痰涎壅盛。

【注意】孕妇慎用。

Tongren Pill of Bezoar*

Name of Chinese Phonetic Alphabet Tong Ren Niu Huang Qing Xin Wan

Formula Angelicae Sinensis Radix, Chuanxiong Rhizoma, Glycyrrhizae Radix et Rhizoma, Dioscoreae Rhizoma, Scutellariae Radix, Paeoniae Radix Alba, Ophiopogonis Radix, Atractylodis Macrocephalae Rhizoma (fried with bran), Medicata Massa Fermentata (fried with bran), Typhae Pollen (fried), Jujubae Fructus (removed nucleus), Asini Corii Colla, Poria, Ginseng Radix et Rhizoma, Saposhnikoviae Radix, Zingiberis Rhizoma, Bupleuri Radix, Cinnamomi Cortex, Ampelopsis Radix, Platycodonis Radix, Sojae Semen Germinatum, Armeniacae Semen Amarum (fried), Bovis Calculus, Moschus, Bubali Cornu Pulvis Concentratio, Saigae Tataricae Cornu and Borneolum Syntheticum.

Actions and Indications Tonifying *qi*, nourishing blood, settling fright, tranquilizing the mind, resolving phlegm and extinguishing wind. It is indicated for stagnant heat in the chest, fright, vexation, dizziness, dizzy vision, apoplectic dysphasia, deviated eyes and mouth, hemiplegia, alalia, coma and obstruction of phlegm due to dual insufficiency of *qi* and blood, phlegm-heat harassment upward.

Warning It should be used carefully for pregnant women.

* 牛黄

回生第一丹胶囊

【处方】当归、血竭、麝香、土鳖虫、朱砂、乳香（醋炙）、自然铜（煅醋淬）。

【功能主治】活血散瘀，消肿止痛。用于跌打损伤，伤筋动骨，皮肤青肿，血瘀疼痛。

【注意】孕妇忌服。

Hui Sheng Capsule for Traumatic Injury

Name of Chinese Phonetic Alphabet Hui Sheng Di Yi Dan Jiao Nang

Formula Angelicae Sinensis Radix, Draconis Sanguis, Moschus, Eupolyphaga seu Steleophaga, Cinnabaris, Olibanum (prepared with vinegar) and Pyritum (calcined and quenched by vinegar).

Actions and Indications Activating blood, dissipating stasis, reducing swelling, alleviating pain. It is used for traumatic injury marked by swelling, pain and blood-stasis.

Warning It is contraindicated for pregnant women.

回春如意胶囊

【处方】鹿茸、熟地黄、狗肾、锁阳、羊肾、菟丝子、山药、何首乌、槐角、巴戟天、枸杞子、肉苁蓉、黄精、黄芪、狗脊、补骨脂。

【功能主治】补血养血，助肾壮阳，益精生髓，强筋壮骨。用于头晕健忘，体虚乏力，肾虚耳鸣，腰膝酸痛，阳痿早泄。

Huichun Capsule for Tonifying Kidney

Name of Chinese Phonetic Alphabet Hui Chun Ru Yi Jiao Nang

Formula Cervi Cornu Pantotrichum, Rehmanniae Radix Praeparata, Canis Ren, Cynomorii Caulis Carnosus, Carprinus Testis, Cuscutae Semen, Dioscoreae Rhizoma, Polygoni Multiflori Radix, Sophorae Fructus, Morindae Officinalis Radix, Lycii Fructus, Cistanches Caulis Carnosus, Polygonati Rhizoma, Astragali Radix, Cibotii Rhizoma and Psoraleae Fructus.

Actions and Indications Tonifying blood, invigorating the kidney-*yang* and vital essence, strengthening the sinews and bone. It is used for dizziness, amnesia, fatigue, general debility, tinnitus, soreness and pain of waist and knees, impotence and ejaculation praecox.

朱砂安神丸

【处方】朱砂、黄连、地黄、当归、甘草。

【功能主治】清心养血，镇惊安神。用于胸中烦热，心悸不宁，失眠多梦。

Cinnabar* Bolus for Tranquilizing Mind

Name of Chinese Phonetic Alphabet Zhu Sha An Sheng Wan

Formula Cinnabaris, Coptidis Rhizoma, Rehmanniae Radix, Angelicae Sinensis Radix and Glycyrrhizae Radix et Rhizoma.

Actions and Indications Clearing heart-fire, nourishing blood, settling fright to tranquilize the mind. It is used for heat vexation in the chest, palpitation, restlessness, insomnia and profuse dreaming.

*朱砂

优福宁胶囊

【处方】本品为狼毒经提取加工制成的胶囊剂。

【功能主治】抗结核药。主治各型肺结核，也可用于其他结核，适用于对某些抗结核药过敏、耐药及合并肝病的结核病患者。

You Fu Ning Capsule for Relieving Tuberculosis

Name of Chinese Phonetic Alphabet You Fu Ning Jiao Nang

Formula Euphorbiae Ebracteolatae Radix (extract).

Actions and Indications Anti-tuberculosis. It is indicated for various pulmonary tuberculosis, also for cases with allergy of antituberculotic or drug resistance accompanied by liver diseases.

仲景胃灵片

【处方】肉桂、延胡索、牡蛎、小茴香、砂仁、高良姜、白芍、炙甘草。

【功能主治】温中散寒，健胃止痛。用于脾胃虚弱，食欲不振，寒凝胃痛，脘腹胀满，呕吐酸水或清水。

Zhongjing Fortifying Stomach Tablet

Name of Chinese Phonetic Alphabet Zhong Jing Wei Ling Pian

Formula Cinnamomi Cortex, Corydalis Rhizoma, Ostreae Concha, Foeniculi Fructus, Amomi Fructus, Alpiniae Officinarum Rhizoma, Paeoniae Radix Alba and Glycyrrhizae Radix et Rhizoma Praeparata cum Melle.

Actions and Indications Warming the middle and dissipating cold, fortifying the stomach and relieving pain. It is indicated for poor appetite, stomachache, abdominal distention and fullness, acid vomiting or watery vomiting due to dual deficiency of the spleen and stomach.

伤风停胶囊

【处方】麻黄、荆芥、白芷、苍术（炒）、陈皮、甘草。

【功能主治】发散风寒。用于外感风寒，恶寒发热，头痛，鼻塞，鼻流清涕，肢体酸重，喉痒咳嗽，咳嗽痰清稀，舌质淡红，苔薄白，脉浮紧，以及上呼吸道感染、鼻炎等见上述证候者。

Relieving Common Cold Capsule

Name of Chinese Phonetic Alphabet Shang Feng Ting Jiao Nang

Formula Ephedrae Herba, Schizonepetae Herba, Angelicae Dahuricae Radix, Atractylodis Rhizoma (fried), Citri Reticulatae Pericarpium and Glycyrrhizae Radix et Rhizoma.

Actions and Indications Dispersing wind-cold. It is indicated for common cold, marked by aversion to cold, fever, headache, nasal congestion, clear nasal discharge, aching and heavy sensation of limbs, itch-throat and cough, thin phlegm, pale red tongue, thin-white tongue fur, superficial and tight pulse due to external contraction of wind-cold and also used for upper respiratory infection and rhinitis with the above mentioned symptoms.

伤疖膏

【处方】黄芩、连翘、生天南星、白芷、冰片、薄荷脑、水杨酸甲酯。

【功能主治】清热，解毒，消肿，镇痛。用于各种疖痛脓肿，乳腺炎、静脉炎及其他皮肤创伤。

【注意】皮肤如有过敏现象可停用。

Medicated Adhesive Plaster for Settling Pain

Name of Chinese Phonetic Alphabet Shang Jie Gao

Formula Scutellariae Radix, Forsythiae Fructus, Arisaematis Rhizoma (raw), Angelicae Dauricae Radix, Borneolum Syntheticum, Menthol and Methyl Salicylate.

Actions and Indications Clearing heat and detoxicating, dispersing swelling and settling pain. It is used for furuncle and abscess with swelling and pain, mastitis, phlebitis and skin injury.

Warning In case of allergic reaction, suspend the application.

伤科接骨片

【处方】红花、三七、没药（炙）、冰片、海星（炙）、鸡骨（炙）、土鳖虫、朱砂、马钱子粉、自然铜（煅）、乳香（炙）、甜瓜子。

【功能主治】活血化瘀，消肿止痛，舒筋壮骨。用于跌打损伤，闪腰岔气，伤筋动骨，瘀血肿痛，损伤红肿。对骨折患者需经复位后配合使用。

【注意】孕妇忌服；10岁以下儿童禁服。

Bone-knitting Tablet

Name of Chinese Phonetic Alphabet Shang Ke Jie Gu Pian

Formula Carthami Flos, Notoginseng Radix et Rhizoma, Myrrha (prepared), Borneolum Syntheticum, Asterias (prepared), Galli Os (prepared), Eupolyphaga seu Steleophaga, Cinnabaris, Strychni Semen Pulvis, Pyritum (calcined), Olibanum (prepared) and Melo Semen.

Actions and Indications Activating blood, resolving stasis, reducing swelling, alleviating pain, relaxing sinews, strengthening bone. It is used for traumatic injury, sudden lumbar sprain, swelling and blood-stasis. The preparation is also used as associated treatment for reposition of fracture.

Warning It is contraindicated for pregnant women and children under 10 years old.

伤痛宁膏

【处方】黄柏、红花、延胡索、白芷、儿茶、樟脑、薄荷脑、冰片、水杨酸甲酯。

【功能主治】活血散瘀，消肿止痛。用于关节扭伤，肌肉拉伤，韧带挨伤等急性软组织损伤。

【注意】凡对橡胶膏过敏或皮肤糜烂、破裂者不宜贴用。孕妇慎用，腰部忌用。

Traumatic Pain Alleviating Adhesive Plaster

Name of Chinese Phonetic Alphabet Shang Tong Ning Gao

Formula Phellodendri Chinensis Cortex, Carthami Flos, Corydalis Rhizoma, Angelicae Dahuricae Radix, Catechu, Camphora, Menthol, Borneolum Syntheticum and Methyl Salicylate.

Actions and Indications Activating blood, dissipating stasis, reducing swelling, alleviating pain. It is used for traumatic sprain of joints, muscle injury due to traction, strain of ligament.

Warning It is contraindicated for cases with hypersensitivity on adhesive plaster and skin erosion, and use on the lumbar part. It should be used cautiously for pregnant women.

伤湿止痛膏

【处方】薄荷脑、冰片、樟脑、芸香浸膏、颠茄流浸膏、水杨酸甲酯等。

【功能主治】祛风湿，活血止痛。用于风湿关节、肌肉痛，扭伤。

【注意】外用，孕妇慎用。

Rheumatalgia-relieving Plaster

Name of Chinese Phonetic Alphabet Shang Shi Zhi Tong Gao

Formula Menthol, Borneolum Syntheticum, Camphora, Cymbopogonis Distantis Extractum, Belladonnae Extractum, Methyl Salicylate, etc.

Actions and Indications Dispelling wind-damp, activating blood, alleviating pain. It is used for rheumatic arthralgia, muscular pain and sprain.

Warning It is for external use only and should be used cautiously for pregnant women.

伊痛舒注射液

【处方】细辛、当归、川芎、羌活、独活、防风、白芷。

【功能主治】祛风散寒胜湿，活血祛瘀镇痛。用于多种原因引起的头痛，牙痛，神经痛，风湿痛及肌纤维炎，骨关节、胃肠、胆、肾疾患，癌症引起的疼痛。按中医辨证用药，尤其对寒邪和瘀血所致的痛证有较好的效果。

Pain-soothing Injection

Name of Chinese Phonetic Alphabet Yi Tong Shu Zhu She Ye

Formula Asari Radix et Rhizoma, Angelicae Sinensis Radix, Chuanxiong Rhizoma, Notopterygii Rhizoma et Radix, Angelicae Pubescentis Radix, Saposhnikoviae Radix and Angelicae Dahuricae Radix.

Actions and Indications Dispelling wind and dampness, dissipating cold, activating blood, dispelling stasis and settling pain. It is indicated for headache, toothache, neuralgia and rheumatalgia due to various causes. It is also used for pains due to myofibrositis, joints, stomach, intestine, gallbladder, nephrosis and cancer. According to syndrome differentiation of traditional Chinese medicine, it is especially used for pain due to cold and static blood.

华佗风痛宝片

【处方】九层风、大风艾、两面针、三七茎叶等。

【功能主治】驱风祛湿，通络，消肿止痛。用于风湿痹痛，肢体屈伸不利，筋脉拘挛，关节肿痛、变形及风湿性关节炎、肩周炎。

Hua Tuo Tablet for Relieving Impediment Syndrome

Name of Chinese Phonetic Alphabet Hua Tuo Feng Tong Bao Pian

Formula Spatholobi Caulis, Blumae Balsamiferae Folium et Ramulus, Zanthoxyli Radix, Notoginseng Caulis et Folium, etc.

Actions and Indications Dispelling wind and dampness, dredging collaterals, dispersing swelling and alleviating pain. It is used for wind-dampness impediment syndrome marked by immobility of limbs, spasm, swelling and pain of the joints, joint deformity, rheumatic arthritis, periarthritis of the shoulder.

华佗再造丸

【处方】本品为川芎、吴茱萸、冰片等药经加工制成的浓缩水蜜丸。

【功能主治】活血化瘀，化痰通络，行气止痛。用于瘀血或痰湿闭阻经络之中风瘫痪，拘挛麻木，口眼歪斜，言语不清。

【注意】孕妇忌服。

Hua Tuo Pill for Relieving Paralysis

Name of Chinese Phonetic Alphabet Hua Tuo Zai Zao Wan

Formula Chuanxiong Rhizoma, Euodiae Fructus, Borneolum Syntheticum, etc.

Actions and Indications Activating blood, resolving stasis and phlegm, dredging collaterals, moving *qi*, alleviating pain. It is used for paralysis, spasm and numbness of limbs, deviated eyes and mouth and alalia due to apoplexy.

Warning It is contraindicated for pregnant women.

华蟾素片

【处方】本品为干蟾皮经适宜的加工制成的片剂。

【功能主治】解毒，消肿，止痛。用于中、晚期肿瘤，慢性乙型肝炎。

Hua Chan Su Tablet

Name of Chinese Phonetic Alphabet Hua Chan Su Pian

Formula Bufonis Cutis.

Actions and Indications Detoxicating, dispersing swelling, relieving pain. It is used for middle or late stage of tumor, chronic hepatitis B.

血安胶囊

【处方】本品为棕榈的干燥成熟果实经乙醇浸渍提取所得干浸膏粉。

【功能主治】止血、收敛、调经。月事不准，经血过量，崩漏，淋漓不止，产后恶露不尽。

Blood-easing Capsule

Name of Chinese Phonetic Alphabet Xue An Jiao Nang

Formula Trachycarpi Fructus (powder of dried extract).

Actions and Indications Relieving hemorrhage, astringent, regulating menstruation. It is used for irregular menstruation, hypermenorrhea, metrorrhagia, postpartum lochiorrhagia.

血府逐瘀胶囊

【处方】柴胡、当归、地黄、赤芍、红花、桃仁、枳壳（麸炒）、甘草、川芎、牛膝、桔梗。

【功能主治】活血祛瘀，行气止痛。用于淤血内阻，头痛或胸痛，内热瞀闷，失眠多梦，心悸怔忡，急躁善怒。

【注意】忌食辛冷。孕妇忌服。

Blood-stasis-removing Capsule

Name of Chinese Phonetic Alphabet Xue Fu Zhu Yu Jiao Nang

Formula Bupleuri Radix, Angelicae Sinensis Radix, Rehmanniae Radix, Paeoniae Radix Rubra, Carhami Flos, Persicae Semen, Aurantii Fructus (fried with bran), Glycyrrhizae Radix et Rhizoma, Chuanxiong Rhizoma, Achyranthis Bidentatae Radix and Platycodonis Radix.

Actions and Indications Activating blood, dispelling stasis, moving *qi* to alleviate pain. It is used for headache, chest pain, insomnia, profuse dreaming, palpitation, fearful throbbing and impetuosity due to blood-stasis and accumulation of internal heat.

Warning It is contraindicated for pregnant women; pungent and cold foods should be avoided.

血宝胶囊

【处方】熟地黄、当归、附子、紫河车等。

【功能主治】补阴培阳，益肾健脾。用于再生障碍性贫血，白细胞缺乏症，原发性血小板减少症，紫癜。

Blood Treasure Capsule

Name of Chinese Phonetic Alphabet Xue Bao Jiao Nang

Formula Rehmanniae Radix Praeparata, Angelicae Sinensis Radix. Aconiti Lateralis Radix Praeparata, Hominis Placenta, etc.

Actions and Indications Tonifying *yin* and *yang*, fortifying the kidney and spleen. It is used for aplastic anemia, aleukemia, thrombopenia essentialis and purpura.

血美安胶囊

【处方】猪蹄甲、地黄、赤芍。

【功能主治】清热养阴，凉血活血。用于原发性血小板减少性紫癜血热伤阴夹瘀证，症见皮肤紫癜、鼻衄、妇女月经过多、口渴、烦热、盗汗等。

【注意】孕妇忌服。虚寒者慎用。服药期间忌辛、辣食物。

Xue Mei An Capsule

Name of Chinese Phonetic Alphabet Xue Mei An Jiao Nang

Formula Suillus Ungui, Rehmanniae Radix and Paeoniae Radix Rubra.

Actions and Indications Clearing heat, nourishing *yin*, cooling blood, activating blood. It is indicated for primary thrombocytopenic purpura, dermal purpura, epistaxis, menorrhagia, thirst, heat vexation and night sweating due to blood-heat damage *yin*.

Warning It is contraindicated for pregnant women and should be used cautiously for cases with deficiency-cold constitution. Pungent foods should be avoided during medication.

血栓心脉宁

【处方】川芎、槐角、丹参、水蛭、毛冬青、牛黄、麝香、人参茎叶皂苷、冰片、蟾酥。

【功能主治】芳香开窍，活血散瘀。用于脑血栓、冠心病、心绞痛属气滞血瘀证者。

【注意】孕妇忌服。

Relieving Cerebral Thrombosis Capsule

Name of Chinese Phonetic Alphabet Xue Shuan Xin Mai Ning

Formula Chuanxiong Rhizoma, Sophorae Fructus, Salviae Miltiorrhizae Radix et Rhizoma, Hirudo, Ilicis Pubescentis Radix, Bovis Calculus, Moschus, Ginseng Caulis et Folium Saponin, Borneolum Syntheticum and Bufonis Venenum.

Actions and Indications Inducing resuscitation, activating blood, dissipating stasis. It is indicated for cerebral thrombosis, coronary heart disease and angina pectoris attributed to *qi*-stagnation and blood-stasis syndrome.

Warning It is contraindicated for pregnant women.

血速升颗粒

【处方】黄芪、当归、阿胶、鸡血藤、淫羊藿、山楂。

【功能主治】益气温阳，养血活血。用于气血亏虚引起的贫血及各种失血疾患。

【注意】感冒发烧时忌服。

Relieving Anemia Soluble Granules

Name of Chinese Phonetic Alphabet Xue Su Sheng Ke Li

Formula Astragali Radix, Angelicae Sinensis Radix, Asini Corii Colla, Spatholobi Caulis, Epimedii Folium and Crataegi Fructus.

Actions and Indications Tonifying *qi* and warming *yang*, nourishing and activating blood. It is used for various anemia due to dual depletion of *qi* and blood; blood loss.

Warning It is contraindicated for cases with common cold, fever.

血康口服液

【处方】本品为肿节风经加工制成的口服液。

【功能主治】活血化瘀，消肿散结，凉血止血。用于血热妄行，皮肤紫斑；原发性及继发性血小板性紫癜。

【注意】服药后个别患者如有轻度恶心、嗜睡现象，继续服药后可自行消失。

Relieving Thrombocytic Purpura Oral Liquid

Name of Chinese Phonetic Alphabet Xue Kang Kou Fu Ye

Formula Sarcandrae Herba.

Actions and Indications Activating blood, resolving stasis, reducing swelling, dissipating mass, cooling blood and relieving hemorrhage. It is indicated for primary and secondary thrombocytic purprua caused by frenetic movement of blood due to heat.

Warning After administration, mild nausea and somnolence occur occasionally but disappear spontaneously.

血滞通胶囊

【处方】本品为薤白经加工制成的胶囊。

【功能主治】通阳散结，行气导滞。用于高脂血症血瘀痰阻所致的胸闷、乏力、腹胀。

Relieving Hyperlipemia Capsule

Name of Chinese Phonetic Alphabet Xue Zhi Tong Jiao Nang

Formula Allii Macrostemonis Bulbus.

Actions and Indications Activating *yang* and dissipating mass, moving *qi* and removing stagnation. It is indicated for chest distress, fatigue and abdominal distention due to hyperlipemia, blood-stasis and stragnation of phlegm.

血塞通注射液

【处方】本品为三七总皂苷制成的灭菌水溶液。

【功能主治】活血祛瘀，通脉活络，抑制血小板聚集和增加脑血流量。用于脑络瘀阻，中风偏瘫，心脉瘀阻，胸痹心痛；脑血管病后遗症，冠心病心绞痛属上述证候者。

Inhibiting Platelet Aggregation Injection

Name of Chinese Phonetic Alphabet Xue Sai Tong Zhu She Ye

Formula Notoginseng Radix et Rhizoma (total saponin).

Actions and Indications Activating blood, dispelling stasis, dredging vessels, activating collaterals, inhibiting platelet aggregation, increasing cerebral blood flow. It is indicated for apoplexy, hemiparalysis due to stagnation of cerebral collaterals; cardialgia, sequela of cerebrovascular disease, coronary heart disease and angina pectoris with the above mentioned symptoms.

舟车丸

【处方】牵牛子（炒）、大黄、甘遂（醋制）、红大戟（醋制）、芫花（醋制）、青皮（醋制）、陈皮、木香、轻粉。

【功能主治】行气利水。用于蓄水腹胀，四肢浮肿，胸腹胀满，停饮喘急，大便秘结，小便短少。

【注意】孕妇及久病气虚者忌服。

Edema-relieving Pill

Name of Chinese Phonetic Alphabet Zhou Ju Wan

Formula Pharbitidis Semen (fried), Rhei Radix et Rhizoma, Kansui Radix (prepared with vinegar), Knoxiae Radix (prepared with vinegar), Genkwa Flos (prepared with vinegar), Citri Reticulatae Pericarpium Viride (prepared with vinegar), Citri Reticulatae Pericarpium, Aucklandiae Radix and Calomelas.

Actions and Indications Activating *qi* and inducing diuresis. It is indicated for abdominal fullness due to water-retention; edema of extremities, distention and fullness of the chest and abdomen, dyspnea, constipation, scanty urine.

Warning It is contraindicated for pregnant women and cases with deficiency of *qi* due to prolonged illness.

创灼膏

【处方】炉甘石（煅）、石膏粉（煅）、白及粉、冰片、对羟基苯甲酸乙酯、凡士林、羊毛脂、液状石蜡。

【功能主治】排脓，去腐，生皮。用于烧伤，烫伤，挫伤，褥疮，手术后创口感染，冻疮溃烂，慢性湿疹及常见疮疖。

【注意】外用药。溃烂初期禁用。

Soft Extract for Relieving Burn and Scald

Name of Chinese Phonetic Alphabet Chuang Zhuo Gao

Formula Calamina (calcined), Gypsum Fibrosum Pulvis (calcined), Bletillae Rhizoma Pulvis, Borneolum Syntheticum, Ethyl p-hydroxybenzoate, Vaseline, Lanolinom and Liquid Paraffin.

Actions and Indications Draining pus, removing necrosis, promoting skin regeneration. It is used for burn, scald, contusion, bedsore, wound infection after operation, chilblain ulceration, chronic eczema, sore and furuncle.

Warning It is for external use only and contraindicated for initial ulceration.

全天麻胶囊

【处方】本品为天麻经加工成细粉制成的胶囊剂。

【功能主治】平肝息风止痉。用于头痛眩晕，肢体麻木，小儿惊风，癫痫抽搐，破伤风症。

Gastrodia* Capsule

Name of Chinese Phonetic Alphabet Quan Tian Ma Jiao Nang

Formula Gastrodiae Rhizoma.

Actions and Indications Pacifying the liver, extinguishing wind and relieving spasm. It is used for obstinate headache, vertigo, numbness of extremities, infantile convulsion, epilepsy, spasm, tetanus.

* 天麻

全龟胶囊

【处方】本品为龟科动物乌龟经加工制成的胶囊。

【功能主治】滋阴补肾。用于肺肾不足引起的骨蒸劳热，腰膝酸软，流注，流痰。

Tortoise Meat and Shell Capsule

Name of Chinese Phonetic Alphabet Quan Gui Jiao Nang

Formula Testudinis Totus Preaparata.

Actions and Indications Enriching *yin*, tonifying the kidney. It is used for tidal fever, soreness and weakness of waist and knees, deep multiple abscess and tuberculosis of bone and joint due to dual insufficiency of the lung and kidney.

产灵丸

【处方】人参、白术（麸炒）、当归、何首乌（黑豆酒炙）、苍术、八角茴香、川芎、川乌（银花、甘草炙）、细辛、两头尖、白芷、草乌（银花、甘草炙）、木香、桔梗、血竭、甘草（蜜炙）、防风、荆芥穗、麻黄。

【功能主治】益气养血，散寒止痛。用于产后气血虚弱，感受风寒引起的周身疼痛，头目眩晕，恶心呕吐，四肢浮肿。

【注意】孕妇忌服。

Tonic Bolus for Puerperal *Qi* and Blood Deficiency

Name of Chinese Phonetic Alphabet Chan Ling Wan

Formula Ginseng Radix et Rhizoma, Atractylodis Macrocephalae Rhizoma (fried with bran), Angelicae Sinensis Radix, Polygoni Multiflori Radix (prepared with wine), Atractylodis Rhizoma, Anisi Stellati Fructus, Chuanxiong Rhizoma, Aconiti Radix (prepared with honeysuckle flower and licorice root), Asari Radix et Rhizoma, Anemones Raddeanae Rhizoma, Angelicae Dahuricae Radix, Aconiti Kusnezoffii Radix (prepared with honeysuckle flower and licorice root), Aucklandiae Radix, Platycodonis Radix, Draconis Sanguis, Glycyrrhizae Radix et Rhizoma (prepared with honey), Saposhnikoviae Radix, Schizonepetae Spica and Ephedrae Herba.

Actions and Indications Tonifying *qi*, nourishing blood, dispersing cold, alleviating pain. It is used for puerperal deficiency of *qi* and blood marked by general pain, vertigo, nausea, vomiting, edema of limbs.

Warning It is contraindicated for pregnant women.

产复康颗粒

【处方】本品为益母草、当归、人参、黄芪、何首乌、桃仁、蒲黄、熟地黄、香附、昆布、白术、黑木耳等药味加工制成的颗粒。

【功能主治】补气养血，排瘀生新。用于产后出血过多，气血俱亏。症见腰腿酸软，倦怠无力。

Puerperal Convalescence Soluble Granules

Name of Chinese Phonetic Alphabet Chan Fu Kang Ke Li

Formula Leonuri Herba, Angelicae Sinensis Radix, Ginseng Radix et Rhizoma, Astragali Radix, Polygoni Multiflori Radix, Persicae Semen, Typhae Pollen, Rehmanniae Radix Praeparata, Cyperi Rhizoma, Laminariae et Eckloniae Thallus, Atractylodis Macrocephalae Rhizoma and Auriculariae Sporocarpium.

Actions and Indications Tonifying *qi* and blood, dispelling stasis to promote regeneration. It is indicated for puerperal excessive bleeding due to dual deficiency of *qi* and blood manifested as soreness of waist and weakness of legs, tiredness and fatigue.

灯盏花素注射液

【处方】本品为灯盏花素的灭菌水溶液。

【功能主治】活血化瘀，通络止痛。用于中风后遗症，冠心病，心绞痛。

【注意】脑出血急性期或有出血倾向的患者禁用。

Breviscapine* Injection

Name of Chinese Phonetic Alphabet Deng Zhan Hua Su Zhu She Ye

Formula Breviscapine.

Actions and Indications Activating blood, resolving stasis, dredging collaterals, alleviating pain. It is indicated for sequela of apoplexy, coronary heart disease and angina pectoris.

Warning It is contraindicated for cases at acute stage of cerebral hemorrhage or with hemorrhagic tendency.

＊灯盏花素

灯盏细辛注射液

【处方】灯盏细辛。

【功能主治】活血化瘀，通络止痛。用于中风后遗症，冠心病，心绞痛。

Erigeron* Injection

Name of Chinese Phonetic Alphabet Deng Zhan Xi Xin Zhu She Ye

Formula Erigerontis Herba.

Actions and Indications Activating blood, resolving stasis, dredging collaterals, alleviating pain. It is indicated for sequela of apoplexy, coronary heart and angina pectoris.

＊灯盏细辛

冰黄肤乐软膏

【处方】大黄、姜黄、硫黄、冰片等。

【功能主治】祛风燥湿，清热解毒，杀虫止痒。用于神经性皮炎、湿疹、足癣及银屑病所致的皮肤瘙痒症。

【注意】治疗期间忌酒等辛辣发物。

Borneol* Soft Plaster

Name of Chinese Phonetic Alphabet Bing Huang Fu Le Ruan Gao

Formula Rhei Radix et Rhizoma, Curcumae Rhizoma Longae, Sulfur, Borneolum Syntheticum, etc.

Actions and Indications Dispelling wind and dampness, clearing heat and detoxicating, killing worms and relieving itching. It is indicated for skin itching due to neurodermatitis, eczema, tinea pedis, and psoriasis.

Warning Pungent foods and wine are prohibited during therapeutic periods.

* 冰片

冰硼含片

【处方】冰片、硼砂（煅）、朱砂、玄明粉。

【功能主治】清热解毒，消肿止痛。用于咽喉疼痛，牙龈肿痛，口舌生疮。

Borneol* and Borax** Sucked Tablet

Name of Chinese Phonetic Alphabet Bing Peng Han Pian

Formula Borneolum Syntheticum, Borax (calcined), Cinnabaris and Natrii Sulfas Exsiccatus.

Actions and Indications Clearing heat and detoxicating, dispersing swelling and relieving pain. It is indicated for sore-throat, gingivitis, aphthae.

* 冰片 ** 硼砂

江南卷柏片

【处方】江南卷柏。

【功能主治】清热凉血。用于肌衄，见有皮下散在紫癜、出血点，舌质红，脉细数等血热证候。

Moellendorfs Spikemoss* Tablet

Name of Chinese Phonetic Alphabet Jiang Nan Juan Bai Pian

Formula Selaginellae Moellendorfii Herba (extract).

Actions and Indications Clearing heat, cooling blood. It is used for dermorrhagia marked by scattered subcutaneous purpura, hemorrhagic spots, red tongue, fine and rapid pulse.

* 江南卷柏

壮阳健威丸

【处方】人参、肉苁蓉、鹿茸、鹿角胶、沉香、杜仲（盐水炒）、茯苓、远志（制）、肉桂、甘草（蜜炙）、山药、枸杞子、锁阳、附子（制）、制何首乌、狗肾。

【功能主治】补肾壮阳，生精益髓。用于阳虚畏寒，腰膝酸痛，阳痿。

Strengthening Kidney-*yang* Pill

Name of Chinese Phonetic Alphabet Zhuang Yang Jian Wei Wan

Formula Ginseng Radix et Rhizoma, Cistanches Caulis Carnosus, Cervi Cornu Pantotrichum, Cervi Cornus Colla, Aquilariae Lignum Resinatum, Eucommiae Cortex (fried with salt water), Poria, Polygalae Radix (prepared), Cinnamomi Cortex, Glycyrrhizae Radix et Rhizoma (prepared with honey), Dioscoreae Rhizoma, Lycii Fructus, Cynomorii Caulis Carnosus, Aconiti Lateralis Radix Praeparata, Polygoni Multiflori Radix Praeparata and Canis Ren.

Actions and Indications Tonifying kidney-*yang*, marrow and essence. It is used for cases with fear of cold, soreness and pain of waist and knees, and impotence due to *yang*-deficiency.

壮骨木瓜丸

【处方】玉竹、栀子、木瓜、当归、羌活、独活、陈皮、香加皮、川芎、秦艽、川牛膝、红花、桑寄生、千年健、豹骨汁。

【功能主治】祛风去湿，通经活络。用于筋脉拘急，骨节疼痛，四肢麻木。

【注意】孕妇忌服。

Chinese-quince* Pill for Strengthening Bone

Name of Chinese Phonetic Alphabet Zhuang Gu Mu Gua Wan

Formula Polygonati Odorati Rhizoma, Gardeniae Fructus, Chaenomelis Frucrus, Angelicae Sinensis Radix, Notopterygii Rhizoma et Radix, Angelicae Pubescentis Radix, Citri Reticulatae Pericarpium, Periplocae Cortex, Chuanxiong Rhizoma, Gentianae Macrophyllae Radix, Cyathulae Radix, Carthami Flos,

Taxilli Herba, Homalomenae Rhizoma and Pardi Os Succus.

Actions and Indications Dispelling wind and dampness, unblocking the meridian and activating the collateral. It is indicated for hypertonicity of sinews, arthralgia and numbness of limbs.

Warning It is contraindicated for pregnant women.

*木瓜

壮骨伸筋胶囊

【处方】淫羊藿、熟地黄、鹿衔草、骨碎补（炙）、肉苁蓉、鸡血藤、红参、狗骨、茯苓、威灵仙、豨莶草、葛根、山楂、洋金花、延胡索（醋炙）。

【功能主治】补益肝肾，强筋壮骨，活络止痛。用于肝肾两虚，寒湿阻络所致的神经根型颈椎病。

【注意】不宜超量服用；高血压、心脏病慎用；青光眼和孕妇忌服。

Bone-strengthening Capsule

Name of Chinese Phonetic Alphabet Zhuang Gu Shen Jin Jiao Nang

Formula Epimedii Folium, Rehmanniae Radix Praeparata, Pyrolae Herba, Drynariae Rhizoma (prepared), Cistanches Caulis Carnosus, Spatholobi Caulis, Ginseng Radix et Rhizoma Rubra, Canis Os, Poria, Clematidis Radix et Rhizoma, Siegesbeckiae Herba, Puerariae Lobatae Radix, Crataegi Fructus, Daturae Flos and Corydalis Rhizoma (prepared with vinegar).

Actions and Indications Tonifying the liver and kidney, strengthening the bone and sinews, activating collaterals, alleviating pain. It is used for nerve root cervical spondylopathy due to dual deficiency of the liver and kidney, and stagnation of cold-damp in collaterals.

Warning Over dosage is prohibited. It is contraindicated for glaucoma and pregnant women, and should be used cautiously for cases with hypertension, heart disease.

壮骨药酒

【处方】本品由豹骨、乳香、没药、当归、牛膝、天南星、天麻、血竭、肉桂、熟地黄等药经适宜的加工、炮制，制成的酒剂。

【功能主治】祛风散寒，舒筋活络。用于风寒湿痹，四肢拘挛，半身不遂，腰腿疼痛，跌打损伤。

【注意】孕妇忌服。

Bone-strengthening Medicated Wine

Name of Chinese Phonetic Alphabet Zhuang Gu Yao Jiu

Formula Pardi Os, Olibanum, Myrrha, Angelicae Sinensis Radix, Achyranthis Bidentatae Radix, Arisaematis Rhizoma, Gastrodiae Rhizoma, Draconis Sanguis, Cinnamomi Cortex, Rehmanniae Radix Praeparata, etc.

Actions and Indications Dispelling wind and dissipating cold, relaxing sinews and activating collaterals. It is indicated for wind-cold-damp impediment syndrome, marked by spasm of the limbs, hemiplegia, pain of the waist and legs; and traumatic injury.

Warning It is contraindicated for pregnant women.

壮骨追风酒

【处方】豹骨、鹿角、当归、补骨脂、威灵仙、红花、杜仲、木瓜、续断、何首乌、川牛膝等。

【功能主治】祛风除湿，活血止痛。用于风寒湿痹，四肢麻木，筋骨疼痛，腰膝无力。

【注意】孕妇忌服。

Medicated Wine for Strengthening Bone

Name of Chinese Phonetic Alphabet Zhuang Gu Zhui Feng Jiu

Formula Pardi Os, Cervi Cornu, Angelicae Sinensis Radix, Psoraleae Fructus, Clematidis Radix et Rhizoma, Carthami Flos, Eucommiae Cortex, Chaenomelis Fructus, Dipsaci Radix, Polygoni

Multiflori Radix, Cyathulae Radix, etc.

Actions and Indications Dispelling wind and dampness, activating blood and alleviating pain. It is indicated for wind-cold-damp impediment, numbness of the limbs, ostealgia, weakness of the waist and knees.

Warning It is contraindicated for pregnant women.

壮腰健肾丸

【处方】狗脊（制）、金樱子、黑老虎根、桑寄生（蒸）、鸡血藤、千斤拔、牛大力、菟丝子、女贞子。

【功能主治】壮腰健肾，祛风活络。用于肾亏腰痛，风湿骨痛，膝软无力，神经衰弱，小便频数，遗精梦泄。

【注意】感冒发热者忌服。

Waist-strengthening and Kidney-fortifying Bolus

Name of Chinese Phonetic Alphabet Zhuang Yao Jian Shen Wan

Formula Cibotii Rhizoma(prepared), Rosae Laevigatae Fructus, Kadsurae Coccineae Radix, Taxilli Herba (steamed), Spatholobi Caulis, Flemingiae Philippinensis Radix, Millettae Speciosae Radix, Cuscutae Semen and Ligustri Lucidi Fructus.

Actions and Indications Strengthening the waist, fortifying the kidney, dispelling wind and activating collaterals. It is indicated for lumbago, rheumatalgia, weakness of kness, neurasthenia, frequent urination, nocturnal emission and oneirogmus due to depletion of the kidney.

Warning It is contraindicated for cases with common cold and fever.

壮腰消痛液

【处方】枸杞子、淫羊藿（制）、巴戟天、穿山龙、地龙、威灵仙、狗脊、川牛膝、豨莶草、乌梅、鹿角胶、鹿衔草、木瓜、没药（炒）、海龙、杜仲。

【功能主治】壮腰益肾，疏风祛湿，活络止痛。用于肾虚腰痛，骨质增生引起的疼痛。

【注意】孕妇忌服。

Relieving Lumbago Oral Liquid

Name of Chinese Phonetic Alphabet Zhuang Yao Xiao Tong Ye

Formula Lycii Fructus, Epimedii Folium (prepared), Morindae Officinalis Radix, Dioscoreae Nipponicae Rhizoma, Pheretima, Clematidis Radix et Rhizoma, Cibotii Rhizoma, Cyathulae Radix, Siegesbeckiae Herba, Mume Fructus, Cervi Cornus Colla, Pyrolae Herba, Chaenomelis Fructus, Myrrha (fried), Syngnathus and Eucommiae Cortex.

Actions and Indications Strengthening the loin and nourishing the kidney, dispersing wind and dispelling dampness, activating collaterals and alleviating pain. It is indicated for lumbago due to kidney-deficiency; and algogenesis due to hyperosteogeny.

Warning It is contraindicated for pregnant women.

安中片

【处方】桂枝、延胡索（醋制）、牡蛎（煅）、小茴香、砂仁、高良姜、甘草。

【功能主治】温中散寒，理气止痛，和胃止呕。用于胃脘疼痛，慢性胃炎，胃酸过多，胃及十二指肠溃疡。

【注意】急性胃炎、出血性溃疡禁用。

Warming Middle Energizer Tablet

Name of Chinese Phonetic Alphabet An Zhong Pian

Formula Cinnamomi Ramulus, Corydalis Rhizoma (prepared with vinegar), Ostreae Concha (calcined), Foeniculi Fructus, Amomi Fructus, Alpiniae Officinarum Rhizoma and Glycyrrhizae Radix et Rhizoma.

Actions and Indications Warming the middle and dissipating cold, regulating *qi* to relieve pain, harmonizing the stomach and relieving vomiting. It is indicated for stomach duct pain, chronic gastritis, gastroxia, gastric and duodenal ulcer.

Warning It is contraindicated for cases with acute gastritis and hemorrhagic ulcer.

安尔眠糖浆

【处方】丹参（切片）、首乌藤、大枣。
【功能主治】安神。用于神经衰弱或失眠。

Promoting Peaceful Sleep Syrup

Name of Chinese Phonetic Alphabet An Er Mian Tang Jiang

Formula Salviae Miltiorrhizae Radix et Rhizoma (sliced), Polygoni Multiflori Caulis and Jujubae Fructus.

Actions and Indications Tranquilizing the mind. It is indicated for neurasthenia and insomnia.

安乐片

【处方】柴胡、当归、川芎、茯苓、钩藤、首乌藤、白术（炒）、甘草。
【功能主治】疏肝解郁，定惊安神。用于精神抑郁，惊恐失眠，胸闷不适，纳少神疲，对神经官能症及小儿夜啼、磨牙等症状者亦可使用。

Tranquility Tablet

Name of Chinese Phonetic Alphabet An Le Pian

Formula Bupleuri Radix, Angelicae Sinensis Radix, Chuanxiong Rhizoma, Poria, Uncariae Ramulus cum Uncis, Polygoni Multiflori Caulis, Atractylodis Macrocephalae Rhizoma (fried) and Glycyrrhizae Radix et Rhizoma.

Actions and Indications Soothing the liver, releasing depression and tranquilizing the mind. It is used for depression of spirit, fluster, insomnia, chest distress, impaired appetite, lassitude of spirit, and also used for neurosis, infantile night crying and motar teeth.

安多霖胶囊

【处方】略。
【功能主治】益气补血，扶正解毒。主治气血两虚证。用于肿瘤放、化疗引起的白细胞减少，免疫功能低下，食欲不振，神疲乏力，头晕气短。

Anduolin Capsule

Name of Chinese Phonetic Alphabet An Duo Lin Jiao Nang

Formula Omitted.

Actions and Indications Tonifying *qi* and blood, reinforcing the healthy *qi* and detoxifying. It is indicated for the treatment of radiotherapy and chemotherapy in tumor leading to leukopenia, hypofunction of immunologic function, poor appetite, lassitude of spirit, fatigue, dizziness and shortness of breath.

安坤颗粒

【处方】牡丹皮、栀子、当归、白术、白芍、茯苓、女贞子、墨旱莲、益母草。
【功能主治】滋阴清热，健脾养血。用于放环后引起的出血，月经提前、量多或月经紊乱，腰骶酸痛，下腹坠痛，心烦易怒，手足心热。

Menstruation-soothing Granules

Name of Chinese Phonetic Alphabet An Kun Ke Li

Formula Moutan Cortex, Gardeniae Fructus, Angelicae Sinensis Radix, Atractylodis Macrocephalae Rhizoma, Paeoniae Radix Alba, Poria, Ligustri Lucidi Fructus, Ecliptae Herba and Leonuri Herba.

Actions and Indications Enriching *yin*, clearing heat, fortifying the spleen and nourishing blood. It is indicated for bleeding due to putting in contraceptive device, advanced menstruation and hypermenorrhea or menstrual disorder, soreness and pain of lumbosacral portion, bearing-down pain of hypogastrium, vexation, vexing heat in the palms and soles.

安坤赞育丸

【处方】香附（醋制）、鹿茸、阿胶、紫河车、白芍、当归、牛膝、川牛膝、北沙参、没药（醋制）、天冬、补骨脂（盐制）、龙眼肉、茯苓、黄柏、龟甲、锁阳、杜仲（盐制）、秦艽、鳖甲（醋制）、艾叶（炭）、白薇、延胡索（醋制）、山茱萸（酒制）、鹿尾、枸杞子、鸡冠花、黄芪、乳香（醋制）、赤石脂（煅）、鹿角胶、菟丝子、肉苁蓉（酒制）、鸡血藤、桑寄生、琥珀、甘草、人参、乌药、丝绵（炭）、血余炭、白术（麸炒）、西红花、地黄、砂仁、沉香、酸枣仁（炒）、续断、陈皮、橘红、川芎、泽泻、黄芩、青蒿、远志（制）、肉豆蔻（煨）、藁本、红花、柴胡、木香、紫苏叶、熟地黄、丹参。

【功能主治】补气养血，调经止带。用于气血两亏，肝肾不足，形瘦虚羸，神倦体疲，面黄浮肿，心悸失眠，腰酸腿软，午后低热，骨蒸潮热，月经不调，崩漏带下，产后虚弱，瘀血腹痛，大便溏泻。

【注意】孕妇遵医嘱服用。

Bolus of Tonifying *Qi* and Blood to Regulate Menstruation

Name of Chinese Phonetic Alphabet An Kun Zan Yu Wan

Formula Cyperi Rhizoma (prepared with vinegar), Cervi Cornu Pantotrichum, Asini Corii Colla, Homins Placenta, Paeoniae Radix Alba, Angelicae Sinensis Radix, Achyranthis Bidentatae Radix, Cyathulae Radix, Glehniae Radix, Myrrha (prepared with vinegar), Asparagi Radix, Psoraleae Fructus (prepare with salt), Longan Arillus, Poria, Phellodendri Chinensis Cortex, Testudinis Carapax et Plastrum, Cynomorii Caulis Cornousus, Eucommiae Cortex (prepared with salt), Gentianae Macrophyllae Radix, Trionycis Carapax (preared with vinegar), Artemisiae Argyi Folium (carbonated), Cynanchi Atrati Radix et Rhizoma, Corydalis Rhizoma (prepared with vinegar), Corni Fructus (prepared with wine), Cervi Cauda, Lycii Fructus, Celosiae Cristatae Flos, Astragali Radix, Olibanum (prepared with vinegar), Halloysitum Rubrum (calcined), Cervi Cornus Colla, Cuscutae Semen, Cistanches Caulis Carnosus (prepared with wine), Spatholobi Caulis, Taxilli Herba, Succinum, Glycyrrhizae Radix et Rhizoma, Ginseng Radix et Rhizoma, Linderae Radix, Bombycis Incunabulum (carbonate), Crinis Carbonisatrus, Atractylodis Macrocephalae Rhizoma (fried with bran), Croci Stigma, Rehmanniae Radix, Amomi Fructus, Aquilariae Lignum Resinatum, Ziziphi Spinosae Semen (fried), Dipsaci Radix, Citri Reticulatae Pericarpium, Citri Exocarpium Rubrum, Chuanxiong Rhizoma, Alismatis Rhizoma, Scutellariae Radix, Artemisiae Annuae Herba, Myristicae Semen (stewed), Ligustici Rhizoma et Radix, Carthami Flos, Bupleuri Radix, Aucklandiae Radix, Perillae Folium, Rehmanniae Radix Praeparata and Salviae Miltiorrhizae Radix et Rhizoma.

Actions and Indications Tonifying *qi* and blood, regulating menstruation and relieving white vaginal discharge. It is indicated for emaciation of women, lassitude of spirit, tiredness, sallow complexion, facial edema, palpitation, insomnia, soreness of waist and weakness of legs, afternoon low-grade fever, tidal fever, irregular menstruation, metrorrhagia, white vaginal discharge, puerperal debility, abdominal pain and sloppy stool due to dual deficiency of *qi*, blood and insufficiency of the liver and kidney.

Warning The pregnant women should be followed the physician's advice.

安肾丸

【处方】巴戟天（甘草炙）、肉苁蓉（酒炙）、补骨脂（盐炙）、肉桂、川乌（甘草、银花炙）、白术（麸炒）、山药、茯苓、蒺藜（盐炙）、粉萆薢、石斛、桃仁。

【功能主治】补肾散寒。用于肾不纳气，湿寒侵袭引起的梦遗滑精，遗淋白浊，脐腹作痛，精神倦怠，健忘失眠，腰腿酸痛，头晕耳鸣，二便不利。

Tonifying Kidney Pill

Name of Chinese Phonetic Alphabet An Shen Wan

Formula Morindae Officinalis Radix (prepared with licorice root), Cistanches Caulis Carnosus (prepared with wine), Psoraleae Fructus (prepared with salt), Cinnamomi Cortex, Aconiti Radix (prepared with licorice root and honeysuckle flower), Atractylodis

Macrocephalae Rhizoma (fried with bran), Dioscoreae Rhizoma, Poria, Tribuli Fructus (prepared with salt), Dioscoreae Hypoglaucae Rhizoma, Dendrobii Caulis and Persicae Semen.

Actions and Indications Tonifying the kidney, dissipating cold. It is indicated for spermatorrhea, cloudy urine, umbilical and abdominal pain, tiredness, amnesia, insomnia, soreness and pain of waist and legs, dizziness, tinnitus and difficulty in urination and defecation due to kidney falling to receive *qi* and invasion of damp-cold.

安胃疡胶囊

【处方】本品为甘草提取物，含黄酮类化合物不少于80%。

【功能主治】补中益气，解毒生肌。用于治胃及十二指肠球部溃疡，对虚寒型和气滞型患者有较好疗效，并可用于溃疡愈合后的维持治疗。

Peptic Ulcer-relieving Capsule

Name of Chinese Phonetic Alphabet An Wei Yang Jiao Nang

Formula Glycyrrhizae Extractum and Flavonones compound not less than 80%.

Actions and Indications Tonifying *qi*, detoxifying, promoting tissue regeneration. It is indicated for gastric and duodenal bulbar ulcer. The medicine possesses better curative effect for types of deficiency-cold and *qi*-stagnation, and as a maintenance treatment after the ulcer healing.

安宫牛黄丸

【处方】牛黄、水牛角浓缩粉、麝香、珍珠、朱砂、雄黄、黄连、黄芩、栀子、郁金、冰片。

【功能主治】清热解毒，震惊开窍。用于热病，邪入心包，高热惊厥，神昏谵语。

【注意】孕妇慎用。

Angong Bezoar* Pill

Name of Chinese Phonetic Alphabet An Gong Niu Huang Wan

Formula Bovis Calculus, Bubali Cornu Pulvis Concentratio, Moschus, Margarita, Cinnabaris, Realgar, Coptidis Rhizoma, Scutellariae Radix, Gardeniae Fructus, Curcumae Radix and Borneolum Syntheticum.

Actions and Indications Clearing heat and detoxifying, settling fright, inducing resuscitation. It is indicated for heat disease, pathogens entering the pericardium, high fever, convulsion, coma and delirious speech.

Warning It is used cautiously for pregnant women.

*牛黄

安宫降压丸

【处方】郁金、黄连、栀子、黄芩、天麻、珍珠母、黄芪、白芍、党参、麦冬、五味子（炙）、川芎、牛黄、冰片、水牛角浓缩粉。

【功能主治】清热镇惊，平肝降压。用于胸中郁热，肝阳上亢引起的头目眩晕，项强脑胀，心悸多梦，烦躁起急，高血压症。

Angong Pill for Lowering Blood Pressure

Name of Chinese Phonetic Alphabet An Gong Jiang Ya Wan

Formula Curcumae Radix, Coptidis Rhizoma, Gardeniae Fructus, Scutellariae Radix, Gastrodiae Rhizoma, Margaritifera Concha, Astragali Radix, Paeoniae Radix Alba, Codonopsis Radix, Ophiopogonis Radix, Schisandrae Chinensis Fructus (prepared), Chuanxiong Rhizoma, Bovis Calculus, Borneolum Syntheticum and Bubali Cornu Pulvis Concentratio.

Actions and Indications Clearing heat, settling fright, pacifying the liver, lowering blood pressure. It is used for vertigo, neck rigidity, palpitation, profuse dreaming, vexation and hypertension due to stagnation of heat in the chest and ascendant hyperactivity of liver-*yang*.

安神补心丸

【处方】丹参、五味子（蒸）、石菖蒲、安神膏。

【功能主治】养心安神。用于心悸失眠，头昏耳鸣。

Tranquility Pill

Name of Chinese Phonetic Alphabet An Shen Bu Xin Wan

Formula Salviae Miltiorrhizae Radix et Rhizoma, Schisandrae Chinensis Fructus (steamed), Acori Tatarinowii Rhizoma and Anshen Extractum.

Actions and Indications Nourishing the heart, tranquilizing the mind. It is indicated for palpitation, insomnia, dizziness and tinnitus.

安神补脑液

【处方】鹿茸、制何首乌、淫羊藿、干姜、甘草、大枣、维生素 B_1。

【功能主治】生精补髓，增强脑力。用于神经衰弱，失眠，健忘，头痛。

Mind-tranquilizing Oral Liquid

Name of Chinese Phonetic Alphabet An Shen Bu Nao Ye

Formula Cervi Cornu Pantotrichum, Polygoni Multiflori Radix Praeparata, Epimedii Folium, Zingiberis Rhizoma, Glycyrrhizae Radix et Rhizoma, Jujubae Fructus and Vitamin B_1.

Actions and Indications Engendering the essence, tonifying marrow, enhancing the nervous force. It is indicated for neurasthenia, insomnia, amnesia and headache.

安神宝冲剂

【处方】酸枣仁、枸杞子、合欢花。

【功能主治】补肾益精，养心安神。用于失眠健忘，眩晕耳鸣，腰膝酸软等症。

Tranquility Soluble Granules

Name of Chinese Phonetic Alphabet An Shen Bao Chong Ji

Formula Ziziphi Spinosae Semen, Lycii Fructus and Albiziae Flos.

Actions and Indications Tonifying the kidney and essence, nourishing the heart and tranquilizing the mind. It is used for insomnia, amnesia, vertigo, tinnitus, soreness and weakness of waist and knees.

安神健脑液

【处方】人参、五味子（醋炙）、麦冬、枸杞子、丹参。

【功能主治】益气养血，滋阴生津，养心安神。用于气血两亏，阴津不足所致的失眠多梦，神疲健忘，头昏头痛，心悸乏力，口干津少。

【注意】感冒忌服。

Oral Liquid of Tranquilization

Name of Chinese Phonetic Alphabet An Shen Jian Nao Ye

Formula Ginseng Radix et Rhizoma, Schisandrae Chinensis Fructus (prepared with vinegar), Ophiopogonis Radix, Lycii Fructus and Salviae Miltiorrhizae Radix et Rhizoma.

Actions and Indications Tonifying *qi*, nourishing blood and *yin*, engendering fluid, nourishing the heart and tranquilizing the mind. It is used for insomnia, profuse dreaming, lassitude of spirit, amnesia, dizziness, headache, palpitation, fatigue, dry mouth and shortage of fluid due to dual depletion of *qi* and blood and insufficiency of *yin*-fluid.

Warning It is contraindicated for cases with common cold.

安脑丸

【处方】人工牛黄、猪胆汁粉、朱砂、冰片、水牛角浓缩粉、珍珠、黄芩、黄连、栀子、雄黄、郁金、石膏、赭石、珍珠母、薄荷脑。

【功能主治】清热解毒，豁痰开窍，镇惊息风。用于高热神昏、烦躁谵语、抽搐痉厥、中风窍闭、头痛眩晕。用于高血压及一切急性炎症伴有的高热不退。

Coma-relieving Pill

Name of Chinese Phonetic Alphabet An Nao Wan

Formula Bovis Calculus Artifactus, Suillus Bilis Pulvis, Cinnabaris, Borneolum Syntheticum, Bubali Cornu Pulvis Concentratio, Margarita, Scutellariae Radix, Coptidis Rhizoma, Gardeniae Fructus, Realgar, Curcumae Radix, Gypsum Fibrosum, Haematitum, Margaritifera Concha and Menthol.

Actions and Indications Clearing heat and detoxifying, dispelling phlegm, inducing resuscitation, settling fright and extinguishing wind. It is used for high fever, coma, vexation, delirious speech, spasm, apoplexy, headache and vertigo, and is also used for hypertension, acute inflammation complicated with unabatement of high fever.

安替可胶囊

【处方】蟾皮、当归。

【功能主治】软坚散结，解毒定痛，养血活血。用于食管癌瘀毒证，与放疗合用可增强对食管癌的治疗。

【注意】心脏病患者和孕妇慎用。

An Ti Ke Capsule

Name of Chinese Phonetic Alphabet An Ti Ke Jiao Nang

Formula Bufonis Cutis and Angelicae Sinensis Radix.

Actions and Indications Dispersing mass, detoxifying, settling pain, nourishing and activating blood. The preparation possesses action to enhance the curative effect with radiotherapy for carcinoma of esophagus.

Warning It should be used cautiously for pregnant women and cases with heart disease.

关节止痛膏

【处方】辣椒流浸膏、颠茄流浸膏、薄荷油、水杨酸甲酯、樟脑、碘、碘化钾、盐酸苯海拉明。

【功能主治】活血，消炎，镇痛，对局部血管有扩张作用。用于风湿性关节痛，关节扭伤。

【注意】本品含刺激性药物，忌贴于创伤处，有皮肤病者慎用。

Relieving Rheumatic Arthralgia Plaster

Name of Chinese Phonetic Alphabet Guan Jie Zhi Tong Gao

Formula Capsici Extractum, Belladonnae Extractum, Menthae Haplocalycis Oleum, Methyl Salicylate, Camphora, Iodine, Potassium Iodide and Diphenhydramine Hydrochloride.

Actions and Indications Activating blood, antiphlogistic, settling pain and dilating topical blood vessels. It is indicated for rheumatic arthralgia, sprain of the joints .

Warning It contains irritant drug and can't be attached to injury area and should be used carefully for cases with dermatosis.

关节解痛膏

【处方】辣椒、白芷、细辛、姜黄、肉桂、生川乌、生草乌、骨碎补、五加皮、红花、天南星、半夏、闹羊花、防风、独活、羌活、桑枝、海风藤、芥子、防己、凤仙透、骨草、伸筋草、威灵仙、冰片、薄荷脑、水杨酸甲酯、樟脑、麝香草酚、二甲苯、麝香、颠茄流浸膏、盐酸苯海拉明。

【功能主治】驱风除湿，活血止痛。用于风寒湿痹，关节痛，神经痛、腰痛，肌肉酸痛，扭伤。

【注意】孕妇慎用。

Relieving Arthralgia Plaster

Name of Chinese Phonetic Alphabet Guan Jie

Jie Tong Gao

Formula Capsici Fructus, Angelicae Dahuricae Radix, Asari Radix et Rhizoma, Curcumae Rhizoma Longae, Cinnamomi Cortex, Aconiti Radix, Aconiti Kusnezoffii Radix, Drynariae Rhizoma, Acanthopanacis Cortex, Carthami Flos, Arisaematis Rhizoma, Pinelliae Rhizoma, Rhododendri Mollis Flos, Saposhnikoviae Radix, Angelicae Pubescentis Radix, Notopterygii Rhizoma et Radix, Mori Ramulus, Piperis Kadsurae Caulis, Sinapis Semen, Stephaniae Tetrandrae Radix, Impatientis Balsaminae Herba, Lycopodii Herba, Clematidis Radix et Rhizoma, Borneolum Syntheticum, Menthol, Methyl Salicylate, Camphora, Thymol, Xylene, Moschus, Belladonnae Extractum and Diphenhydramine Hydrochloride.

Actions and Indications Dispelling wind and dampness, activating blood and alleviating pain. It is indicated for wind-cold-damp impediment syndrome, marked by arthralgia, neuralgia, lumbago, soreness and pain of the muscles, and sprain.

Warning It should be used carefully for pregnant women.

羊痫疯丸

【处方】白矾、郁金、金礞石（煅）、全蝎、黄连、乌梅。

【功能主治】息风止惊，清心安神。用于癫痫。

Relieving Epilepsy Pill

Name of Chinese Phonetic Alphabet Yang Xian Feng Wan

Formula Alumen, Curcumae Radix, Micae Lapis Aureus (calcined), Scorpio, Coptidis Rhizoma and Mume Fructus.

Actions and Indications Extinguishing wind and settling fright, clearing heart-fire and tranquilizing. It is indicated for epilepsy.

导赤丸

【处方】连翘、黄连、栀子（姜炒）、关木通、玄参、天花粉、赤芍、大黄、黄芩、滑石。

【功能主治】清热泻火，利尿通便。用于口舌生疮，咽喉疼痛，心胸烦热，小便短赤，大便秘结。

Dao Chi Pill

Name of Chinese Phonetic Alphabet Dao Chi Wan

Formula Forsythiae Fructus, Coptidis Rhizoma, Gardeniae Fructus (fried with ginger), Aristochiae Manshuriensis Caulis, Scrophulariae Radix, Trichosanthis Radix, Paeoniae Radix Rubra, Rhei Radix et Rhizoma, Scutellariae Radix and Talcum.

Actions and Indications Clearing heat and purging fire, inducing diuresis and relaxing the bowels. It is indicated aphthae, sore-throat, vexing heat in the chest, scanty and dark urine, constipation.

导便栓

【处方】猪胆膏、醋酸洗必泰。

【功能主治】润肠通便。用于肠燥便秘。

Inducing Defecation Suppository

Name of Chinese Phonetic Alphabet Dao Bian Shuan

Formula Suillus Fel Extractum and Chlorhexidine Acetate.

Actions and Indications Moistening the intestines to relax the bowels. It is used for constipation due to intestinal dryness.

阳和解凝膏

【处方】鲜牛蒡草（或干品）、鲜凤仙透骨草（或干品）、生川乌、桂枝、大黄、当归、生草乌、生附子、地龙、僵蚕、赤芍、白芷、白蔹、白及、川芎、续断、防风、荆芥、五灵脂、木香、香橼、陈皮、肉桂、乳香、没药、苏合香、麝香。

【功能主治】温阳化湿，消肿散结。用于阴疽瘰疬。

【注意】外用。

Scrofula-subsiding Plaster

Name of Chinese Phonetic Alphabet Yang He Jie Ning Gao

Formula Herba Arctii(raw), Impatientis Balsaminae Herba(raw), Aconiti Radix (raw), Cinnamomi Ramulus, Rhei Radix et Rhizoma, Angelicae Sinensis Radix, Aconiti Kusnezoffii Radix (raw), Aconiti Lateralis Radix (raw), Pheretima, Bombyx Batryticatus, Paeoniae Radix Rubra, Angelicae Dahuricae Radix, Ampelopsis Radix, Bletillae Rhizoma, Chuanxiong Rhizoma, Dipsaci Radix, Saposhnikoviae Radix, Schizonepetae Herba, Trogopterori Faeces, Aucklandiae Radix, Citri Fructus, Citri Reticulatae Pericarpium, Cinnamomi Cortex, Olibanum, Myrrha, Styrax and Moschus.

Actions and Indications Warming *yang* and resolving dampness, dispersing swelling and dissipating mass. It is used for deep-rooted carbuncle and scrofula.

Warning It is for external use only.

阴虚胃痛冲剂

【处方】北沙参、麦冬、石斛、川楝子、甘草（炙）、玉竹、白芍。

【功能主治】养阴益胃，缓中止痛。用于胃阴不足引起的胃脘隐隐灼痛，口干舌燥，纳呆，干呕，以及慢性胃炎、消化性溃疡见上述症状者。

Stomachache-relieving Soluble Granules

Name of Chinese Phonetic Alphabet Yin Xu Wei Tong Chong Ji

Formula Glehniae Radix, Ophiopogonis Radix, Dendrobii Caulis, Toosendan Fructus, Glycyrrhizae Radix et Rhizoma (prepared), Polygonati Odorati Rhizoma and Paeoniae Radix Alba.

Actions and Indications Nourishing *yin* and the stomach, relaxing the middle energizer to alleviate pain. It is indicated for dull and scorching pain in the stomach due to insufficiency of stomach-*yin*; dry tongue and mouth, poor appetite, dry retching, and chronic gastritis, peptic ulcer with the above mentioned symptoms.

防风通圣丸

【处方】防风、荆芥穗、薄荷、麻黄、大黄、芒硝、栀子、滑石、桔梗、石膏、川芎、当归、白芍、黄芩、连翘、甘草、白术（炒）。

【功能主治】解表通里，清热解毒。用于外寒内热，表里俱实，恶寒壮热，头痛咽干，小便短赤，大便秘结，瘰疬初起，风疹湿疮。

【注意】孕妇慎用。

Divaricate Saposhnikovia* Pill for Releasing Exterior Syndrome

Name of Chinese Phonetic Alphabet Fang Feng Tong Sheng Wan

Formula Saposhnikoviae Radix, Schizonepetae Spica, Menthae Haplocalycis Herba, Ephedrae Herba, Rhei Radix et Rhizoma, Natrii Sulfas, Gardeniae Fructus,Talcum, Platycodonis Radix, Gypsum Fibrosum, Chuanxiong Rhizoma, Angelicae Sinensis Radix, Paeoniae Radix Alba, Scutellariae Radix, Forsythiae Fructus, Glycyrrhizae Radix et Rhizoma and Atractylodis Macrocephalae Rhizoma (fried).

Actions and Indications Releasing exterior, dredging interior, clearing heat and detoxicating. It is used for cases with aversion to cold, high fever, headache, dry pharynx, scanty dark urine, constipation, initial stage of scrofula, rubella and eczema due to exterior cold and interior heat, dual excess of the exterior and interior.

Warning It should be used carefully for pregnant women.

*防风

如意金黄散

【处方】姜黄、大黄、黄柏、苍术、厚朴、陈皮、甘草、生天南星、白芷、天花粉。

【功能主治】消肿止痛。用于疮疡肿毒，丹毒流注，跌扑损伤。

Ru Yi Powder for Traumatic Injury

Name of Chinese Phonetic Alphabet Ru Yi Jin Huang San

Formula Curcumae Longae Rhizoma, Rhei Radix et Rhizoma, Phellodendri Chinensis Cortex, Atractylodis Rhizoma, Magnoliae Officinalis Cortex, Citri Reticulatae Pericarpium, Glycyrrhizae Radix et Rhizoma, Arisaematis Rhizoma (raw), Angelicae Dahuricae Radix and Trichosanthis Radix.

Actions and Indications Dispersing swelling and relieving pain. It is used for furuncle with swelling and pain, erysipelas, deep multiple abscess and traumatic injury.

妇女痛经丸

【处方】延胡索（醋制）、五灵脂（醋炒）、丹参、蒲黄（炭）。

【功能主治】活血，调经，止痛。用于瘀血凝滞，小腹胀痛，经期腹痛。

【注意】孕妇忌服。

Dysmenorrhea-promoting Pill

Name of Chinese Phonetic Alphabet Fu Nü Tong Jing Wan

Formula Corydalis Rhizoma (prepared with vinegar), Trogopterori Faeces (fried with vinegar), Salviae Miltiorrhizae Radix et Rhizoma and Typhae Pollen (carbonated).

Actions and Indications Activating blood, regulating menstruation, allevating pain. It is indicated for dysmenorrhea due to blood-stasis.

Warning It is contraindicated for pregnant women.

妇乐冲剂

【处方】忍冬藤、大血藤、甘草、牡丹皮、大青叶、蒲公英、赤芍、延胡索（制）、川楝子、大黄（制）。

【功能主治】清热凉血，消肿止痛。用于盆腔炎，附件炎，子宫内膜炎等引起的带下、腹痛。

【注意】孕妇慎用。

Leukorrhea-relieving Soluble Granules

Name of Chinese Phonetic Alphabet Fu Le Chong Ji

Formula Lonicerae Japonicae Caulis, Sargentodoxae Caulis, Glycyrrhizae Radix et Rhizoma, Moutan Cortex, Isatidis Folium, Taraxaci Herba, Paeoniae Radix Rubra, Corydalis Rhizoma (prepared), Toosendan Fructus and Rhei Radix et Rhizoma (prepared).

Actions and Indications Clearing heat, cooling blood, reducing swelling, alleviating pain. It is used for leukorrhea, abdominal pain due to pelvic inflammation, adnexitis and endometritis.

Warning It should be used cautiously for pregnant women.

妇宁康片

【处方】人参、枸杞子、当归、熟地黄、赤芍、山茱萸、知母、黄柏、牡丹皮、石菖蒲、远志、茯苓、菟丝子、淫羊藿、巴戟天、蛇床子、狗脊、五味子。

【功能主治】补肾助阳，调整冲任，益气养血，安神解郁。用于妇女更年期综合征及月经不调，阴道干燥，精神抑郁不安。

Relieving Menopausal Syndrome Tablet

Name of Chinese Phonetic Alphabet Fu Ning Kang Pian

Formula Ginseng Radix et Rhizoma, Lycii Fructus, Angelicae Sinensis Radix, Rehmanniae Radix Praeparata, Paeoniae Radix Rubra, Corni Fructus, Anemarrhenae Rhizoma, Phellodendri Chinensis Cortex, Moutan Cortex, Acori Tatarinowii

Rhizoma, Polygalae Radix, Poria, Cuscutae Semen, Epimedii Folium, Morindae Officinalis Radix, Cnidii Fructus, Cibotii Rhizoma and Schisandrad Chinensis Fructus.

Actions and Indications Tonifying kidney-*yang*, regulating thoroughfare and conception vessels, tonifying *qi* and nourishing blood, tranquilizing the mind. It is used for menopausal syndrome, irregular menstruation, dryness of vagina, depression of spirit and restlessness.

妇炎平胶囊

【处方】苦参、蛇床子、苦木、珍珠层粉、冰片、盐酸小檗碱、枯矾、薄荷脑、硼酸。

【功能主治】清热解毒，燥湿止带，杀虫止痒。用于湿热下注，带脉失约，赤白带下，阴痒，以及滴虫、霉菌、细菌引起的阴道炎、外阴炎。

【注意】孕妇慎用；月经期至经净3天内停用，切忌内服。

Relieving Vaginitis Capsule

Name of Chinese Phonetic Alphabet Fu Yan Ping Jiao Nang

Formula Sophorae Flavescentis Radix, Cnidii Fructus, Picrasmae Ramulus et Folium, Margaritae Concha Strati Pulvis, Borneolum Syntheticum, Berberine hydrochloride, Alumen Usta, Menthol and Borate.

Actions and Indications Clearing heat and detoxicating, drying dampness and relieving vaginal discharge, killing worms and relieving itching. It is indicated for downward attack of damp-heat and irregular belt vessel, marked by red-white vaginal discharge, pruritus vulvae, vaginitis and vulvitis due to trichomonad, fungus and bacterium.

Warning It should be used carefully for pregnant women; suspend medicine during menstrual period and three days after menstrual period; it's prohibited for internal use.

妇炎灵胶囊

【处方】紫珠叶、硼酸、苦参、樟脑、仙鹤草、白矾、百部、冰片、蛇床子、苯甲溴铵。

【功能主治】清热燥湿，杀虫止痒。用于湿热下注引起的阴部瘙痒、灼痛、赤白带下，或兼见尿频、尿急、尿痛等症，以及霉菌性、滴虫性、细菌性阴道炎见上述证候者。

Relieving Gynecological Inflammation Capsule

Name of Chinese Phonetic Alphabet Fu Yan Ling Jiao Nang

Formula Callicarpae Formosanae Folium, Borate, Sophorae Flavescentis Radix, Camphora, Agrimoniae Herba, Alumen, Stemonae Radix, Borneolum Syntheticum, Cnidii Fructus and Benzoic Ammonium Bromide.

Actions and Indications Clearing heat, drying dampness, killing worms, relieving itching. It is used for pruritus vulvae, scoching pain, red-white vaginal discharge or complicated by urinary urgency, urinary frequency, urodynia, mycotic, trichomonal and bacterial vaginitis with the above mentioned symptoms.

妇炎净胶囊

【处方】苦玄参、地胆草、当归、鸡血藤、两面针等。

【功能主治】清热祛湿，行气止痛。用于湿热带下、月经不调、痛经，以及附件炎，盆腔炎，子宫内膜炎。

Gynecological Inflammation Relieving Capsule

Name of Chinese Phonetic Alphabet Fu Yan Jing Jiao Nang

Formula Picriae Herba, Elephantopi Herba, Angelicae Sinensis Radix, Spatholobi Caulis, Zanthoxyli Radix, etc.

Actions and Indications Clearing heat and

draining dampness, moving *qi* and alleviating pain. It is indicated for vaginal discharge due to damp-heat; irregular menstruation, dysmenorrhea, annexitis, pelvic inflammation, and endometritis.

妇炎康片

【处方】赤芍、土茯苓、苦参、延胡索（醋制）、丹参、莪术（醋炙）、当归、川楝子（炒）、黄柏、芡实（炒）、山药、三棱（醋炙）、香附（醋炙）。

【功能主治】活血化瘀，软坚散结，清热解毒，消炎镇痛。适用于慢性附件炎、盆腔炎、阴道炎、膀胱炎、慢性阑尾炎、尿路感染。

Relieving Gynecological Inflammation Tablet

Name of Chinese Phonetic Alphabet Fu Yan Kang Pian

Formula Paeoniae Radix Rubra, Smilacis Glabrae Rhizoma, Sophorae Flavescentis Radix, Corydalis Rhizoma (prepared with vinegar), Salviae Miltiorrhizae Radix et Rhizoma, Curcumae Rhizoma (prepared with vinegar), Angelicae Sinensis Radix, Toosendan Fructus (fried), Phellodendri Chinensis Cortex, Euryales Semen (fried), Dioscoreae Rhizoma, Sparganii Rhizoma (prepared with vinegar) and Cyperi Rhizoma (prepared with vinegar).

Actions and Indications Activating blood, resolving stasis, dissipating mass, clearing heat, detoxifying, anti-inflammation, settling pain. It is indicated for chronic adenxitis, pelvic inflammation, vaginitis, cystitis, chronic appendicitis and urinary tract infection.

妇炎康复颗粒

【处方】败酱草、薏苡仁、川楝子、柴胡、陈皮、黄芩等。

【功能主治】清热利湿，化瘀止痛。用于湿热瘀阻所致妇女带下，色黄质黏稠，味臭，少腹、腰骶疼痛，舌暗苔黄腻等症，以及慢性盆腔炎见上述证候者。

【注意】明显脾胃虚弱者慎用。

Relieving Leukorrheal Disease Soluble Granules

Name of Chinese Phonetic Alphabet Fu Yan Kang Fu Ke Li

Formula Patriniae Herba, Coicis Semen, Toosendan Fructus, Bupleuri Radix, Citri Reticulatae Pericarpium, Scutellariae Radix, etc.

Actions and Indications Clearing heat and draining dampness, resolving stasis and alleviating pain. It is indicated for leukorrheal disease, marked by yellow and sticky, thick vaginal discharge with bad odor, pain in the lower abdomen and lumbosacral pain, dark tongue with yellow slimy fur due to stagnation damp-heat, also for chronic pelvic inflammation with the above mentioned symptoms.

Warning It should be used carefully for cases with obvious deficiency of the spleen and stomach.

妇宝冲剂

【处方】地黄、忍冬藤、续断、杜仲叶（盐水炒）、麦冬、莲房（炭）、川楝子（炒）、白芍（酒炒）、延胡索（醋制）、甘草、侧柏叶（炒）、红藤。

【功能主治】益肾和血，理气止痛。用于妇女盆腔炎、附件炎等引起的小腹胀痛，腰酸，白带，经漏。

Relieving Gynecopathy Soluble Granules

Name of Chinese Phonetic Alphabet Fu Bao Chong Ji

Formula Rehmanniae Radix, Lonicerae Japonicae Caulis, Dipsaci Radix, Eucommiae Folium (fried with salt water), Ophiopogonis Radix, Nelumbinis Receptaculum (carbonated), Toosendan Fructus (fried), Paeoniae Radix Alba (fried with wine), Corydalis Rhizoma (prepared with vinegar), Glycyrrhizae Radix et Rhizoma, Platycladi Cacumen (fried) and Sargentodoxae Caulis.

Actions and Indications Tonifying the kidney

and harmonizing blood, regulating *qi* and relieving pain. It is used for distention and pain in the lower abdomen, soreness of the waist, leukorrhagia and menstrual dripping due to pelvic inflammation or adnexitis.

妇科十味片

【处方】香附（醋炙）、川芎、当归、延胡索（醋炙）、白术、甘草、大枣、白芍、赤芍、熟地黄、碳酸钙。

【功能主治】舒肝理气，养血调经。用于肝郁血虚，月经不调，行经腹痛，闭经。

Ten Medicinals Tablet for Regulating Menstruation

Name of Chinese Phonetic Alphabet Fu Ke Shi Wei Pian

Formula Cyperi Rhizoma (prepared with vinegar), Chuanxiong Rhizoma, Angelicae Sinensis Radix, Corydalis Rhizoma (prepared with vinegar), Atractylodis Macrocephalae Rhizoma, Glycyrrhizae Radix et Rhizoma, Jujubae Fructus, Paeoniae Radix Alba, Paeoniae Radix Rubra, Rehmanniae Radix Praeparata and Calcium Carbonate.

Actions and Indications Soothing the liver and regulating *qi*, tonifying blood to regulate menstruation. It is indicated for irregular menstruation, dysmenorrhea and amenorrhea due to liver depression and blood deficiency.

妇科万应膏

【处方】苏木、川芎、青皮、白蔹、干姜、石南藤、胡芦巴（炒）、泽兰、小茴香、茺蔚子、九香虫、艾叶、白芷、拳参、红花、当归、桉油。

【功能主治】温经散寒，活血化瘀，理气止痛。用于宫寒血滞引起的月经不调，经期腹痛，腹冷经闭，腰疼带下。

【注意】孕妇禁用。

Medicated Plaster for Regulating Menstruation

Name of Chinese Phonetic Alphabet Fu Ke Wan Ying Gao

Formula Sappan Lignum, Chuanxiong Rhizoma, Citri Reticulatae Pericarpium Viride, Ampelopsis Radix, Zingiberis Rhizoma, Photiniae Serrulatae Caulis et Folium, Trigonellae Semen (fried), Lycopi Herba, Foeniculi Fructus, Leonuri Fructus, Aspongopus, Artemisiae Argyi Folium, Angelicae Dahuricae Radix, Bistortae Rhizoma, Carthami Flos, Angelicae Sinensis Radix and Eucalypti Oleum.

Actions and Indications Warming the meridians, dissipating cold, activating blood, resolving stasis, regulating *qi*, alleviating pain. It is used for irregular menstruation, dysmenorrhea, amenorrhea, lumbago and vaginal discharge due to uterus-coldness and blood-stagnation.

Warning It is contraindicated for pregnant women.

妇科千金片

【处方】千斤拔、单面针、金樱根、穿心莲、功劳木、党参、鸡血藤。

【功能主治】清热除湿，补益气血。用于带下病；也用于盆腔炎、子宫内膜炎、宫颈炎。

Philippine Flemingia* and Cherokee Rose Root** Tablet for Leukorrheal Disease

Name of Chinese Phonetic Alphabet Fu Ke Qian Jin Pian

Formula Flemingiae Philippinensis Radix, Zanthoxyli Dissiti Fructus seu Semen, Rosae Laevigatae Radix, Andrographis Herba, Mahoniae Caulis, Codonopsis Radix and Spatholobi Caulis.

Actions and Indications Clearing heat and dispelling dampness, tonifying *qi* and blood. It is indicated for leukorrheal disease, also for pelvic inflammation, endometritis and cervicitis.

* 千斤拔 ** 金樱根

妇科白带膏

【处方】白术（炒）、苍术、党参、陈皮、山药、甘草、荆芥、车前子、柴胡、白芍。

【功能主治】健脾舒肝，除湿止带。用于脾虚湿盛，白带连绵，腰腿酸痛。

Thick Paste of Leukorrhea-arresting

Name of Chinese Phonetic Alphabet Fu Ke Bai Dai Gao

Formula Atractylodis Macrocephalae Rhizoma (fried), Atractylodis Rhizoma, Codonopsis Radix, Citri Reticulatae Pericarpium, Dioscoreae Rhizoma, Glycyrrhizae Radix et Rhizoma, Schizonepetae Herba, Plantaginis Semen, Bupleuri Radix and Paeoniae Radix Alba.

Actions and Indications Fortifying the spleen, soothing the liver, eliminating dampness and arresting leukorrhea. It is indicated for leukorrhagia, soreness and pain of waist and legs due to deficiency of the spleen and abundance of dampness.

妇科回生丸

【处方】人参、白术（麸炒）、苍术、茯苓、甘草、青皮（醋炙）、陈皮、熟地黄、当归、白芍、川芎、桃仁（去皮）、红花、木香、香附（醋炙）、乌药、延胡索（醋炙）、三棱（麸炒）、蒲黄、五灵脂（醋炙）、苏木、乳香（醋炙）、没药（醋炙）、牛膝、大黄、地榆（炭）、米醋、山茱萸（酒炙）、黑豆、高良姜、羌活、木瓜。

【功能主治】通经化瘀，止痛。用于气虚血亏，瘀血凝滞引起的经期不准，经闭，癥瘕血块，腹部痞胀，身体消瘦，四肢困倦，产后恶露不尽。

【注意】孕妇忌服。

Relieving Gynecopathy Bolus

Name of Chinese Phonetic Alphabet Fu Ke Hui Sheng Wan

Formula Ginseng Radix et Rhizoma, Atractylodis Macrocephalae Rhizoma (fried with bran), Atractylodis Rhizoma, Poria, Glycyrrhizae Radix et Rhizoma, Citri Reticulatae Pericarpium Viride (prepared with vinegar), Citri Reticulatae Pericarpium, Rehmanniae Radix Praeparata, Angelicae Sinensis Radix, Paeoniae Radix Alba, Chuanxiong Rhizoma, Persicae Semen (removed seed coat), Carthami Flos, Aucklandiae Radix, Cyperi Rhizoma (prepared with vinegar), Linderae Radix, Corydalis Rhizoma (prepared with vinegar), Sparganii Rhizoma (fried with bran), Typhae Pollen, Trogopterori Faeces (prepared with vinegar), Sappan Lignum, Olibanum (prepared with vinegar), Myrrha (prepared with vinegar), Achyranthis Bidentatae Radix, Rhei Radix et Rhizoma, Sanguisorbae Radix (carbonated), Oryzi-Acetum, Corni Fructus (prepared with wine), Sojae Semen Nigrum, Alpiniae Officinarum Rhizoma, Notopterygii Rhizoma et Radix and Chaenomelis Fructus.

Actions and Indications Regulating menstruation and resolving stasis, relieving pain. It is uesd for irregular menstruation, amenorrhea, emaciation, abdominal mass,tiredness of limbs and postpartum lochiorrhagia due to dual deficiency of *qi* and blood and blood-stasis.

Warning It is contraindicated for pregnant women.

妇科得生丸

【处方】益母草、白芍、当归、木香、羌活、柴胡。

【功能主治】解郁和肝，化瘀调经。用于肝郁不舒，气凝血滞引起的月经不准，行经腹痛，胸满胁痛，午后身热，倦怠食少。

Gynecopathy-relieving Bolus

Name of Chinese Phonetic Alphabet Fu Ke De Sheng Wan

Formula Leonuri Herba, Paeoniae Radix Alba, Angelicae Sinensis Radix, Aucklandiae Radix, Notopterygii Rhizoma et Radix and Bupleuri Radix.

Actions and Indications Releasing depression, harmonizing the liver, resolving stasis, regulating menstruation. It is used for irregular menstrual cycle, dysmenorrhea, hypochondriac fullness and pain, afternoon fever, tiredness and anorexia due to depression of liver-*qi*, stagnation of *qi* and blood.

妇康宁片

【处方】白芍、香附、当归、三七、艾叶（炭）、麦冬、党参、益母草。

【功能主治】调经养血，理气止痛。用于气血两亏，经期腹痛。

【注意】孕妇忌服。

Dysmenorrhea-relieving Tablet

Name of Chinese Phonetic Alphabet Fu Kang Ning Pian

Formula Paeoniae Radix Alba, Cyperi Rhizoma, Angelicae Sinensis Radix, Notoginseng Radix et Rhizoma, Artemisiae Argyi Folium (carbonated), Ophiopogonis Radix, Codonopsis Radix and Leonuri Herba.

Actions and Indications Regulating menstruation and nourishing blood, regulating *qi* and relieving pain. It is indicated for dysmenorrhea due to dual deficiency of *qi* and blood.

Warning It is contraindicated for pregnant women.

红灵散

【处方】麝香、雄黄、朱砂、硼砂、金礞石（煅）、硝石（精制）、冰片。

【功能主治】祛暑，开窍，避瘟，解毒。用于中暑昏厥，头晕胸闷，恶心呕吐，腹痛泄泻。

【注意】孕妇忌用。

Exorcising Seasonal Disease Powder

Name of Chinese Phonetic Alphabet Hong Ling San

Formula Moschus, Realgar, Cinnabaris, Borax, Micae Lapis Aureus (calcined), Nitrum (refined) and Borneolum Syntheticum.

Actions and Indications Dispelling summer-heat, inducing resuscitation, exorcising seasonal disease and detoxifying. It is used for summer-heat stroke, coma, dizziness, chest distress, nausea, vomiting, abdominal pain and diarrhea.

Warning It is contraindicated for pregnant women.

红药气雾剂

【处方】三七、白芷、土鳖虫、川芎、当归、红花、冰片、薄荷脑等。

【功能主治】活血逐瘀，消肿止痛。用于跌打损伤，局部瘀血肿胀，筋骨疼痛。

【注意】皮肤破损慎用。

Hong Yao Spray

Name of Chinese Phonetic Alphabet Hong Yao Qi Wu Ji

Formula Notoginseng Radix et Rhizoma, Angelicae Dahuricae Radix, Eupolyphaga seu Steleophaga, Chuanxiong Rhizoma, Angelicae Sinensis Radix, Carthami Flos, Borneolum Syntheticum, Menthol, etc.

Actions and Indications Activating blood, eliminating stasis, reducing swelling, alleviating pain. It is used for traumatic injury, topical blood-stasis and swelling, ostealgia.

Warning It should be used cautiously for cases with wound of skin.

红棉散

【处方】枯矾、炉甘石、冰片、麝香等。

【功能主治】化毒收敛，止痒消肿。用于肝经郁热，耳内生疮，流脓痛痒，小儿胎热耳疳。

【注意】忌食辛辣发物。

Relieving Otopathy Powder

Name of Chinese Phonetic Alphabet Hong Mian San

Formula Alumen Usta, Calamina, Borneolum

Syntheticum, Moschus, etc.

Actions and Indications Astringing and detoxicating, relieving itching and dispersing swelling in the ears. It is used for sore in the ears, otopyosis and ulcered ear of children due to accumulation of heat in the liver meridian.

Warning Pungent foods should be avoided.

七画

麦味地黄丸

【处方】麦冬、五味子、熟地黄、山茱萸（制）、牡丹皮、山药、茯苓、泽泻。

【功能主治】滋肾养肺。用于肺肾阴亏引起的潮热盗汗，咽干咳血，眩晕耳鸣，腰膝酸软，消渴。

Bolus of Lily-turf * and Chinese Foxglove**

Name of Chinese Phonetic Alphabet Mai Wei Di Huang Wan

Formula Ophiopogonis Radix, Schisandrae Chinensis Fructus, Rehmanniae Radix Praeparata, Corni Fructus (prepared), Moutan Cortex, Dioscoreae Rhizoma, Poria and Alismatis Rhizoma.

Actions and Indications Enriching the kidney and lung. It is indicated for tidal fever, night sweating, dry throat, hemoptysis, vertigo, tinnitus, soreness of waist and weakness of knees, and wasting-thirst.

* 麦冬 ** 地黄

坎离砂

【处方】当归、川芎、防风、透骨草、铁屑。

【功能主治】祛风散寒，活血止痛。用于风寒湿痹，四肢麻木，关节疼痛，脘腹冷痛。

【注意】外用。

Kanlisha Powder for Relieving Wind-cold-damp Impediment

Name of Chinese Phonetic Alphabet Kan Li Sha

Formula Angelicae Sinensis Radix, Chuanxiong Rhizoma, Saposhnikoviae Radix, Speranskiae Tuberculatae Herba and Ferum Squamae.

Actions and Indications Expelling wind and dissipating cold, activating blood to relieve pain. It is used for wind-cold-damp impediment syndrome marked by numbness of limbs, arthralgia, cold pain of stomach duct and abdomen.

Warning It is for external use only.

杜仲冲剂

【处方】杜仲、杜仲叶。

【功能主治】补肝肾，强筋骨，安胎，降血压。用于肾虚腰痛，腰膝无力，胎动不安，先兆流产，高血压症。

Gutta-percha-tree* Soluble Granules

Name of Chinese Phonetic Alphabet Du Zhong Chong Ji

Formula Eucommiae Cortex and Eucommiae Folium.

Actions and Indications Tonifying the liver and kidney, strengthening the sinews and bone, preventing abortion and lowering blood pressure. It is used for lumbago, weakness of waist and knees, threathened abortion and hypertension due to deficiency of kidney.

* 杜仲

杜仲壮骨丸

【处方】杜仲、白术、乌梢蛇、人参、桑枝、三七、金铁锁、木瓜、狗骨胶、细辛、续断、石南藤、川芎、附片、淫羊藿、当归、黄芪、大血藤、秦艽、防风、威灵仙、独活、豹骨、寻骨风。

【功能主治】益气健脾，养肝壮腰，活血通络，强筋健骨，祛风除湿。用于治疗风湿痹痛，筋骨无力，屈伸不利，腰膝疼痛，畏寒喜温。

【注意】服药期间忌食酸、生冷食物。孕妇忌服。

Gutta-percha-tree* Pill for Strengthening Bone

Name of Chinese Phonetic Alphabet Du Zhong Zhuang Gu Wan

Formula Eucommiae Cortex, Atractylodis Macrocephalae Rhizoma, Zaocys, Ginseng Radix et Rhizoma, Mori Ramulus, Notoginseng Radix et Rhizoma, Psammosilenes Tunicoidis Radix, Chaenomelis Fructus, Canis Os Colla, Asari Radix et Rhizoma,Dipsaci Radix, Photiniae Serrulatae Herba, Chuanxiong Rhizoma, Aconiti Lateralis Radix Praeparata (sliced), Epimedii Folium, Angelicae Sinensis Radix, Astragali Radix, Sargentodoxae Caulis, Gentianae Macrophyllae Radix, Saposhnikoviae Radix, Clematidis Radix et Rhizoma, Angelicae Pubescentis Radix, Pardi Os and Aristolochiae Mollissimae Rhizoma seu Herba.

Actions and Indications Tonifying *qi*, fortifying the spleen, nourishing the liver, strengthening the waist, activating blood and collateral, dispelling wind and dampness. It is indicated for rheumatalgia, weakness of sinew and bone, immobility of limbs, pain of waist and knees, fear of cold and joy of warmth.

Warning During medication, sour and uncooked foods are prohibited. It is contraindicated for pregnant women.

*杜仲

杜仲补天素片

【处方】杜仲（盐水炒）、菟丝子（制）、肉苁蓉、远志（制）、当归（酒制）、莲子、泽泻、牡丹皮、白芍、淫羊藿、黄芪、熟地黄、山药、茯苓、白术、陈皮、砂仁、女贞子、金樱子、山茱萸、巴戟天、柏子仁、党参、枸杞子、甘草。

【功能主治】温肾养心，壮腰安神。用于肾气不足，心肾不交引起的腰脊酸软，夜多小便，神经衰弱。

【注意】感冒伤风，应暂时停服。

Gutta-percha-tree* Tablet for Warming Kidney

Name of Chinese Phonetic Alphabet Du Zhong Bu Tian Su Pian

Formula Eucommiae Cortex (fried with salt water), Cuscutae Semen (prepared), Cistanches Caulis Carnosus, Polygalae Radix (prepared), Angelicae Sinensis Radix (prepared with wine), Nelumbinis Semen, Alismatis Rhizoma, Moutan Cortex, Paeoniae Radix Alba, Epimedii Folium, Astragali Radix, Rehmanniae Radix Praeparata, Dioscoreae Rhizoma, Poria, Atractylodis Macrocephalae Rhizoma, Citri Reticulatae Pericarpium, Amomi Fructus, Ligustri Lucidi Fructus. Rosae Laevigatae Fructus, Corni Fructus, Morindae Officinalis Radix, Platycladi Semen, Codonopsis Radix, Lycii Fructus and Glycyrrhizae Radix et Rhizoma.

Actions and Indications Warming the kidney, nourishing the heart, strengthening the waist and tranquilizing the mind. It is used for soreness and weakness of waist, frequent urination at night and neurasthenia due to insufficiency of kidney-*qi* and non-interaction between the heart and kidney.

Warning Suspend the medicine in case of common cold.

*杜仲

杜仲补腰合剂

【处方】杜仲、党参、当归、枸杞子、牛膝、补骨脂、熟地黄、菟丝子、香菇、猪腰子。

【功能主治】补肝肾，益气血，强腰膝。用于肝肾不足，气血亏虚引起的腰腿疼痛，疲劳无力，精神不振，小便频数。

Gutta-percha-tree *Mixture

Name of Chinese Phonetic Alphabet Du Zhong Bu Yao He Ji

Formula Eucommiae Cortex, Codonopsis Radix, Angelicae Sinensis Radix, Lycii Fructus, Achyranthis Bidentatae Radix, Psoraleae Fructus, Rehmanniae Radix Praeparata, Cuscutae Semen, Lentini Sporocarpium

Edodis and Suillus Ren.

Actions and Indications Tonifying the liver and kidney, *qi* and blood, strengthening the waist and knees. It is used for lumbago and scelalgia, tiredness, fatigue, lassitude of spirit and frequent urination due to dual insufficiency of the liver and kidney and dual depletion of *qi* and blood.

* 杜仲

杞菊地黄丸

【处方】枸杞子、菊花、熟地黄、山茱萸（制）、牡丹皮、山药、茯苓、泽泻。

【功能主治】滋肾养肝。用于肝肾阴亏，眩晕耳鸣，羞明畏光，迎风流泪，视物昏花。

Bolus of Barbary Wolfberry* with Chrysanthemum** and Chinese Foxglove***

Name of Chinese Phonetic Alphabet Qi Ju Di Huang Wan

Formula Lycii Fructus, Chrysanthemi Flos, Rehmanniae Radix Praeparata, Corni Fructus (prepared), Moutan Cortex, Dioscoreae Rhizoma, Poria and Alismatis Rhizoma.

Actions and Indications Enriching the kidney and liver. It is indicated for vertigo, photophobia, overflow of tear induced by wind and blurred vision due to dual *yin*-depletion of the liver and kidney.

* 枸杞 ** 菊花 *** 地黄

克伤痛搽剂

【处方】当归、川芎、红花、丁香、生姜、樟脑、松节油。

【功能主治】活血化瘀，消肿止痛。主治急性软组织扭挫伤。

【注意】外用药。

Sprain-relieving Liniment

Name of Chinese Phonetic Alphabet Ke Shang Tong Cha Ji

Formula Angelicae Sinensis Radix, Chuanxiong Rhizoma, Carthami Flos, Caryophylli Flos, Zingiberis Rhizoma Recens, Camphora and Terebinthinae Oleum.

Actions and Indications Activating blood, resolving stasis, reducing swelling, alleviating pain. It is used for acute sprain and contusion of soft tissue.

Warning It is for external use only.

克泻灵片

【处方】苦豆草总生物碱。

【功能主治】清热解毒，祛风燥湿。用于湿热泄泻，痢疾。

Diarrhea-relieving Tablet

Name of Chinese Phonetic Alphabet Ke Xie Ling Pian

Formula Total Aloperines.

Actions and Indications Clearing heat and detoxicating, dispelling wind and drying dampness. It is indicated for diarrhea and dysentery of damp-heat type.

克泻胶囊

【处方】番石榴叶、黄连、茯苓等。

【功能主治】清热利湿，消食止泻。用于湿热或兼食滞所致泄泻。症见：泻下急迫，肛门灼热，泻下粪便呈稀水状，或黏腻，或臭如败卵夹有不化之物，脘腹痞满，嗳腐吞酸，呕吐，舌红，苔黄腻或白腻，脉滑数。

【注意】有明显脱水者，应注意采用综合治疗措施。

Diarrhea-relieving Capsule

Name of Chinese Phonetic Alphabet Ke Xie Jiao Nang

Formula Psidii Guajavae Folium, Coptidis Rhizoma, Poria, etc.

Actions and Indications Clearing heat and draining dampness, promoting digestion and relieving diarrhea. It is indicated for diarrhea due to damp-heat or companied by food stagnation, manifested as urgent diarrhea, scorching heat in the anus, watery or sticky stool with bad smell, fullness and stuffiness in the stomach and abdomen, belching and acid regurgitation, vomiting, red tongue, yellow or white greasy fur, slippery rapid pulse.

Warning For cases with obvious dehydration, comprehensive treatment should be applied.

克银丸

【处方】土茯苓、白鲜皮、北豆根、拳参。

【功能主治】清热解毒，祛风止痒。用于皮损基底红，便秘，尿黄属血热型银屑病。

【注意】忌食辛辣厚味食物。

Relieving Psoriasis Honeyed Bolus

Name of Chinese Phonetic Alphabet Ke Yin Wan

Formula Smilacis Glabrae Rhizoma, Dictamni Cortex, Menispermi Rhizoma and Bistortae Rhizoma.

Actions and Indications Clearing heat and detoxicating, dispelling wind and relieving itching. It is indicated for psoriasis with constipation and yellow urine attributive to blood-heat type.

Warning Pungent foods and greasy diet should be avoided.

克痢痧胶囊

【处方】白芷、苍术、石菖蒲、细辛、荜茇、鹅不食草、猪牙皂、雄黄、丁香、硝石、白矾、冰片。

【功能主治】解毒，理气止泻。用于泄泻，痢疾和痧气（中暑）。

【注意】孕妇禁用。

Relieving Dysentery Capsule

Name of Chinese Phonetic Alphabet Ke Li Sha Jiao Nang

Formula Angelicae Dahuricae Radix, Atractylodis Rhizoma, Acori Tatarinowii Rhizoma, Asari Radix et Rhizoma, Piperis Longi Fructus, Centipedae Herba, Gleditsiae Fructus Abnomalis, Realgar, Caryophylli Flos, Nitrum, Alumen and Borneolum Syntheticum.

Actions and Indications Detoxicating, regulating *qi* and relieving diarrhea. It is used for diarrhea, dysentery, summer-heat stroke.

Warning It is contraindicated for pregnant women.

芙朴感冒冲剂

【处方】芙蓉叶、厚朴、陈皮、牛蒡子（炒）。

【功能主治】清热解毒，宣肺利咽，理气。用于风热或风热夹湿感冒引起的发热头痛，咽痛，肢体酸痛，鼻塞，胃纳减退。

Cottonrose Hibiscus* and Magnolia Bark** Soluble Granules for Relieving Common Cold

Name of Chinese Phonetic Alphabet Fu Pu Gan Mao Chong Ji

Formula Hibisci Mutabilis Folium, Magnoliae Officinalis Cortex, Citri Reticulatae Pericarpium and Arctii Fructus (fried).

Actions and Indications Clearing heat and detoxicating, diffusing the lung and soothing the throat, regulating *qi*. It is indicated for common cold attributive to wind-heat type or wind-heat accompanied with dampness, marked by fever, headache, sore-throat, soreness and pain of limbs, nasal congestion, poor appetite.

* 芙蓉叶 ** 厚朴

花红冲剂

【处方】一点红、白花蛇舌草、鸡血藤、桃金娘根、白背桐、地桃花、菥蓂。

【功能主治】清热解毒，燥湿止带，祛瘀止痛。用于湿热下注，带下黄稠，子宫内膜炎、附件炎、盆腔炎属于湿热带下者。

Spreading Hedyotis* and Snake Strawberry** Soluble Granules

Name of Chinese Phonetic Alphabet Hua Hong Chong Ji

Formula Duchesneae Indicae Herba, Hedyotis Diffusae Herba, Spatholobi Caulis, Rhodomyrti Tomentosae Radix, Malloti Apeltae Folium, Urenae Lobatae Radix seu Herba and Thlaspis Herba.

Actions and Indications Clearing heat, detoxifying, drying dampness, relieving vaginal discharge, dispelling stasis, alleviating pain. It is used for yellow and thick vaginal discharge, endometritis, adnexitis and pelvic inflammation due to downward pour of damp-heat.

* 白花蛇舌草 ** 一点红

苁蓉通便口服液

【处方】肉从蓉、何首乌、枳实（麸炒）、蜂蜜。

【功能主治】滋阴补肾，润肠通便。主治中、老年人，病后、产后等虚性便秘及习惯性便秘。

Broomrape* Oral Liquid for Relaxing Bowels

Name of Chinese Phonetic Alphabet Cong Rong Tong Bian Kou Fu Ye

Formula Cistanches Caulis Carnosus, Polygoni Multiflori Radix, Aurantii Fructus Immaturus (fried with bran) and Mel.

Actions and Indications Enriching *yin*, tonifying the kidney, moistening the intestines to relax the bowels. It is mainly used for constipation of the middle age and aged, and after illness or childbirth, and habitual constipation.

* 肉苁蓉

芩连片

【处方】黄芩、连翘、黄连、黄柏、赤芍、甘草。

【功能主治】清热解毒，消肿止痛。用于脏腑蕴热，头痛目赤，口鼻生疮，热痢腹痛，湿热带下，疮疖肿痛。

Baical Skullcap* and Weeping Forsythia** Tablet for Clearing Heat

Name of Chinese Phonetic Alphabet Qin Lian Pian

Formula Scutellariae Radix, Forsythiae Fructus, Coptidis Rhizoma, Phellodendri Chinensis Cortex, Paeoniae Radix Rubra and Glycyrrhizae Radix et Rhizoma.

Actions and Indications Clearing heat and detoxicating, dispersing swelling and relieving pain. It is used for headache, conjunctival congestion, aphthae, dysentery, abdominal pain, white vaginal discharge, abscess and deep-rooted boil due to accumulation of heat in the viscera.

* 黄芩 ** 连翘

芩翘口服液

【处方】黄芩、连翘、荆芥等。

【功能主治】疏风清热，解毒利咽，消肿止痛。用于急喉痹（急性咽炎）、风热乳蛾（急性充血性扁桃体炎）属内有郁热、外感风热证者。症见咽痛或吞咽痛，咽干灼热，口渴多饮，咳嗽，痰黄，便干，尿黄，舌质红，苔薄白或黄，脉浮数有力。

Baical Skullcap* and Weeping Forsythia** Oral Liquid

Name of Chinese Phonetic Alphabet Qin Qiao Kou Fu Ye

Formula Scutellariae Radix, Forsythiae Fructus, Schizonepetae Herba, etc.

Actions and Indications Dispersing wind and clearing heat, detoxicating and soothing the throat, dispersing swelling and relieving pain. It is used for acute pharyngitis and acute congestive tonsillitis attributive to internal heat and exogenous wind-heat syndrome, manifested as sore-throat, odynophagia, dry throat and scorching hot, thirst, polydipsia, cough, yellow phlegm, dry stool, yellow urine, red tongue body, thin white or yellow fur, floating, rapid and powerful pulse.

* 黄芩 ** 连翘

芩暴红止咳颗粒

【处方】满山红、暴马子皮、黄芩。

【功能主治】清热化痰，止咳平喘。用于急性支气管炎及慢性支气管炎急性发作。

Soluble Granules of Baical Skullcap* Amur Lilae** and Daurian Rhododendron*** for Suppressing Cough

Name of Chinese Phonetic Alphabet Qin Bao Hong Zhi Ke Ke Li

Formula Rhododendri Daurici Folium, Syringae Cortex and Scutellariae Radix.

Actions and Indications Clearing heat and resolving phlegm, suppressing cough and dyspnea. It is indicated for acute bronchitis and acute attack of chronic bronchitis.

* 黄芩 ** 暴马子皮 *** 满山红

苍苓止泻口服液

【处方】苍术、茯苓、金银花、柴胡、葛根、黄芩等。

【功能主治】清热除湿，运脾止泻。用于湿热所致的小儿泄泻，症见水样或蛋花样粪便、发热、腹胀、舌红苔黄，以及小儿轮状病毒性肠炎见以上症状者。

【注意】脱水及病重患儿注意补液等综合治疗。

Chinese Atractylodes *and Indian Bread** Oral liquid for Relieving Diarrhea

Name of Chinese Phonetic Alphabet Cang Ling Zhi Xie Kou Fu Ye

Formula Atractylodis Rhizoma, Poria, Lonicerae Japonicae Flos, Bupleuri Radix, Puerariae Lobatae Radix, Scutellariae Radix, etc.

Actions and Indications Clearing heat and dispelling dampness, activating the spleen and relieving diarrhea. It is indicated for infantile diarrhea due to damp-heat, manifested as watery stool, or egg-soup-like-stool, fever, abdominal distention, red tongue and yellow fur, and for infantile rotaviral enteritis with the above mentioned symptoms.

Warning For severe cases with dehydration, fluid infusion and comprehensive treatment should be applied.

* 苍术 ** 茯苓

芪枣冲剂

【处方】黄芪、大枣、茯苓、鸡血藤干膏。

【功能主治】益气补血，健脾和胃。用于白细胞减少症及病后体虚，以及肝脏亏损所致的免疫力下降等症。

Milkvetch* and Chinese Date** Soluble Granules

Name of Chinese Phonetic Alphabet Qi Zao Chong Ji

Formula Astragali Radix, Jujubae Fructus, Poria and Spatholobi Caulis Extractum.

Actions and Indications Tonifying *qi* and blood, fortifying the spleen and harmonizing the stomach. It is indicated for leukopenia and debility after illness, and hypofunction of immunologic function due to liver depletion.

* 黄芪 ** 大枣

苏合丸

【处方】苏合香、丁香、安息香、乳香、木香、檀香、八角茴香、香附（酒醋制）、白术（土炒）、诃子（去核）、荜茇、朱砂、冰片。

【功能主治】祛风镇痛，通窍除痰。用于中风痰厥，昏迷不省，小儿受惊吐乳，风痰腹痛吐泻。

【注意】孕妇禁服。

Storax* Pill

Name of Chinese Phonetic Alphabet Su He Wan

Formula Styrax, Caryophylli Flos, Benzoinum, Olibanum, Aucklandiae Radix, Santali Albi Lignum, Anisi Stellati Fructus, Cyperi Rhizoma (prepared with wine and vinegar), Atractylodis Macrocephalae Rhizoma (fried with earth), Chebulae Fructus (removed nucleus), Piperis Longi Fructus, Cinnabaris and Borneolum Syntheticum.

Actions and Indications Dispelling wind, settling pain, inducing resuscitation, eliminating phlegm. It is used for apoplexy, coma, infantile vomiting of milk due to fright; abdominal pain, vomiting and diarrhea due to wind-phlegm.

Warning It is contraindicated for pregnant women.

* 苏合香

苏合香丸

【处方】苏合香、安息香、冰片、水牛角浓缩粉、麝香、檀香、沉香、丁香、香附、木香、乳香（制）、荜茇、白术、诃子肉、朱砂。

【功能主治】芳香开窍，行气止痛。用于中风，中暑，痰厥昏迷，心胃气痛。

【注意】孕妇禁服。

Storax* Bolus

Name of Chinese Phonetic Alphabet Su He Xiang Wan

Formula Styrax, Benzoinum, Borneolum Syntheticum, Bubali Cornu Pulvis Concentratio, Moschus, Santali Albi Lignum, Aquilariae Lignum Resinatum, Caryophylli Flos, Cyperi Rhizoma, Aucklandiae Radix, Olibanum (prepared), Piperis Longi Fructus, Atractylodis Macrocephalae Rhizoma, Chebulae Fructus and Cinnabaris.

Actions and Indications Inducing resuscitation, moving *qi* and alleviating pain. It is indicated for apoplexy, summer-heat stroke, phlegm syncope, pain due to dual *qi*-stagnation in heart and stomach.

Warning It is contraindicated for pregnant women.

* 苏合香

苏南山肚痛丸

【处方】白芍、陈皮、木香、香附（制）、甘草、丹参、郁金、没药（炒）、血竭、川楝子、乳香（炒）。

【功能主治】行气止痛。用于肚痛，食滞腹痛，胃气痛，月经痛，小肠疝气痛，胁痛。

【注意】孕妇忌服。

Su Nan Shan Pill for Abdominal Pain

Name of Chinese Phonetic Alphabet Su Nan Shan Du Tong Wan

Formula Paeoniae Radix Alba, Citri Reticulatae Pericarpium, Aucklandiae Radix, Cyperi Rhizoma (prepared), Glycyrrhizae Radix et Rhizoma, Salviae Miltiorrhizae Radix et Rhizoma, Curcumae Radix, Myrrha (fried), Draconis Sangui, Toosendan Fructus and Olibanum (fired).

Actions and Indications Moving *qi* to alleviate pain. It is used for abdominal pain due to indigestion, stomach pain, dysmenorrhea, hernia and hypochondriac pain.

Warning It is contraindicated for pregnant women.

杏仁止咳糖浆

【处方】杏仁水、百部流浸膏、远志流浸膏、陈皮流浸膏、桔梗流浸膏、甘草流浸膏。

【功能主治】化痰止咳。用于痰浊阻肺，咳嗽痰多，急、慢性支气管炎。

Apricot Seed* Syrup for Relieving Cough

Name of Chinese Phonetic Alphabet Xing Ren Zhi Ke Tang Jiang

Formula Armeniacae Aqua Amarum, Stemonae Extractum, Polygalae Extractum, Citri Reticulatae

Extractum, Platycodonis Extractum and Glycyrrhizae Extractum.

Actions and Indications Resolving phlegm and relieving cough. It is indicated for cough with profuse phlegm, acute and chronic bronchitis due to stagnation of phlegm turbidity in the lung.

＊苦杏仁

更年宁

【处方】柴胡、黄芩、白芍、墨旱莲、人参、党参、郁金、香附（醋炙）、当归、薄荷、川芎、玄参、茯苓、法半夏、石菖蒲、牡丹皮、陈皮、干姜、白术（麸炒）、丹参、王不留行（炒）、女贞子（酒炙）。

【功能主治】疏肝解郁，益气养血，健脾安神。用于更年期引起的心悸气短，烦躁易怒，眩晕失眠，阵热汗出，胸乳胀痛，月经紊乱。

Menopausal-syndrome-relieving Bolus

Name of Chinese Phonetic Alphabet Geng Nian Ning

Formula Bupleuri Radix, Scutellariae Radix, Paeoniae Radix Alba, Ecliptae Herba, Ginseng Radix et Rhizoma, Codonopsis Radix, Curcumae Radix, Cyperi Rhizoma (prepared with vinegar), Angelicae Sinensis Radix, Menthae Haplocalycis Herba, Chuanxiong Rhizoma, Scrophulariae Radix, Poria, Pinelliae Rhizoma Praeparatum, Acori Tatarinowii Rhizoma, Moutan Cortex, Citri Reticulatae Pericarpium, Zingiberis Rhizoma, Atractylodis Macrocephalae Rhizoma (fried with bran), Salviae Miltiorrhizae Radix et Rhizoma, Vaccariae Semen (fried) and Ligustri Lucidi Fructus (prepared with wine).

Actions and Indications Soothing the liver, relieving depression, tonifying *qi*, nourishing blood, fortifying the spleen, tranquilizing the mind. It is used for palpitation, shortness of breath, vexation, vertigo, insomnia, paroxysmal fever, sweating, mastalgia and menstrual disorder due to climacterium.

更年宁心胶囊

【处方】熟地黄、黄连、白芍等。

【功能主治】滋阴清热，安神除烦。用于妇女更年期综合征阴虚火旺证，症见：潮热面红，自汗盗汗，心烦不宁，失眠多梦，头晕耳鸣，腰膝酸软，手足心热。

Menopausal-syndrome Relieving Capsule

Name of Chinese Phonetic Alphabet Geng Nian Ning Xin Jiao Nang

Formula Rehmanniae Radix Praeparata, Coptidis Rhizoma, Paeoniae Radix Alba, etc.

Actions and Indications Enriching *yin*, clearing heat and tranquilizing the mind. It is indicated for menopausal syndrome due to *yin*-deficiency with effulgent fire, and manifested as tidal fever, flushed complexion, spontaneous sweating, night sweating, vexation, insomnia, profuse dreaming, dizziness, tinnitus, soreness and weakness of waist and knees and vexing heat in the palms and soles.

更年安片

【处方】本品为熟地黄、生地黄、玄参、何首乌、麦冬、牡丹皮、泽泻、茯苓、五味子、珍珠母、磁石、钩藤、夜交藤、浮小麦、仙茅等药经加工制成的片剂。

【功能主治】滋阴清热，除烦安神。用于更年期出现的潮热汗出，眩晕，耳鸣，失眠，烦躁不安，血压不稳。

Relieving Climacteric Symptoms Tablet

Name of Chinese Phonetic Alphabet Geng Nian An Pian

Formula Rehmanniae Radix Praeparata, Rehmanniae Radix, Scrophulariae Radix, Polygoni Multiflori Radix, Ophiopogonis Radix, Moutan Cortex, Alismatis Rhizoma, Poria, Schisandrae

Chinensis Fructus, Margaritifera Concha, Magnetitum, Uncariae Ramulus cum Uncis, Polygoni Multiflori Caulis, Tritici Aestivi Fructus Natantia, Curculiginis Rhizoma, etc.

Actions and Indications Enriching *yin*, clearing heat, relieving vexation, tranquilizing the mind. It is used for climacterium marked by tidal fever, sweating, vertigo, tinnitus, insomnia, vexation, fluctuation of blood pressure.

尪痹冲剂

【处方】地黄、熟地黄、续断、附子（制）、独活、骨碎补、桂枝、淫羊藿、防风、威灵仙、皂角刺、羊骨、白芍、狗脊（制）、知母、伸筋草、红花。

【功能主治】补肝肾，强筋骨，祛风湿，通经络。用于久痹体虚，关节疼痛或局部肿大、僵硬畸形，屈伸不利及类风湿性关节炎见有上述证候者。

【注意】孕妇慎用。

Relieving Impediment Syndrome Soluble Granules

Name of Chinese Phonetic Alphabet Wang Bi Chong Ji

Formula Rehmanniae Radix, Rehmanniae Radix Praeparata, Dipsaci Radix, Aconiti Lateralis Radix Praeparata, Angelicae Pubescentis Radix, Drynariae Rhizoma, Cinnamomi Ramulus, Epimedii Folium, Saposhnikoviae Radix, Clematidis Radix et Rhizoma, Gleditsiae Spina, Caprinus Os, Paeoniae Radix Alba, Cibotii Rhizoma(prepared), Anemarrhenae Rhizoma, Lycopodii Herba and Carthami Flos.

Actions and Indications Tonifying the liver and kidney, strengthening the sinews and bone, dispelling wind and dampness, freeing meridians and collaterals. It is indicated for chronic impediment syndrome and arthralgia, local swelling, stiffness and deformation, immobility of pulling and stretching, and rheumatoid arthritis with the above mentioned symptoms.

Warning It should be used carefully for pregnant women.

抗骨质增生丸

【处方】熟地黄、鸡血藤、淫羊藿、骨碎补、狗脊（盐制）、女贞子（盐炒）、肉苁蓉（蒸）、牛膝、莱菔子（炒）。

【功能主治】补腰肾，强筋骨，活血，利气，止痛。用于增生性脊椎炎，颈椎综合征，骨刺等骨质增生症。

Anti-hyperosteogeny Pill

Name of Chinese Phonetic Alphabet Kang Gu Zhi Zeng Sheng Wan

Formula Rehmanniae Radix Praeparata, Spatholobi Caulis, Epimedii Folium, Psoraleae Fructus, Cibotii Rhizoma(prepared with salt), Ligustri Lucidi Fructus (fried with salt), Cistanches Caulis Carnosus (steamed), Achyranthis Bidentatae Radix and Raphani Semen (fried).

Actions and Indications Tonifying the kidney, strengthening the sinews and bone, activating blood, moving *qi* and alleviating pain. It is used for hyperplastic spondylitis, cervical vertebrae syndrome, bony spur.

抗骨增生胶囊

【处方】熟地黄、肉苁蓉、狗脊、女贞子、淫羊藿等。

【功能主治】补腰肾，强筋骨，活血，止痛。用于增生性脊椎炎，颈椎综合征，骨刺。

Anti-hyperosteogeny Capsule

Name of Chinese Phonetic Alphabet Kang Gu Zeng Sheng Jiao Nang

Formula Rehmanniae Radix Praeparata, Cistanches Caulis Carnosus, Cibotii Rhizoma, Ligustri Lucidi Fructus, Epimedii Folium. etc.

Actions and Indications Tonifying the kidney, strengthening the sinews and bone, activating blood, alleviating pain. It is indicated for hyperplastic spondylitis, cervical vertebrae syndrome, bony spur.

抗骨髓炎片

【处方】金银花、蒲公英、苦地丁、半枝莲、白头翁、白花蛇舌草。

【功能主治】清热解毒，散瘀消肿。用于附骨疽及骨髓炎属热毒血瘀者。

【注意】孕妇慎用。

Relieving Osteomyelitis Tablet

Name of Chinese Phonetic Alphabet Kang Gu Sui Yan Pian

Formula Lonicerae Japonicae Flos, Taraxaci Herba, Corydalis Bungeanae Herba, Scutellariae Barbatae Herba, Pulsatillae Radix and Hedyotis Diffusae Herba.

Actions and Indications Clearing heat and detoxicating, dissipating stasis and dispersing swelling. It is indicated for osteomyelitis attributed to heat-toxin and static blood.

Warning It should be used cautiously for pregnant women.

抗宫炎片

【处方】广东紫珠干浸膏、益母草干浸膏、乌药干浸膏。

【功能主治】清湿热，止带下。用于因慢性宫颈炎引起的赤白带下，宫颈糜烂，出血。

【注意】孕妇忌服。

Relieving Cervicitis Tablet

Name of Chinese Phonetic Alphabet Kang Gong Yan Pian

Formula Callicarpae Kwangtungensis Extractum, Leonuri Extractum and Linderae Extractum.

Actions and Indications Clearing damp-heat and relieving vaginal discharge. It is indicated for red-white vaginal discharge, erosion of cervix and bleeding due to chronic cervicitis.

Warning It is contraindicated for pregnant women.

抗扁桃腺炎合剂

【处方】板蓝根、山豆根、连翘、青果、黄芩、大黄、玄参、麦冬。

【功能主治】泻热解毒，清利咽喉。用于急性扁桃体炎，咽喉炎。

Relieving Tonsillitis Mixture

Name of Chinese Phonetic Alphabet Kang Bian Tao Xian Yan He Ji

Formula Isatidis Radix, Sophorae Tonkinensis Radix et Rhizoma, Forsythiae Fructus, Canarii Fructus, Scutellariae Radix, Rhei Radix et Rhizoma, Scrophulariae Radix and Ophiopogonis Radix.

Actions and Indications Purging heat and detoxicating, soothing the throat. It is indicated for acute tonsillitis, laryngopharyngitis.

抗栓保心片

【处方】丹参、白芍、刺五加、山楂、郁金。

【功能主治】活血化瘀，通络止痛，益气降脂。用于气血瘀滞所致的胸闷、憋痛、心悸等症及冠心病，心绞痛，心律不齐，高血脂符合上述证候者。

Heart-protecting Tablet

Name of Chinese Phonetic Alphabet Kang Shuan Bao Xin Pian

Formula Salviae Miltiorrhizae Radix et Rhizoma, Paeoniae Radix Alba, Acanthopanacis Senticosi Radix et Rhizoma seu Caulis, Crataegi Fructus and Curcumae Radix.

Actions and Indications Activating blood, resolving stasis, dredging collaterals, alleviating pain, tonifying *qi*, downbearing lipid. It is used for chest distress, chest pain, palpitation and coronary heart disease, angina pectoris, arrhythmia and hyperlipemia with the above mentioned symptoms.

抗衰灵膏

【处方】黄芪、白术、枸杞子、地黄、桑椹、菟丝子、茯神、熟地黄、芡实、麦冬、党参、莲子、黄精、山茱萸、何首乌、甘草、五味子、山药、玉竹、柏子仁、紫河车、龙眼肉、葡萄干、丹参、黑豆、乌梅。

【功能主治】滋补肝肾，健脾养血，宁心安神，润肠通便。用于头昏眼花，精力衰竭，失眠健忘，各种原因引起的身体虚弱。

【注意】脾胃寒湿、脘痞纳呆、舌苔厚腻、大便溏薄者慎用。

Debility-counteracting Thick Paste

Name of Chinese Phonetic Alphabet Kang Shuai Ling Gao

Formula Astragali Radix, Atractylodis Macrocephalae Rhizoma, Lycii Fructus, Rehmanniae Radix, Mori Fructus, Cuscutae Semen, Poria Sclerotium Circum Pini Radicem, Rehmanniae Radix Praeparata, Euryales Semen, Ophiopogonis Radix, Codonopsis Radix, Nelumbinis Semen, Polygonati Rhizoma, Corni Fructus, Polygoni Multiflori Radix, Glycyrrhizae Radix et Rhizoma, Schisandrae Chinensis Fructus, Dioscoreae Rhizoma, Polygonati Odorati Rhizoma, Platycladi Semen, Hominis Placenta, Longan Arillus, Vitis Viniferae Fructus Siccus, Salviae Miltiorrhizae Radix et Rhizoma, Sojae Semen Nigrum and Mume Fructus.

Actions and Indications Tonifying the liver and kidney, fortifying the spleen and nourishing blood, tranquilizing the mind, moistening the intestines to relax bowels. It is used for dizziness, dim eyesight, declination of energy, insomnia, amnesia and physical debility due to various causes.

Warning It should be used carefully for cases with cold-damp of spleen-stomach, loss of appetite, thick and greasy tongue fur and sloppy stool.

抗病毒胶囊

【处方】板蓝根、忍冬藤、山豆根、鱼腥草、重楼、绵马贯众、白芷、青蒿、射干。

【功能主治】清热解毒。用于病毒性上呼吸道感染（病毒性感冒）。

【注意】临床症状较重、病程较长或合并有细菌感染的患者，应加服其他治疗药。

Relieving Viral Cold Capsule

Name of Chinese Phonetic Alphabet Kang Bing Du Jiao Nang

Formula Isatidis Radix, Lonicerae Japonicae Caulis, Sophorae Tonkinensis Radix et Rhizoma, Houttuyniae Herba, Paridis Rhizoma, Dryopteridis Crassirhizomatis Rhizoma, Angelicae Dahuricae Radix, Artemisiae Annuae Herba and Belamcandae Rhizoma.

Actions and Indications Clearing heat and detoxicating. It is used for viral upper respiratory infection (viral common cold).

Warning In case with worse clinical symptoms and longer course of illness or complicated with bacterial infection, other treatments should be applied.

护肝片

【处方】保肝浸膏、五味子浸膏、猪胆膏粉、绿豆粉。

【功能主治】疏肝理气，健脾消食。具有降低转氨酶作用。用于慢性肝炎及早期肝硬化。

Liver-protecting Tablet

Name of Chinese Phonetic Alphabet Hu Gan Pian

Formula Bao gan Extractum, Schisandrae Chinensis Extractum, Suillus Fel Extractum Pulvis and Phaseoli Radiati Pulvis.

Actions and Indications Soothing the liver and regulating *qi*, fortifying the spleen and promoting digestion, decreasing aminotransferase. It is indicated for chronic hepatitis and early stage of cirrhosis.

连翘败毒散

【处方】金银花、连翘、大黄、紫花地丁、蒲公英、栀子、白芷、黄芩、赤芍、浙贝母、桔梗、玄参、关木通、防风、白鲜皮、甘草、蝉蜕、天花粉。

【功能主治】清热解毒，消肿止痛。用于疮疖溃烂，发热，流脓流水，丹毒疱疹，疥癣痛痒。

【注意】孕妇忌服。

Weeping Forsythia* Powder for Detoxicating

Name of Chinese Phonetic Alphabet Lian Qiao Bai Du San

Formula Lonicerae Japonicae Flos, Forsythiae Fructus, Rhei Radix et Rhizoma, Violae Herba, Taraxaci Herba, Gardeniae Fructus, Angelicae Dahuricae Radix, Scutellariae Radix, Paeoniae Radix Rubra, Fritillariae Thunbergii Bulbus, Platycodonis Radix, Scorphulariae Radix, Aristolochiae Manshuriensis Caulis, Saposhnikoviae Radix, Dictamni Cortex, Glycyrrhizae Radix et Rhizoma, Cicadae Periostracum and Trichosanthis Radix.

Actions and Indications Clearing heat and detoxicating, dispersing swelling and relieving pain. It is used for ulcerous sore and furuncle with fever, pus-discharge, erysipelas, herpes, scabies and tinea.

Warning It is contraindicated for pregnant women.

*连翘

医痫丸

【处方】生白附子、天南星（制）、半夏（制）、猪牙皂、僵蚕（炒）、乌梢蛇（制）、蜈蚣、全蝎、白矾、雄黄、朱砂。

【功能主治】祛风化痰，定痫止搐。用于诸痫时发，二目上窜，口吐涎沫，抽搐昏迷。

【注意】不宜多服，孕妇禁用。

Epilepsy-relieving Pill

Name of Chinese Phonetic Alphabet Yi Xian Wan

Formula Typhonii Rhizoma, Arisaematis Rhizoma (prepared), Pinelliae Rhizoma (prepared), Gleditsiae Fructus Abnormalis, Bombyx Batryticatus (fried), Zaocys (prepared), Scolopendra, Scorpio, Alumen, Realgar and Cinnabaris.

Actions and Indications Dispelling wind and resolving phlegm, relieving epilepsy and convulsion. It is indicated for accidental attack of epilepsy, marked staring of eyes, vomitus of salivary foam, convulsion and loss of consciousness.

Warning Over dosage is prohibited and is contraindicated for pregnant women.

男宝胶囊

【处方】鹿茸、海马、阿胶、牡丹皮、黄芪、驴肾、狗肾、枸杞子、人参、当归、杜仲、菟丝子、肉桂、附子、白术、巴戟天、茯苓、麦冬、锁阳、肉苁蓉、仙茅、牛膝、玄参、熟地黄、山茱萸、淫羊藿、补骨脂、覆盆子、胡芦巴、续断、甘草。

【功能主治】壮阳补肾。用于肾阳不足引起的性欲淡漠，阳痿滑泄，腰腿酸痛，精神萎靡，食欲不振等症。

Masculine Treasure Capsule

Name of Chinese Phonetic Alphabet Nan Bao Jiao Nang

Formula Cervi Cornu Pantotrichum, Hippocampus, Asini Corii Colla, Moutan Cortex, Astragali Radix, Asini Ren, Canis Ren, Lycii Fructus, Ginseng Radix et Rhizoma, Angelicae Sinensis Radix, Eucommiae Cortex, Cuscutae Semen, Cinnamomi Cortex, Aconiti Lateralis Radix Praeparata, Atractylodis Macrocephalae Rhizoma, Morindae Officinalis Radix, Poria, Ophiopogonis Radix, Cynomorii Caulis Carnosus, Cistanches Caulis Carnosus, Curculiginis Rhizoma, Achyranthis Bidentatae Radix, Scrophulariae Radix, Rehmanniae Radix Praeparata, Corni Fructus, Epimedii Folium, Psoraleae Fructus, Rubi Fructus, Trigonellae Semen, Dipsaci Radix and Glycyrrhizae Radix et Rhizoma.

Actions and Indications Tonifying kidney-*yang*. It is used for low sexual desire, impotence, spermatorrhea, soreness and pain of waist and legs, listlessness of spirit and poor appetite due to insufficiency of kidney-*yang*.

男康片

【处方】白花蛇舌草、赤芍、熟地黄、肉苁蓉、甘草（蜜炙）、蒲公英、鹿衔草、败酱草、黄柏、红花、鱼腥草、淫羊藿、覆盆子、白术、黄芪、菟丝子、紫花地丁、野菊花、当归。

【功能主治】补肾益精，活血化瘀，利湿解毒。用于治疗肾精亏损，瘀血阻滞，湿热蕴结引起的慢性前列腺炎。

Relieving Chronic Prostatitis Tablet

Name of Chinese Phonetic Alphabet Nan Kang Pian

Formula Hedyotis Diffusae Herba, Paeoniae Radix Rubra, Rehmanniae Radix Praeparata, Cistanches Caulis Carnosus, Glycyrrhizae Radix et Rhizoma (prepared with honey), Taraxaci Herba, Pyrolae Herba, Patriniae Herba, Phellodendri Chinensis Cortex, Carthami Flos, Houttuyniae Herba, Epimedii Folium, Rubi Fructus, Atractylodis Macrocephalae Rhizoma, Astragali Radix, Cuscutae Semen, Violae Herba, Chrysanthemi Indici Flos and Angelicae Sinensis Radix.

Actions and Indications Tonifying the kidney and essence, activating blood and resolving stasis, draining dampness and detoxifying. It is indicated for chronic prostatitis due to depletion of kidney-essence, blood-stasis and accumulation of damp-heat.

利心丸

【处方】貂心、茯苓、地黄、天冬、防己、牡丹皮、琥珀、朱砂。

【功能主治】补心安神。用于风湿性心脏病，心动过速，心律不齐，心力衰竭。

Cardiotonic Bolus

Name of Chinese Phonetic Alphabet Li Xin Wan

Formula Martis Zibellinae Cor, Poria, Rehmanniae Radix, Asparagi Radix, Stephaniae Tetrandrae Radix, Moutan Cortex, Succinum and Cinnabaris.

Actions and Indications Tonifying the heart, tranquilizing the mind. It is indicated for rheumatic heart disease, tachycardia, arrhythmia and heart failure.

利肝片

【处方】金钱草、猪胆汁。

【功能主治】清肝、利胆。用于急、慢性传染性肝炎，胆囊炎以及肝脏分泌功能障碍。

Relieving Hepatitis Tablet

Name of Chinese Phonetic Alphabet Li Gan Pian

Formula Lysimachiae Herba and Suillus Bilis.

Actions and Indications Clearing liver-and-gall-bladder-fire. It is used for acute and chronic infective hepatitis, cholecystitis and secretory functional disturbance of the liver.

利肝隆冲剂

【处方】板蓝根、茵陈、郁金、五味子、甘草、当归、黄芪、刺五加浸膏。

【功能主治】疏肝解郁，清热解毒。用于急、慢性肝炎，迁延性肝炎，慢性活动性肝炎，对血清谷丙转氨酶、麝香香草酚浊度、黄疸指数均有显著的降低作用，对乙型肝炎表面抗原转阴有较好的效果。

Relieving Hepatitis Soluble Granules

Name of Chinese Phonetic Alphabet Li Gan Long Chong Ji

Formula Isatidis Radix, Artemisiae Scopariae Herba, Curcumae Radix, Schisandrae Chinensis Fructus, Glycyrrhizae Radix et Rhizoma, Angelicae Sinensis Radix, Astragali Radix and Acanthopanacis Senticosi Extractum.

Actions and Indications Soothing the liver and releasing depression, clearing heat and detoxicating. It is indicated for acute and chronic hepatitis, persistent hepatitis, chronic active hepatitis. The preparation can decrease the serum glutamic pyruvic transaminase, thymol turbidity and icteric index, also possesses desirable effects for surface antigen negative transformation of hepatitis B.

利肺片

【处方】百部、百合、五味子、枇杷叶、白及、牡蛎、甘草、冬虫夏草、蛤蚧粉。

【功能主治】驱痨补肺，镇咳化痰。用于肺痨咳嗽咯痰，咯血，气虚哮喘，慢性气管炎。

Relieving Cough and Asthma Tablet

Name of Chinese Phonetic Alphabet Li Fei Pian

Formula Stemonae Radix, Lilii Bulbus, Schisandrae Chinensis Fructus, Eriobotryae Folium, Bletillae Rhizoma, Ostreae Concha, Glycyrrhizae Radix et Rhizoma, Cordyceps and Gecko Pulvis.

Actions and Indications Relieving consumption and tonifying the lung, settling cough and resolving phlegm. It is indicated for pulmonary tuberculosis, marked by cough and spitting phlegm, hemoptysis, asthma due to *qi*-deficiency; chronic trachitis.

利咽解毒冲剂

【处方】板蓝根、金银花、连翘、麦冬、桔梗、大青叶、僵蚕、薄荷、玄参、黄芩、山楂（焦）、地黄、天花粉、川贝母、牛蒡子（炒）、大黄。

【功能主治】清肺利咽，解毒退热。用于急、慢性扁桃体炎，咽喉肿痛，口疮痄腮症。

【注意】忌食辛辣及过咸食物。

Soothing Throat Soluble Granules

Name of Chinese Phonetic Alphabet Li Yan Jie Du Chong Ji

Formula Isatidis Radix, Lonicerae Japonicae Flos, Forsythiae Fructus, Ophiopogonis Radix, Platycodonis Radix, Isatidis Folium, Bombyx Batryticatus, Menthae Haplocalycis Herba, Scrophulariae Radix, Scutellariae Radix, Crataegi Fructus (charred), Rehmanniae Radix, Trichosanthis Radix, Fritillariae Cirrhosae Bulbus, Arctii Fructus (fired) and Rhei Radix et Rhizoma.

Actions and Indications Clearing lung-heat and soothing the throat, detoxicating and reducing fever. It is used for acute and chronic tonsillitis, sore-throat, aphthae and mumps.

Warning Pungent and over salty foods are prohibited.

利胆片

【处方】大黄、金银花、金钱草、木香、知母、大青叶、柴胡、白芍、黄芩、芒硝、茵陈。

【功能主治】清热止痛。用于胆道疾患，胁肋及腹部疼痛，拒按，大便不通，小便短黄，身热头痛，呕吐不食。

【注意】孕妇慎服。

Relieving Gallbladder Disorder Tablet

Name of Chinese Phonetic Alphabet Li Dan Pian

Formula Rhei Radix et Rhizoma, Lonicerae Japonicae Flos, Lysimachiae Herba, Aucklandiae Radix, Anemarrhenae Rhizoma, Isatidis Folium, Bupleuri Radix, Paeoniae Radix Alba, Scutellariae Radix, Natrii Sulfas and Artemisiae Scopariae Herba.

Actions and Indications Clearing heat and alleviating pain. It is indicated for biliary tract diseases, marked by hypochondriac and abdominal pain, tenderness, difficulty in bowel movement, scanty yellow urine, fever and headache, vomiting and anorexia.

Warning It should be used carefully for pregnant women.

利胆排石片

【处方】金钱草、茵陈、黄芩、木香、郁金、大黄、槟榔、枳实（麸炒）、芒硝（精制）、厚朴（姜制）。

【功能主治】清热利湿，利胆排石。用于胆道结石，胆道感染，胆囊炎。

【注意】体弱、肝功能不良者慎用；孕妇禁用。

Relieving Cholelithes Tablet

Name of Chinese Phonetic Alphabet Li Dan Pai Shi Pian

Formula Lysimachiae Herba, Artemisiae Scopariae Herba, Scutellariae Radix, Aucklandiae Radix, Curcumae Radix, Rhei Radix et Rhizoma, Arecae Semen, Aurantii Fructus Immaturus (fried with bran), Natrii Sulfas (prepared) and Magnoliae Officinalis Cortex (prepared with ginger).

Actions and Indications Clearing heat and draining dampness, draining bile and removing stone. It is indicated for biliary calculi, infection of biliary tract and cholecystitis.

Warning It should be used carefully for general debility and hepatic insufficiency, and is contraindicated for pregnant women.

利脑心胶囊

【处方】丹参、川芎、葛根、地龙、赤芍、红花、郁金、制何首乌、泽泻、枸杞子、远志、酸枣仁（炒）、九节菖蒲、牛膝、甘草。

【功能主治】活血祛瘀，行气化痰，通络止痛。用于气滞血瘀，痰浊阻络，胸痹刺痛、绞痛，固定不移，入夜更甚，心悸不宁，头晕头痛，以及冠心病，心肌梗死，脑动脉硬化，脑血栓等见上述证候者。

Soothing Brain and Heart Capsule

Name of Chinese Phonetic Alphabet Li Nao Xin Jiao Nang

Formula Salviae Miltiorrhizae Radix et Rhizoma, Chuanxiong Rhizoma, Puerariae Lobatae Radix, Pheretima, Paeoniae Radix Rubra, Carthami Flos, Curcumae Radix, Polygoni Multiflori Radix Praeparata, Alismatis Rhizoma, Lycii Fructus, Polygalae Radix, Ziziphi Spinosae Semen (fried), Anemones Altaicae Rhizoma, Achyranthis Bidentatae Radix and Glycyrrhizae Radix et Rhizoma.

Actions and Indications Activating blood, dispelling stasis, moving *qi*, resolving phlegm, dredging collaterals, alleviating pain. It is used for chest impediment syndrome with fixed stabbing pain in chest which is even more serious at night, palpitaion, restlessness, dizziness and headache due to *qi*-stagnation, blood-stasis and phlegm-turbidity stagnation, and also used for coronary heart disease, myocardial infarction, cerebral arteriosclerosis and cerebral thrombosis with the above mentioned symptoms.

利鼻片

【处方】黄芩、苍耳子、辛夷、白芷、薄荷、细辛、蒲公英。

【功能主治】清热解毒、祛风开窍。用于鼻渊、鼻塞流涕。

Relieving Sinusitis Tablet

Name of Chinese Phonetic Alphabet Li Bi Pian

Formula Scutellariae Radix, Xanthii Fructus, Magnoliae Flos, Angelicae Dahuricae Radix, Menthae Haplocalycis Herba, Asari Radix et Rhizoma and Taraxaci Herba.

Actions and Indications Clearing heat and detoxicating, dispelling wind and opening the orifices. It is used for sinusitis, nasal congestion, rhinorrhea.

余甘子喉片

【处方】余甘子、冰片、薄荷脑。

【功能主治】清热润燥，利咽止痛。用于燥热伤津引起的咽喉干燥疼痛。

Emblic Myrobalan* Sucked Tablet

Name of Chinese Phonetic Alphabet Yu Gan Zi Hou Pian

Formula Phyllanthi Fructus, Borneolum Syntheticum and Menthol.

Actions and Indications Clearing heat, moistening dryness, soothing the throat, alleviating pain. It is used for dry throat and sore-throat due to consumption of fluid.

*余甘子

坐珠达西

【处方】寒水石、天竺黄、船形乌头、西红花、肉豆蔻、草果、熊胆、牛黄、麝香等。

【功能主治】疏肝，健胃，清热，愈溃疡，消肿。用于胃脘嘈杂，灼痛，肝热痛，消化不良，呃逆，急腹痛，食物中毒，浮肿。

【注意】忌用酸、腐、生冷、油腻食物。

Zuozhu Daxi Pill

Name of Chinese Phonetic Alphabet Zuo Zhu Da Xi

Formula Gypsum Rubrum, Bambusae Concretio Silicea, Aconiti Navicularis Herba, Croci Stigma, Myristicae Semen, Tsaoko Fructus, Ursi Fel, Bovis Calculus, Moschus, etc.

Actions and Indications Soothing the liver, fortifying the stomach, clearing heat, healing ulcer and dispersing swelling. It is used for gastric upset, scorching pain, hepatalgia, dyspepsia, hiccup, acute abdominal pain, food poisoning, edema.

Warning Sour, rotten, uncooked, cold and oily foods are prohibited.

肝达康片

【处方】柴胡（醋炙）、白芍（醋炙）、当归（酒炙）、茜草、白术（麸炒）、茯苓、鳖甲（醋炙）、党参、白茅根、枳实（麸炒）、青皮（炒）、砂仁、地龙（炒）、甘草等。

【功能主治】疏肝健脾，化瘀通络。适用于慢性乙型肝炎（慢性活动性及慢性迁延性肝炎）具肝郁脾虚兼血瘀证候者，证候特点为：疲乏纳差，胁痛腹胀，大便溏薄，胁下痞块，舌色淡或色暗有瘀点，脉弦缓或涩。

【注意】孕妇慎用。

Liver-soothing Tablet

Name of Chinese Phonetic Alphabet Gan Da Kang Pian

Formula Bupleuri Radix (prepared with vinegar), Paeoniae Radix Alba (prepared with vinegar), Angelicae Sinensis Radix (prepared with wine), Rubiae Radix, Atractylodis Macrocephalae Rhizoma (fried with bran), Poria, Trionycis Carapax (prepared with vinegar), Codonopsis Radix, Imperatae Rhizoma, Aurantii Fructus Immaturus (fried with bran), Citri Reticulatae Pericarpium Viride (fried), Amomi Fructus, Pheretima (fried), Glycyrrhizae Radix et Rhizoma, etc.

Actions and Indications Soothing the liver and tonifying the spleen, resolving stasis and dredging the collaterals. It is used for chronic hepatitis B (chronic active hepatitis and chronic persistent hepatitis) with syndrome of liver depression and spleen deficiency and blood stasis, and manifested as fatigue, poor appetite, hypochondriac pain and abdominal fullness, sloppy stool, hypochondriac mass, pale tongue or dull tongue with ecchymosis, string like and moderate or rough pulse.

Warning It should be used carefully for pregnant women.

肝苏颗粒

【处方】扯根菜。

【功能主治】降酶，保肝，退黄，健脾。用于慢性活动性肝炎、乙型肝炎，也可用于急性病毒性肝炎。

Liver Resuscitation Granules

Name of Chinese Phonetic Alphabet Gan Su Ke Li

Formula Lysimachiae Clethroidis Radix seu Herba.

Actions and Indications Lowering transaminase, protecting the liver, relieving jaundice, fortifying the spleen. It is indicated for chronic active hepatitis, hepatitis B, also used for acute viral hepatitis.

肝郁调经膏

【处方】白芍、佛手、郁金、玫瑰花、代代花、牡丹皮、川楝子、香附（制）、当归、丹参、葛根、泽泻。

【功能主治】疏肝解郁，清肝泻火，养血调经。用于肝郁所致的月经失调、痛经、乳房胀痛，不孕症。

Regulating Menstruation Liquid Extract

Name of Chinese Phonetic Alphabet Gan Yu Tiao Jing Gao

Formula Paeoniae Radix Alba, Citri Sarcodactylis Fructus, Curcumae Radix, Rosae Rugosae Flos, Citri Amarae Flos Immaturus, Moutan Cortex, Toosendan Fructus, Cyperi Rhizoma (prepared), Angelicae Sinensis Radix, Salviae Miltiorrhizae Radix et Rhizoma, Puerariae Lobatae Radix and Alismatis Rhizoma.

Actions and Indications Soothing the liver and clearing liver-fire, nourishing blood to regulate menstruation. It is indicated for irregular menstruation, dysmenorrhea, distention and pain of the breast and sterility due to liver depression.

肝肾滋

【处方】枸杞子、黄芪、党参、麦冬、阿胶。

【功能主治】益肝明目，滋阴补肾。用于肾阴不足，气血两亏，目眩昏暗，心烦失眠，肢倦乏力，腰腿酸软。

【注意】高血压患者慎用。

Tonifying Liver and Kidney Liquid

Name of Chinese Phonetic Alphabet Gan Shen Zi

Formula Lycii Fructus, Astragali Radix, Codonopsis Radix, Ophiopogonis Radix and Asini Corii Colla.

Actions and Indications Tonifying the liver to improving vision, enriching kidney-*yin*. It is used for blurred vision, vexation, insomnia, tiredness of limbs, fatigue and soreness of waist and weakness of legs due to insufficiency of kidney-*yin* and dual depletion of *qi* and blood.

Warning It should be used carefully for hypertension.

肝炎灵注射液

【处方】山豆根提取物。

【功能主治】降低转氨酶，提高机体免疫力。用于慢性、活动性肝炎。

Tonkines Sophora* Injection for Relieving Hepatitis

Name of Chinese Phonetic Alphabet Gan Yan Ling Zhu She Ye

Formula Sophorae Tonkinensis Radix et Rhizoma.

Actions and Indications Decreasing transaminase and improving immunity. It is indicated for chronic, active hepatitis.

* 山豆根

肝炎康复丸

【处方】茵陈、郁金、板蓝根、当归、菊花、金钱草、丹参、滑石、拳参。

【功能主治】清热解毒，利湿化郁。用于急性黄疸型肝炎，迁延性及慢性肝炎。

Relieving Hepatitis Bolus

Name of Chinese Phonetic Alphabet Gan Yan Kang Fu Wan

Formula Artemisiae Scopariae Herba, Curcumae Radix, Isatidis Radix, Angelicae Sinensis Radix, Chrysanthemi Flos, Lysimachiae Herba, Salviae Miltiorrhizae Radix et Rhizoma, Talcum and Bistortae Rhizoma.

Actions and Indications Clearing heat and detoxicating, draining dampness. It is indicated for acute icterohepatitis, persistent hepatitis and chronic hepatitis.

肝复乐片

【处方】党参、鳖甲（醋制）、重楼、黄芪、陈皮、土鳖虫、大黄、桃仁、半枝莲、败酱草、茯苓、薏苡仁、郁金、苏木、牡蛎、茵陈、关木通、香附（制）、沉香、柴胡、白术（炒）。

【功能主治】健脾理气，化瘀软坚，清热解毒。适用于以肝郁脾虚为主证的原发性肝癌，症见上腹肿块，胁肋疼痛，神疲乏力，食少纳呆，脘腹胀满，心烦易怒，口苦咽干。

【注意】少数患者开始服药后出现腹泻，多可自行缓解。

Relieving Primary Hepatic Carcinoma Tablet

Name of Chinese Phonetic Alphabet Gan Fu Le Pian

Formula Codonopsis Radix, Trionycis Carapax (prepared with vinegar), Paridis Rhizoma, Astragali Radix, Citri Reticulatae Pericarpium, Eupolyphaga seu Steleophaga, Rhei Radix et Rhizoma, Persicae Semen, Scutellariae Barbatae Herba, Patriniae Herba, Poria, Coicis Semen, Curcumae Radix, Sappan Lignum, Ostreae Concha, Artemisiae Scopariae Herba, Aristolochiae Manshuriensis Caulis, Cyperi Rhizoma (prepared), Aquilariae Lignum Resinatum, Bupleuri Radix and Atractylodis Macrocephalae Rhizoma (fried).

Actions and Indications Fortifying the spleen, regulating *qi*, resolving stasis, softening mass, clearing heat, detoxifying. It is indicated for primary hepatic carcinoma manifested as upper abdominal mass, hypochondriac pain, lassitude of spirit, hypodynamia, poor appetite, abdominal fullness, irritability, bitter mouth and dry throat due to depression of the liver and deficiency of the spleen.

Warning After medication, diarrhea occurs occasionally and is spontaneously relieved.

肛泰栓

【处方】盐酸小檗碱、人工麝香、冰片等。

【功能主治】凉血止血，清热解毒，燥湿敛疮，消肿止痛。用于内痔、外痔、混合痔出现的便血，肿胀，疼痛。

Suppository for Hemorrhoids

Name of Chinese Phonetic Alphabet Gang Tai Shuan

Formula Berberine Hydrochloride, Moschus Artifactus, Borneolum Syntheticum, etc.

Actions and Indications Cooling blood and relieving bleeding, clearing heat and detoxicating, drying dampness and astringing sore, dispersing swelling and alleviating pain. It is indicated for hematochezia, swelling, distention and pain due to internal hemorrhoid, external hemorrhoid and mixed hemorrhoid.

肚痛丸

【处方】豆蔻（去壳）、干姜、砂仁、荜茇、厚朴（姜制）、罂粟壳、肉桂、枳实（麸炒）、木香、乌药。

【功能主治】温中散寒，理气止痛。用于停寒气滞，腹中冷痛，胸肋胀闷，呕逆吐酸。

【注意】孕妇禁用，忌食辛辣油腻之物。

Relieving Abdominal Pain Pill

Name of Chinese Phonetic Alphabet Du Tong Wan

Formula Amomi Fructus Rotundus (removed shell), Zingiberis Rhizoma, Amomi Fructus, Piperis Longi Fructus, Magnoliae Officinalis Cortex (prepared with ginger), Papaveris Pericarpium, Cinnamomi Cortex, Aurantii Fructus Immaturus (fried with bran), Aucklandiae Radix and Linderae Radix.

Actions and Indications Warming the middle and dissipating cold, regulating *qi* and relieving pain. It is indicated for cold pain in the abdomen, hypochondriac distention, hiccup and acid vomiting due to stagnation of cold and *qi*.

Warning It is contraindicated for pregnant

women, pungent and oily foods should be avoided.

肠炎宁片

【处方】地锦草、黄毛耳草、樟树根、香薷、枫树叶。

【功能主治】清热利湿，行气。用于急、慢性胃肠炎，腹泻，细菌性痢疾，小儿消化不良。

Gastroenteritis-promoting Tablet

Name of Chinese Phonetic Alphabet Chang Yan Ning Pian

Formula Euphorbiae Humifusae Herba, Hedyotis Chrysotrichae Herba, Litseae Rubescentis Radix, Moslae Herba and Liquidambaris Folium.

Actions and Indications Clearing heat and draining dampness, moving *qi*. It is indicated for acute and chronic gastroenteritis, diarrhea, bacillary dysentery and infantile dyspepsia.

肠胃适胶囊

【处方】十大功劳叶、鸡骨香、黄连须、救心应、两面针、防己。

【功能主治】清热利湿，调中止泻，解毒。用于湿热腹泻，腹痛，急性肠胃炎。

【注意】慢性虚寒性泻痢者慎用。

Soothing Stomach and Intestine Capsule for Relieving Diarrhea

Name of Chinese Phonetic Alphabet Chang Wei Shi Jiao Nang

Formula Mahoniae Folium, Crotonis Crassifolii Radix, Coptidis Radix Fibrosae , Ilicis Rotundae Cortex, Zanthoxyli Radix and Stephaniae Tetrandrae Radix.

Actions and Indications Clearing heat and draining dampness, regulating the middle and relieving diarrhea, detoxicating. It is indicated for diarrhea due to damp-heat; abdominal pain, acute gastroenteritis.

Warning It should be used carefully for cases with chronic diarrhea and dysentery due to deficiency-cold.

龟甲胶

【处方】本品为龟甲经煎煮、浓缩制成的固体胶。

【功能主治】滋阴，养血，止血。用于阴虚潮热，骨蒸盗汗，腰膝酸软，血虚萎黄，崩漏带下。

Tortoise Shell and Plastron Glue*

Name of Chinese Phonetic Alphabet Gui Jia Jiao

Formula Testudinis Carapacis et Plastri Colla.

Actions and Indications Enriching *yin*, tonifying blood and relieving bleeding. It is indicated for tidal fever, night sweating, soreness and weakness of waist and knees, sallow complexion, metrorrhagia and white vaginal discharge due to *yin*-deficiency.

*龟甲胶

龟蛇酒

【处方】活乌龟、眼镜蛇（去头、内脏）、银环蛇（去头、内脏）、党参、杜仲、大枣、枸杞子、当归、锁阳、黄芪、肉桂、牛膝、川芎、桑寄生、乌梢蛇（去头、内脏）。

【功能主治】滋阴补肾，益气活血，舒筋通络，祛风除湿。用于老年体弱，头昏眼花，腰酸膝软，阳痿尿频，四肢麻木，关节酸痛。

Medicated Wine of Tortoise and Snake

Name of Chinese Phonetic Alphabet Gui She Jiu

Formula Testudinis Totus (living body), Naja (removed head and internal organs), Bungarus Multicinctus (removed head and internal organs), Codonopsis Radix, Eucommiae Cortex, Jujubae Fructus, Lycii Fructus, Angelicae Sinensis Radix, Cynomorii Caulis Carnosus, Astragali Radix, Cinnamomi Cortex, Achyranthis Bidentatae Radix, Chuanxiong Rhizoma, Taxilli Herba and Zaocys (removed head and internal organs).

Actions and Indications Enriching *yin*, tonifying the kidney, activating blood, relaxing sinews and activating collaterals, dispelling wind and dampness. It is used for senile debility, dizziness, dim eyesight, soreness of waist and weakness of legs, impotence, frequent urination, numbness of limbs and arthralgia.

龟鹿二仙膏

【处方】龟甲、鹿角、党参、枸杞子。

【功能主治】温肾益精，补气养血。用于久病肾虚，精血不足引起的腰膝酸软，遗精阳痿。

【注意】脾胃虚弱者慎用。

Thick Paste of Tortoise Shell* and Deerhorn**

Name of Chinese Phonetic Alphabet Gui Lu Er Xian Gao

Formula Testudinis Carapax et Plastrum. Cervi Cornu, Codonopsis Radix and Lycii Fructus.

Actions and Indications Warming the kidney and enriching essence, tonifying *qi* and blood. It is used for soreness and weakness of waist and knees, nocturnal emission and impotence due to prolonged illness, deficiency of the kidney and dual insufficiency of essence and blood.

Warning It should be used carefully for cases with dual hypofunction of the spleen and stomach.

*龟甲 **鹿角

龟鹿补肾丸

【处方】菟丝子（炒）、淫羊藿（蒸）、续断（蒸）、锁阳（蒸）、狗脊（蒸）、酸枣仁（炒）、何首乌（制）、甘草（蜜炙）、陈皮（蒸）、鹿角胶（炒）、熟地黄、龟甲胶（炒）、金樱子（蒸）、黄芪（蜜炙）、山药（炒）、覆盆子（蒸）。

【功能主治】壮筋骨，益气血，补肾壮阳。用于身体虚弱，精神疲乏，腰腿酸软，头昏目眩，肾亏精冷，性欲减退，夜多小便，健忘失眠。

Tortoise Shell Glue* and Deerhorn Glue** Bolus

Name of Chinese Phonetic Alphabet Gui Lu Bu Shen Wan

Formula Cuscutae Semen (fried), Epimedii Folium (steamed), Dipsaci Radix (steamed), Cynomorii Caulis Carnosus (steamed), Cibotii Rhizoma(steamed), Ziziphi Spinosae Semen (fried), Polygoni Multiflori Radix Praeparata, Glycyrrhizae Radix et Rhizoma (prepared with honey), Citri Reticulatae Pericarpium (steamed), Cervi Cornus Colla (fried), Rehmanniae Radix Praeparata, Testudinis Carapacis et Plastri Colla (fried), Rosae Laevigatae Fructus (steamed), Astragali Radix (prepared with honey), Dioscoreae Rhizoma (fried) and Rubi Fructus (steamed).

Actions and Indications Strengthening the sinews and bone, tonifying *qi*, blood and kidney-*yang*. It is used for debility of constitution, lassitude of spirit, soreness and weakness of waist and legs, dizziness, dizzy vision, sperm-coldness, sexual hypoesthesia, frequent urination at night, amnesia and insomnia.

*龟甲胶 **鹿角胶

龟龄集

【处方】本品为人参、鹿茸、海马、枸杞子、丁香、穿山甲、雀脑、牛膝、锁阳、熟地黄、补骨脂、菟丝子、杜仲、石燕、肉苁蓉、甘草、天冬、淫羊藿、大青盐、砂仁等经加工制成的胶囊剂。

【功能主治】强身补脑，固肾补气，增进食欲。用于肾亏阳弱，记忆减退，夜梦精溢，腰酸腿软，气虚咳嗽，五更溏泻，食欲不振。

【注意】忌生冷刺激性食物；孕妇禁用；伤风感冒时停服。

Guiling Tonic Capsule

Name of Chinese Phonetic Alphabet Gui Ling Ji

Formula Ginseng Radix et Rhizoma, Cervi Cornu Pantotrichum, Hippocampus, Lycii Fructus, Caryophylli Flos, Manis Squama, Passeris Encephalon, Achyranthis Bidentatae Radix, Cynomorii Caulis

Carnosus, Rehmanniae Radix Praeparata, Psoraleae Fructus, Cuscutae Semen, Eucommiae Cortex, Spiriferis Fossilia, Cistanches Caulis Carnosus, Glycyrrhizae Radix et Rhizoma, Asparagi Radix, Epimedii Folium, Sal, Amomi Fructus, etc.

Actions and Indications Strengthening the body, tonifying the brain, tonifying the kidney and *qi*, improving appetite. It is used for hypomnesis, oneirogmus, soreness of waist and weakness of legs, cough, fifth-watch diarrhea and poor appetite due to weakness of kidney-*yang*.

Warning It is contraindicated for pregnant women and cold, uncooked and irritant foods should be avoided; in case of common cold, suspend the administration.

辛夷鼻炎丸

【处方】辛夷、薄荷、紫苏叶、甘草、广藿香、苍耳子、鹅不食草、板蓝根、山白芷、防风、鱼腥草、菊花、三叉苦。

【功能主治】祛风清热，消肿解毒。用于治疗鼻炎（包括过敏性鼻炎，慢性鼻炎），神经性头痛，感冒流涕，鼻塞不通。

Biond Magnolia* Pill for Relieving Rhinitis

Name of Chinese Phonetic Alphabet XinYi Bi Yan Wan

Formula Magnoliae Flos, Menthae Haplocalycis Herba, Perillae Folium, Glycyrrhizae Radix et Rhizoma, Pogostemonis Herba, Xanthii Fructus, Centipedae Herba, Isatidis Radix, Inulae Cappae Radix, Saposhnikoviae Radix, Houttuyniae Herba, Chrysanthemi Flos and Euodiae Leptae Folium.

Actions and Indications Dispelling wind and clearing heat, dispersing swelling and detoxicating. It is indicated for rhinitis (including allergic rhinitis, chronic rhinitis), nervous headache, common cold, rhinorrhea, nasal congestion.

* 辛夷

辛芩颗粒

【处方】细辛、黄芩、荆芥、防风、白芷、苍耳子、黄芪、白术、桂枝、石菖蒲。

【功能主治】益气固表，祛风通窍，用于肺气虚证之鼻鼽（过敏性鼻炎）、鼻窒。

Chinese Wild Ginger* and Baical Skullcap** Granules

Name of Chinese Phonetic Alphabet Xin Qin Ke Li

Formula Asari Radix et Rhizoma, Scutellariae Radix, Schizonepetae Herba, Saposhnikoviae Radix, Angelicae Dahuricae Radix, Xanthii Fructus, Astragali Radix, Atractylodis Macrocephalae Rhizoma, Cinnamomi Ramulus and Acori Tatarinowii Rhizoma.

Actions and Indications Replenishing *qi* and securing the exterior, dispelling wind and dredging orifices. It is indicated for allergic rhinitis, chronic rhinitis.

* 细辛 ** 黄芩

辛芳鼻炎胶囊

【处方】辛夷、白芷、黄芩、柴胡、川芎、桔梗、薄荷、菊花、荆芥穗、枳壳（炒）、防风、细辛、龙胆、蔓荆子（炒）、水牛角浓缩粉。

【功能主治】发表散风，清热解毒，宣肺通窍。用于慢性鼻炎，鼻窦炎。

【注意】孕妇慎服。

Biond Magnolia* Capsule for Relieving Rhinitis

Name of Chinese Phonetic Alphabet Xin Fang Bi Yan Jiao Nang

Formula Magnoliae Flos, Angelicae Dahuricae Radix, Scutellariae Radix, Bupleuri Radix, Chuanxiong Rhizoma, Platycodonis Radix, Menthae Haplocalycis Herba, Chrysanthemi Flos, Schizonepetae Spica, Aurantii Fructus (fried), Saposhnikoviae Radix, Asari Radix et Rhizoma, Gentianae Radix et Rhizoma, Viticis

Fructus (fried) and Bubali Cornu Pulvis Concentratio.

Actions and Indications Exterior effusing and dispersing wind, clearing heat and detoxicating, diffusing the lung and dredging the orifices. It is indicated for chronic rhinitis, sinusitis.

Warning It should be used carefully for pregnant women.

*辛夷

快胃片

【处方】海螵蛸、白矾（煅）、延胡索（醋制）、白及、甘草。

【功能主治】消炎生肌，制酸止痛。用于胃溃疡，十二指肠溃疡，浅表性胃炎，胃窦炎。

【注意】低酸性胃病、胃阴不足者慎用。

Stomach-soothing Tablet

Name of Chinese Phonetic Alphabet Kuai Wei Pian

Formula Sepiae Endoconcha, Alumen (calcined), Corydalis Rhizoma (prepared with vinegar), Bletillae Rhizoma and Glycyrrhizae Radix et Rhizoma.

Actions and Indications Antiphlogistic and promoting tissue regeneration, antiacid to relieve pain. It is indicated for gastric ulcer, duodenal ulcer, superficial gastritis, antrum gastrititis.

Warning It should be used carefully for cases with low-acidity gastropathy and *yin*-insufficiency of the stomach.

沙棘颗粒

【处方】本品为沙棘制成的颗粒剂。

【功能主治】止咳祛痰，消食化滞，活血散瘀。用于咳嗽痰多，消化不良，食积腹痛，跌打瘀肿，瘀血经闭。

Sand Thorn* Soluble Granules

Name of Chinese Phonetic Alphabet Sha Ji Ke Li

Formula Hippophae Fructus.

Actions and Indications Relieving cough and dispelling phlegm, promoting digestion and removing food stagnation, activating blood and dipersing blood-stasis. It is indicated for cough with profuse phlegm, dyspepsia, retention of food and abdominal pain, traumatic injury and amenorrhea.

*沙棘

沉香化气丸

【处方】沉香、木香、广藿香、香附（醋制）、砂仁、陈皮、莪术（醋制）、六神曲（炒）、麦芽（炒）、甘草。

【功能主治】理气疏肝，消积和胃。用于肝胃气滞，脘腹胀痛，胸膈痞满，不思饮食，嗳气反酸。

【注意】孕妇慎服。

Chinese Eaglewood* Pill for Relieving *Qi*-stagnation

Name of Chinese Phonetic Alphabet Chen Xiang Hua Qi Wan

Formula Aquilariae Lignum Resinatum, Aucklandiae Radix, Pogostemonis Herba, Cyperi Rhizoma (prepared with vinegar), Amomi Fructus, Citri Reticulatae Pericarpium, Curcumae Rhizoma (prepared with vinegar), Medicata Massa Fermentata (fried), Hordei Fructus Germinatus (fried) and Glycyrrhizae Radix et Rhizoma.

Actions and Indications Regulating *qi*, soothing the liver, promoting digestion, harmonizing the stomach. It is used for abdominal fullness and pain, chest stuffiness, anorexia, eructation and acid regurgitation due to dual stagnation of *qi* in the liver and stomach.

Warning It should be used cautiously for pregnant women.

*沉香

沉香化滞丸

【处方】沉香、牵牛子（炒）、枳实（炒）、五灵脂（制）、山楂（炒）、枳壳（炒）、陈皮、香附（制）、厚朴（制）、莪术（制）、砂仁、三棱（制）、木香、青皮、大黄。

【功能主治】理气化滞。用于饮食停滞，胸腹胀满。

【注意】孕妇忌服。

Qi-stagnation-resolving Pill of Chinese Eaglewood*

Name of Chinese Phonetic Alphabet Chen Xiang Hua Zhi Wan

Formula Aquilariae Lignum Resinatum, Pharbitidis Semen (fried), Aurantii Fructus Immaturus (fried), Trogopterori Faeces (prepared), Crataegi Fructus (fried), Aurantii Fructus (fried), Citri Reticulatae Pericarpium, Cyperi Rhizoma (prepared), Magnoliae Officinalis Cortex (prepared), Curcumae Rhizoma (perpared), Amomi Fructus, Sparganii Rhizoma (prepared), Aucklandiae Radix, Citri Reticulatae Pericarpium Viride and Rhei Radix et Rhizoma.

Actions and Indications Regulating *qi*, resolving stagnation. It is used for food stagnation and abdominal fullness.

Warning It is contraindicated for pregnant women.

*沉香

沉香舒气丸

【处方】木香、砂仁、沉香、青皮（醋炙）、厚朴（姜炙）、香附（醋炙）、乌药、枳壳（去瓤麸炒）、草果、豆蔻、片姜黄、郁金、延胡索（醋炙）、五灵脂（醋炙）、柴胡、山楂（炒）、槟榔、甘草。

【功能主治】舒气化郁，和胃止痛。用于肝郁气滞、肝胃不和引起的胃脘胀痛，两肋胀满疼痛或刺痛，烦躁易怒，呕吐吞酸，呃逆嗳气，倒饱嘈杂，不思饮食。

【注意】孕妇慎服。

Soothing *Qi* Pill of Chinese Eaglewood*

Name of Chinese Phonetic Alphabet Chen Xiang Shu Qi Wan

Formula Aucklandiae Radix, Amomi Fructus, Aquilariae Lignum Resinatum, Citri Reticulatae Pericarpium Viride (prepared with vinegar), Magnoliae Officinalis Cortex (prepared with ginger), Cyperi Rhizoma (prepared with vinegar), Linderae Radix, Aurantii Fructus (removed pulp and fried with bran), Tsaoko Fructus, Amomi Fructus Rotundus, Wenyujin Rhizoma Concisum, Curcumae Radix, Corydalis Rhizoma (prepared with vinegar), Trogopterori Faeces (prepared with vinegar), Bupleuri Radix, Crataegi Fructus (fried), Arecae Semen and Glycyrrhizae Radix et Rhizoma.

Actions and Indications Soothing *qi*, relieving depression, harmonizing the stomach, alleviating pain. It is used for fullness and pain in stomach duct, hypochondriac fullness and pain or stabbing pain, vexation, vomiting, acid regurgitation, hiccup, eructation, gastric upset and anorexia due to stagnation of *qi* and disharmony of the liver and stomach.

Warning It should be used carefully for pregnant women.

*沉香

沈阳红药片

【处方】三七、川芎、白芷、当归、红花、延胡索、土鳖虫。

【功能主治】活血止痛，祛瘀生新。用于跌打损伤，筋骨肿痛，亦可用于血瘀阻络的风湿麻木。

【注意】孕妇忌服，经期停服。

Shen Yang Hong Yao Tablet

Name of Chinese Phonetic Alphabet Shen Yang Hong Yao Pian

Formula Notoginseng Radix et Rhizoma, Chuanxiong Rhizoma, Angelicae Dahuricae Radix, Angelicae Sinensis Radix, Carthami Flos, Corydalis Rhizoma and Eupolyphaga seu Steleophaga.

Actions and Indications Activating blood, alleviating pain, dispelling stasis, promoting tissue regeneration. It is used for traumatic injury with swelling and pain, rheumatic numbness due to blood-stasis.

Warning It is contraindicated for pregnant

women, suspend medication during menstrual period.

补中益气丸

【处方】黄芪（蜜炙）、党参、甘草（蜜炙）、白术、当归、升麻、柴胡、陈皮、生姜、大枣。

【功能主治】补中益气，升阳举陷。用于脾胃虚弱，中气下陷，体倦乏力，食少腹胀，久泻，脱肛，子宫脱垂。

Tonifying Middle-*qi* Pill

Name of Chinese Phonetic Alphabet Bu Zhong Yi Qi Wan

Formula Astragali Radix (prepared with honey), Codonopsis Radix, Glycyrrhizae Radix et Rhizoma (prepared with honey), Atractylodis Macrocephalae Rhizoma, Angelicae Sinensis Radix, Cimicifugae Rhizoma, Bupleuri Radix, Citri Reticulatae Pericarpium, Zingiberis Rhizoma Recens and Jujubae Fructus.

Actions and Indications Tonifying the middle and *qi*, upraising the middle *qi*. It is used for fatigue, poor appetite and abdominal distention, chronic diarrhea, prolapse of the rectum and prolapse of uterus due to dual deficiency of the spleen and stomach and sunken middle-*qi*.

补心气口服液

【处方】本品为黄芪、人参、石菖蒲、薤白等药经加工制成的口服液。

【功能主治】补益心气，理气止痛。用于气短、心悸、乏力、头晕等心气虚损型胸痹心痛。

Tonifying Heart-*qi* Oral Liquid

Name of Chinese Phonetic Alphabet Bu Xin Qi Kou Fu Ye

Formula Astragali Radix, Ginseng Radix et Rhizoma, Acori Tatarinowii Rhizoma, Allii Macrostemonis Bulbus, etc.

Actions and Indications Tonifying heart-*qi*, regulating qi and relieving pain. It is indicated for chest impediment syndrome and cardialgia due to heart-*qi* deficiency and marked by shortness of breath, palpitation, fatigue and dizziness.

补肾宁片

【处方】羊鞭、枸杞子、淫羊藿、肉苁蓉、人参、海马。

【功能主治】温肾助阳，益气固本。用于肾阳虚衰所致阳痿，对妇女更年期综合征也有一定疗效。

【注意】阴虚内热者慎用。

Kidney-tonifying Tablet

Name of Chinese Phonetic Alphabet Bu Shen Ning Pian

Formula Carprinus Testis et Penis, Lycii Fructus, Epimedii Folium, Cistanches Caulis Carnosus, Ginseng Radix et Rhizoma and Hippocampus.

Actions and Indications Warming kidney-*yang*, tonifying *qi*. It is used for impotence due to deficiency of kidney-*yang*. It possesses certain curative effect for menopausal syndrome.

Warning It should be used carefully for cases with *yin*-deficiency with internal heat.

补肾防喘片

【处方】地黄、熟地黄、淫羊藿（羊油炙）、补骨脂（盐炙）、菟丝子（盐炙）、山药、陈皮、附片。

【功能主治】温阳补肾。用于预防和治疗支气管哮喘的季节性发作，慢性支气管炎咳喘。

Preventing and Treating Bronchial Asthma Tablet

Name of Chinese Phonetic Alphabet Bu Shen Fang Chuan Pian

Formula Rehmanniae Radix, Rehmanniae Radix Praeparata, Epimedii Folium (prepared with sheep suet), Psoraleae Fructus (prepared with salt), Cuscutae

Semen (prepared with salt), Dioscoreae Rhizoma, Citri Reticulatae Pericarpium and Aconiti Lateralis Radix Praeparata (sliced).

Actions and Indications Warming *yang* and tonifying the kidney. It is used for preventing and treating seasonal attack of bronchial asthma and cough due to chronic bronchitis.

补肾固齿丸

【处方】本品为地黄、丹参等药经加工制成的水丸。

【功能主治】补肾固齿，活血解毒。用于肾虚血热型牙周病，牙齿酸软，咀嚼无力，松动移位，牙龈出血。

Securing Teeth Pill

Name of Chinese Phonetic Alphabet Bu Shen Gu Chi Wan

Formula Rehmanniae Radix, Salviae Miltiorrhizae Radix et Rhizoma, etc.

Actions and Indications Tonifying the kidney, securing the teeth, activating blood and detoxifying. It is used for periodontal disease (kidney-deficiency and blood-heat type), soreness of teeth, weakness of chew, movable tooth, tooth displacement and gingival bleeding.

补肾益寿胶囊

【处方】红参、珍珠、灵芝、制何首乌、枸杞子、淫羊藿、丹参、甘草、黄精。

【功能主治】补肾益气。用于肾气不足引起的失眠，耳鸣，腰酸，健忘，倦怠，胸闷气短，夜尿频数，性功能减退。

Tonifying Kidney-*qi* Capsule

Name of Chinese Phonetic Alphabet Bu Shen Yi Shou Jiao Nang

Formula Ginseng Radix et Rhizoma Rubra, Margarita, Ganoderma, Polygoni Multiflori Radix Praeparata, Lycii Fructus, Epimedii Folium, Salviae Miltiorrhizae Radix et Rhizoma, Glycyrrhizae Radix et Rhizoma and Polygonati Rhizoma.

Actions and Indications Tonifying kidney-*qi*. It is used for insomnia, tinnitus, soreness of waist, amnesia, tiredness, chest distress, shortness of breath, frequent urination at night and sexual hypoesthesia due to insufficiency of kidney-*qi*.

补肾益脑片

【处方】鹿茸（去毛）、红参、茯苓、山药（炒）、熟地黄、当归、川芎、补骨脂（盐制）、牛膝、枸杞子、玄参、麦冬、五味子、酸枣仁（炒）、远志（蜜炙）、朱砂。

【功能主治】补肾益气，养血生精。用于气血两虚，肾虚精亏，心悸气短，失眠健忘，遗精盗汗，腰腿酸软，耳鸣耳聋。

【注意】感冒发热者忌用。

Tonifying Kidney and Brain Tablet

Name of Chinese Phonetic Alphabet Bu Shen Yi Nao Pian

Formula Cervi Cornu Pantotrichum (removed hair), Ginseng Radix et Rhizoma Rubra, Poria, Dioscoreae Rhizoma (fried), Rehmanniae Radix Praeparata, Angelicae Sinensis Radix, Chuanxiong Rhizoma, Psoraleae Fructus (prepared with salt), Achyranthis Bidentatae Radix, Lycii Fructus, Scrophulariae Radix, Ophiopogonis Radix, Schisandrae Chinensis Fructus, Ziziphi Spinosae Semen (fried), Polygalae Radix (prepared with honey) and Cinnabaris.

Actions and Indications Tonifying the kidney and *qi*, nourishing blood and essence. It is used for palpitation, shortness of breath, insomnia, amnesia, nocturnal emission, night sweating, soreness and weakness of waist and legs, tinnitus and deafness due to dual deficiency of *qi* and blood, and deficiency of the kidney and essence.

Warning It is contraindicated for cases with common cold and fever.

补肾强身片

【处方】淫羊藿、菟丝子、金樱子、女贞子、狗脊（烫）。

【功能主治】补肾强身。用于肾阳不足引起的腰酸足软，头晕耳鸣，眼花心悸，阳痿遗精。

Kidney-tonifying Tablet for Impotence

Name of Chinese Phonetic Alphabet Bu Shen Qiang Shen Pian

Formula Epimedii Folium, Cuscutae Semen, Rosae Laevigatae Fructus, Ligustri Lucidi Fructus and Cibotii Rhizoma(scalded).

Actions and Indications Tonifying the kidney, strengthening the body. It is used for soreness of waist and weakness of legs, dizziness, tinnitus, dim eyesight, palpitation, impotence and nocturnal emission due to insufficiency of kidney-*yang*.

补脑丸

【处方】当归、胆南星、酸枣仁（炒）、益智（盐炒）、枸杞子、柏子仁（炒）、龙骨（煅）、石菖蒲、肉苁蓉（蒸）、五味子（酒炖）、核桃仁、天竺黄、远志（制）、琥珀、天麻。

【功能主治】滋补精血，健脑益智，安神镇惊，化痰息风。用于迷惑健忘，记忆减退，头昏耳鸣，心烦失眠，心悸不宁，癫痫头痛，神烦胸闷。

Mind-invigorating Pill

Name of Chinese Phonetic Alphabet Bu Nao Wan

Formula Angelicae Sinensis Radix, Arisaema cum Bile, Ziziphi Spinosae Semen (fried), Alpineae Oxyphyllae Fructus (fried with salt), Lycii Fructus, Platycladi Semen (fried), Draconis Os (calcined), Acori Tatarinowii Rhizoma, Cistanches Caulis Carnosus (steamed), Schisandrae Chinensis Fructus (stewed with wine), Juglandis Semen , Bumbusae Concretio Silicea, Polygalae Radix (prepared), Succinum and Gastrodiae Rhizoma.

Actions and Indications Tonifying essence and blood, strengthening the mental state, settling fright, resolving phlegm and extinguishing wind. It is used for amnesia, hypomnesia, dizziness, tinnitus, vexation, insomnia, palpitation, restlessness, epilepsy, headache and chest distress.

补益蒺藜丸

【处方】黄芪（蜜炙）、白术（麸炒）、山药、茯苓、白扁豆、芡实（麸炒）、当归、沙苑子、菟丝子、陈皮。

【功能主治】健脾补肾，益气明目。用于脾肾不足，眼目昏花，视物不清，腰酸气短。

【注意】忌食辛辣食物。

Tonic Bolus of Caltrop*

Name of Chinese Phonetic Alphabet Bu Yi Ji Li Wan

Formula Astragali Radix (prepared with honey), Atractylodis Macrocephalae Rhizoma (fried with bran), Dioscoreae Rhizoma, Poria, Lablab Semen Album, Euryales Semen (fried with bran), Angelicae Sinensis Radix, Astragali Complanati Semen, Cuscutae Semen and Citri Reticulatae Pericapium.

Actions and Indications Fortifying the spleen and kidney, tonifying *qi* to improve vision. It is indicated for blurred vision, soreness of waist and shortness of breath due to dual insufficency of the spleen and kidney.

Warning The pungent food is prohibited.

* 蒺藜

补脾益肠丸

【处方】黄芪、党参（米炒）、砂仁、白芍、当归（土炒）、白术（土炒）、肉桂、延胡索（制）、荔枝核、干姜（炮）、甘草（炙）、防风、木香、补骨脂（盐制）、赤石脂（煅）。

【功能主治】补中益气，健脾和胃，涩肠止泻，止痛止血，生肌消肿。临床表现为腹泻腹痛、腹胀、肠鸣、黏液血便或阳虚便秘，以及溃疡性结肠炎、结肠过敏见有上述证候者。

【注意】感冒发热者慎用。服药期间忌食生冷、辛辣、油腻之物。

Tonifying Spleen and Intestine Pill

Name of Chinese Phonetic Alphabet Bu Pi Yi Chang Wan

Formula Astragali Radix, Codonopsis Radix (fried with rice), Amomi Fructus, Paeoniae Radix Alba, Angelicae Sinensis Radix (fried with earth), Atractylodis Macrocephalae Rhizoma (fried with earth), Cinnamomi Cortex, Corydalis Rhizoma (prepared), Litchi Semen, Zingiberis Rhizoma Praeparatum, Glycyrrhizae Radix et Rhizoma (prepared), Saposhnikoviae Radix, Aucklandiae Radix, Psoraleae Fructus (prepared with salt) and Halloysitum Rubrum (calcined).

Actions and Indications Tonifying the middle and *qi*, fortifying the spleen, harmonizing the stomach, astringing the intestines, arresting diarrhea, relieving pain and bleeding, promoting tissue regeneration and dispersing swelling. It is used for cases with clinical manifestations including diarrhea, abdominal pain, abdominal distention, borborygmus, mucous bloody stool or constipation due to *yang*-deficiency; ulcerative colitis and irritable colon.

Warning It should be used carefully for cases with common cold and fever. During medication, uncooked, cold, pungent and oily foods are prohibited.

启脾丸

【处方】人参、白术（炒）、茯苓、甘草、陈皮、山药、莲子（炒）、山楂（炒）、六神曲（炒）、麦芽（炒）、泽泻。

【功能主治】健脾和胃。用于脾胃虚弱，消化不良，腹胀便溏。

Fortifying Spleen Pill for Improving Dyspepsia

Name of Chinese Phonetic Alphabet Qi Pi Wan

Formula Ginseng Radix et Rhizoma, Atractylodis Macrocephalae Rhizoma (fried), Poria, Glycyrrhizae Radix et Rhizoma, Citri Reticulatae Pericarpium, Dioscoreae Rhizoma, Nelumbinis Semen (fried), Grataegi Fructus (fried), Medicata Massa Fermentata (fried), Hordei Fructus Germinatus (fried) and Alismatis Rhizoma.

Actions and Indications Fortifying the spleen and harmonizing the stomach. It is used for dyspepsia, abdominal distention and sloppy stool due to hypofunction of the spleen and stomach.

良附丸

【处方】高良姜、香附（醋制）。

【功能主治】温胃理气。用于寒凝气滞，胃脘痛，吐酸，胸腹胀满。

Lesser Galangal* and Nut-grass** Pill

Name of Chinese Phonetic Alphabet Liang Fu Wan

Formula Alpiniae Officinarum Rhizoma and Cyperi Rhizoma (prepared with vinegar).

Actions and Indications Warming the stomach and regulating *qi*. It is indicated for stomach duct pain, acid vomiting, abdominal distention and fullness due to stagnation of *qi* and cold.

* 高良姜 ** 香附

灵丹草颗粒

【处方】本品为臭灵丹经加工制成的颗粒剂。

【功能主治】清热疏风，解毒利咽，止咳祛痰。用于风热邪毒，咽喉肿痛，肺热咳嗽，急性咽炎，扁桃体炎，上呼吸道感染见上述证候者。

Wingedtooth Laggera* Soluble Granules

Name of Chinese Phonetic Alphabet Ling Dan Cao Ke Li

Formula Laggerae Herba.

Actions and Indications Clearing heat and dispelling wind, detoxicating and soothing throat, relieving cough and dispelling phlegm. It is indicated for sore-throat, cough due to lung-heat; acute pharyngitis and acute tonsillitis due to wind-heat pathogens; and also used for upper respiratory tract infection with the above mentioned symptoms.

*臭灵丹

灵芝胶囊

【处方】本品为灵芝制成的胶囊。

【功能主治】宁心安神，健脾和胃。用于失眠健忘，身体虚弱，神经衰弱，慢性支气管炎；亦可用于冠心病的辅助治疗。

Glossy Ganoderma* Capsule

Name of Chinese Phonetic Alphabet Ling Zhi Jiao Nang

Formula Ganoderma.

Actions and Indications Tranquilizing the mind, fortifying the spleen and harmonizing the stomach. It is used for insomnia, amnesia, physical debility, neurasthenia, chronic bronchitis, and also used for accessory treatment of coronary heart disease.

*灵芝

灵猫香解毒丸

【处方】珍珠、牛黄、蟾酥、冰片、雄黄、药用灵猫香。

【功能主治】清热解毒，消肿止痛。用于喉蛾，咽喉疼痛，烂喉丹痧，痈肿，疔疮，乳痈，无名肿痛。

【注意】孕妇忌服。

Civet* Pill for Detoxicating

Name of Chinese Phonetic Alphabet Ling Mao Xiang Jie Du Wan

Formula Margarita, Bovis Calculus, Bufonis Venenum, Borneolum Syntheticum, Realgar and Zibethum.

Actions and Indications Clearing heat and detoxicating, dispersing swelling and relieving pain. It is used for tonsillitis, sore-throat, scarlet fever with pharyngitis, deep-rooted boil, abscess, swelling and pain of unknown origin.

Warning It is contraindicated for pregnant women.

*灵猫香

局方至宝丸

【处方】水牛角浓缩粉、牛黄、玳瑁粉、琥珀粉、麝香、安息香、朱砂、雄黄、冰片。

【功能主治】清热解毒，开窍镇惊。用于温邪入里，逆传心胞引起的高热痉厥，烦躁不安，神昏谵语，以及小儿急热惊风。

【注意】孕妇忌服。

Officinal Treasure Pill

Name of Chinese Phonetic Alphabet Ju Fang Zhi Bao Wan

Formula Bubali Cornu Pulvis Concentratio, Bovis Calculus, Eretmochelydis Carapax Pulvis, Succini Pulvis, Moschus, Benzoinum, Cinnabaris, Realgar and Borneolum Syntheticum.

Actions and Indications Clearing heat and detoxifying, inducing resuscitation, settling fright. It is used for high fever, spasm, vexation, restlessness, coma, delirious speech and infantile acute convulsion due to warm pathogens entering interior and reverse transmission to the pericardium.

Warning It is contraindicated for pregnant woman.

尿毒清颗粒

【处方】大黄、黄芪、甘草、茯苓、白术、制何首乌、川芎、菊花、丹参、姜半夏等。

【功能主治】通腑降浊，健脾利湿，活血化瘀。用于慢性肾功能衰竭，氮质血症期和尿毒症早期、中医辨证属脾虚湿浊证和脾虚血瘀证者。本品可降低血肌酐、尿素氮，稳定肾功能，延缓透析时间，对改善肾贫血，提高血钙、降低血磷也有一定作用。

Relieving Uremia Soluble Granules

Name of Chinese Phonetic Alphabet Niao Du Qing Ke Li

Formula Rhei Radix et Rhizoma, Astragali Radix, Glycyrrhizae Radix et Rhizoma, Poria, Atractylodis Macrocephalae Rhizoma, Polygoni Multiflori Radix Preparata, Chuanxiong Rhizoma, Chrysanthemi Flos, Salviae Miltiorrhizae Radix et Rhizoma, Pinelliae Rhizoma Praeparatum cum Zingibere et Alumine, etc.

Actions and Indications Freeing *fu*-organ and downbearing turbid, fortifying the spleen and draining dampness, activating blood and resolving stasis. It is indicated for chronic renal failure, azotemic stage, early stage of uremia attributive to spleen-deficiency and dampness turbid syndrome, spleen-deficiency and blood stasis syndrome. The preparation can decrease blood creatinine, urea nitrogen, stabilize renal function, delay dialyse time and has the effect of improving renal anemia, increasing blood calcium and decreasing serium inorganic phosphorus to certain extent.

尿感宁冲剂

【处方】海金沙藤、金钱草、凤尾草、紫花地丁。

【功能主治】清热解毒，通淋利尿，抗菌消炎。用于急、慢性尿路感染。

Relieving Urinary Tract Infection Soluble Granules

Name of Chinese Phonetic Alphabet Niao Gan Ning Chong Ji

Formula Lygodii Caulis, Lysimachiae Herba, Pteridis Multifidae Herba and Violae Herba.

Actions and Indications Clearing heat and detoxicating, relieving strangury and inducing urine, antibacterial and antiphlogistic. It is indicated for acute, chronic urinary tract infection.

阿胶三宝膏

【处方】阿胶、大枣、黄芪。

【功能主治】补气血，健脾胃。用于气短心悸，崩漏下血，脾虚食少，体虚浮肿。

Soft Extract of Ass-hide Gelatin* and Chinese Date**

Name of Chinese Phonetic Alphabet E Jiao San Bao Gao

Formula Asini Corii Colla, Jujubae Fructus and Astragali Radix.

Actions and Indications Tonifying *qi* and blood, fortifying the spleen and stomach. It is indicated for shortness of breath, palpitation, metrorrhagia, poor appetite, general debility, edema.

* 阿胶 ** 枣

阿胶补血膏

【处方】阿胶、熟地黄、党参、黄芪、枸杞子、白术。

【功能主治】滋阴补血，补中益气，健脾润肺。用于久病体弱，血亏目昏，虚痨咳嗽。

Ass-hide Gelatin* Soft Extract for Tonifying Blood

Name of Chinese Phonetic Alphabet E Jiao Bu Xue Gao

Formula Asini Corii Colla, Rehmanniae Radix Praeparata, Codonopsis Radix, Astragali Radix, Lycii Fructus and Atractylodis Macrocephalae Rhizoma.

Actions and Indications Enriching *yin*, tonifying *qi* and blood, tonifying middle energizer, fortifying the spleen and moistening the lung. It is indicated for general debility due to chronic disease; blood deficiency, blurred vision, cough due to consumptive disease.

* 阿胶

阿胶胶囊

【处方】本品为驴皮经煎煮、浓缩制成的固体胶。

【功能主治】补血滋阴，润燥，止血。用于血虚萎黄，眩晕心悸，肌痿无力，心烦不眠，肺燥咳嗽，劳咳咯血，吐血尿血，便血崩漏，妊娠胎漏。

Ass-hide Gelatin* Capsule

Name of Chinese Phonetic Alphabet E Jiao Jiao Nang

Formula Asini Corii Colla.

Actions and Indications Tonifying blood and enriching *yin*, moistening dryness, relieving bleeding. It is used for sallow complexion, vertigo, palpitation, myoatrophy, fatigue, insomnia, cough due to lung-dryness, hemoptysis, hematemesis, hematuria, hematochezia, metrorrhagia, vaginal bleeding during pregnancy.

* 阿胶

附子理中丸

【处方】附子（制）、党参、白术（炒）、干姜、甘草。

【功能主治】温中健脾。用于脾胃虚寒，脘腹冷痛，呕吐泄泻，手足不温。

【注意】孕妇慎用。

Szechuan Aconite* Bolus for Warming Middle Energizer

Name of Chinese Phonetic Alphabet Fu Zi Li Zhong Wan

Formula Aconiti Lateralis Radix (prepared), Codonopsis Radix, Atractylodis Macrocephalae Rhizoma (fried), Zingiberis Rhizoma and Glycyrrhizae Radix et Rhizoma.

Actions and Indications Warming the middle energizer and fortifying the spleen. It is indicated for abdominal cold and pain, vomiting, diarrhea and cold limbs due to deficiency-cold of the spleen and stomach.

Warning It should be used carefully for pregnant women.

* 附子

附桂风湿膏

【处方】生姜、鲜葱、生附子、当归、地黄、乳香、肉桂、苍术、没药、杜仲、川牛膝、独活、千年健、川芎、干姜、厚朴、羌活、骨碎补、桂枝、防风、甘草、生南星、木香、白芷、丁香、锁阳、韭菜子、陈皮、麻黄、北细辛、生草乌、淫羊藿、吴茱萸、生白附子、山柰、薄荷脑、冰片、肉桂油、水杨酸甲酯等。

【功能主治】祛风除湿，散寒止痛。用于四肢麻木，腰腿疼痛，跌打损伤。

【注意】孕妇慎用。

Szechuan Aconite* and Cassia Bark** Plaster for Dispelling Wind-dampness

Name of Chinese Phonetic Alphabet Fu Gui Feng Shi Gao

Formula Zingiberis Rhizoma Recens, Allii Fistulosi Folium, Aconiti Lateralis Radix (raw), Angelicae Sinensis Radix, Rehmanniae Radix, Olibanum, Cinnamomi Cortex, Atractylodis Rhizoma, Myrrha, Eucommiae Cortex, Cyathulae Radix, Angelicae Pubescentis Radix, Homalomenae Rhizoma, Chuanxiong Rhizoma, Zingiberis Rhizoma, Magnoliae Officinalis Cortex, Notopterygii Rhizoma et Radix, Drynariae Rhizoma, Cinnamomi Ramulus, Saposhnikoviae Radix, Glycyrrhizae Radix et Rhizoma, Arisaematis Rhizoma, Aucklandiae Radix, Angelicae Dahuricae Radix, Caryophylli Flos, Cynomorii Caulis Carnosus, Allii Tuberosi Semen, Citri Reticulatae Pericarpium, Ephedrae Herba, Asari Mandshurici Herba, Aconiti Kusnezoffii Radix (raw), Epimedii Folium, Euodiae Fructus, Typhonii Radix (raw), Kaempferiae Rhizoma, Menthol, Borneolum Syntheticum, Cinnamomi Oleum, Methyl Salicylate, etc.

Actions and Indications Dispelling wind and dampness, dissipating cold and alleviating pain. It is used for numbness of the limbs, pain of the waist and legs and traumatic injury.

Warning It should be used carefully for pregnant women.

* 附子 ** 肉桂

妙灵丸

【处方】天竺黄、胆南星、生石膏、僵蚕、桔梗、薄荷、浙贝母、桑叶、黄芩、苦杏仁、朱砂、连翘、金银花、地黄、甘草、蝉蜕、钩藤、冰片、麝香。

【功能主治】清热解表，化痰镇惊。用于小儿外感风热，痰热壅盛出现的发热头痛，咳嗽痰多，烦躁不安，咽喉肿痛，甚则高热神昏、惊风抽搐。

Miraculous Effectiveness Pill

Name of Chinese Phonetic Alphabet Miao Ling Wan

Formula Bambusae Concretio Silicea, Arisaema cum Bile, Gypsum Fibrosum, Bombyx Batryticatus, Platycodonis Radix, Menthae Haplocalycis Herba, Fritillariae Thunbergii Bulbus, Mori Folium, Scutellariae Radix, Armeniacae Semen Amarum, Cinnabaris, Forsythiae Fructus, Lonicerae Japonicae Flos, Rehmanniae Radix, Glycyrrhizae Radix et Rhizoma, Cicadae Periostracum, Uncariae Ramulus cum Uncis, Borneolum Syntheticum and Moschus.

Actions and Indications Clearing heat and releasing the exterior, resolving phlegm and settling fright. It is indicated for infant with manifestations as fever, headache, productive cough, vexation, sore-throat, even high fever, coma, convulsion, and spasm due to exogenous wind-heat and prevailing phlegm-heat.

鸡苏丸

【处方】陈皮、橘红、法半夏、葶苈子、瓜蒌子（蜜炙）、紫苏子（炒）、紫苏叶、桑白皮（蜜炙）、苦杏仁（炒）、桔梗、前胡、马兜铃（蜜炙）、款冬花、紫菀、远志（制）、百合、天冬、麦冬、北沙参、知母、五味子（醋蒸）、麻黄、黄芩、白芍、石膏、甘草。

【功能主治】清肺平喘，润燥止咳，化痰。用于肺热咳喘，气急鼻煽，燥咳痰黏，咽干鼻燥，劳嗽咳血，颧红盗汗，痰黏难咯，胸膈满闷。

Ji Su Bolus for Relieving Cough

Name of Chinese Phonetic Alphabet Ji Su Wan

Formula Citri Reticulatae Pericarpium, Citri Exocarpium Rubrum, Pinelliae Rhizoma Praeparatum, Lepidii Semen, Trichosanthis Semen (prepared with honey), Perillae Fructus, (fried), Perillae Folium, Mori Cortex (prepared with honey), Armeniacae Semen Amarum (fried), Platycodonis Radix, Peucedani Radix, Aristolochiae Fructus (prepared with honey), Farfarae Flos, Asteris Radix et Rhizoma, Polygalae Radix (prepared), Lilii Bulbus, Asparagi Radix, Ophiopogonis Radix, Glehniae Radix, Anemarrhenae Rhizoma, Schisandrae Chinensis Fructus (steamed by vinegar), Ephedrae Herba, Scutellariae Radix, Paeoniae Radix Alba, Gypsum Fibrosum and Glycyrrhizae Radix et Rhizoma.

Actions and Indications Clearing lung-fire and pacifying dyspnea, moistening dryness and relieving cough, resolving phlegm. It is used for cough and dyspnea due to lung-heat; faring of nares, sticky phlegm, dry throat and nose, hemoptysis, flushed zygomatic region, night sweating, difficult expectoration, chest distress.

鸡骨草胶囊

【处方】三七、人工牛黄、猪胆汁、牛至、鸡骨草、白芍、大枣、栀子、茵陈、枸杞子。

【功能主治】疏肝利胆，清热解毒。用于急、慢性肝炎和胆囊炎属肝胆湿热证者。

Chinese Prayer-beads* Capsule for Relieving Hepatitis

Name of Chinese Phonetic Alphabet Ji Gu Cao Jiao Nang

Formula Notoginseng Radix et Rhizoma, Bovis Calculus Artifactus, Suillus Bilis, Origani Vulgaris Herba, Abri Herba, Paeoniae Radix Alba, Jujubae Fructus, Gardeniae Fructus, Artemisiae Scopariae Herba and Lycii Fructus.

Actions and Indications Soothing the liver and draining bile, clearing heat and detoxicating. It is indicated for acute, chronic hepatitis and cholecystitis attributive to damp-heat in the liver and gallbladder.

* 鸡骨草

鸡胆口服液

【处方】鸡胆浸膏。

【功能主治】镇咳和祛痰。用于由上呼吸道感染和急、慢性支气管炎引起的咳嗽和咳痰。

Oral Liquid of Chicken Gall*

Name of Chinese Phonetic Alphabet Ji Dan Kou Fu Ye

Formula Galli Fel Extractum.

Actions and Indications Settling cough and dispelling phlegm. It is indicated for productive cough due to infection of the upper respiratory tract, acute, chronic bronchitis.

纯阳正气丸

【处方】广藿香、半夏（制）、青木香、陈皮、丁香、肉桂、苍术、白术、茯苓、朱砂、硝石（精制）、硼砂、雄黄、金礞石（煅）、麝香、冰片。

【功能主治】温中散寒。用于暑天感寒受湿，腹痛吐泻，胸膈胀满，头痛恶寒，肢体酸重。

【注意】孕妇禁用。

Chun Yang Pill

Name of Chinese Phonetic Alphabet Chun Yang Zheng Qi Wan

Formula Pogostemonis Herba, Pinelliae Rhizoma (prepared), Aristolochiae Radix, Citri Reticulatae Pericarpium, Caryophylli Flos, Cinnamomi Cortex, Atractylodis Rhizoma, Atractylodis Macrocephalae Rhizoma, Poria, Cinnabaris, Nitrum (refined), Borax, Realgar, Micae Lapis Aureus (calcined), Moschus and Borneolum Syntheticum.

Actions and Indications Warming the middle and dissipating cold. It is indicated for abdominal pain, vomiting, diarrhea, hypochondric distention and fullness, headache and aversion to cold, soreness and heavy sensation of extremities due to invasion of cold-damp in summer.

Warning It is contraindicated for pregnant women.

驴胶补血冲剂

【处方】阿胶、黄芪、党参、熟地黄、白术、当归。

【功能主治】滋阴补血，健脾益气，调经养血。用于久病体虚，血亏气虚，妇女血虚、经闭、经少。

Ass-hide Gelatin* Soluble Granules for Tonifying Blood

Name of Chinese Phonetic Alphabet Lu Jiao Bu Xue Chong Ji

Formula Asini Corii Colla, Astragali Radix, Codonopsis Radix, Rehmanniae Radix Praeparata, Atractylodis Macrocephalae Rhizoma and Angelicae Sinensis Radix.

Actions and Indications Enriching *yin*, tonifying *qi* and blood, fortifying the spleen, regulating menstruation. It is indicated for amenorrhea and scant menstruation in women due to chronic disease or general debility and dual deficiency of *qi* and blood.

* 阿胶

八画

青石冲剂

【处方】本品为麻黄、桂枝、白芍、干姜、细辛、甘草等药味经加工制成的冲剂。

【功能主治】解表，化饮，清热止咳，平喘祛痰。用于表寒里饮化热所致的咳喘，症见恶寒发热，咳嗽喘促，痰稀色白、量多或淡黄，舌淡红、苔滑润、脉浮数或滑数。或用于上呼吸道感染，急、慢性支气管炎有上述证候者。

【注意】干咳、虚咳者忌服。

Qing Shi Soluble Granules

Name of Chinese Phonetic Alphabet Qing Shi Chong Ji

Formula Ephedrae Herba, Cinnamomi Ramulus, Paeoniae Radix Alba, Zingiberis Rhizoma, Asari Radix et Rhizoma, Glycyrrhizae Radix et Rhizoma, etc.

Actions and Indications Releasing the exterior, resolving retained fluid, clearing heat and suppressing cough, calming panting and dispelling phlegm. It is indicated for productive cough due to exterior cold and interior retained fluid transforming into heat, manifested as aversion to cold, fever, cough and dyspnea, thin and white, profuse or slight yellow phlegm, slight red tongue, slippery fur, floating rapid or slippery rapid pulse, or for upper respiratory tract infection, acute, chronic bronchitis with the above mentioned symptoms.

Warning It is contraindicated for cases with dry cough and deficiency cough.

青果丸

【处方】青果、金银花、黄芩、北豆根、麦冬、玄参、白芍、桔梗。

【功能主治】清热利咽，消肿止痛。用于咽喉肿痛，失声声哑，口干舌燥，肺燥咳嗽。

【注意】忌食辛辣。

Chinese Olive* Bolus

Name of Chinese Phonetic Alphabet Qing Guo Wan

Formula Canarii Fructus, Lonicerae Japonicae Flos, Scutellariae Radix, Menispermi Rhizoma, Ophiopogonis Radix, Scrophulariae Radix, Paeoniae Radix Alba and Platycodonis Radix.

Actions and Indications Clearing heat, soothing the throat, reducing swelling, alleviating pain. It is used for sore-throat, hoarseness, dry mouth and tongue, cough due to lung-dryness.

Warning Pungent foods should be avoided.

* 青果

青蛾丸

【处方】杜仲（盐炒）、补骨脂（盐炒）、核桃仁（炒）、大蒜。

【功能主治】补肾强腰。用于肾虚腰痛，起坐不利，膝软乏力。

Kidney-tonifying Bolus

Name of Chinese Phonetic Alphabet Qing E Wan

Formula Eucommiae Cortex (fried with salt), Psoraleae Fructus (fried with salt), Juglandis Semen (fried) and Allii Sativi Bulbus.

Actions and Indications Tonifying the kidney to strengthen the waist. It is used for lumbago due to deficiency of the kidney and marked by uneasiness whether sitting or standing, weakness of knees.

表实感冒冲剂

【处方】紫苏叶、葛根、白芷、麻黄、防风、桔梗、生姜、苦杏仁（炒）、甘草、桂枝、陈皮。

【功能主治】发汗解表，祛风散寒。用于感冒病风寒表实证，症见恶寒重，发热轻，无汗，头项强痛，鼻流清涕，咳嗽，痰稀白。

Common Cold (Exterior Excess Type) Relieving Soluble Granules

Name of Chinese Phonetic Alphabet Biao Shi Gan Mao Chong Ji

Formula Perillae Folium, Puerariae Lobatae Radix, Angelicae Dahuricae Radix, Ephedrae Herba, Saposhnikoviae Radix, Platycodonis Radix, Zingiberis Rhizoma Recens, Armeniacae Semen Amarum (fried), Glycyrrhizae Radix et Rhizoma, Cinnamomi Ramulus and Citri Reticulatae Pericarpium.

Actions and Indications Promoting sweating, releasing the exterior, dispelling wind and dissipating cold. It is used for common cold (wind-cold) type with exterior excess syndrome of common cold manifested as severe aversion to wind, mild fever, anhidrosis, headache and painful stiff nape, clear nasal discharge, cough, thin and white phlegm.

表虚感冒冲剂

【处方】桂枝、葛根、白芍、苦杏仁（炒）、生姜、大枣。

【功能主治】散风解肌，和营退热。用于感冒病外感风寒表虚证，症见发热恶风，有汗，头痛项强，咳嗽痰白，干呕，苔薄白，脉浮缓。

Common Cold (Exterior Deficiency Type) Relieving Soluble Granules

Name of Chinese Phonetic Alphabet Biao Xu Gan Mao Chong Ji

Formula Cinnamomi Ramulus, Puerariae Lobatae Radix, Paeoniae Radix Alba, Armeniacae Semen Amarum (fried), Zingiberis Rhizoma Recens and Jujubae Fructus.

Actions and Indications Dispersing wind and releasing the flesh, harmonizing the nutrient and antifebrile. It is used for common cold (wind-cold) type with exterior deficiency syndrome of common cold, manifested as aversion to wind with fever, sweating, headache and painful stiff nape, cough with white phlegm, retching, thin-white tongue fur, moderate pulse.

坤宝丸

【处方】女贞子（酒炙）、覆盆子、菟丝子、枸杞子、何首乌（黑豆酒炙）、龟甲、地骨皮、南沙参、麦冬、酸枣仁（炒）、地黄、白芍、赤芍、当归、鸡血藤、珍珠母、石斛、菊花、墨旱莲、桑叶、白薇、知母、黄芩。

【功能主治】滋补肝肾，镇静安神，养血通络。用于肝肾阴虚引起的月经紊乱，潮热多汗，失眠健忘，心烦易怒，头晕耳鸣，咽干口渴，四肢酸楚，关节疼痛，及妇女更年期综合征而见上述症状者。

Treasure Pill for Menopausal Syndrome

Name of Chinese Phonetic Alphabet Kun Bao Wan

Formula Ligustri Lucidi Fructus (prepared with wine), Rubi Fructus, Cuscutae Semen, Lycii Fructus, Polygoni Multiflori Radix (prepared with wine), Testudinis Carapax et Plastrum, Lycii Cortex, Adenophorae Radix, Ophiopogonis Radix, Ziziphi Spinosae Semen (fried), Rehmanniae Radix, Paeoniae Radix Alba, Paeoniae Radix Rubra, Angelicae Sinensis Radix, Spatholobi Caulis, Margaritifera Concha, Dendrobii Caulis, Chrysanthemi Flos, Ecliptae Herba, Mori Folium, Cynanchi Atrati Radix et Rhizoma, Anemarrhenae Rhizoma and Scutellariae Radix.

Actions and Indications Enriching the liver and kidney, tranquilizing the mind, tonifying blood and activating collaterals. It is indicated for disturbance of menstruation, tidal fever, hyperhidrosis, insomnia, amnesia, vexation, dizziness, tinnitus, dry throat, thirst, soreness of extremities, arthralgia, and menopausal syndrome with the above mentioned symptoms due to dual *yin*-deficiency of the liver and kidney.

枇杷止咳冲剂

【处方】枇杷叶、罂粟壳、百部、白前、桑白皮、桔梗、薄荷脑。

【功能主治】止嗽化痰。用于咳嗽，支气管炎。

Loquat Leaf* Soluble Granules for Relieving Cough

Name of Chinese Phonetic Alphabet Pi Pa Zhi Ke Chong Ji

Formula Eriobotryae Folium, Papaveris Pericarpium, Stemonae Radix, Cynanchi Stauntonii Rhizoma et Radix, Mori Cortex, Platycodonis Radix and Menthol.

Actions and Indications Relieving cough and resolving phlegm. It is indicated for cough and bronchitis.

* 枇杷叶

板蓝根冲剂

【处方】板蓝根。

【功能主治】清热解毒，凉血利咽，消肿。用于扁桃体炎、腮腺炎、咽喉肿痛，防治传染性肝炎，小儿麻疹。

Woad Root* Soluble Granules for Clearing Heat

Name of Chinese Phonetic Alphabet Ban Lan Gen Chong Ji

Formula Isatidis Radix.

Actions and Indications Clearing heat and detoxicating, cooling blood and soothing the throat, dispersing swelling. It is indicated for tonsillitis, parotitis, sore-throat, preventing infective hepatitis and infantile measles.

* 板蓝根

松龄血脉康胶囊

【处方】葛根珍珠层粉等。

【功能主治】平肝潜阳，镇心安神。用于高血压病见有头痛眩晕、急躁易怒、心悸失眠等属肝阳上亢证者。

Song Ling Capsule for Relieving Hypertension

Name of Chinese Phonetic Alphabet Song Ling Xue Mai Kang Jiao Nang

Formula Puerariae Lobatae Radix and Margaritae Concha Strati Pulvis.

Actions and Indications Pacifying the liver, subduing *yang*, tranquilizing the mind. It is used for hypertension marked by headache, vertigo, vexation, palpitation and insomnia due to ascendant hyperactivity of liver-*yang*.

枫蓼肠胃康冲剂

【处方】牛耳枫、辣蓼。

【功能主治】理气健胃，除湿化滞。用于急性胃肠炎及其所引起的腹胀、腹痛和腹泻等消化不良。

Calyx-shaped Daphniphyllum* and Smartweed Soluble Granules** for Gastroenteritis

Name of Chinese Phonetic Alphabet Feng Liao Chang Wei Kang Chong Ji

Formula Daphniphylli Calycini Radix and Polygoni Flaccidi Herba.

Actions and Indications Regulating *qi* and fortifying the stomach, dispelling dampness and relieving stagnation. It is indicated for acute gastroenteritis, manifested as abdominal distention, abdominal pain, diarrhea and indigestion.

* 牛耳枫 ** 辣蓼

刺五加片

【处方】本品为刺五加浸膏制成。

【功能主治】益气健脾，补肾安神。用于脾肾阳虚，体虚乏力，食欲不振，腰膝酸痛，失眠多梦。

Manyprickle Acanthopanax* Tablet

Name of Chinese Phonetic Alphabet Ci Wu Jia Pian

Formula Acanthopanacis Senticosi Extractum.

Actions and Indications Tonifying *qi*, fortifying the spleen and kidney, tranquilizing the mind. It is used for physical debility, fatigue, poor appetite, soreness and pain of waist and knees, insomnia and profuse dreaming due to dual *yang*-deficiency of the spleen and kidney.

* 刺五加

苦甘冲剂

【处方】麻黄、薄荷、蝉蜕、金银花、黄芩、苦杏仁、桔梗、浙贝母、甘草。

【功能主治】疏风清热，宣肺化痰，止咳平喘。用于风热感冒及肺热引起的恶风、发热、头痛、咽痛、咳嗽、气喘。

Apricot Seed* and Licorice** Soluble Granules

Name of Chinese Phonetic Alphabet Ku Gan Chong Ji

Formula Ephedrae Herba, Menthae Haplocalycis Herba, Cicadae Periostracum, Lonicerae Japonicae Flos, Scutellariae Radix, Armeniacae Semen Amarum, Platycodonis Radix, Fritillariae Thunbergii Bulbus and Glycyrrhizae Radix et Rhizoma.

Actions and Indications Dispersing wind and clearing heat, diffusing the lung and resolving phlegm, relieving cough and calming dyspnea. It is indicated for aversion to wind, fever, headache, sore-throat, cough and dyspnea due to common cold of wind-heat and lung-heat.

* 苦杏仁 ** 甘草

苦胆草片

【处方】本品为坚龙胆的浸膏片。

【功能主治】清热燥湿，泻火。用于目赤口燥，咽喉肿痛。

Rigescent Gentian* Tablet

Name of Chinese Phonetic Alphabet Ku Dan Cao Pian

Formula Gentianae Extractum.

Actions and Indications Clearing heat and drying dampness, purging fire. It is used for conjunctival congestion, dry mouth, sore-throat.

* 坚龙胆

苦黄注射液

【处方】苦参、大黄等。

【功能主治】清热利湿，疏肝退黄。主治湿热黄疸，适用于黄疸型病毒性肝炎患者的退黄。

Shrubby Sophora* and Rhubarb** Injection for Relieving Jaundice

Name of Chinese Phonetic Alphabet Ku Huang Zhu She Ye

Formula Sophorae Flavescentis Radix, Rhei Radix et Rhizoma, etc.

Actions and Indications Clearing heat and draining dampness, soothing the liver and relieving jaundice. It is indicated for jaundice due to damp-heat; and also used for relieving jaundice of icteric viral hepatitis.

* 苦参 ** 大黄

苓桂咳喘宁胶囊

【处方】茯苓、法半夏、桂枝等。

【功能主治】温肺化饮，止咳平喘。主治外感风寒，痰湿阻肺，症见咳嗽痰多，喘息胸闷，气短，适用于急、慢性支气管炎见上述证候者。

【注意】服药期间忌食生冷食物，孕妇慎用。

Indian Bread* and Cassia Twig** for Relieving Cough and Dyspnea Capsule

Name of Chinese Phonetic Alphabet Ling Gui Ke Chuan Ning Jiao Nang

Formula Poria, Pinelliae Rhizoma Praeparatum, Cinnamomi Ramulus, etc.

Actions and Indications Warming the lung and resolving retained fluid, relieving cough and calming dyspnea. It is indicated for external contraction of wind-cold, stagnation of phlegm-damp in the lung, manifested as cough with profuse phlegm, dyspnea and chest distress, shortness of breath, also for acute, chronic bronchitis with the above mentioned symptoms.

Warning Uncooked and cold foods are prohibited during medication and it should be used carefully for pregnant women.

* 茯苓 ** 桂枝

枣仁安神颗粒

【处方】酸枣仁（炒）、丹参、五味子（醋炙）。

【功能主治】补心养肝，安神益智。用于心肝血虚，神经衰弱引起的失眠健忘，头昏头痛。

Sour Jujube★ Soluble Granules for Tranquilization

Name of Chinese Phonetic Alphabet Zao Ren An Shen Ke Li

Formula Ziziphi Spinosae Semen (fried), Salviae Miltiorrhizae Radix et Rhizoma and Schisandrae Chinensis Fructus (prepared with vinegar).

Actions and Indications Tonifying the heart, nourishing the liver, tranquilizing the mind. It is used for neurasthenia, insomnia, amnesia, dizziness and headache due to dual blood-deficiency of the heart and liver.

* 酸枣仁

矽肺宁片

【处方】虎杖、岩白菜素等。

【功能主治】活血散结，清热化痰，止咳平喘。用于矽肺、煤矽肺等引起的咳嗽、胸闷、胸痛、气短、乏力。

【注意】服药期间不宜用冷饮、辛辣之品。

Relieving Silicosis Tablet

Name of Chinese Phonetic Alphabet Xi Fei Ning Pian

Formula Polygoni Cuspidati Rhizoma et Radix , Bergenin, etc.

Actions and Indications Activating blood and dispersing mass, clearing heat and resolving phlegm, suppressing cough and dyspnea. It is indicated for cough, chest upset, pectoralgia, shortness of breath and fatigue due to silicosis, anthracosilicosis.

Warning Cold drink and pungent foods are prohibited during medication.

奇应内消膏

【处方】天南星、乳香（制）、没药、山柰、重楼、姜黄。

【功能主治】行气活血，消肿止痛，用于跌打扭伤等所致的急性闭合性软组织损伤，局部肿胀，疼痛。

【注意】出血性损伤，皮肤破损部分禁用，皮肤易过敏者忌用。孕妇及3岁以下小儿慎用。

Qi Ying Plaster for Traumatic Injury

Name of Chinese Phonetic Alphabet Qi Ying Nei Xiao Gao

Formula Arisaematis Rhizoma, Olibanum (prepared), Myrrha, Kaempferiae Rhizoma, Paridis Rhizoma and Curcumae Rhizoma Longae.

Actions and Indications Moving *qi*, activating blood, reducing swelling, alleviating pain. It is used for acute closed soft tissue injury due to traumatic injury and marked with topical swelling and pain.

Warning It is contraindicated for hemorrhagic injury, wound of skin and dermal hypersensitivity, and should be used cautiously for pregnant women and children under 3 years old.

拔毒膏

【处方】金银花、连翘、大黄、桔梗、地黄、栀子、黄柏、黄芩、赤芍、当归、川芎、白芷、白蔹、木鳖子、蓖麻子、玄参、穿山甲、苍术、蜈蚣、樟脑、没药、儿茶、乳香、红粉、血竭、轻粉。

【功能主治】清热解毒，活血消肿。多用于治疗疖疔痈发、有头疽之初期或化脓期。

Drawing Out Toxin Ointment

Name of Chinese Phonetic Alphabet Ba Du Gao

Formula Lonicerae Japonicae Flos, Forsythiae

Fructus, Rhei Radix et Rhizoma, Platycodonis Radix, Rehmanniae Radix, Gardeniae Fructus, Phellodendri Chinensis Cortex, Scutellariae Radix, Paeoniae Radix Rubra, Angelicae Sinensis Radix, Chuanxiong Rhizoma, Angelicae Dahuricae Radix, Ampelopsis Radix, Momordicae Semen, Ricini Semen, Scrophulariae Radix, Manis Squma, Atractylodis Rhizoma, Scolopendra, Camphora, Myrrha, Catechu, Olibanum, Hydrargyri Oxydum Rubrum, Draconis Sanguis and Calomelas.

Actions and Indications Clearing heat and detoxicating, activating blood and dispersing swelling. It is used for furuncle, deep-rooted boil, abscess, initial stage or stadium suppuration of carbuncle.

拨云退翳丸

【处方】密蒙花、蒺藜（盐炒）、菊花、木贼、蛇蜕、蝉蜕、荆芥穗、蔓荆子、薄荷、当归、川芎、黄连、地骨皮、花椒、楮实子、天花粉、甘草。

【功能主治】散风明目，消障退翳。用于目翳外障，视物不清，隐痛流泪。

Wind-dispersing and Nebula-removing Bolus

Name of Chinese Phonetic Alphabet Bo Yun Tui Yi Wan

Formula Buddlejae Flos, Tribuli Fructus (fried with salt), Chrysanthemi Flos, Equiseti Hiemalis Herba, Serpentis Periostracum, Cicadae Periostracum, Schizonepetae Spica, Viticis Fructus, Menthae Haplocalycis Herba, Angelicae Sinensis Radix, Chuanxiong Rhizoma, Coptidis Rhizoma, Lycii Cortex, Zanthoxyli Pericarpium, Broussonetiae Fructus, Trichosanthis Radix and Glycyrrhizae Radix et Rhizoma.

Actions and Indications Dispersing wind and improving vision, dispersing corneal opacity, removing nebula. It is indicated for nebula, external ophthalmopathy, blurred vision, dull pain of eyes and lacrimation.

拨云散

【处方】牛黄、麝香、冰片、朱砂、琥珀、硇砂、硼砂、炉甘石（煅）。

【功能主治】清热解毒，明目退翳。用于暴发火眼，眼边赤烂，云翳遮睛。

Wind-dispering and Nebula-removing Powder

Name of Chinese Phonetic Alphabet Bo Yun San

Formula Bovis Calculus, Moschus, Borneolum Syntheticum, Cinnabaris, Cutis Succinum, Sal Ammoniacum, Borax and Calamina (calcined).

Actions and Indications Clearing heat and detoxicating, removing nebula to improve vision. It is used for sudden conjunctivitis, blepharitis marginalis, corneal macula.

软脉灵口服液

【处方】熟地黄、五味子、枸杞子、牛膝 、茯苓、制何首乌、白芍、柏子仁、远志、黄芪（炙）、陈皮、淫羊藿、当归、川芎、丹参、人参。

【功能主治】滋补肝肾，益气活血。用于肝肾阴虚，气虚血瘀证之早期脑动脉硬化，冠心病，心肌炎，中风后遗症。

Relieving Cerebral Arteriosclerosis Oral Liquid

Name of Chinese Phonetic Alphabet Ruan Mai Ling Kou Fu Ye

Formula Rehmanniae Radix Praeparata, Schisandrae Chinensis Fructus, Lycii Fructus, Achyranthis Bidentatae Radix, Poria, Polygoni Multiflori Radix Praeparata, Paeoniae Radix Alba, Platycladi Semen, Polygalae Radix, Astragali Radix (prepared), Citri Reticulatae Pericarpium, Epimedii Folium, Angelicae Sinensis Radix, Chuanxiong Rhizoma, Salviae Miltiorrhizae Radix et Rhizoma and Ginseng Radix et Rhizoma.

Actions and Indications Enriching the liver and

kidney, tonifying *qi*, activating blood. It is used for early stage of cerebral arteriosclerosis, coronary heart disease, myocarditis and sequela of apoplexy due to dual *yin*-deficiency of the liver and kidney, deficiency of *qi* and blood-stasis.

齿痛冰硼散

【处方】硼砂、硝石、冰片。

【功能主治】散郁火，止牙痛。用于火热内闭引起的牙龈肿痛，口舌生疮。

【注意】不可内服，忌食辛辣食物。

Relieving Toothache Powder

Name of Chinese Phonetic Alphabet Chi Tong Bing Peng San

Formula Borax, Nitrum and Borneolum Syntheticum.

Actions and Indications Dissipating fire, relieving toothache. It is used for gingivitis, aphthae due to internal fire.

Warning Oral use is prohibited. Pungent foods should be avoided.

虎力胶囊

【处方】制草乌、三七、断节参等。

【功能主治】驱风除湿，舒筋活络，行瘀，消肿定痛。用于风湿麻木，筋骨疼痛，跌打损伤，创伤流血。

【注意】孕妇慎用。

Hu Li Capsule for Relieving Rheumatic Numbness

Name of Chinese Phonetic Alphabet Hu Li Jiao Nang

Formula Aconiti Kusnezoffii Radix Cocta, Notoginseng Radix et Rhizoma, Cynanchi Wallichii Radix, etc.

Actions and Indications Dispelling wind and dampness, relaxing sinews and activating collaterals, moving stasis, dispersing swelling and alleviating pain. It is used for numbness due to wind-damp; pain of sinews and bone, traumatic injury and bleeding.

Warning It should be used carefully for pregnant women.

虎驹乙肝胶囊

【处方】虎杖、蚂蚁、柴胡、茵陈、板蓝根、枸杞子、黄芪、三七、丹参、五味子、大枣。

【功能主治】疏肝健脾，利湿清热，活血化瘀。用于慢性乙型肝炎肝郁脾虚兼湿热瘀滞症，症见胁肋胀满疼痛，脘痞腹胀，胃纳不佳，四肢倦怠，小便色黄。

Bushy Knotweed* Capsule for Relieving Hepatitis B

Name of Chinese Phonetic Alphabet Hu Ju Yi Gan Jiao Nang

Formula Polygoni Cuspidati Rhizoma et Radix , Formica Fusca, Bupleuri Radix, Artemisiae Scopariae Herba, Isatidis Radix, Lycii Fructus, Astragali Radix, Notoginseng Radix et Rhizoma, Salviae Miltiorrhizae Radix et Rhizoma, Schisandrae Chinensis Fructus and Jujubae Fructus.

Actions and Indications Soothing the liver and fortifying the spleen, draining dampness and clearing heat, activating blood and resolving stasis. It is indicated for chronic hepatitis B of liver depression and spleen deficiency accompanied by damp-heat-stasis stagnation syndrome, manifested as hypochondriac distention and pain, abdominal distention, anorexia, fatigue of limbs, yellow urine.

* 虎杖

肾石通冲剂

【处方】金钱草、王不留行（炒）、萹蓄、丹参、延胡索（醋制）、鸡内金（烫）、木香、瞿麦、牛膝、海金沙。

【功能主治】清热利湿，活血止痛，化石，排石。用于肾结石，肾盂结石，输尿管结石。

Removing Kidney Stone Soluble Granules

Name of Chinese Phonetic Alphabet Shen Shi Tong Chong Ji

Formula Lysimachiae Herba, Vaccariae Semen (fried), Polygoni Avicularis Herba, Salviae Miltiorrhizae Radix et Rhizoma, Corydalis Rhizoma (prepared with vinegar), Galli Gigerii Endothelium Corneum (scalded), Aucklandiae Radix, Dianthi Herba, Achyranthis Bidentatae Radix and Lygodii Spora.

Actions and Indications Clearing heat and draining dampness, activating blood to alleviate pain, resolving and removing stone. It is indicated for calculus of the kidney, pyelolithiasis and ureterolith.

肾炎四味片

【处方】细梗胡枝子、黄芩、石韦、黄芪。

【功能主治】活血化瘀，清热解毒，补肾益气。用于慢性肾炎。

Four Medicinals Tablet for Nephritis

Name of Chinese Phonetic Alphabet Shen Yan Si Wei Pian

Formula Lespedezae Virgatae Herba, Scutellariae Radix, Pyrrosiae Folium and Astragali Radix.

Actions and Indications Activating blood and resolving stasis, clearing heat and detoxicating, tonifying the kidney and replenishing *qi*. It is indicated for chronic nephritis.

肾炎消肿片

【处方】桂枝、泽泻、陈皮、香加皮、苍术、茯苓、姜皮、大腹皮、黄柏、花椒、冬瓜皮、益母草等。

【功能主治】健脾渗湿，通阳利水。用于急、慢性肾炎。临床表现为肢体浮肿，晨起面肿甚，午后腿肿较重，按之凹陷，身体重困，尿少，脘胀食少，舌苔白腻，脉沉缓。

Reducing Nephritic Edema Tablet

Name of Chinese Phonetic Alphabet Shen Yan Xiao Zhong Pian

Formula Cinnamomi Ramulus, Alismatis Rhizoma, Citri Reticulatae Pericarpium, Periplocae Cortex, Atractylodis Rhizoma, Poria, Zingiberis Rhizomatis Epidermis, Arecae Pericarpium, Phellodendri Chinensis Cortex, Zanthoxyli Pericarpium, Benincasae Pericarpium, Leonuri Herba, etc.

Actions and Indications Fortifying the spleen and draining dampness, unblocking *yang* and inducing diuresis. It is indicated for acute, chronic nephritis, manifested as edema, facial edema severely in the morning, legs edema seriously in the afternoon, the pit occurrence when pressed, bodily heaviness, oliguria, stomach distention and anorexia, white slimy tongue fur, sunken and slow pulse.

肾炎康复片

【处方】西洋参、人参、地黄、杜仲（炒）、山药、白花蛇舌草、黑豆、土茯苓、益母草、丹参、泽泻、白茅根、桔梗。

【功能主治】益气养阴，补肾健脾，清除余毒。主治慢性肾小球肾炎，属于气阴两虚，脾肾不足，表现为神疲乏力，腰酸腿软，面浮肢肿，头晕耳鸣；蛋白尿，血尿。

【禁忌】服药期间忌辛、辣、肥甘等刺激性食物，禁房事。

Relieving Nephritis Tablet

Name of Chinese Phonetic Alphabet Shen Yan Kang Fu Pian

Formula Panacis Quinquefolii Radix, Ginseng Radix et Rhizoma, Rehmanniae Radix, Eucommiae Cortex (fried), Dioscoreae Rhizoma, Hedyotis Diffusae Herba, Sojae Semen Nigrum, Smilacis Glabrae Rhizoma, Leonuri Herba, Salviae Miltiorrhizae Radix et Rhizoma, Alismatis Rhizoma, Imperatae Rhizoma and Platycodonis Radix.

Actions and Indications Replenishing *qi* and nourishing *yin*, tonifying the kidney and fortifying the spleen, eliminating remaining toxin. It is indicated for chronic glomerulonephritis, attributive to dual deficiency of *qi* and *yin* and dual insufficiency of the spleen and kidney, manifested as lassitude of spirit and fatigue, aching of the waist and weakness of the legs, edema of the face and limbs, dizziness and tinnitus, proteinuria, hematuria.

Warning Irritative foods including pungent, fat, sweet and sexual intercourse are prohibited during medication.

肾炎舒片

【处方】苍术、茯苓、白茅根、防己、生晒参等。

【功能主治】益肾健脾，利水消肿。用于治疗脾肾阳虚肾炎引起的浮肿腰痛，头晕，乏力。

Nephritis-relieving Tablet

Name of Chinese Phonetic Alphabet Shen Yan Shu Pian

Formula Atractylodis Rhizoma, Poria, Imperatae Rhizoma, Stephaniae Tetrandrae Radix, Ginseng Radix et Rhizoma Exsiccatus, etc.

Actions and Indications Tonifying the kidney and fortifying the spleen, inducing diuresis and dispersing edema. It is indicated for edema, lumbago, dizziness, fatigue due to nephritis of dual *yang*-deficiency of the spleen and kidney.

肾炎温阳片

【处方】人参、黄芪、附子（盐制）、党参、茯苓、肉桂、香加皮、木香、大黄、白术、葶苈子等。

【功能主治】温肾健脾，化气行水。用于慢性肾炎，症见脾肾阳虚，全身浮肿，面色苍白，脘腹胀满，纳少便溏，神倦尿少。

Relieving Chronic Nephritis Tablet

Name of Chinese Phonetic Alphabet Shen Yan Wen Yang Pian

Formula Ginseng Radix et Rhizoma, Astragali Radix, Aconiti Lateralis Radix (prepared with salt), Codonopsis Radix, Poria, Cinnamomi Cortex, Periplocae Cortex, Aucklandiae Radix, Rhei Radix et Rhizoma, Atractylodis Macrocephalae Rhizoma, Lepidii Semen, etc.

Actions and Indications Warming the kidney and fortifying the spleen, resolving *qi* and moving water. It is indicated for chronic nephritis, manifested as general edema, pale complexion, abdominal distention and fullness, anorexia and sloppy stool, lassitude of spirit and dysuria due to *yang*-deficiency of the spleen and kidney.

肾炎解热片

【处方】本品为白茅根、连翘、荆芥、苦杏仁（炒）、陈皮、大腹皮、泽泻（盐制）、茯苓、桂枝、车前子（炒）、赤小豆、生石膏、蒲公英、蝉蜕等药经加工制成的片剂。

【功能主治】疏解风热，宣肺利水。用于急性肾炎，见有发热不恶寒或热重寒轻，头面眼睑浮肿，咽喉肿痛或口干咽燥，肢体酸痛，小便短赤，舌苔薄黄，脉浮数等属风热证者。

Relieving Acute Nephritis Tablet

Name of Chinese Phonetic Alphabet Shen Yan Jie Re Pian

Formula Imperatae Rhizoma, Forsythiae Fructus, Schizonepetae Herba, Armeniacae Semen Amarum (fried), Citri Reticulatae Pericarpium, Arecae Pericarpium, Alismatis Rhizoma (prepared with salt), Poria, Cinnamomi Ramulus, Plantaginis Semen (fried), Vignae Semen, Gypsum Fibrosum, Taraxaci Herba, Cicadae Periostracum, etc.

Actions and Indications Releasing wind-heat, diffusing the lung and inducing diuresis. It is indicated for acute nephritis, manifested as fever without aversion to cold or with heat prevailing to cold, facial edema, edema of the eyelid, sore-throat or dry mouth and throat, aching pain of the limbs, scanty dark urine, thin yellow fur, floating and rapid pulse attributive to wind-heat syndrome.

肾骨胶囊

【处方】本品为牡蛎经加工制成的胶囊。

【功能主治】促进骨质形成，维持神经传导、肌肉收缩、毛细血管正常渗透压，保持血液酸碱平衡。用于儿童、成年人或老年人缺钙引起的骨质疏松、骨质增生、骨痛、肌肉痉挛，小儿佝偻症。

【注意】饭后立即服。

Strengthening Bone Capsule

Name of Chinese Phonetic Alphabet Shen Gu Jiao Nang

Formula Ostreae Concha Praeparata.

Actions and Indications Promoting the osteosis, maintaining the nerve conduction, muscular contraction, normal osmotic pressure of capillary and maintaining the acid-base balance of blood. It is indicated for osteoporosis, hyperosteogeny, ostealgia, myospasm and rickets due to calciprivia in children, adult and the aged.

Warning Take the capsule after meal immediately.

肾复康胶囊

【处方】土茯苓、槐花、白茅根、益母草、藿香。

【功能主治】清热利尿，益肾化浊。用于热淋涩痛，急性肾炎水肿，慢性肾炎紧急性发作。

Renal Rehabilitation Capsule

Name of Chinese Phonetic Alphabet Shen Fu Kang Jiao Nang

Formula Smilacis Glabrae Rhizoma, Sophorae Flos, Imperatae Rhizoma, Leonuri Herba and Agastaches Herba.

Actions and Indications Clearing heat and inducing diuresis, tonifying the kidney and resolving turbidity. It is indicated for heat strangury, acute nephritic edema, chronic nephritis with acute attack.

肾衰宁胶囊

【处方】太子参、黄连、半夏（制）、陈皮、茯苓、大黄、丹参、牛膝、红花、甘草。

【功能主治】益气健脾，活血化瘀，通腑泄浊。用于脾失运化，瘀浊阻滞所引起的腰痛疲倦，面色萎黄，恶心呕吐，食欲不振，小便不利，大便黏滞及多种原因引起的慢性肾功能不全见上述证候者。

Renal-failure-relieving Capsule

Name of Chinese Phonetic Alphabet Shen Shuai Ning Jiao Nang

Formula Pseudostellariae Radix, Coptidis Rhizoma, Pinelliae Rhizoma (prepared), Citri Reticulatae Pericarpium, Poria, Rhei Radix et Rhizoma, Salviae Miltiorrhizae Radix et Rhizoma, Achyranthis Bidentatae Radix, Carthami Flos and Glycyrrhizae Radix et Rhizoma.

Actions and Indications Replenishing *qi* and fortifying the spleen, activating blood and resolving stasis, discharging turbidity. It is indicated for lumbago and lassitude, sallow complexion, nausea and vomiting, poor appetite, dysuria, viscous stool due to the spleen failing in transportation and transformation, stagnation of turbidity, and chronic renal insufficiency due to various causes with the above mentioned symptoms.

肾衰康灌肠液

【处方】黄芪、大黄、丹参、红花。

【功能主治】清热解毒，益气利尿，活血化瘀。用于急性肾功能衰竭。

Enema for Renal Failure

Name of Chinese Phonetic Alphabet Shen Shuai Kang Guan Chang Ye

Formula Astragali Radix, Rhei Radix et Rhizoma, Salviae Miltiorrhizae Radix et Rhizoma and Carthami Flos.

Actions and Indications Clearing heat and

detoxicating, replenishing *qi* and inducing diuresis, activating blood and resolving stasis. It is indicated for acute renal failure.

肾康宁片

【处方】黄芪、丹参、茯苓、泽泻、益母草、附片、锁阳、山药。

【功能主治】温肾，益气，活血，渗湿。用于慢性肾炎，肾气亏损，肾功能不全所引起的腰酸、疲乏、畏寒及夜尿增多。

Chronic Nephritis Relieving Tablet

Name of Chinese Phonetic Alphabet Shen Kang Ning Pian

Formula Astragali Radix, Salviae Miltiorrhizae Radix et Rhizoma, Poria, Alismatis Rhizoma, Leonuri Herba, Aconiti Lateralis Radix Praeparata (sliced), Cynomorii Caulis Carnosus and Dioscoreae Rhizoma.

Actions and Indications Warming the kidney, tonifying *qi*, activating blood and draining dampness. It is indicated for aching of the waist, fatigue, fear of cold and increase of nocturia due to chronic nephritis, depletion of kidney-*qi* and renal insufficiency.

肾舒冲剂

【处方】白花蛇舌草、大青叶、瞿麦、萹蓄、海金沙藤、淡竹叶、黄柏、茯苓、地黄、甘草。

【功能主治】清热解毒，利水通淋。用于尿道炎，膀胱炎，急、慢性肾盂肾炎。

Relieving Pyelonephritis Soluble Granules

Name of Chinese Phonetic Alphabet Shen Shu Chong Ji

Formula Hedyotis Diffusae Herba, Isatidis Folium, Dianthi Herba, Polygoni Avicularis Herba, Lygodii Caulis, Lophatheri Herba, Phellodendri Chinensis Cortex, Poria, Rehmanniae Radix and Glycyrrhizae Radix et Rhizoma.

Actions and Indications Clearing heat and detoxicating, inducing diuresis and relieving strangury. It is indicated for urethritis, cystitis, acute, chronic pyelonephritis.

明目地黄丸

【处方】熟地黄、山茱萸（制）、牡丹皮、山药、茯苓、泽泻、枸杞子、菊花、当归、白芍、蒺藜、石决明（煅）。

【功能主治】滋肾，养肝，明目。用于肝肾阴虚，目涩畏光，视物模糊，迎风流泪。

Chinese Fox-glove* Bolus for Improving Vision

Name of Chinese Phonetic Alphabet Ming Mu Di Huang Wan

Formula Rehmanniae Radix Praeparata, Corni Fructus (prepared), Moutan Cortex, Dioscoreae Rhizoma, Poria, Alismatis Rhizoma, Lycii Fructus, Chrysanthemi Flos, Angelicae Sinensis Radix, Paeoniae Radix Alba, Tribuli Fructus and Haliotidis Concha (calcined).

Actions and Indications Enriching the kidney and liver, improving vision. It is indicated for dry eyes, photophobia and overflow of tear induced by wind due to dual *yin*-deficiency of the liver and kidney.

* 地黄

明目蒺藜丸

【处方】黄连、川芎、白芷、蒺藜（盐水炙）、地黄、荆芥、旋覆花、菊花、薄荷、蔓荆子（微炒）、黄柏、连翘、密蒙花、防风、赤芍、栀子（姜水炙）、当归、甘草、决明子（炒）、黄芩、蝉蜕、石决明、木贼。

【功能主治】清热散风，明目退翳。用于上焦火盛引起的暴发火眼，云雾移睛，羞明，眼边赤烂，红肿痛痒，迎风流泪。

Caltrop* Pill for Improving Vision

Name of Chinese Phonetic Alphabet Ming Mu Ji Li Wan

Formula Coptidis Rhizoma, Chuanxiong Rhizoma, Angelicae Dahurica Radix, Tribuli Fructus (prepared with salt water), Rehmanniae Radix, Schizonepetae Herba, Inulae Flos, Chrysanthemi Flos, Menthae Haplocalycis Herba, Viticis Fructus (slightly fried), Phellodendri Chinensis Cortex, Forsythiae Fructus, Buddlejae Flos, Saposhnikoviae Radix, Paeoniae Radix Rubra, Gardeniae Fructus (prepared with ginger water), Angelicae Sinensis Radix, Glycyrrhizae Radix et Rhizoma, Cassiae Semen (fired), Scutellariae Radix, Cicadae Periostracum, Haliotidis Concha and Equiseti Hiemalis Herba.

Actions and Indications Clearing heat and dissipating wind, removing nebula to improve vision. It is used for sudden conjunctivitis, vitreous opacity, photophobia, blepharitis marginalis, pain, swelling and itching of the eyes and epiphora due to excess-fire of the upper energizer.

*蒺藜

明珠口服液

【处方】决明子、何首乌、珍珠母等。

【功能主治】滋补肝肾，养血和血，渗湿明目。用于肝肾阴虚之中心性浆液性视网膜病变，症见视力下降，视物变形。

Oral Liquid for Improving Vision

Name of Chinese Phonetic Alphabet Ming Zhu Kou Fu Ye

Formula Cassiae Semen, Polygoni Multiflori Radix, Margaritifera Concha, etc.

Actions and Indications Enriching the liver and kidney, nourishing and harmonizing blood to improve vision. It is indicated for central serous retinopathy due to dual *yin*-deficiency of the liver and kidney, and marked by hypopsia, metamorphopsia.

昆明山海棠片

【处方】本品为昆明山海棠加工制成的浸膏片。

【功能主治】祛风除湿，舒筋活络，清热解毒。用于类风湿性关节炎，红斑狼疮。

【注意】肾功能不全者慎用。

Glaucousback Threewingnut* Tablet for Relieving Rheumatoid Arthritis

Name of Chinese Phonetic Alphabet Kun Ming Shan Hai Tang Pian

Formula Tripterygii Hypoglauci Cortex.

Actions and Indications Dispelling wind and dampness, relaxing sinews and activating collaterals, clearing heat and detoxicating. It is indicated for rheumatoid arthritis, lupus erythematosus.

Warning It should be used carefully for cases with renal insufficiency.

*昆明山海棠

罗汉果玉竹冲剂

【处方】罗汉果 玉竹。

【功能主治】养阴润肺，止咳生津。用于肺燥咳嗽，咽喉干痛。

Grosvenor Siraitia* and Solomon's Seal** Soluble Granules

Name of Chinese Phonetic Alphabet Luo Han Guo Yu Zhu Chong Ji

Formula Siraitiae Fructus and Polygonati Odorati Rhizoma.

Actions and Indications Nourishing *yin*, moistening the lung, relieving cough, engendering fluid. It is used for cough and sore-throat due to lung-dryness.

*罗汉果 **玉竹

国公酒

【处方】本品为当归、川芎、独活、牛膝、佛手、玉竹、陈皮等药经加工制成的酒剂。

【功能主治】散风祛湿，舒筋活络。用于经络不和、风寒湿痹引起的手足麻木，半身不遂，口眼歪斜，腰腿酸痛，下肢痿软，行步无力。

【注意】孕妇忌服。

Guo Gong Medicated Wine

Name of Chinese Phonetic Alphabet Guo Gong Jiu

Formula Angelicae Sinensis Radix, Chuanxiong Rhizoma, Angelicae Pubescentis Radix, Achyranthis Bidentatae Radix, Citri Sarcodactylis Fructus, Polygonati Odorati Rhizoma, Citri Reticulatae Pericarpium, etc.

Actions and Indications Dissipating wind and dispelling dampness, relaxing sinews and activating collaterals. It is used for numbness of the hands and feet, hemiplegia, deviated eye and mouth, aching pain of the waist and legs and wilting of the lower limbs due to disharmony of meridian and collateral and attack of wind-cold-damp.

Warning It is contraindicated for pregnant women.

国产血竭胶囊

【处方】本品为国产血竭经加工制成的胶囊剂。

【功能主治】活血散瘀，定痛止血，敛疮生肌。用于跌打损伤，淤血作痛，妇女气血凝滞，外伤出血，脓疮久不收口。

【注意】孕妇忌服。

Dragon's Blood Palm* Capsule

Name of Chinese Phonetic Alphabet Guo Chan Xue Jie Jiao Nang

Formula Draconis Sanguis.

Actions and Indications Activating blood, dissipating stasis, alleviating pain, relieving hemorrhage, astringing sore and promoting tissue regeneration. It is used for injury due to fall and strike; stagnation of *qi* and blood in women, bleeding due to external injury; unhealed sore.

Warning It is contraindicated for pregnant women.

* 血竭

固本咳喘片

【处方】党参、白术（麸炒）、茯苓、麦冬、甘草（蜜炙）、五味子（醋制）、补骨脂（盐水炒）。

【功能主治】益气固表，健脾补肾。用于慢性支气管炎，肺气肿，支气管哮喘，支气管扩张。

Bronchitis-relieving Tablet

Name of Chinese Phonetic Alphabet Gu Ben Ke Chuan Pian

Formula Codonopsis Radix, Atractylodis Macrocephalae Rhizoma (fried with bran), Poria, Ophiopogonis Radix, Glycyrrhizae Radix et Rhizoma (prepared with honey), Schisandrae Chinensis Fructus (prepared with vinegar) and Psoraleae Fructus (fried with salt water).

Actions and Indications Replenishing *qi* and securing the superficies, fortifying the spleen and tonifying the kidney. It is indicated for chronic bronchitis, pulmonary emphysema, bronchial asthma and bronchiectasis.

固本统血冲剂

【处方】锁阳、菟丝子、肉桂、巴戟天、黄芪、山药、附子、枸杞子、党参、淫羊藿。

【功能主治】温肾健脾，填精益气。用于阳气虚损、血失固摄。症见畏寒肢冷，腰酸乏力，尿清便溏，皮下紫斑，其色淡暗，或其他出血。可用于具上述症候表现的轻型原发性血小板减少性紫癜。

Blood-controlling Soluble Granules

Name of Chinese Phonetic Alphabet Gu Ben Tong Xue Chong Ji

Formula Cynomorii Caulis Carnosus, Cuscutae Semen, Cinnamomi Cortex, Morindae Officinalis Radix, Astragali Radix, Dioscoreae Rhizoma, Aconiti

Lateralis Radix Praeparata, Lycii Fructus, Codonopsis Radix and Epimedii Folium.

Actions and Indications Warming the kidney, fortifying the spleen, tonifying *qi*. It is used for fear of cold, cold limbs, soreness of waist, fatigue, clear urine, sloppy stool, subcutaneous suggillation or bleeding, also used for primary thrombocytopenic purpura with the above mentioned symptoms.

固本益肠片

【处方】党参、黄芪、延胡索等。

【功能主治】健脾温肾，涩肠止泻。用于脾虚或脾肾阳虚所致慢性腹泻，症见慢性腹痛腹泻、大便清稀或有黏液，及黏液血便、食少腹胀、腰酸乏力、形寒肢冷、舌淡苔白、脉虚。

【注意】忌生冷、辛辣、油腻食物。湿热下痢非本方所宜。

Relieving Diarrhea Tablet

Name of Chinese Phonetic Alphabet Gu Ben Yi Chang Pian

Formula Codonopsis Radix, Astragali Radix, Corydalis Rhizoma, etc.

Actions and Indications Fortifying the spleen, warming the kidney, astringing the intestine and checking diarrhea. It is indicated for chronic diarrhea due to *yang*-deficiency of the spleen or kidney, and manifested as abdominal pain, chronic diarrhea, clear and loose stool or mucous stool, or mucous bloody stool, poor appetite, abdominal fullness, soreness of waist, fatigue, cold limbs, pale tongue with white fur, vacuous pulse.

Warning It is contraindicated for dysentery of damp-heat type；cold, uncooked, pungent and oily foods should be avoided.

固肾生发丸

【处方】熟地黄、枸杞子、羌活、何首乌、川芎、木瓜、女贞子、当归、桑椹、丹参、党参、黑芝麻。

【功能主治】固肾养血，益气祛风。用于斑秃、全秃、普秃及肝肾之症状性脱发。

Kidney-strengthening and hair-engendering Bolus

Name of Chinese Phonetic Alphabet Gu Shen Sheng Fa Wan

Formula Rehmanniae Radix Praeparata, Lycii Fructus, Notopterygii Rhizoma et Radix, Polygoni Multiflori Radix, Chuanxiong Rhizoma, Chaenomelis Fructus, Ligustri Lucidi Fructus, Angelicae Sinensis Radix, Mori Fructus, Salviae Miltiorrhizae Radix et Rhizoma, Codonopsis Radix and Sesami Semen Nigrum.

Actions and Indications Securing the kidney, tonifying *qi* and blood, dispelling wind. It is used for alopecia areata, total alopecia, alopecia universalis and symptomatic alopecia.

固肾定喘丸

【处方】熟地黄、附子（制）、牡丹皮、牛膝、砂仁、车前子、茯苓、肉桂、山药、益智（盐制）、泽泻、金樱子（肉）、补骨脂（盐制）。

【功能主治】温肾纳气，健脾利水。用于脾肾虚型及肺肾气虚型的慢性支气管炎，肺气肿，先天性哮喘，老人虚喘。

Relieving Congenital Asthma Pill

Name of Chinese Phonetic Alphabet Gu Shen Ding Chuan Wan

Formula Rehmanniae Radix Praeparata, Aconiti Lateralis Radix Praeparata, Moutan Cortex, Achyranthis Bidentatae Radix, Amomi Fructus, Plantaginis Semen, Poria, Cinnamomi Cortex, Dioscoreae Rhizoma, Alpiniae Oxyphyllae Fructus (prepared with salt), Alismatis Rhizoma, Rosae Laevigatae Fructus, Psoraleae Fructus (prepared with salt).

Actions and Indications Warming the kidney and improving inspiration, fortifying the spleen and inducing diuresis. It is indicated for chronic bronchitis, pulmonary emphysema, congenital asthma, deficiency-asthma of the aged, attributive to dual deficiency of the spleen and kidney, and dual *qi*-deficiency of the lung and kidney.

固经丸

【处方】黄柏（盐炒）、黄芩（酒炒）、椿皮（炒）、香附（醋制）、白芍（炒）、龟甲（制）。

【功能主治】滋阴清热，固经止带。用于阴虚血热，月经先期、量多、色紫黑，赤白带下。

Menstruation-securing Pill

Name of Chinese Phonetic Alphabet Gu Jing Wan

Formula Phellodendri Chinensis Cortex (fried with salt), Scutellariae Radix (fried with wine), Ailanthi Cortex (fried), Cyperi Rhizoma (prepared with vinegar), Paeoniae Radix Alba (fried) and Testudinis Carapax et Plastrum (prepared).

Actions and Indications Enriching *yin*, clearing heat, regulating menstruation and arresting leucorrhea. It is used for advanced menstruation, profuse menstruation, red and white vaginal discharge.

和中理脾丸

【处方】党参、白术（麸炒）、苍术（米泔炙）、茯苓、甘草、陈皮、法半夏、木香、砂仁、枳壳（去瓤麸炒）、厚朴（姜炙）、豆蔻、香附（醋炙）、广藿香、山楂、六神曲（麸炒）、麦芽（炒）、莱菔子（炒）。

【功能主治】理脾和胃。用于脾胃不和引起的胸膈痞闷，脘腹胀满，恶心呕吐，不思饮食，大便不调。

Spleen-regulating Bolus

Name of Chinese Phonetic Alphabet He Zhong Li Pi Wan

Formula Codonopsis Radix, Atractylodis Macrocephalae Rhizoma (fried with bran), Atractylodis Rhizoma (prepared with rice swilled water), Poria, Glycyrrhizae Radix et Rhizoma, Citri Reticulatae Pericarpium, Pinelliae Rhizoma Praeparatum, Aucklandiae Radix, Amomi Fructus, Aurantii Fructus (removed pulp and fried with bran), Magnoliae Officinalis Cortex (prepared with ginger), Amomi Fructus Rotundus, Cyperi Rhizoma (prepared with vinegar), Pogostemonis Herba, Crataegi Fructus, Medicata Massa Fermentata (fried with bran), Hordei Fructus Germinatus (fried) and Raphani Semen (fried).

Actions and Indications Regulating the spleen, harmonizing the stomach. It is used for hypochondriac stuffiness and depression, abdominal fullness, nausea, vomiting, anorexia and disorder of bowels movement due to disharmony of the spleen and stomach.

和胃片

【处方】蒲公英、洋金花、川芎、瓦楞子（煅）、郁金、赤芍、丹参、甘草、黄芩。

【功能主治】疏肝清热，凉血活血，祛瘀生新，和胃止痛。用于消化性溃疡及胃痛腹胀，嗳气反酸，恶心呕吐。

【注意】青光眼、外感初起的喘咳患者禁用；心脏病或高血压患者、肝肾功能不正常或体弱者以及孕妇慎用。

Harmonizing Stomach Tablet

Name of Chinese Phonetic Alphabet He Wei Pian

Formula Taraxaci Herba, Daturae Flos, Chuanxiong Rhizoma, Arcae Concha (calcined), Curcumae Radix, Paeoniae Radix Rubra, Salviae Miltiorrhizae Radix et Rhizoma, Glycyrrhizae Radix et Rhizoma and Scutellariae Radix.

Actions and Indications Soothing the liver, clearing heat, cooling and activating blood, dispelling stasis, promoting tissue regeneration, harmonizing the stomach, alleviating pain. It is indicated for peptic ulcer, stomachache, abdominal fullness, eructation, acid regurgitation, nausea and vomiting.

Warning It is contraindicated for glaucoma, initial stage of asthma and cough due to external contraction. It should be used cautiously for heart disease or hypentension, hepatic and renal dysfunction or physical debility and pregnant women.

和胃平肝丸

【处方】沉香、佛手、木香、檀香、砂仁、豆蔻、枳壳（麸炒）、厚朴（姜炙）、川楝子、延胡索（醋炙）、陈皮、片姜黄、白芍、茯苓。

【功能主治】舒气平肝，和胃止痛。用于肝胃不和，气郁结滞引起的两肋胀满，倒饱嘈杂，气逆作呕，胃脘刺痛，饮食无味。

Stomach-harmonizing and Liver-pacifying Bolus

Name of Chinese Phonetic Alphabet He Wei Ping Gan Wan

Formula Aquilariae Lignum Resinatum, Citri Sarcodactylis Fructus, Aucklandiae Radix, Santali Albi Lignum, Amomi Fructus, Amomi Fructus Rotundus, Aurantii Fructus (fried with bran), Magnoliae Officinalis Cortex (prepared with ginger), Toosendan Fructus, Corydalis Rhizoma (prepared with vinegar), Citri Reticulatae Pericarpium, Wenyujin Rhizoma Concisum, Paeoniae Radix Alba and Poria.

Actions and Indications Soothing *qi*, pacifying the liver, harmonizing the stomach, alleviating pain. It is used for hypochondriac fullness, gastric upset, vomiting due to *qi* counterflow; stabbing pain in stomach duct and poor appetite due to disharmony of the liver and stomach and stagnation of *qi*.

和络舒肝胶囊

【处方】白术（炒）、白芍、三棱、香附（制）、莪术、当归、木瓜、大黄、红花、鳖甲（炙）、桃仁、郁金、茵陈、海藻、昆布、玄参、地黄、熟地黄、虎杖、土鳖虫、柴胡、制何首乌、凌霄花、蜣螂、五灵脂、黑豆、半边莲。

【功能主治】疏肝理气，清化湿热，活血化瘀，滋养肝肾。用于慢性迁延性肝炎，慢性活动性肝炎及早期肝硬化。

【注意】孕妇慎用。

Relieving Hepatitis Capsule

Name of Chinese Phonetic Alphabet He Luo Shu Gan Jiao Nang

Formula Atractylodis Macrocephalae Rhizoma (fried), Paeoniae Radix Alba, Sparganii Rhizoma, Cyperi Rhizoma (prepared), Curcumae Rhizoma, Angelicae Sinensis Radix, Chaenomelis Fructus, Rhei Radix et Rhizoma, Carthami Flos, Trionycis Carapax (prepared), Persicae Semen, Curcumae Radix, Artemisiae Scopariae Herba, Sargassum, Larminariae et Eckloniae Thallus, Scorphulariae Radix, Rehmanniae Radix, Rehmanniae Radix Praeparata, Polygoni Cuspidati Rhizoma et Radix , Eupolyphaga seu Steleophaga, Bupleuri Radix, Polygoni Multiflori Radix Praeparata, Campsis Flos, Catharsius, Trogopterori Faeces, Sojae Semen Nigrum and Lobeliae Chinensis Herba.

Actions and Indications Soothing the liver, regulating *qi*, clearing damp-heat, activating blood, resolving stasis, nourishing the liver and kidney. It is indicated for chronic persistent hepatitis, chronic active hepatitis and early stage of cirrhosis.

Warning It is used cautiously for pregnant women.

知柏地黄浓缩丸

【处方】知母、黄柏、熟地黄、山茱萸（制）、牡丹皮、山药、茯苓、泽泻。

【功能主治】滋阴降火。用于阴虚火旺，潮热盗汗，口干咽痛，耳鸣遗精，小便短赤。

Pill of Concentrative Common Anemarrhena* Chinese Corktree** and Chinese Fox-glove***

Name of Chinese Phonetic Alphabet Zhi Bai Di Huang Nong Suo Wan

Formula Anemarrhenae Rhizoma, Phellodendri Chinensis Cortex, Rehmanniae Radix Praeparata, Corni Fructus (prepared), Moutan Cortex, Discoreae Rhizoma, Poria and Alismatis Rhizoma.

Actions and Indications Enriching *yin* and downbearing fire. It is indicated for tidal fever, night sweating, dry mouth, sore-throat, tinnitus, nocturnal emission and scanty and yellow urine due to *yin*-deficiency with effulgent fire.

* 知母 ** 黄柏 *** 地黄

制金柑丸

【处方】金橘、佛手、砂仁、肉桂、沉香、豆蔻、木香、延胡索（制）、梅花、郁金、香附（制）、青皮、橘络、紫苏梗、川楝子、白术、甘草、玫瑰花、香橼、小茴香、陈皮、枳壳、乌药、党参、白芍。

【功能主治】疏肝理气，和胃止痛。用于肝胃气痛，胸胁胀满，不思饮食。

Prepared Kumquat* Bolus

Name of Chinese Phonetic Alphabet Zhi Jin Gan Wan

Formula Fortunellae Fructus, Citri Sarcodactylis Fructus, Amomi Fructus, Cinnamomi Cortex, Aquilariae Lignum Resinatum, Amomi Fructus Rotundus, Aucklandiae Radix, Corydalis Rhizoma (prepared), Mume Flos, Curcumae Radix, Cyperi Rhizoma (prepared), Citri Reticulatae Pericarpium Viride, Citri Tangerinea Vascular Fascis, Perillae Caulis, Toosendan Fructus, Atractylodis Macrocephalae Rhizoma, Glycyrrhizae Radix et Rhizoma, Rosae Rugosae Flos, Citri Fructus, Foeniculi Fructus, Citri Reticulatae Pericarpium, Aurantii Fructus, Linderae Radix, Codonopsis Radix and Paeoniae Radix Alba.

Actions and Indications Soothing the liver, regulating *qi*, harmonizing the stomach, alleviating pain. It is used for pain due to dual *qi*-stagnation of the liver and stomach; fullness of hypochondrium and anorexia.

* 金橘

季德胜蛇药片

【处方】本品由七叶一枝花、蟾蜍皮、蜈蚣、地锦草等药，经加工制成的片剂。

【功能主治】清热，解毒，消肿止痛。用于毒蛇、毒虫咬伤。

Ji De Sheng Tablet for Poisonous Snake-bite

Name of Chinese Phonetic Alphabet Ji De Sheng She Yao Pian

Formula Paridis Rhizoma, Bufonis Cutis, Scolopendra, Euphorbiae Humifusae Herba, etc.

Actions and Indications Clearing heat and detoxicating, dispersing swelling, relieving pain. It is used for poisonous snake and pest bite.

乳宁颗粒

【处方】柴胡、当归、香附（醋制）、丹参等。

【功能主治】疏肝养血，理气解郁，用于乳腺增生病气滞证。对乳房两胁疼痛，乳房结节压痛，经前疼痛加重或月经不调。

Relieving Hyperplasia of Mammary Gland Granules

Name of Chinese Phonetic Alphabet Ru Ning Ke Li

Formula Bupleuri Radix, Angelicae Sinensis Radix, Cyperi Rhizoma (prepared with vinegar), Salviae Miltiorrhizae Radix et Rhizoma, etc.

Actions and Indications Soothing the liver, nourishing blood, regulating *qi*, releasing depression. It is used for hyperplasia of mammary gland, attributed to *qi*-stagnation syndrome. It also used for improving the symptoms of distending pain in breast, tenderness in mammary nodule, premenstrual pain in breast and irregular menstruation.

乳块消片

【处方】橘叶、丹参、皂角刺、地龙、川楝子、王不留行。

【功能主治】疏肝理气，活血化瘀，消散乳块。用于肝气郁结，气滞血瘀，乳腺增生，乳房胀痛。

【注意】孕妇忌服。

Relieving Hyperplasia of Mammary Gland and Mastalgia Tablet

Name of Chinese Phonetic Alphabet Ru Kuai Xiao Pain

Formula Citri Reticulatae Folium, Salviae Miltiorrhizae Radix et Rhizoma, Gleditsiae Spina, Pheretima, Toosendan Fructus and Vaccariae Semen.

Actions and Indications Soothing the liver, regulating *qi*, activating blood, resolving stasis, dissipating mammary mass. It is used for hyperplasia of mammary glands, fullness and pain of breast due to stagnation of liver-*qi* and blood-stasis.

Warning It is contraindicated for pregnant women.

乳泉冲剂

【处方】王不留行、穿山甲（炙）、天花粉、甘草（炙）、当归、漏芦。

【功能主治】通经，活血，下乳。用于产后乳少。

【注意】孕妇忌用。

Improving Puerperal Oligogalactia Soluble Granules

Name of Chinese Phonetic Alphabet Ru Quan Chong Ji

Formula Vaccariae Semen, Manis Squma (prepared), Trichosanthis Radix, Glycyrrhizae Radix et Rhizoma (prepared), Angelicae Sinensis Radix and Rhapontici Radix.

Actions and Indications Regulating menstruation, activating blood, promoting lactation. It is indicated for puerperal oligogalactia.

Warning It is contraindicated for pregnant women.

乳核散结片

【处方】当归、黄芪、光慈姑、漏芦、柴胡、郁金、昆布、海藻、淫羊藿、鹿衔草。

【功能主治】疏肝解郁，软坚散结，理气活血。用于治疗乳腺囊增生，乳痛症，乳腺纤维腺瘤和男性乳房发育。

Mastalgia-relieving Tablet

Name of Chinese Phonetic Alphabet Ru He San Jie Pian

Formula Angelicae Sinensis Radix, Astragali Radix, Tulipae Edulis Bulbus, Rhapontici Radix, Bupleuri Radix, Curcumae Radix, Laminariae et Eckloniae Thallus, Sargassum, Epimedii Folium and Pyrolae Herba.

Actions and Indications Soothing the liver, releasing depression, softening and dissipating mass, regulating *qi*, activating blood. It is indicated for cystic hyperplasia of breast, mastalgia, fibroadenoma of breast and mammary development in male.

乳疾灵冲剂

【处方】牡蛎、海藻、昆布、鸡血藤、淫羊藿、菟丝子、青皮、赤芍、丹参、柴胡、香附（醋炙）、王不留行（炒）。

【功能主治】舒肝解郁，散结消肿。用于乳腺增生症，属肝气郁结，痰瘀阻滞证候者，症见乳腺肿块，胀满疼痛。

【注意】孕妇忌服。

Relieving Hyperplasia of Mammary Gland Soluble Granules

Name of Chinese Phonetic Alphabet Ru Ji Ling Chong Ji

Formula Ostreae Concha, Sargassum, Larminariae et Eckloniae Thallus, Spatholobi Caulis, Epimedii Folium, Cuscutae Semen, Citri Reticulatae Pericarpium Viride, Paeoniae Radix Rubra, Salviae Miltiorrhizae Radix et Rhizoma, Bupleuri Radix, Cyperi Rhizoma (prepared with vinegar) and Vaccariae Semen (fried).

Actions and Indications Soothing the liver, releasing depression, dissipating mass, reducing swelling. It is used for hyperplasia of mammary gland, attributed to stagnation of liver-*qi* and retention of phlegm and manifested as mammary mass with swelling and pain.

Warning It is contraindicated for pregnant women.

乳康片

【处方】牡蛎、乳香、瓜蒌、海藻、黄芪、没药、天冬、夏枯草、三棱、玄参、白术、浙贝母、莪术、丹参、鸡内金（炒）。

【功能主治】疏肝解郁，理气止痛，活血破瘀，消积化痰，软坚散结，补气健脾。用于乳腺增生病。

【注意】孕妇慎服。

Hyperplasia of Mammary Gland Relieving Tablet

Name of Chinese Phonetic Alphabet Ru Kang Pian

Formula Ostreae Concha, Olibanum, Trichosanthis Fructus, Sargassum, Astragali Radix, Myrrha, Asparagi Radix, Prunellae Spica, Sparganii Rhizoma, Scrophulariae Radix, Atractylodis Macrocephalae Rhizoma, Fritillariae Thunbergii Bulbus, Curcumae Rhizoma, Salviae Miltiorrhizae Radix et Rhizoma and Galli Gigerii Endothelium Corneum (fried).

Actions and Indications Soothing the liver, releasing depression, regulating *qi* to alleviate pain, activating blood, resolving stasis, dispersing stagnation, resolving phlegm, dissipating mass, tonifying *qi*, fortifying the spleen. It is used for hyperplasia of mammary gland.

Warning It should be used cautiously for pregnant women.

乳增宁片

【处方】本品为艾叶、淫羊藿、天冬、柴胡等药经提取制成的片剂。

【功能主治】疏肝解郁，调理冲任。用于肝郁气滞、冲任失调引起的乳痛症及乳腺增生。

Relieving Mastalgia Tablet

Name of Chinese Phonetic Alphabet Ru Zeng Ning Pian

Formula Artemisiae Argyi Folium, Epimedii Folium, Asparagi Radix, Bupleuri Radix, etc.

Actions and Indications Soothing the liver, relieving depression, regulating the thoroughfare and conception vessels. It is indicated for mastalgia and hyperplasia of mammary glands due to stagnation of liver-*qi* and disharmony of the thoroughfare and conception vessels.

乳癖消片

【处方】鹿角、蒲公英、鸡血藤、三七、海藻、玄参、红花等。

【功能主治】软坚散结，活血消痈，清热解毒。用于乳癖结块，乳痈初起，乳腺囊性增生病及乳腺炎前期。

【注意】孕妇慎服。

Dissipating Breast Nodule Tablet

Name of Chinese Phonetic Alphabet Ru Pi Xiao Pian

Formula Cervi Cornu, Taraxaci Herba, Spatholobi Caulis, Notoginseng Radix et Rhizoma, Sargassum, Scrophulariae Radix, Carthami Flos, etc.

Actions and Indications Softening and dissipating mass, activating blood, clearing heat, detoxifying. It is used for breast nodule, initial stage of acute mastitis, cystic hyperplasia of breast and early stage of mastitis.

Warning It should be used cautiously for pregnant women.

金贝痰咳清颗粒

【处方】浙贝母、金银花、前胡、苦杏仁等。

【功能主治】清肺止咳，化痰平喘。用于痰热证所致的咳嗽、痰黄黏稠、喘息，以及慢性支气管炎急性发作见于上述症状者。

Honeysuckle Flower* and Thunberg Fritillary** Granule for Relieving Cough

Name of Chinese Phonetic Alphabet Jin Bei Tan Ke Qing Ke Li

Formula Fritillariae Thunbergii Bulbus, Lonicerae Japonicae Flos, Peucedani Radix, Armeniacae Semen Amarum, etc.

Actions and Indications Clearing lung-heat and relieving cough, resolving phlegm and calming dyspnea. It is indicated for cough with yellow, sticky and thick phlegm and dyspnea due to phlegm-heat syndrome; and also for acute attack of chronic bronchitis with the above mentioned symptoms.

*金银花 **川贝母

金水宝胶囊

【处方】本品为虫草菌粉经加工制成的胶囊剂。

【功能主治】补肾保肺，秘精益气。用于慢性支气管炎（久咳，盗汗，痰少或痰白而黏），高血脂症（身重乏力，头晕目眩，肢麻肢胀，胸脘气闷，或体胖痰多），性功能低下症及老年人腰膝酸软，神疲畏寒，属于肺肾两虚，精气不足者。

Treasure Capsule of Fungus Cordyceps

Name of Chinese Phonetic Alphabet Jin Shui Bao Jiao Nang

Formula Cordyceps (Fungus) Pulvis.

Actions and Indications Tonifying the kidney, lung and *qi*. It is indicated for chronic bronchitis marked by prolonged cough, night sweating, few phlegm or white sticky phlegm, for hyperlipemia marked by heavy body sensation, fatigue, dizziness, dizzy vision, numbness of extremities, chest distress or obesity with profuse phlegm; for hypofunction of sexual function and senile soreness and weakness of waist and knees, lassitude of spirit and fear of cold attributed to dual deficiency of the lung and kidney and insufficiency of *qi*.

金龙胶囊

【处方】鲜守宫、鲜金钱白花蛇、鲜蕲蛇。

【功能主治】破瘀结，解郁通络。用于原发性肝癌血瘀郁结证，症见右肋下积块，胸胁疼痛，神疲乏力，腹胀，纳差等。

【注意】服药期间出现过敏者，应及时停药。

Jin Long Capsule for Primary Liver Cancer

Name of Chinese Phonetic Alphabet Jin Long Jiao Nang

Formula Gekko Chinensis (fresh), Bungarus Parvus (fresh) and Agkistrodon (fresh).

Actions and Indications Expelling mass, releasing stagnation, activating collaterals. It is used for primary liver cancer marked by right inferior hypochondriac mass and pain, lassitude of spirit, hypodynamia, abdominal fullness, poor appetite.

Warning In case of allergic reaction, suspend the medication timely.

金龙舒胆颗粒

【处方】金钱草、龙胆、柴胡、黄芩、大黄、滑石、莪术、青皮。

【功能主治】清热利胆，舒肝理气。适用于湿热型及湿热兼气滞型的急、慢性胆囊炎。

【处方】孕妇禁服。

Christina Loosestrife* and Scabrous Gentian**Soluble Granules for Relieving Cholecystitis

Name of Chinese Phonetic Alphabet Jin Long Shu Dan Ke Li

Formula Lysimachiae Herba, Gentianae Radix et Rhizoma, Bupleuri Radix, Scutellariae Radix, Rhei Radix et Rhizoma, Talcum, Curcumae Rhizoma and

Citri Reticularae Pericarpium Viride.

Actions and Indications Clearing heat and draining bile, soothing the liver and regulating *qi*. It is indicated for acute and chronic cholecystitis due to damp-heat accompanied by *qi* stagnation.

Warning It is contraindicated for pregnant women.

* 金钱草 ** 龙胆

金刚藤糖浆

【处方】金刚藤。

【功能主治】清热解毒，消肿散结。用于附件炎和附件炎性包块及妇科多种炎症。

Chinese Greenbrier* Syrup

Name of Chinese Phonetic Alphabet Jin Gang Teng Tang Jiang

Formula Smilacis Bockii Rhizoma.

Actions and Indications Clearing heat and detoxicating, dispersing swelling and mass. It is indicated for annexitis, adnexal mass and inflammation of gynecology.

* 金刚藤

金花消痤丸

【处方】栀子（炒）、金银花、黄芩（炒）、黄连、桔梗、薄荷、黄柏、甘草、大黄（酒炙）。

【功能主治】清热泻火，解毒消肿。用于肺胃热盛所致的痤疮（粉刺），口舌生疮，胃火牙痛，咽喉肿痛，目赤，便秘，尿黄赤。

【注意】孕妇慎用。

Jin Hua Pill for Acne-eliminating

Name of Chinese Phonetic Alphabet Jin Hua Xiao Cuo Wan

Formula Gardeniae Fructus (fried), Lonicerae Japonicae Flos, Scutellariae Radix (fried), Coptidis Rhizoma, Platycodonis Radix, Menthae Haplocalycis Herba, Phellodendri Chinensis Cortex, Glycyrrhizae Radix et Rhizoma and Rhei Radix et Rhizoma (prepared with wine).

Actions and Indications Clearing heat and purging fire, detoxicating and dispersing swelling. It is used for acne, aphthae, toothache, sore-throat, conjunctival congestion, constipation and yellowish dark urine due to excessive heat in the lung and stomach.

Warning It should be used cautiously for pregnant women.

金芪降糖片

【处方】黄连、黄芪、金银花。

【功能主治】清热益气。主治气虚兼内热之消渴病，症见口渴喜饮，易饥多食，气短乏力；用于轻、中型非胰岛素依赖型糖尿病。

Hypoglycemic Tablet of Honeysuckle Flower* and Milkvetch**

Name of Chinese Phonetic Alphabet Jin Qi Jiang Tang Pian

Formula Coptidis Rhizoma, Astragali Radix and Lonicerae Japonicae Flos.

Actions and Indications Clearing heat, tonifying *qi*. It is indicated for wasting-thirst disease attributed to *qi*-deficiency with internal heat and manifested as thirst, polydipsia, polyphagia, shortness of breath and fatigue. And also used for mild and middle degree non-insulin-dependent diabetes.

* 金银花 ** 黄芪

金利油软胶囊

【处方】黑芝麻、麻黄、甘草、秦皮、柴胡、制草乌、沉香、秦艽、黄连、苦杏仁。

【功能主治】宣肺平喘，温肾纳气，利尿通淋。主治哮喘（慢性支气管哮喘）症见喘咳而痰多色白，胸憋气短，喘甚自汗者；癃闭（老年性前列腺增生），症见夜尿频急，排尿不畅，小腹坠胀，腰酸乏力，精神疲惫者。

Jinliyou Soft Capsule for Asthma

Name of Chinese Phonetic Alphabet Jin Li You Ruan Jiao Nang

Formula Sesami Semen Nigrum, Ephedrae Herba, Glycyrrhizae Radix et Rhizoma, Fraxini Cortex, Bupleuri Radix, Aconiti Kusnezoffii Radix Cocta, Aquilariae Lignum Resinatum, Gentianae Macrophyllae Radix, Coptidis Rhizoma and Armeniacae Semen Amarum.

Actions and Indications Diffusing the lung, pacifying dyspnea, warming the kidney, absorbing *qi*, inducing diuresis and relieving stranguria. It is mainly indicated for asthma (chronic bronchial asthma) manifested as dyspnea with profuse white sputum, chest distress and spontaneous sweating; also used for difficult urination (senile hyperplasia of prostate) manifested as frequent and urgent urination at night, bearing down fullness of lower abdomen, soreness of waist, fatigue and lassitude of spirit.

金佛止痛丸

【处方】白芍、延胡索、三七、郁金、佛手、姜黄、甘草。

【功能主治】行气止痛，舒肝和胃，祛瘀生新。用于胃脘气痛，经痛，消化道溃疡，慢性胃炎引起疼痛。

【注意】孕妇及月经过多者忌服。

Turmeric* and Finger Citron** Pill for Alleviating Pain

Name of Chinese Phonetic Alphabet Jin Fo Zhi Tong Wan

Formula Paeoniae Radix Alba, Corydalis Rhizoma, Notoginseng Radix et Rhizoma, Curcumae Radix, Citri Sarcodactylis Fructus, Curcumae Longae Rhizoma and Glycyrrhizae Radix et Rhizoma.

Actions and Indications Moving *qi*, alleviating pain, soothing the liver, harmonizing the stomach, dispelling stasis, promoting tissue regeneration. It is used for pain of stomach duct, dysmenorrhea, ulcer of digestive tract and pain due to chronic gastritis.

Warning It is contraindicated for pregnant women and cases with hypermenorrhea .

*郁金 **佛手

金鸡虎补丸

【处方】狗脊、牛大力、黑老虎根、骨碎补、大枣、鸡血藤、桑寄生（盐酒制）、金樱子（盐制）、千斤拔。

【功能主治】补气补血，舒筋活络，健肾固精。用于肾阳不足，水气凝滞引起的四肢麻痹，腰膝酸痛，夜尿频数，梦遗滑精。

Jin Ji Hu Emission-arresting Bolus

Name of Chinese Phonetic Alphabet Jin Ji Hu Bu Wan

Formula Cibotii Rhizoma, Millettae Speciosae Radix, Kadsurae Coccineae Radix, Drynariae Rhizoma, Jujubae Fructus, Spatholobi Caulis, Taxilli Herba (prepared with salt and wine), Rosae Laevigatae Fructus (prepared with salt) and Flemingiae Philippinensis Radix.

Actions and Indications Tonifying *qi* and blood, relaxing sinews and activating collaterals, fortifying the kidney to arrest emission. It is used for numbness of limbs, soreness and pain of waist and knees, frequent urination at night, oneirogmus and spermatorrhea due to insufficiency of kidney-*yang*.

金鸡胶囊

【处方】金樱根、鸡血藤、千斤拔、功劳木、两面针、穿心莲。

【功能主治】清热解毒，健脾除湿，通络活血。用于附件炎、子宫内膜炎、盆腔炎属湿热下注证者。

【注意】孕妇慎用。

Cherokee Rose Root* and Millettia** Capsule

Name of Chinese Phonetic Alphabet Jin Ji Jiao

Nang

Formula Rosae Laevigatae Radix, Spatholobi Caulis, Flemingiae Philippinensis Radix, Mahoniae Caulis, Zanthoxyli Radix and Andrographis Herba.

Actions and Indications Clearing heat and detoxicating, fortifying the spleen and dispelling dampness, dredging collaterals and activating blood. It is indicated for annexitis, endometritis and pelvic inflammation attributive to lower downward attack of damp-heat.

Warning It should be used carefully for pregnant women.

* 金樱根 ** 鸡血藤

金鸣片

【处方】本品为地黄、硼砂（煅）、玄参、牛黄、麦冬、冰片、丹参、薄荷脑、乌梅、珍珠粉、玄明粉等药经加工制成的片剂。

【功能主治】清热生津，利咽。用于慢性咽炎，慢性喉炎，咽喉肿痛，声哑失声，咽干，喉痒。

Jin Ming Tablet for Sore-throat

Name of Chinese Phonetic Alphabet Jin Ming Pian

Formula Rehmanniae Radix, Borax (calcined), Scrophularia Radix, Bovis Calculus, Ophiopogonis Radix, Borneolum Syntheticum, Salviae Miltiorrhizae Radix et Rhizoma, Menthol, Mume Fructus, Margaritae Pulvis, Natrii Sulfas Exsiccatus, etc.

Actions and Indications Clearing heat, engendering fluid, soothing the throat. It is used for chronic pharyngitis, chronic laryngitis, sore-throat, hoarseness, dry throat, throat itching.

金果饮糖浆

【处方】地黄、玄参、西青果、蝉蜕、麦冬、胖大海、南沙参、太子参、陈皮、薄荷油适量。

【功能主治】养阴生津，清热利咽，润肺。用于急慢性咽喉炎（喉痹），也可用于放疗引起的咽干不适。

Myrobalan* Syrup

Name of Chinese Phonetic Alphabet Jin Guo Yin Tang Jiang

Formula Rehmanniae Radix, Scrophulariae Radix, Chebulae Fructus Immaturus, Cicadae Periostracum, Ophiopogonis Radix, Sterculiae Lychnophorae Semen, Adenophorae Radix, Pseudostellariae Radix, Citri Reticulatae Pericarpium and Menthae Haplocalycis Oleum.

Actions and Indications Nourishing *yin*, engendering fluid, clearing heat, soothing the throat, moistening the lung. It is used for acute, chronic laryngopharyngitis, dry throat due to radiotherapy.

* 西青果

金泽冠心胶囊

【处方】泽泻、雪胆。

【功能主治】降血脂，增加心肌营养性血流量，降低心肌耗氧量。用于冠心病、心绞痛和高脂血症。

Oriental Waterplantain* Capsule for Coronary Heart Disease

Name of Chinese Phonetic Alphabet Jin Ze Guan Xin Jiao Nang

Formula Alismatis Rhizoma and Hemsleyae Radix.

Actions and Indications Decreasing blood-lipid, increasing nutritional volume of blood flow of myocardium, decreasing oxygen consumption of myocardium. It is indicated for coronary heart disease, angina pectoris and hyperlipemia.

* 泽泻

金荞麦片

【处方】本品为金荞麦浸膏片。

【功能主治】清热解毒，排脓祛瘀，祛痰止咳平喘。用于急、慢性气管炎，喘息型慢性气管炎，支气管哮喘及细菌性痢疾。

Dibotrys Buckwheat★ Tablet

Name of Chinese Phonetic Alphabet Jin Qiao Mai Pian

Formula Fagopyri Dibotryis Rhizoma (extract).

Actions and Indications Clearing heat and detoxicating, draining pus and eliminatinsg stasis, dispelling phlegm, relieving cough and dyspnea. It is used for acute, chronic bronchitis and asthmatic chronic tracheitis, bronchial asthma and bacillary dysentery.

* 金荞麦

金胆片

【处方】龙胆、金钱草、虎杖、猪胆膏。

【功能主治】利胆消炎。用于急、慢性胆囊炎，胆石症以及胆道感染。

【注意】孕妇慎用。

Christina Loosestrife★and Scabrous Gentian★★ Tablet for Cholecystitis

Name of Chinese Phonetic Alphabet Jin Dan Pian

Formula Gentianae Radix et Rhizoma, Lysimachiae Herba, Polygoni Cuspidati Rhizoma et Radix and Suillus Fel Extractum.

Actions and Indications Draining bile and antiphlogistic. It is indicated for acute or chronic cholecystitis, cholelithiasis and infection of biliary tract.

Warning It should be used carefully for pregnant women.

* 金钱草 ** 龙胆

金莲花润喉片

【处方】金莲花。

【功能主治】清热解毒，消肿止痛，利咽爽口。用于咽喉肿痛，牙龈肿胀，口舌生疮，上呼吸道感染、咽炎、扁桃体炎。

Trollius★ Tablet for Soothing Throat

Name of Chinese Phonetic Alphabet Jin Lian Hua Run Hou Pian

Formula Trollii Flos.

Actions and Indications Clearing heat and detoxicating, dispersing swelling and relieving pain, soothing the throat. It is indicated for sore-throat, gingivitis, aphthae and upper respiratory tract infection, pharyngitis, tonsillitis.

* 金莲花

金莲清热冲剂

【处方】金莲花、大青叶、生石膏、地黄、玄参、苦杏仁（炒）。

【功能主治】清热解毒，止咳祛痰。主治外感热证。症见高热、口渴、咽干、咽痛、咳嗽、痰稠，亦适用于流行性感冒、上呼吸道感染见有上述证候者。

【注意】虚寒泄泻不宜服用。

Trollius★ Soluble Granules

Name of Chinese Phonetic Alphabet Jin Lian Qing Re Chong Ji

Formula Trollii Flos, Isatidis Folium, Gypsum Fibrosum, Rehmanniae Radix, Scrophulariae Radix and Armeniacae Semen Amarum (fried).

Actions and Indications Clearing heat and detoxicating, relieving cough and dispelling phlegm. It is indicated for syndrome of heat with external contraction, manifested as high fever, thirst, dry throat, sore-throat, cough, thick phlegm, also used for influenza, upper respiratory tract infection with the above mentioned symptoms.

Warning It should be used cautiously for cases with deficiency-cold diarrhea.

* 金莲花

金匮肾气丸

【处方】肉桂、附子（制）、熟地黄、山茱萸

（制）、牡丹皮、山药、茯苓、泽泻。

【功能主治】温补肾阳，化气运水。用于肾虚水肿，腰膝酸软，小便不利，畏寒肢冷。

Jingui Bolus for Tonifying Kidney-*yang*

Name of Chinese Phonetic Alphabet Jin Kui Shen Qi Wan

Formula Cinnamomi Cortex, Aconiti Lateralis Radix Praeparata, Rehmanniae Radix Praeparata, Corni Fructus (prepared), Moutan Cortex, Dioscoreae Rhizoma, Poria and Alismatis Rhizoma.

Actions and Indications Warming and tonifying kidney-*yang*. It is used for soreness and cold of waist and knees, edema, oliguria or profuse urination, phlegm-fluid retention, dyspnea, cough and wasting-thirst due to insufficiency of kidney-*yang*.

金银花露

【处方】金银花。

【功能主治】清热解毒。用于暑热口渴，疮疖，小儿胎毒。

Honeysuckle Flower* Distillate

Name of Chinese Phonetic Alphabet Jin Yin Hua Lu

Formula Lonicerae Japonicae Flos.

Actions and Indications Clearing heat and detoxicating. It is used for thirst due to summer heat; sore and furuncle, fetal toxin.

* 金银花

金锁固精丸

【处方】沙苑子（炒）、芡实（蒸）、莲须、龙骨（煅）、牡蛎（煅）、莲子。

【功能主治】固肾涩精。用于肾虚不固，遗精滑泄，神疲乏力，四肢酸软，腰痛耳鸣。

Emission-arresting Bolus

Name of Chinese Phonetic Alphabet Jin Suo Gu Jing Wan

Formula Astragali Complanati Semen (fried) Euryales Semen (steamed), Nelumbinis Stamen, Draconis Os (calcined), Ostreae Concha (calcined) and Nelumbinis Semen.

Actions and Indications Securing the kidney and arresting emission. It is used for nocturnal emission, spermatorrhea, lassitude of spirit, fatigue, soreness and weakness of extremities, lumbago and tinnitus.

金嗓开音丸

【处方】金银花、连翘、玄参、板蓝根、赤芍、黄芩、桑叶、菊花、前胡、牛蒡子、泽泻、苦杏仁（去皮）、胖大海、蝉蜕、木蝴蝶、僵蚕（麸炒）。

【功能主治】清热解毒，疏风利咽。用于风热邪毒引起的咽喉肿痛，声音嘶哑，急性、亚急性咽炎及喉炎。

Throat-soothing and Hoarseness-relieving Pill

Name of Chinese Phonetic Alphabet Jin Sang Kai Yin Wan

Formula Lonicerae Japonicae Flos, Forsythiae Fructus, Scrophulariae Radix, Isatidis Radix, Paeoniae Radix Rubra, Scutellariae Radix, Mori Folium, Chrysanthemi Flos, Peucedani Radix, Arctii Fructus, Alismatis Rhizoma, Armeniacae Semen Amarum (removed seed coat), Sterculiae Lychnophorae Semen, Cicadae Periostracum, Oroxyli Semen and Bombyx Batryticatus (fried with bran).

Actions and Indications Clearing heat and detoxicating, dispersing wind and soothing the throat. It is indicated for sore-throat, hoarseness, acute, sub-acute pharyngitis, laryngitis.

金嗓利咽丸

【处方】茯苓、法半夏、枳实（炒）、青皮（炒）、胆南星、橘红、砂仁、豆蔻、槟榔、合欢皮、神曲（炒）、紫苏梗、生姜、蝉蜕、木蝴蝶、厚朴（制）。

【功能主治】燥湿化痰，舒肝理气。用于咽部不适，咽部异物感，声带肥厚属于痰湿内阻，肝郁气滞型者。

Honeyed Bolus for Soothing Throat

Name of Chinese Phonetic Alphabet Jin Sang Li Yan Wan

Formula Poria, Pinelliae Rhizoma Praeparatum, Aurantii Fructus Immaturus (fried), Citri Reticulatae Pericarpium Viride (fried), Arisaema cum Bile, Citri Exocarpium Rubrum, Amomi Fructus, Amomi Fructus Rotundus, Arecae Semen, Albiziae Cortex, Medicata Massa Fermentata (fried), Perillae Caulis, Zingiberis Rhizoma Recens, Cicadae Periostracum, Oroxyli Semen and Magnoliae Officinalis Cortex (prepared).

Actions and Indications Drying dampness, resolving phlegm, releasing liver-*qi*. It is used for feeling of foreign body in the throat, hypertrophy of vocal cord due to stagnation of phlegm-damp and liver-*qi*.

金嗓清音丸

【处方】玄参、地黄、麦冬、黄芩、牡丹皮、赤芍、川贝母、泽泻、薏苡仁（炒）、石斛、僵蚕（麸炒）、薄荷、胖大海、蝉蜕、木蝴蝶、甘草。

【功能主治】养阴清肺，化痰利咽。用于阴虚肺热而致的咽喉肿痛，慢性咽炎、喉炎。

Honeyed Bolus for Relieving Laryngopharyngitis

Name of Chinese Phonetic Alphabet Jin Sang Qing Yin Wan

Formula Scrophulariae Radix, Rehmanniae Radix, Ophiopogonis Radix, Scutellariae Radix, Moutan Cortex, Paeoniae Radix Rubra, Fritillariae Cirrhosae Bulbus, Alismatis Rhizoma, Coicis Semen (fried), Dendrobii Caulis, Bombyx Batryticatus (fried with bran), Menthae Haplocalycis Herba, Sterculiae Lychnophorae Semen, Cicadae Periostracum, Oroxyli Semen and Glycyrrhizae Radix et Rhizoma.

Actions and Indications Nourishing *yin*, clearing lung-heat, resolving phlegm, soothing the throat. It is used for sore-throat, chronic pharyngitis and chronic laryngitis.

金嗓散结丸

【处方】马勃、莪术（醋炒）、金银花、桃仁（去皮）、玄参、三棱（醋炒）、板蓝根、鸡内金（炒）、红花、丹参、麦冬、浙贝母、泽泻、木蝴蝶、蝉蜕、蒲公英。

【功能主治】清热解毒，活血化瘀，利湿化痰。用于热毒蓄结、气滞血瘀而形成的慢喉暗，声音嘶哑。

Aphonia-relieving Pill

Name of Chinese Phonetic Alphabet Jin Sang San Jie Wan

Formula Lasiosphaera seu Calvatia, Curcumae Rhizoma (fried with vinegar), Lonicerae Japonicae Flos, Persicae Semen (removed seed coat), Scrophulariae Radix, Sparganii Rhizoma (fried with vinegar), Isatidis Radix, Galli Gigerii Enthothelium Corneum (fired), Carthami Flos, Salviae Miltiorrhizae Radix et Rhizoma, Ophiopogonis Radix, Fritillariae Thunbergii Bulbus, Alismatis Rhizoma, Oroxyli Semen, Cicadae Periostracum and Taraxaci Herba.

Actions and Indications Clearing heat and detoxicating, activating blood and resolving stasis, draining dampness and resolving phlegm. It is used for chronic aphonia and hoarseness due to heat accumulation, *qi*-stagnation and blood-stasis.

金酸萍糖浆

【处方】阴行草、酸模、浮萍。

【功能主治】清热解毒，利湿退黄，有恢复肝功能、降低转氨酶的作用。用于急性黄疸型肝炎，慢性肝炎，重症肝炎。

Jin Suan Ping Syrup for Relieving Hepatitis

Name of Chinese Phonetic Alphabet Jin Suan Ping Tang Jiang

Formula Siphonostegiae Chinensis Herba, Rumicis Acetosae Radix and Spirodelae Herba.

Actions and Indications Clearing heat and detoxicating, draining dampness and relieving jaundice. It possesses the effect to recover hepatic function and decreasing transaminase. It is indicated for acute icteric hepatitis, chronic and severe hepatitis.

金樱子膏

【处方】金樱子。

【功能主治】补肾固精。用于肾虚所致遗精、遗尿、白带过多。

Thick Paste of Cherokee Rose* Fruit

Name of Chinese Phonetic Alphabet Jin Ying Zi Gao

Formula Rosae Laevigatae Fructus.

Actions and Indications Tonifying the kidney, arresting emission. It is used for nocturnal emission, enuresis and profuse white vaginal discharge due to deficiency of the kidney.

* 金樱子

狗皮膏

【处方】生川乌、生草乌、羌活、独活、青风藤、香加皮、防风、威灵仙、苍术、蛇床子、麻黄、高良姜、小茴香、肉桂、当归、赤芍、木瓜、苏木、大黄、松节油、续断、川芎、白芷、乳香、没药、冰片、樟脑、丁香。

【功能主治】祛风散寒，活血止痛。用于风寒湿邪气、气滞血瘀引起的四肢麻木，腰腿疼痛，筋脉拘挛，跌打损伤，闪腰岔气，脘腹冷痛，行经腹痛，湿寒带下。

【注意】外用，孕妇忌贴腰部、腹部。

Gou Pi Plaster for Traumatic Injury

Name of Chinese Phonetic Alphabet Gou Pi Gao

Formula Aconiti Radix (raw), Aconiti Kusnezoffii Radix (raw), Notopterygii Rhizoma et Radix, Angelicae Pubescentis Radix, Sinomenii Caulis, Periplocae Cortex, Saposhnikoviae Radix, Clematidis Radix et Rhizoma, Atractylodis Rhizoma, Cnidii Fructus, Ephedrae Herba, Alpiniae Officinarum Rhizoma, Foeniculi Fructus, Cinnamomi Cortex, Angelicae Sinensis Radix, Paeoniae Radix Rubra, Chaenomelis Fructus, Sappan Lignum, Rhei Radix et Rhizoma, Pini Lignum Nodi, Dipsaci Radix, Chuanxiong Rhizoma, Angelicae Dahuricae Radix, Olibanum, Myrrha, Borneolum Syntheticum, Camphora and Caryophylli Flos

Actions and Indications Dispelling wind and dissipating cold, activating blood to relieve pain. It is used for numbness of the limbs, pain of the waist and the legs, spasm of the sinews, traumatic injury, sudden lumbar sprain, cold pain of the stomach duct and abdomen, dysmenorrhea and vaginal discharge.

Warning It is for external use only and contraindicated for pregnant women to spread on the waist and abdominal regions.

肤阴洁液

【处方】苦豆草、岗松、黄柏等。

【功能主治】清热解毒，泻火燥湿，杀虫止痒。用于阴痒、带下，症见外阴阴道灼热瘙痒，阴道分泌物增多，黄稠而臭等症，以及滴虫性、霉菌性、非特异性阴道炎见上述证候者。

Cleaning Vagina Washings

Name of Chinese Phonetic Alphabet Fu Yin Jie Ye

Formula Astragali Melilotoidis Herba, Baeckeae Frutescentis Herba, Phellodendri Chinensis Cortex, etc.

Actions and Indications Clearing heat and detoxicating, purging fire and drying dampness, killing worms to relieve itching. It is indicated for pruritus vulvae, vaginal discharge, manifested as burning heat sensation and itching of vulva vagina, increase of vaginal secretion with yellow color, sticky and bad odor, and trichomonal vaginitis, colpomycosis and nonspecific vaginitis with the above mentioned symptoms.

肺宁冲剂

【处方】本品为返魂草制成的冲剂。

【功能主治】清热祛痰，镇咳平喘。用于肺内感染，慢性支气管炎，喘息性支气管炎，急性呼吸道感染。

Relieving Pulmonary Infection Soluble Granules

Name of Chinese Phonetic Alphabet Fei Ning Chong Ji

Formula Senecionis Cannabifolii Herba.

Actions and Indications Clearing heat and dispelling phlegm, settling cough and calming dyspnea. It is indicated for intrapulmonary infection, chronic bronchitis, asthmatic bronchitis, acute respiratory tract infection.

肿节风片

【处方】本品为肿节风浸膏片。

【功能主治】消肿散结、清热解毒。用于肺炎，阑尾炎，蜂窝织炎，大剂量用于肿瘤。

Tablet of Glabrous Sarcandra*

Name of Chinese Phonetic Alphabet Zhong Jie Feng Pian

Formula Sarcandrae Herba (extract).

Actions and Indications Dispersing swelling and mass, clearing heat and detoxicating. It is indicated for pneumonia, appendicitis, phlegmon and large dose for tumor.

*肿节风

肥儿丸

【处方】肉豆蔻（煨）、木香、六神曲（炒）、麦芽（炒）、胡黄连、槟榔、使君子。

【功能主治】健胃消积，驱虫。用于小儿消化不良，虫积腹痛，面黄肌瘦，食少腹胀泄泻。

Fortifying Stomach Pill for Children Dyspepsia

Name of Chinese Phonetic Alphabet Fei Er Wan

Formula Myristicae Semen (roasted), Aucklandiae Radix, Medicata Massa Fermentata (fried), Hordei Fructus Germinatus (fried), Picrorhizae Rhizoma, Arecae Semen and Quisqualis Semen.

Actions and Indications Fortifying the stomach and relieving stagnation, expelling worms. It is used for children dyspepsia, abdominal fullness due to intestinal worms, sallow complexion, emaciation, poor appetite, abdominal distention and diarrhea.

肥儿疳积颗粒

【处方】使君子（炒去壳）、莲子、芡实、牵牛子（炒）、茯苓、苍术（炒）、鸡内金（炒）、乌梅（炒）、车前子、薏苡仁（炒）、苦楝皮、槟榔（炒）、白芍（酒炙）、芜荑、蓼实子、山药（炒）、麦芽、蓝花参、雷丸（炒）、甘草、白术、百部。

【功能主治】健脾和胃，平肝杀虫。用于脾弱肝滞，面黄肌瘦，消化不良。

Relieving Children Malnutrition Granules

Name of Chinese Phonetic Alphabet Fei Er Gan Ji Ke Li

Formula Quisqualis Fructus (fried, removed shell), Nelumbinis Semen, Euryales Semen, Pharbitidis Semen (fried), Poria, Atractylodis Rhizoma (fried), Galli Gigerii Endothelium Corneum (fried), Mume Fructus (fried), Plantaginis Semen, Coicis Semen (fried), Meliae Cortex, Arecae Semen (fried), Paeoniae Radix Alba (perpaerd with wine), Ulmi Macrocarpae

Fructus, Polygoni Hydropiperis Fructus, Dioscoreae Rhizoma (fried), Hordei Fructus Germinatus, Wahlenbergiae Marginatae Herba, Omphalia (fried), Glycyrrhizae Radix et Rhizoma, Atractylodis Macrocephalae Rhizoma and Stemonae Radix.

Actions and Indications Fortifying the spleen and harmonizing the stomach, pacifying the liver and killing worms. It is used for sallow complexion, emaciation and dyspepsia due to hypofunction of the spleen and stagnation of liver-*qi*.

鱼腥草注射液

【处方】本品为鲜鱼腥草经加工制成的灭菌水溶液。

【功能主治】清热，解毒，利湿。用于痰热咳嗽，白带，尿路感染，痈疖。

Fishword* Injection

Name of Chinese Phonctic Alphabet Yu Xing Cao Zhu She Ye

Formula Houttuyniae Herba.

Actions and Indications Clearing heat and detoxicating, draining dampness. It is used for cough due to phlegm-heat; white vaginal discharge, urinary tract infection, carbuncle and furuncle.

* 鱼腥草

鱼鳔丸

【处方】鱼鳔（滑石烫）、熟地黄、泽泻、山药、茯苓、山茱萸（酒炙）、鹿角胶、鹿角霜、巴戟天（去心甘草炙）、肉苁蓉（酒炙）、枸杞子、菟丝子、沙苑子、五味子（醋炙）、覆盆子、车前子（盐炙）、莲须、赤石脂（煅醋淬）、地黄、地骨皮、石斛、天冬、麦冬、杜仲炭、牛膝、石菖蒲、远志（甘草炙）、柏子仁、酸枣仁（炒）、白术（麸炒）、当归、木香、花椒。

【功能主治】补肝肾、益精血。用于肝肾不足，气血两虚，症见腰膝酸软无力，头晕耳鸣，失眠健忘，梦遗滑精，阳痿早泄，骨蒸潮热。

Fish Swim-bladder* Pill

Name of Chinese Phonetic Alphabet Yu Biao Wan

Formula Piscis Colla (scalded by talc), Rehmanniae Radix Praeparata, Alismatis Rhizoma, Dioscoreae Rhizoma, Poria, Corni Fructus (prepared with wine), Cervi Cornus Colla, Cervi Cornu Degelatinatum, Morindae Officinalis Radix (removed core and prepared with licorice root), Cistanches Caulis Carnosus (prepared with wine), Lycii Fructus, Cuscutae Semen, Astragali Complanati Semen, Schisandrae Chinensis Fructus (prepared with vinegar), Rubi Fructus, Plantaginis Semen (prepared with salt), Nelumbinis Stamen, Halloysitum Rubrum (calcined and quenched by vinegar), Rehmanniae Radix, Lycii Cortex, Dendrobii Caulis, Asparagi Radix, Ophiopogonis Radix, Eucommiae Cortex Carbonisatus, Achyranthis Bidentatae Radix, Acori Tatarinowii Rhizoma, Polygalae Radix (prepared with licorice root), Platycodi Semen, Ziziphi Spinosae Semen (fried), Atractylodis Macrocephalae Rhizoma (fried with bran), Angelicae Sinensis Radix, Aucklandiae Radix and Zanthoxyli Pericarpium.

Actions and Indications Tonifying the liver and kidney, enriching essence and blood. It is used for soreness and weakness of waist and knees, dizziness, tinnitus, insomnia, amnesia, oneirogmus, spermatorrhea, impotence, ejaculatio praecox and tidal fever due to dual insufficiency of the liver and kidney, and dual deficiency of *qi* and blood.

* 鱼鳔

鱼鳞病片

【处方】白鲜皮、威灵仙、地黄、苍术、防风、蝉蜕、火麻仁、红花、桂枝、当归、川芎、甘草、苦参、麻黄、地肤子。

【功能主治】养血，祛风，通络。用于鱼鳞病。

【注意】孕妇忌服。

Ichthyosis-relieving Tablet

Name of Chinese Phonetic Alphabet Yu Lin

Bing Pian

Formula Dictamni Cortex, Clematidis Radix et Rhizoma, Rehmanniae Radix, Atractylodis Rhizoma, Saposhnikoviae Radix, Cicadae Periostracum, Cannabis Fructus, Carthami Flos, Cinnamomi Ramulus, Angelicae Sinensis Radix, Chuanxiong Rhizoma, Glycyrrhizae Radix et Rhizoma, Sophorae Flavescentis Radix, Ephedrae Herba and Kochiae Fructus.

Actions and Indications Nourishing blood, dispelling wind, dredging the collaterals. It is indicated for ichthyosis.

Warning It is contraindicated for pregnant women.

炙甘草合剂

【处方】甘草（蜜炙）、生姜、人参、地黄、桂枝、阿胶、麦冬、黑芝麻、大枣。

【功能主治】益气滋阴，通阳复脉。用于气虚血少，心动悸，脉结代。

Prepared Licorice* Mixture

Name of Chinese Phonetic Alphabet Zhi Gan Cao He Ji

Formula Glycyrrhizae Radix et Rhizoma Praeparata cum Melle, Zingiberis Rhizoma Recens, Ginseng Radix et Rhizoma, Rehmanniae Radix, Cinnamomi Ramulus, Asini Corii Colla, Ophiopogonis Radix, Sesami Semen Nigrum and Jujubae Fructus.

Actions and Indications Enriching *qi* and *yin*, unblocking *yang* and restoring normal pulse beat. It is used for fearful throbbing and bound and intermittent pulse due to deficiency of *qi* and blood.

* 甘草

周氏回生丸

【处方】五倍子、檀香、木香、沉香、丁香、甘草、千金子霜、红大戟（醋制）、山慈菇、六神曲（麸炒）、麝香、雄黄、冰片、朱砂。

【功能主治】祛暑散寒，解毒，化湿止痛。用于寒霍乱，干霍乱，痧胀。

【注意】孕妇忌服。

Zhous *Hui Sheng* Pill

Name of Chinese Phonetic Alphabet Zhou Shi Hui Sheng Wan

Formula Galla Chinensis, Santali Albi Lignum, Aucklandiae Radix, Aquilariae Lignum Resinatum, Caryophylli Flos, Glycyrrhizae Radix et Rhizoma, Euphorbiae Semen Pulveratum, Knoxiae Radix (prepared with vinegar), Cremastrae seu Pleiones Psedobulbus, Medicate Massa Fermentata (fried with bran), Moschus, Realgar, Borneolum Syntheticum and Cinnabaris.

Actions and Indications Dispelling summer-heat and dissipating cold, detoxicating, resolving dampness and relieving pain. It is indicated for acute diarrhea and vomiting, dry cholera morbus and exanthem syndrome.

Warning It is contraindicated for pregnant women.

京万红

【处方】地榆、地黄、当归、穿山甲、黄连、桃仁、白芷、木鳖子、棕榈、乳香、没药、半边莲、白蔹、黄柏、紫草、金银花、红花、大黄、苦参、五倍子、槐角、木瓜、苍术、罂粟壳、赤芍、黄芩、川芎、胡黄连、栀子、乌梅、冰片、血余炭、血竭、土鳖虫。

【功能主治】活血消肿，祛瘀止痛，解毒排脓，去腐生肌。用于水、火、电灼伤烫伤，疮疡肿痛，皮肤损伤，创面溃烂。

Jing Wan Hong Soft Plaster

Name of Chinese Phonetic Alphabet Jing Wan Hong

Formula Sanguisorbae Radix, Rehmanniae Radix, Angelicae Sinensis Radix, Manis Squma, Coptidis Rhizoma, Persicae Semen, Angelicae Dahuricae Radix, Momordicae Semen, Trachycarpi Petiolus, Olibanum, Myrrha, Lobelia Chinensis Herba, Ampelopsis Radix, Phellodendri Chinensis Cortex, Arnebiae Radix, Lonicerae Japonicae Flos, Carthami

Flos, Rhei Radix et Rhizoma, Sophorae Flavescentis Radix, Galla Chinensis, Sophorae Fructus, Chaenomelis Fructus, Atractylodis Rhizoma, Papaveris Pericarpium, Paeoniae Radix Rubra, Scutellariae Radix, Chuanxiong Rhizoma Picrorhizae Rhizoma, Gardeniae Fructus, Mume Fructus, Borneolum Syntheticum, Crinis Carbonisatus, Draconis Sanguis and Eupolyphaga seu Steleophaga.

Actions and Indications Activating blood, reducing swelling, dispelling stasis, alleviating pain, detoxifying, discharging pus, removing necrosis, promoting tissue regeneration. It is used for scald by water, fire of electricity, sore and ulcer of skin, dermal injury.

京万红痔疮膏

【处方】地榆、地黄、当归、桃仁、黄连、木鳖子、罂粟壳、血余炭、棕榈、半边莲、土鳖虫、穿山甲、白蔹、黄柏、紫草、金银花、红花、大黄、苦参、五倍子、槐角、木瓜、苍术、白芷、赤芍、黄芩、胡黄连、川芎、栀子、乌梅、冰片、血竭、乳香、没药。

【功能主治】清热解毒，化瘀止痛，收敛止血。用于初期内痔、肛裂、肛周炎、混合痔等。

Jing Wan Hong Ointment for Hemorrhoid

Name of Chinese Phonetic Alphabet Jing Wan Hong Zhi Chuang Gao

Formula Sanguisorbae Radix, Rehmanniae Radix, Angelicae Sinensis Radix, Persicae Semen, Coptidis Rhizoma, Momordicae Semen, Papaveris Pericarpium, Crinis Carbonisatus, Trachycarpi Petiolus, Lobeliae Chinensis Herba, Eupolyphaga seu Steleophaga, Manis Squama, Ampelopsis Radix, Phellodendri Chinensis Cortex, Arnebiae Radix, Lonicerae Japonicae Flos, Carthami Flos, Rhei Radix et Rhizoma, Sophorae Flavescentis Radix, Galla Chinensis, Sophorae Fructus, Chaenomelis Fructus, Atractylodis Rhizoma, Angelicae Dahuricae Radix, Paeoniae Radix Rubra, Scutellariae Radix, Picrorhizae Rhizoma, Chuanxiong Rhizoma, Gardeniae Fructus, Mume Fructus, Borneolum Syntheticum, Draconis Sanguis, Olibanum and Myrrha.

Actions and Indications Activating blood and dispersing swelling, dispelling stasis and alleviating pain, detoxicating and discharging pus, removing necrosis and promoting tissue regeneration. It is indicated for scald by boiling water, fire and electricity, swelling, painful sore and ulcer, skin injury, ulceration of wound.

京制咳嗽痰喘丸

【处方】前胡、白前、苦杏仁（去皮炒）、桑叶、麻黄、半夏曲（麸炒）、桔梗、川贝母、紫苏子（炒）、化橘红（盐炙）、紫菀、款冬花（蜜炙）、旋覆花、浮海石（煅）、马兜铃（蜜炙）、茯苓、甘草（蜜炙）、远志（炒焦）、石膏、细辛、五味子（醋炙）、桂枝、浙贝母、白芍（酒炙）、葶苈子、射干、百部（蜜炙）、薤白、黄芩、党参、大枣、煅蛤壳粉、青黛、罂粟壳（蜜炙）、生姜、枇杷叶。

【功能主治】散风清热，宣肺止咳，祛痰定喘。用于外感风邪，痰热阻肺，咳嗽痰盛，气促哮喘，喉中作痒，胸膈满闷，老年痰喘。

Jing Zhi Pill for Relieving Cough and Asthma

Name of Chinese Phonetic Alphabet Jing Zhi Ke Sou Tan Chuan Wan

Formula Peucedani Radix, Cynanchi Stauntonii Rhizoma et Radix, Armeniacae Semen Amarum (removed seed coat and fried), Mori Folium, Ephedrae Herba, Pinelliae Massa Fermentata (fried with bran), Platycodonis Radix, Fritillariae Cirrhosae Bulbus, Perillae Fructus (fried), Citri Grandis Exocarpium (prepared with salt), Asteris Radix et Rhizoma, Farfarae Flos (prepared with honey), Inulae Flos, Pumex (calcined), Aristolochiae Fructus (prepared with honey), Poria, Glycyrrhizae Radix et Rhizoma (prepared with honey), Polygalae Radix (fried), Gypsum Fibrosum, Asari Radix et Rhizoma, Schisandrae Chinensis Fructus (prepared with vinegar), Cinnamomi Ramulus, Fritillariae Thunbergii Bulbus, Paeoniae Radix Alba (prepared with wine), Lepidii Semen, Belamcandae Rhizoma, Stemonae Radix (prepared with honey), Allii Macrostemonis Bulbus, Scutellariae Radix, Codonopsis Radix, Jujubae Fructus, Meretricis Concha Praeparata

Pulvis, Indigo Naturalis, Papaveris Pericarpium (prepared with honey), Zingiberis Rhizoma Recens and Eriobotryae Folium.

Actions and Indications Dispersing wind and clearing heat, diffusing the lung and alleviating cough, dispelling phlegm and calming asthma. It is used for external contraction of wind pathogen and stagnation of phlegm-heat in the lung, marked by cough with profuse phlegm, shortness of breath and asthma, itching in the throat, chest distress, phlegm dyspnea of the aged.

夜宁糖浆

【处方】合欢皮、甘草、首乌藤、大枣、女贞子、灵芝、浮小麦。

【功能主治】安神，养心。用于神经衰弱，头晕失眠，血虚多梦。

Night Tranquility Syrup

Name of Chinese Phonetic Alphabet Ye Ning Tang Jiang

Formula Albiziae Cortex, Glycyrrhizae Radix et Rhizoma, Polygoni Multiflori Caulis, Jujubae Fructus, Ligustri Lucidi Fructus, Ganoderma and Tritici Aestivi Fructus Natantia.

Actions and Indications Tranquilizing the mind and nourishing the heart. It is used for neurasthenia, dizziness, insomnia, profuse dreaming.

河车大造丸

【处方】紫河车、熟地黄、天冬、麦冬、杜仲（盐炒）、牛膝（盐炒）、黄柏（盐炒）、龟甲（制）。

【功能主治】滋阴清热，补肾益肺。用于肺肾两亏，虚劳咳嗽，骨蒸潮热，盗汗遗精，腰膝酸软。

Human Placenta Bolus

Name of Chinese Phonetic Alphabet He Che Da Zao Wan

Formula Hominis Placenta, Rehmanniae Radix Praeparata, Asparagi Radix, Ophiopogonis Radix, Eucommiae Cortex (fried with salt), Achyranthis Bidentatae Radix (fried with salt), Phellodendri Chinensis Cortex (fried with salt) and Testudinis Carapax et Plastrum (prepared).

Actions and Indications Enriching *yin*, clearing heat, tonifying the kidney and lung. It is indicated for consumptive disease, cough, tidal fever, night sweating, nocturnal emission, soreness and weakness of waist and knees due to dual deficiency of the lung and kidney.

河车补丸

【处方】紫河车、人参、五味子（醋炙）、续断、牛膝、天冬、熟地黄、麦冬、陈皮、牡蛎、干姜、黄柏。

【功能主治】滋肾阴，补元气。用于肾阴不足，元气亏损引起的身体消瘦，精神疲倦，腰酸腿软，自汗盗汗。

【注意】阳虚者忌用。

Tonic Bolus of Human Placenta

Name of Chinese Phonetic Alphabet He Che Bu Wan

Formula Hominis Placenta, Ginseng Radix et Rhizoma, Schisandrae Chinensis Fructus (prepared with vinegar), Dipsaci Radix, Achyranthis Bidentatae Radix, Asparagi Radix, Rehmanniae Radix Praeparata, Ophiopogonis Radix, Citri Reticulatae Pericarpium, Ostreae Concha, Zingiberis Rhizoma and Phellodendri Chinensis Cortex.

Actions and Indications Enriching kidney-*yin*, tonifying source *qi*. It is indicated for emaciation, lassitude of spirit, soreness of waist and weakness of legs, spontaneous sweating and night sweating due to insufficiency and depletion of kidney-*yin* and source *qi*.

Warning It is contraindicated for cases with *yang*-deficiency.

泻肝安神丸

【处方】龙胆、黄芩、栀子（姜炙）、珍珠母、牡蛎、龙骨、柏子仁、酸枣仁（炒）、当归、地黄、麦冬、远志（去心甘草炙）、蒺藜（去刺盐炙）、茯苓、车前子（盐炙）、泽泻（盐炙）、甘草。

【功能主治】清肝泻火，重镇安神。用于失眠，心烦，惊悸及神经衰弱。

Tranquilizing Pill

Name of Chinese Phonetic Alphabet Xie Gan An Shen Wan

Formula Gentianae Radix et Rhizoma, Scutellariae Radix, Gardeniae Fructus (prepared with ginger), Margaritifera Concha, Ostreae Concha, Draconis Os, Platycladi Semen, Ziziphi Spinosae Semen (fried), Angelicae Sinensis Radix, Rehmanniae Radix, Ophiopogonis Radix, Polygalae Radix (removed core and prepared with licorice root), Tribuli Fructus (removed thorn and prepared with salt), Poria, Plantaginis Semen (prepared with salt), Alismatis Rhizoma (prepared with salt) and Glycyrrhizae Radix et Rhizoma.

Actions and Indications Clearing liver-fire, tranquilizing the mind. It is used for insomnia, vexation, fright, palpitation and neurasthenia.

泻痢消胶囊

【处方】黄连（酒炙）、苍术（炒）、白芍（酒炙）、木香、吴茱萸（盐炙）、厚朴（姜炙）、槟榔、茯苓、陈皮、泽泻、枳壳（炒）、甘草。

【功能主治】清热燥湿，行气止痛，化浊止痢。用于湿热泻痢，泄泻急迫，大便黄褐色或便脓血，肛门灼热，腹痛，里急后重，心烦，口渴，小便黄赤，舌质红，苔薄黄或黄腻，脉濡数。如急性肠炎，结肠炎，痢疾等见上述证候者。

Relieving Dysentery Capsule

Name of Chinese Phonetic Alphabet Xie Li Xiao Jiao Nang

Formula Coptidis Rhizoma (prepared with wine), Atractylodis Rhizoma (fried), Paeoniae Radix Alba (prepared with wine), Aucklandiae Radix, Euodiae Fructus (prepared with salt), Magnoliae Officinalis Cortex (prepared with ginger), Arecae Semen, Poria, Citri Reticulatae Pericarpium, Alismatis Rhizoma, Aurantii Fructus (fried) and Glycyrrhizae Radix et Rhizoma.

Actions and Indications Clearing heat and drying dampness, moving *qi* to alleviate pain, resolving turbid and relieving dysentery. It is indicated for dysentery due to damp-heat; urgent diarrhea, yellowish brown stool or stool containing pus and blood, scorching heat in the anus, abdominal pain, tenesmus, vexation, thirst, yellowish dark urine, red tongue, thin yellow fur or yellow greasy fur, rapid pulse, also for acute enteritis, colitis and dysentery with the above mentioned symptoms.

泌石通冲剂

【处方】槲叶干浸膏、滑石粉。

【功能主治】清热逐湿，行气化瘀。用于气滞血瘀型及湿热下注型肾结石或输尿管结石，适用于结石在 1.0cm 以下者。

【注意】出现胃脘不适、头晕、血压升高者应停药。孕妇慎用。

Relieving Renal Calculus Soluble Granules

Name of Chinese Phonetic Alphabet Mi Shi Tong Chong Ji

Formula Visci Folium Extractum and Talci Pulvis.

Actions and Indications Clearing heat and eliminating dampness, moving *qi* and resolving stasis. It is indicated for renal calculus or ureter stone due to *qi*-stagnation and blood-stasis and downward attack of damp-heat with the stone diameter lower than 1.0cm.

Warning In case of uncomfortable stomach, dizziness or raise of blood pressure, suspend medication immediately. It should be used carefully for pregnant women.

泽桂癃爽胶囊

【处方】泽兰、皂角刺、肉桂。

【功能主治】行瘀散结，化气利水。用于膀胱瘀阻型前列腺增生症。

【注意】宜饭后服用。

Shiny Bugleweed* and Cassia Bark** for Hyperplasia of Prostate Capsule

Name of Chinese Phonetic Alphabet Ze Gui Long Shuang Jiao Nang

Formula Lycopi Herba, Gleditsiae Spina and Cinnamomi Cortex.

Actions and Indications Removing stasis and dissipating mass, resolving *qi* and inducing diuresis. It is indicated for hyperplasia of prostate of obstructed bladder type.

Warning It should be taken after meal.

* 泽兰 ** 肉桂

治伤胶囊

【处方】本品为生关白附、防风、羌活、天南星、白芷经加工制成的胶囊。

【功能主治】祛风散结，消肿止痛。用于跌打损伤所致之外伤红肿，内伤胁痛。

【注意】孕妇忌服。

Relieving Traumatic Injury Capsule

Name of Chinese Phonetic Alphabet Zhi Shang Jiao Nang

Formula Aconiti Coreani Radix (fresh), Saposhnikoviae Radix, Notopterygii Rhizoma et Radix, Arisaematis Rhizoma and Angelicae Dahuricae Radix.

Actions and Indications Dispelling wind, dissipating mass, reducing swelling, alleviating pain. It is used for topical red and swelling due to traumatic injury; hypochondriac pain due to internal injury.

Warning It is contraindicated for pregnant women.

治红丸

【处方】陈皮、黄芩、百合、铁树叶、石斛、地黄、京墨、关木通、橘络、甘草、大蓟、浙贝母、鲜荷叶、荷叶（炭）、棕榈炭、牡丹皮、侧柏叶（炭）、地黄（炭）。

【功能主治】清热，凉血，止血。用于吐血，便血，咳嗽痰中带血。

Hematemesis-relieving Bolus

Name of Chinese Phonetic Alphabet Zhi Hong Wan

Formula Citri Reticulatae Pericarpium, Scutellariae Radix, Lilii Bulbus, Cordylines Fruticosae Folium, Dendrobii Caulis, Rehmanniae Radix, Chinese Ink, Aristolochiae Manshuriensis Caulis, Citri Tangerinea Vascular Fascis, Glycyrrhizae Radix et Rhizoma, Cirsii Japonici Herba, Fritillariae Thunbergii Bulbus, Nelumbinis Folium (fresh), Nelumbinis Folium (carbonated), Trachycarpi Petiolus Carbonisatus, Moutan Cortex, Platycladi Cacumen (carbonated) and Rehmanniae Radix (carbonated).

Actions and Indications Clearing heat, cooling blood, relieving bleeding. It is used for hematemesis, hematochezia, cough with blood-stained phlegm.

治糜灵栓

【处方】黄柏、苦参、儿茶、枯矾、冰片。

【功能主治】清热燥湿，解毒消炎，祛腐生肌。用于子宫颈糜烂，感染性阴道炎，滴虫性阴道炎。

Relieving Cervical Erosion Suppository

Name of Chinese Phonetic Alphabet Zhi Mi Ling Shuan

Formula Phellodendri Chinensis Cortex, Sophorae Flavescentis Radix, Catechu, Alumen Usta and Borneolum Syntheticum.

Actions and Indications Clearing heat and drying dampness, detoxicating and antiphlogistic, removing necrosis and promoting tissue regeneration. It is indicated for cervical erosion, infective and trichomonal vaginitis.

宝咳宁冲剂

【处方】紫苏叶、桑叶、前胡、浙贝母、麻黄、桔梗、天南星（炙）、陈皮、苦杏仁（去皮炒）、黄芩、青黛、天花粉、枳壳（去瓤麸炒）、山楂（炒）、甘草、牛黄。

【功能主治】清热解表，止嗽化痰。用于小儿感冒风寒内热停食引起的头痛身热，咳嗽痰盛，气促作喘，咽喉肿痛，烦躁不安。

Cough-relieving Soluble Granules for Children

Name of Chinese Phonetic Alphabet Bao Ke Ning Chong Ji

Formula Perillae Folium, Mori Folium, Peucedani Radix, Fritillariae Thunbergii Bulbus, Ephedrae Herba, Platycodonis Radix, Arisaematis Rhizoma (prepared), Citri Reticulatae Pericarpium, Armeniacae Semen Amarum (removed seed coat and fried), Scutellariae Radix, Indigo Naturalis, Trichosanthis Radix, Aurantii Fructus (removed pulp and fried with bran), Crataegi Fructus (fried), Glycyrrhizae Radix et Rhizoma and Bovis Calculus.

Actions and Indications Clearing heat and releasing the exterior, relieving cough and resolving phlegm. It is indicated for common cold (wind-cold) type of children and retention of food, marked by headache, generalized fever, productive cough, shortness of breath, sore-throat, vexation.

定坤丸

【处方】西洋参、白术、茯苓、熟地黄、当归、白芍、川芎、黄芪、阿胶、五味子（醋炙）、鹿茸（去毛）、肉桂、艾叶（炒炭）、杜仲（炒炭）、续断、佛手、陈皮、厚朴（姜炙）、柴胡、香附（醋炙）、延胡索（醋炙）、牡丹皮、琥珀、龟甲（沙烫醋淬）、地黄、麦冬、黄芩。

【功能主治】补气养血，舒郁调经，用于冲任虚损，气血两亏，身体瘦弱，月经不调，经期紊乱，行经腹痛，崩漏不止，腰酸腿软。

【注意】孕妇忌服。

Ding Kun Honeyed Pill

Name of Chinese Phonetic Alphabet Ding Kun Wan

Formula Panacis Quinquefolii Radix, Atractylodis Macrocephalae Rhizoma, Poria, Rehmanniae Radix Praeparata, Angelicae Sinensis Radix, Paeoniae Radix Alba, Chuanxiong Rhizoma, Astragali Radix, Asini Corii Colla, Schisandrae Chinensis Fructus (prepared with vinegar), Cervi Cornu Pantotrichum (removed hair), Cinnamomi Cortex, Artemisiae Argyi Folium (carbonated), Eucommiae Cortex (carbonated), Dipsaci Radix, Citri Sarcodactylis Fructus, Citri Reticulatae Pericarpium, Magnoliae Officinalis Cortex (prepared with ginger), Bupleuri Radix, Cyperi Rhizoma (prepared with vinegar), Corydalis Rhizoma (prepared with vinegar), Moutan Cortex, Succinum, Testudinis Carapax et Plastrum (scalded by heated soil and quenched by vinegar), Rehmanniae Radix, Ophiopogonis Radix and Scutellariae Radix.

Actions and Indications Tonifying *qi* and nourishing blood, regulating menstruation. It is indicated for emaciation, irregular menstruation, dysmenorrhea, metrorrhagia and metrostaxis, soreness of the waist and weakness of the legs due to depletion of thoroughfare and the conception vessels and dual deficiency of *qi* and blood.

Warning It is contraindicated for pregnant women.

定喘膏

【处方】血余炭、洋葱头、附子、生川乌、天南星、干姜。

【功能主治】止咳定喘。用于气促喘息，冬季加重，胸膈满闷，咳嗽痰盛。

Dyspnea-relieving Plaster

Name of Chinese Phonetic Alphabet Ding Chuan Gao

Formula Crinis Carbonisatus, Allii Cepae Bulbus, Aconiti Lateralis Radix Praeparata, Aconiti Radix (raw),

Arisaematis Rhizoma and Zingiberis Rhizoma.

Actions and Indications Relieving cough and calming dyspnea. It is indicated for dyspnea that is more severe in winter, chest distress, cough with profuse phlegm.

定搐化风丸

【处方】全蝎、僵蚕（麸炒）、蝉蜕、防风、羌活、麻黄、桔梗、半夏（制）、黄连、大黄、甘草、人工牛黄、朱砂、麝香、冰片。

【功能主治】清热镇惊，散风化痰。用于小儿脏腑积热，关窍闭塞引起的急热惊风，痰涎壅盛，昏睡，神志不清，牙关紧闭，四肢抽搐，颈项强直，二目直视。

Infant Convulsion Relieving Pill

Name of Chinese Phonetic Alphabet Ding Chu Hua Feng Wan

Formula Scorpio, Bombyx Batryticatus(fried with bran), Cicadae Periostracum, Saposhnikoviae Radix, Notopterygii Rhizoma et Radix, Radix Ephedrae, Platycodonis Radix, Pinelliae Rhizoma (prepared), Coptidis Rhizoma, Rhei Radix et Rhizoma, Glycyrrhizae Radix et Rhizoma, Bovis Calculus Artifactus, Cinnabaris, Moschus and Borneolum Syntheticum.

Actions and Indications Clearing heat, settling fright, dissipating wind and resolving phlegm. It is indicated for acute convulsion of heat type, obstruction of phlegm, unconsciousness, lockjaw, spasm of limbs, neck rigidity and orthophoria due to accumulation of heat in the viscera of infant and blockade of orifices.

降气定喘丸

【处方】麻黄、葶苈子、紫苏子、白皮、芥子、陈皮。

【功能主治】降气定喘，除痰止咳。用于慢性支气管炎，支气管哮喘，咳嗽气促。

Relieving Bronchitis and Asthma Pill

Name of Chinese Phonetic Alphabet Jiang Qi Ding Chuan Wan

Formula Ephedrae Herba, Lepidii Semen, Perillae Fructus, Euonymi Tengyuehensi Cortex, Sinapis Semen and Citri Reticulatae Pericarpium.

Actions and Indications Directing *qi* downward and calming dyspnea, dispelling phlegm and relieving cough. It is indicated for chronic bronchitis, bronchial asthma, cough and shortness of breath.

降压袋泡茶

【处方】夏枯草、决明子、茺蔚子、钩藤、黄芩、茶叶。

【功能主治】清热泻火，平肝明目。用于高血压病属肝火亢盛的头痛、眩晕。

Hypertension-relieving Tea

Name of Chinese Phonetic Alphabet Jiang Ya Dai Pao Cha

Formula Prunellae Spica, Cassiae Semen, Leonuri Fructus, Uncariae Ramulus cum Uncis, Scutellariae Radix and Camelliae Sinensis Folium Gemmae.

Actions and Indications Clearing heat, purging fire, pacifying the liver, improving vision. It is used for hypertension due to hyperactivity of liver-fire and marked by headache, vertigo.

降脂灵片

【处方】制何首乌、枸杞子、黄精、山楂、决明子。

【功能主治】补肝益肾，养血，明目，降脂。用于肝肾阴虚，头晕，目昏，须发早白，高血脂症。

Decreasing Blood Lipid Tablet

Name of Chinese Phonetic Alphabet Jiang Zhi Ling Pian

Formula Polygoni Multiflori Radix Praeparata,

Lycii Fructus, Polygonati Rhizoma, Crataegi Fructus and Cassiae Semen.

Actions and Indications Tonifying the liver and kidney, nourishing blood, improving vision and decreasing blood lipid. It is indicated for dizziness, blurred vision premature graying of beard and hair, and hyperlipemia due to dual *yin*-deficiency of the liver and kidney.

降糖甲片

【处方】黄芪、黄精（酒炙）、地黄、太子参、天花粉。

【功能主治】补中益气，养阴生津。用于气阴两虚型消渴症（非胰岛素依赖型糖尿病）。

Hypoglycemic Tablet A

Name of Chinese Phonetic Alphabet Jiang Tang Jia Pian

Formula Astragali Radix, Polygonati Rhizoma (prepared with wine), Rehmanniac Radix, Pseudostellariae Radix and Trichosanthis Radix.

Actions and Indications Tonifying middle energizer and *qi*, nourishing *yin* to engender fluid. It is indicated for wasting-thirst (non-insulin-dependent diabetes) attributed to dual deficiency of *qi* and *yin*.

降糖舒胶囊

【处方】熟地黄、枸杞子、葛根、人参、黄芪、刺五加等。

【功能主治】滋阴补肾，生津止渴。用于糖尿病及糖尿病引起的全身综合征。

【注意】忌食辛辣。

Downbearing Blood Sugar Capsule

Name of Chinese Phonetic Alphabet Jiang Tang Shu Jiao Nang

Formula Rehmanniae Radix Praeparata, Lycii Fructus, Puerariae Lobatae Radix, Ginseng Radix et Rhizoma, Astragali Radix, Acanthopanacis Senticosi Radix et Rhizoma seu Caulis, etc.

Actions and Indications Enriching kidney-*yin*, engendering fluid and quenching thirst. It is indicated for diabetes and general syndrome induced by diabetes.

Warning Pungent foods are prohibited.

参贝北瓜膏

【处方】北瓜清膏、党参、浙贝母、南沙参、干姜。

【功能主治】平喘化痰，润肺止咳，益气。用于哮喘气急，肺虚咳嗽，痰多。

Bellflower* Thunberg Fritillary** and Pumpkin*** Soft Extract

Name of Chinese Phonetic Alphabet Shen Bei Bei Gua Gao

Formula Cucurbitae Kintogae Extractum, Codonopsis Radix, Fritillariae Thunbergii Bulbus, Adenophorae Radix and Zingiberis Rhizoma.

Actions and Indications Calming dyspnea and resolving phlegm, moistening the lung and relieving cough, replenishing *qi*. It is indicated for asthma and dyspnea, cough with profuse phlegm due to lung-deficiency.

* 党参 ** 浙贝母 *** 北瓜

参芍片

【处方】本品为白芍、人参茎叶皂苷等经加工制成的片剂。

【功能主治】活血化瘀，益气止痛。适用于气虚血瘀所致的胸闷、胸痛、心悸、气短。

【注意】妇女经期及孕妇慎用。

Ginseng* and White Peony** Tablet

Name of Chinese Phonetic Alphabet Shen Shao Pian

Formula Paeoniae Radix Alba, Ginseng Caulis et Folium (saponin), etc.

Actions and Indications Activating blood, resolving stasis, tonifying *qi*, alleviating pain. It is used for chest distress, chest pain, palpitation and shortness of breath due to *qi*-deficiency and blood-stasis.

Warning It should be used cautiously for women during menstrual period, and pregnant women.

* 人参 ** 白芍

参麦注射液

【处方】红参、麦冬。

【功能主治】益气固脱，养阴生津，生脉。用于治疗气阴两虚型之休克、冠心病、病毒性心肌炎、慢性肺心病、粒细胞减少症。能提高肿瘤病人的免疫功能，并能减少化疗药物所引起的毒副反应。

Ginseng* and Lily-turf** Injection

Name of Chinese Phonetic Alphabet Shen Mai Zhu She Ye

Formula Ginseng Radix et Rhizoma Rubra and Ophiopogonis Radix.

Actions and Indications Tonifying *qi* to arrest collapse, nourishing *yin* to engender fluid, restoring normal pulse beat. It is indicated for shock, coronary heart disease, viral myocarditis, chronic cor pulmonale and granulocytopenia due to dual deficiency of *qi* and *yin*. Increasing the immunologic funcion and reducing the toxic and side effects of chemotherapy treatment.

* 人参 ** 麦冬

参芪五味子片

【处方】五味子、党参、黄芪、酸枣仁（炒）。

【功能主治】健脾益气，宁心安神。用于心悸气短，动则气喘易汗，少寐多梦，倦怠乏力，健忘。

Bellflower* Milkvetch** and Five-flavor-fruit*** Pill

Name of Chinese Phonetic Alphabet Shen Qi Wu Wei Zi Pian

Formula Schisandrae Chinensis Fructus, Codonopsis Radix, Astragali Radix and Ziziphi Spinosae Semen (fried).

Actions and Indications Fortifying the spleen, tonifying *qi*, tranquilizing the mind. It is indicated for palpitation, shortness of breath, dyspnea, hidrosis, profuse dreaming, tiredness, fatigue and amnesia.

* 党参 ** 黄芪 *** 五味子

参芪降糖片

【处方】本品为人参茎叶皂苷、五味子、黄芪、山药、地黄、枸杞子等经加工制成的片剂。

【功能主治】益气养阴，滋脾补肾。主治消渴症，用于Ⅱ型糖尿病。

【注意】有实热者禁用。

Hypoglycemic Tablet of Ginseng* and Milkvetch**

Name of Chinese Phonetic Alphabet Shen Qi Jiang Tang Pian

Formula Saponin from Ginseng Caulis et Folium, Schisandrae Chinensis Fructus, Astragali Radix, Dioscoreae Rhizoma, Rehmanniae Radix, Lycii Fructus, etc.

Actions and Indications Tonifying *qi* and nourishing *yin*, enriching the spleen and kidney. It is indicated for wasting-thirst, type Ⅱ diabetes.

Warning It is contraindicated for cases with excess heat.

* 人参 ** 黄芪

参芪糖浆

【处方】党参、黄芪。

【功能主治】补气扶正。用于体弱气虚，四肢无力。

Syrup of Bellflower* and Milkveteh**

Name of Chinese Phonetic Alphabet Shen Qi Tang Jiang

Formula Codonopsis Radix and Astragali Radix.

Actions and Indications Tonifying *qi* and reinforcing the healthy *qi*. It is used for physical debility and *qi*-deficiency, weakness of extremities.

* 党参 ** 黄芪

参苏丸

【处方】党参、紫苏叶、葛根、前胡、茯苓、半夏（制）、陈皮、枳壳（炒）、桔梗、甘草、木香。

【功能主治】疏风散寒，祛痰止咳。用于体弱感受风寒，恶寒发热，头痛鼻塞，咳嗽痰多，胸闷呕逆。

Bellflower* and Purple Perilla Leaf** Pill

Name of Chinese Phonetic Alphabet Shen Su Wan

Formula Codonopsis Radix, Perillae Folium, Puerariae Lobatae Radix, Peucedani Radix, Poria, Pinelliae Rhizoma (prepared), Citri Reticulatae Pericarpium, Aurantii Fructus (fried), Platycodonis Radix, Glycyrrhizae Radix et Rhizoma and Aucklandiae Radix.

Actions and Indications Dispersing wind and cold, dispelling phlegm and relieving cough. It is used for cases with the manifestations of aversion to cold, fever, headache, nasal congestion, productive cough, chest distress and vomiting due to general debility and attack of wind-cold.

* 党参 ** 紫苏叶

参附注射液

【处方】红参、附子（制）。

【功能主治】回阳救逆，益气固脱。主要用于阳气暴脱的厥脱症（感染性、失血性休克等）；也可用于阳虚（气虚）所致的惊悸、怔忡、喘咳、胃疼、泄泻。

Ginseng* and Szechuan Aconite** Injection

Name of Chinese Phonetic Alphabet Shen Fu Zhu She Ye

Formula Ginseng Radix et Rhizoma Rubra and Aconiti Lateralis Radix Praeparata (sliced).

Actions and Indications Restoring *yang* to save from collapse, tonifying *qi* to relieve collapse. It is mainly used for syndrome of syncope due to sudden collapse of *yang* (septic shock, hemorrhagic shock); and it is also used for convulsive palpitation, fearful throbbing, asthmatic cough, stomachache and diarrhea due to sudden loss *yang-qi*.

* 人参 ** 附子

参附强心丸

【处方】本品为人参、附子（制）、桑白皮、猪苓、葶苈子、大黄等制成的丸剂。

【功能主治】益气助阳，强心利水。用于慢性心力衰竭而引起的心悸、气短、胸闷喘促、面肢浮肿等症，属于心肾阳衰者。

【注意】忌服大量钠盐。

Cardiotonic Pill of Ginseng* and Szechuan Aconite**

Name of Chinese Phonetic Alphabet Shen Fu Qiang Xin Wan

Formula Ginseng Radix et Rhizoma, Aconiti Lateralis Radix Praeparata, Mori Cortex, Polyporus, Lepidii Semen, Rhei Radix et Rhizoma, etc.

Actions and Indications Tonifying *qi*, supporting *yang*, strengthening the heart and inducing diuresis. It is indicated for palpitation, shortness of breath, chest distress and edema of face and limbs due to chronic heart failure and dual *yang*-declination of the heart and kidney.

Warning Administration large amount of sodium salt is prohibited.

* 人参 ** 附子

参苓白术散

【处方】人参、茯苓、白术（炒）、山药、白扁豆（炒）、莲子、薏苡仁（炒）、砂仁、桔梗、甘草。

【功能主治】补脾胃，益肺气。用于脾胃虚弱，食少便溏，气短咳嗽，肢倦乏力。

Ginseng* India Bread** and Largehead Atractylodes*** Powder

Name of Chinese Phonetic Alphabet Shen Ling Bai Shu San

Formula Ginseng Radix et Rhizoma, Poria, Atractylodis Macrocephalae Rhizoma (fried), Dioscoreae Rhizoma, Lablab Semen Album (fried), Nelumbinis Semen, Coicis Semen (fried), Amomi Fructus, Platycodonis Radix and Glycyrrhizae Radix et Rhizoma.

Actions and Indications Tonifying the spleen, stomach and replenishing lung-*qi*. It is used for poor appetite and sloppy stool, shortness of breath, cough and fatigue due to hypofunction of the spleen and stomach.

* 人参 ** 茯苓 *** 白术

参茸三鞭丸

【处方】淫羊藿（羊油炙）、补骨脂（盐炙）、阳起石（煅）、覆盆子、金樱子、枸杞子、牛膝、鹿茸、鹿鞭、狗鞭、驴鞭、锁阳、韭菜子、菟丝子、续断、熟地黄、大青盐、人参、肉桂、附子（制）、八角茴香、杜仲（炭）、白术（炒）、地黄、川芎、木香。

【功能主治】补肾助阳，益气生精。用于肾阳不足，肾阴亏虚引起的阳痿滑精，两目昏暗，精神疲倦，腰膝无力。

Ginseng* and Pilose Deerhorn** Bolus

Name of Chinese Phonetic Alphabet Shen Rong San Bian Wan

Formula Epimedii Folium (prepared with sheep suet), Psoraleae Fructus (prepared with salt), Tremolitum (calcined), Rubi Fructus, Rosae Laevigatae Fructus, Lycii Fructus, Achyranthis Bidentatae Radix, Cervi Cornu Pantotrichum, Cervi Penis, Canis Testis et Penis, Asini Testis et Penis, Cynomorii Caulis Carnosus, Allii Tuberosi Semen, Cuscutae Semen, Dipsaci Radix, Rehmanniae Radix Praeparata, Sal, Ginseng Radix et Rhizoma, Cinnamomi Cortex, Aconiti Lateralis Radix Praeparata, Anisi Stellati Fructus, Eucommiae Cortex (canbonated), Atractylodis Macrocephalae Rhizoma (fried), Rehmanniae Radix, Chuanxiong Rhizoma and Aucklandiae Radix.

Actions and Indications Tonifying kidney-*yang*, *qi* and essence. It is used for impotence, spermatorrhea, blurred vision, lassitude of spirit and weakness of waist and knees due to insufficiency of kidney-*yang* and deficiency of kidney-*yin*.

* 人参 ** 鹿茸

参茸卫生丸

【处方】龙眼肉、鹿角、大枣、香附（醋制）、肉苁蓉（酒制）、杜仲（盐制）、当归、猪腰子、牛膝、琥珀、人参、鹿茸、莲子、白芍、牡蛎、枸杞子、龙骨、狗脊（砂烫）、乳香（醋制）、秋石、鹿尾、没药（醋制）、陈皮、白术（麸炒）、熟地黄、砂仁、木香、黄芩、川芎、红花、沉香、续断、地黄、制何首乌、茯苓、紫河车、甘草、桑寄生、党参、酸枣仁（炒）、山茱萸（酒制）、木瓜、黄芪、清半夏、锁阳、肉豆蔻（煨）、补骨脂（盐制）、远志（制）、麦冬、苍术、猪脊髓。

【功能主治】补气益血，兴奋精神。用于身体衰弱，气血两亏所致思虑过度，精神不足，筋骨无力，心脏衰弱，腰膝酸痛，梦遗滑精，自汗盗汗，头昏眼花，妇女血寒，赤白带下，崩漏不止，腰疼腹痛。

Ginseng* and Pilose Deerhorn** Bolus for Debility

Name of Chinese Phonetic Alphabet Shen Rong Wei Sheng Wan

Formula Longan Arillus, Cervi Cornu, Jujubae Fructus, Cyperi Rhizoma (prepared with vinegar), Cistanches Caulis Carnosus (prepared with wine), Eucommiae Cortex (prepared with salt), Angelicae Sinensis Radix, Suillus Ren, Achyranthis Bidentatae Radix, Succinum, Ginseng Radix et Rhizoma, Cervi Cornu Pantotrichum, Nelumbinis Semen, Paeoniae Radix Alba, Ostreae Concha, Lycii Fructus, Draconis Os, Cibotii Rhizoma(scalded by sand), Olibanum (prepared with vinegar), Hominis Urinea Sedimentum et Sal Praeparata, Cervi Cauda, Myrrha (prepared with vinegar), Citri Reticulatae Pericarpium, Atractylodis Macrocephalae Rhizoma (fried with bran), Rehmanniae Radix Praeparata, Amomi Fructus, Aucklandiae Radix, Scutellariae Radix, Chuanxiong Rhizoma, Carthami Flos, Aquilariae Lignum Resinatum, Dipsaci Radix, Rehmanniae Radix, Polygoni Multiflori Radix Praeparata, Poria, Hominis Placenta, Glycyrrhizae Radix et Rhizoma, Taxilli Herba, Codonopsis Radix, Ziziphi Spinosae Semen (fried), Corni Fructus (prepared with wine), Chaenomelis Fructus, Astragali Radix, Pinelliae Rhizoma Praeparatum cum Alumine, Cynomorii Caulis Carnosus, Myristicae Semen (roasted), Psoraleae Fructus (prepared with salt), Polygalae Radix (prepared), Ophiopogonis Radix, Atractylodis Rhizoma and Suillus Spinalis Medulla.

Actions and Indications Tonifying blood and *qi*, exciting the spirit. It is used for general debility, over worry, lassitude of spirit, weakness of heart, sinews and bone, soreness of waist and knees, oneirogmus, spermatorrhea, spontaneous sweating, night sweating, dizziness, dim eyesight, red and white vaginal discharge, metrorrhagia and metrostaxis, lumbago and abdominal pain due to dual depletion of *qi* and blood.

* 人参 ** 鹿茸

参茜固经冲剂

【处方】党参、地黄、槐角、茜草、白术、白芍、蒲黄、山楂、大蓟、小蓟、升麻、女贞子、墨旱莲。

【功能主治】益气养阴，滋肝健脾，和血固经。用于气阴两虚，夹有瘀阻的月经过多，经前心烦，口干，便秘，疲劳，面色少华，脉细数或细弦及功能性子宫出血，子宫肌瘤，放置宫内节育器引起的上述症状者。

【注意】个别病例服药后胃部有不适感。

Soluble Granules of Astringing Menstruation

Name of Chinese Phonetic Alphabet Shen Qian Gu Jing Chong Ji

Formula Codonopsis Radix, Rehmanniae Radix, Sophorae Fructus, Rubiae Radix, Atractylodis Macrocephalae Rhizoma, Paeoniae Radix Alba, Typhae Pollen, Crataegi Fructus, Cirsii Japonici Herba, Cirsii Herba, Cimicifugae Rhizoma, Ligustri Lucidi Fructus and Ecliptae Herba.

Actions and Indications Tonifying *qi*, nourishing *yin*, enriching the liver, fortifying the spleen, harmonizing blood, astringing menstruation. It is used for menorrhagia, premenstrual vexation, dry mouth, constipation, tiredness, lusterless complexion, fine and rapid or fine and string-like pulse, dysfunctional uterine bleeding, hysteromyoma due to dual deficiency of *qi* and *yin*, together with stasis, and the above mentioned symptoms induced by setting of contraceptive ring.

Warning Discomfort of stomach occurs occasionally.

参桂理中丸

【处方】人参、肉桂、附子（制）、干姜、白术（炒）、甘草。

【功能主治】温中散寒，祛湿定痛。用于脾胃虚寒，阳气不足引起的腹痛泄泻，手足厥冷，胃寒呕吐，寒湿疝气，行经腹痛。

【注意】孕妇忌服。

Ginseng* and Cassia Bark** Bolus for Warming Middle Energizer

Name of Chinese Phonetic Alphabet Shen Gui Li Zhong Wan

Formula Ginseng Radix et Rhizoma, Cinnamomi Cortex, Aconiti Lateralis Radix (prepared), Zingiberis Rhizoma, Atractylodis Macrocephalae Rhizoma (fried) and Glycyrrhizae Radix et Rhizoma.

Actions and Indications Warming the middle energizer and dissipating cold, dispelling dampness and relieving pain. It is indicated for abdominal pain, diarrhea, cold limbs, vomiting, hernia and dysmenorrhea due to deficiency-cold of the spleen and stomach and insufficiency of *yang-qi*.

Warning It is contraindicated for pregnant women.

* 人参 ** 肉桂

参桂鹿茸丸

【处方】人参、鹿茸（去毛）、山茱萸（酒炙）、地黄、熟地黄、白芍、龟甲（砂烫醋淬）、鳖甲（砂烫醋淬）、阿胶、杜仲（炒炭）、续断、天冬、茯苓、酸枣仁（炒）、琥珀、艾叶（炒炭）、陈皮、泽泻、没药（醋炙）、乳香（醋炙）、红花、西红花、牛膝（去头）、延胡索（醋炙）、川牛膝（去头）、鸡冠花、赤石脂（煅）、香附（醋炙）、甘草、秦艽、黄芩、白术（麸炒）、木香、砂仁、沉香、当归、川芎、肉桂。

【功能主治】补气益肾，养血调经。用于气虚血亏，肝肾不足引起的体质虚弱，腰膝酸软，头昏耳鸣，自汗盗汗，失眠多梦，肾寒精冷，宫寒带下，月经不调。

【注意】孕妇慎服。忌生冷食物。

Ginseng* Cassia Bark** and Pilose Deerhorn*** Bolus

Name of Chinese Phonetic Alphabet Shen Gui Lu Rong Wan

Formula Ginseng Radix et Rhizoma, Cervi Cornu Pantotrichum (removed hair), Corni Fructus (prepared with wine), Rehmanniae Radix, Rehmanniae Radix Praeparata, Paeoniae Radix Alba, Testudinis Carapax et Plastrum (scalded by sand and quenched by vinegar), Trionycis Carapax (scalded by sand and quenched by vinegar), Asini Corii Colla, Eucommiae Cortex (carbonated), Dipsaci Radix, Asparagi Radix, Poria, Ziziphi Spinosae Semen (fried), Succinum, Artemisiae Argyi Folium (carbonated), Citri Reticulatae Pericarpium, Alismatis Rhizoma, Myrrha (prepared with vinegar), Olibanum (prepared with vinegar), Carthami Flos, Croci Stigma, Achyranthis Bidentatae Radix (removed rhizome), Corydalis Rhizoma (prepared with vinegar), Cyathulae Radix (removed rhizome), Celosiae Cristatae Flos, Halloysitum Rubrum (calcined), Cyperi Rhizoma (prepared with vinegar), Glycyrrhizae Radix et Rhizoma, Gentianae Macrophyllae Radix, Scutellariae Radix, Atractylodis Macrocephalae Rhizoma (fried with bran), Aucklandiae Radix, Amomi Fructus, Aquilariae Lignum Resinatum, Angelicae Sinensis Radix, Chuanxiong Rhizoma and Cinnamomi Cortex.

Actions and Indications Tonifying *qi* and the kidney, nourishing blood, regulating menstruation. It is used for debility of constitution, soreness and weakness of waist and knees, dizziness, tinnitus, spontaneous sweating, night sweating, insomnia, profuse dreaming, sperm-coldness, uterus-coldness, vaginal discharge and irregular menstruation due to dual deficiency of *qi* and blood, and dual insufficiency of the liver and kidney.

Warning It should be used carefully for pregnant women. The Uncooked foods should be avoided.

* 人参 ** 肉桂 *** 鹿茸

九画

珍视明滴眼液

【处方】本品为珍珠层粉水解液制成的滴眼剂。

【功能主治】清热，明目去翳。用于治疗青光眼，防治青少年假性近视眼，并可作为眼的保健用药。

Glaucoma-relieving Eye Drops

Name of Chinese Phonetic Alphabet Zhen Shi Ming Di Yan Ye

Formula Margaritae Concha Strati Pulvis.

Actions and Indications Clearing heat, removing nebula to improve vision. It is indicated for glaucoma and preventing pseudomyopia for teenagers.

珍珠明目液

【处方】珍珠液、冰片。

【功能主治】清热泻火，养肝明目。用于肝虚火旺引起视力疲劳症和慢性结膜炎。长期使用可以保护视力。

Pearl* Eye Drops for Improving Vision

Name of Chinese Phonetic Alphabet Zhen Zhu Ming Mu Ye

Formula Margaritae Liquidum and Borneolum Syntheticum.

Actions and Indications Clearing heat and purging fire, nourishing the liver and improving vision. It is used for asthenopia and chronic conjunctivitis due to liver-deficiency with effulgent fire. Long-time application can protect eyesight.

*珍珠

珍珠胃安丸

【处方】珍珠层粉、甘草、豆豉姜、陈皮、徐长卿。

【功能主治】和中宽胃，行气止痛。用于治疗胃、十二指肠溃疡。

Pearl* Pill for Gastroduodenal Ulcer

Name of Chinese Phonetic Alphabet Zhen Zhu Wei An Wan

Formula Margaritae Concha Strati Pulvis, Glycyrrhizae Radix et Rhizoma, Litseae Cubebae Radix et Rhizoma, Citri Reticulatae Pericarpium and Cynanchi Paniculati Radix et Rhizoma.

Actions and Indications Soothing the stomach, moving *qi*, alleviating pain. It is indicated for gastroduodenal ulcer.

*珍珠

珍珠散

【处方】石决明（煅）、龙骨（煅）、白石脂（煅）、石膏（煅）、珍珠、麝香、冰片。

【功能主治】去腐生肌，收湿敛疮。用于痈疡溃烂，流脓溢水，新肉不生。

【注意】外用药。

Pearl* Powder

Name of Chinese Phonetic Alphabet Zhen Zhu San

Formula Haliotidis Concha (calcined), Draconis Os (calcined), Kaolinum (calcined), Gypsum Fibrosum (calcined), Margarita, Moschus and Borneolum Syntheticum.

Actions and Indications Removing necrosis and promoting tissue regeneration, astringing sore. It is used for ulceration of abscess and sore, irregeneration of granulation.

Warning The preparation is for external use only.

*珍珠

珍黄丸

【处方】珍珠、牛黄、三七、冰片、猪胆汁、薄荷油、黄芩提取物。

【功能主治】清热解毒，消肿止痛。用于咽喉肿痛，疮疡热疖。

Pearl* and Bezoar** Pill

Name of Chinese Phonetic Alphabet Zhen Huang Wan

Formula Margarita, Bovis Calculus, Notoginseng Radix et Rhizoma, Borneolum Syntheticum, Suillus-Bilis, Menthae Haplocalycis Oleum and Scutellariae Radix (extract).

Actions and Indications Clearing heat and detoxicating, dispersing swelling and relieving pain. It is indicated for sore-throat, sore and ulcer.

*珍珠 **牛黄

珍黛散

【处方】珍珠、牛黄、青黛、冰片、滑石。

【功能主治】清热解毒，消炎止痛，生肌收敛。用于口舌生疮，复发性口腔溃疡及疱疹性口腔炎。

Pearl* and Indigo** Powder

Name of Chinese Phonetic Alphabet Zhen Dai San

Formula Margarita, Bovis Calculus, Indigo

Naturalis, Borneolum Syntheticum and Talcum.

Actions and Indications Clearing heat and detoxicating, antiphlogistic and relieving pain, promoting tissue regeneration. It is indicated for aphthae, recurrent ulcerative stomatitis and herpetic ulcerative stomatitis.

*珍珠 **青黛

珊瑚癣净

【处方】复方珊瑚姜酊、水杨酸、甘油、醋酸。

【功能主治】杀菌，止痒。用于脚癣（脚气）、手癣（鹅掌风）、指（趾）甲癣（灰指甲）。

【注意】外用药，切忌入口；严防触及眼、鼻、口腔等黏膜处。皮肤破损处慎用。

Medicated Coral* Aqua for Tinea

Name of Chinese Phonetic Alphabet Shan Hu Xuan Jing

Formula Compound Corallii Japonici Tincture, Salicylic acid, Glycerin and Acetic acid.

Actions and Indications Killing bacteria and relieving itching. It is indicated for tinea pedis, tinea manuum, and tinea of the nail.

Warning Only for external use, cannot be touched by the mucosa of the eyes, nose, mouth; and it shoud be used carefully on the injury area of skin.

*珊瑚

春血安胶囊

【处方】茯苓、柴胡、牛膝、五味子（制）、肉桂、泽泻、三七、附子（制）、山药、黄连、牡丹皮、熟地黄、车前子（盐制）。

【功能主治】益肾固冲，调经止血。用于因肝肾不足，冲任失调所致的月经过多，经期腹痛，青春期功能失调性子宫出血，上环后子宫出血者。

Chun Xue An Capsule

Name of Chinese Phonetic Alphabet Chun Xue An Jiao Nang

Formula Poria, Bupleuri Radix, Achyranthis Bidentatae Radix, Schisandrae Chinensis Fructus (prepared), Cinnamomi Cortex, Alismatis Rhizoma, Notoginseng Radix et Rhizoma, Aconiti Lateralis Radix Praeparata, Dioscoreae Rhizoma, Coptidis Rhizoma, Moutan Cortex, Rehmanniae Radix Praeparata and Plantaginis Semen (prepared with salt).

Actions and Indications Replenishing the kidney, strengthening thoroughfare vessel, regulating menstruation, relieving bleeding. It is used for menorrhagia, menstrual abdominal pain, hebetic dysfunctional uterine bleeding due to insufficiency of the liver and kidney, and insecurity of the thoroughfare and conception vessels. Bleeding due to setting of contraceptive ring.

柏子养心丸

【处方】柏子仁、党参、黄芪（蜜炙）、川芎、当归、茯苓、远志（制）、酸枣仁、肉桂、五味子（蒸）、半夏曲、甘草（蜜炙）、朱砂。

【功能主治】补气，养血，安神。用于心气虚寒，心悸易惊，失眠多梦，健忘。

Chinese Arborvitae* Bolus for Nourishing Heart

Name of Chinese Phonetic Alphabet Bai Zi Yang Xin Wan

Formula Platycladi Semen, Codonopsis Radix, Astragali Radix (prepared with honey), Chuanxiong Rhizoma, Angelicae Sinensis Radix, Poria, Polygalae Radix (prepared), Ziziphi Spinosae Semen, Cinnamomi Cortex, Schisandrae Chinensis Fructus (steamed), Pinelliae Massa Fermentata, Glycyrrhizae Radix et Rhizoma (prepared with honey) and Cinnabaris.

Actions and Indications Tonifying *qi*, nourishing blood and tranquilizing the mind. It is used for palpitation, fright, insomnia, profuse dreaming and amnesia due to deficiency-cold of heart-*qi*.

*侧柏

枸杞药酒

【处方】枸杞子、熟地黄、黄精（蒸）、百合、远志（制）。

【功能主治】滋肾益肝。用于肝肾不足，虚劳羸瘦，腰膝酸软，失眠。

Medicated Wine of Chinese Wolfberry*

Name of Chinese Phonetic Alphabet Gou Qi Yao Jiu

Formula Lycii Fructus, Rehmanniae Radix Praeparata, Polygonati Rhizoma (steamed), Lilii Bulbus and Polygalae Radix (prepared).

Actions and Indications Enriching the kidney and tonifying the liver. It is indicated for emaciation, soreness and weakness of the waist and legs and insomnia due to dual insufficiency of the liver and kidney and consumptive disease.

* 枸杞

荆防合剂

【处方】荆芥、防风、羌活、独活、柴胡、前胡、川芎、枳壳、茯苓、桔梗、甘草。

【功能主治】发汗解表，散风祛湿。用于感冒风寒，头痛身痛，恶寒无汗，鼻塞流涕，咳嗽咽干。

Fineleaf Schizonepeta* and Divaricate Saposhnikovia** Mixture

Name of Chinese Phonetic Alphabet Jing Fang He Ji

Formula Schizonepetae Herba, Saposhnikoviae Radix, Notopterygii Rhizoma et Radix, Angelicae Pubescentis Radix, Bupleuri Radix, Peucedani Radix, Chuanxiong Rhizoma, Aurantii Fructus, Poria, Platycodonis Radix and Glycyrrhizae Radix et Rhizoma.

Actions and Indications Promoting sweating to release the exterior, dispersing wind and dispelling dampness. It is used for common cold (wind-cold) type, marked by headache and generalized pain, aversion to cold, anhidrosis, stuffy nose, rhinorrhea, cough, dry throat.

* 荆芥 ** 防风

荆花胃康丸

【处方】土荆芥、水团花。

【功能主治】理气散寒、清热化痰。用于寒热错杂证，或兼气滞血瘀证的胃脘痛，症见胃脘胀闷疼痛、嗳气、反酸、嘈杂、口苦；以及十二指肠溃疡见于以上证候者。

Wormseed* and Pilular Adina** Stomach-soothing Pill

Name of Chinese Phonetic Alphabet Jing Hua Wei Kang Wan

Formula Chenopodii Ambrosioidis Herba and Adinae Piluliferae Herba.

Actions and Indications Regulating *qi* and dissipating cold, clearing heat and resolving phlegm. It is indicated for stomach duct pain, manifested as stomach duct distention and pain, belching, acid regurgitation, gastric upset and bitter taste in the mouth due to cold-heat complex syndrome or blood-stasis and *qi*-stagnation. And duodenal ulcer with the above mentioned symptoms.

* 土荆芥 ** 水团花

荜铃胃痛冲剂

【处方】荜澄茄、川楝子、延胡索（醋制）、大黄（酒制）、黄连、吴茱萸、香附（醋制）、香橼、佛手、海螵蛸、瓦楞子（煅）。

【功能主治】行气活血，和胃止痛。用于气滞血瘀引起的胃脘痛以及慢性胃炎。

Mountain-pepper* and Szechuan Chinaberry** Soluble Granules

Name of Chinese Phonetic Alphabet Bi Ling Wei Tong Chong Ji

Formula Litseae Fructus, Toosendan Fructus, Corydalis Rhizoma (prepared with vinegar), Rhei Radix et Rhizoma (prepared with wine), Coptidis Rhizoma, Euodiae Fructus, Cyperi Rhizoma (prepared with vinegar), Citri Fructus, Citri Sarcodactylis Fructus, Sepiae Endoconcha and Arcae Concha (calcined).

Actions and Indications Moving *qi*, activating blood, harmonizing the stomach, alleviating pain. It is indicated for pain of stomach duct and chronic gastritis due to *qi*-stagnation and blood-stasis.

* 荜澄茄 ** 川楝子

茵山莲颗粒

【处方】茵陈、半枝莲、五味子、栀子、甘草、板蓝根。

【功能主治】清热解毒利湿。用于慢性迁延性肝炎，慢性活动性肝炎，胆囊炎，胰腺炎，而见湿热蕴毒之症者。

Virgate Wormwood* and Barbed Skullcap** Soluble Granules

Name of Chinese Phonetic Alphabet Yin Shan Lian Ke Li

Formula Artemisiae Scopariae Herba, Scutellariae Barbatae Herba, Schisandrae Chinensis Fructus, Gardeniae Fructus, Glycyrrhizae Radix et Rhizoma and Isatidis Radix.

Actions and Indications Clearing heat, detoxicating and draining dampness. It is indicated for chronic persistent hepatitis, chronic active hepatitis, cholecystitis, pancreatitis, attributive to damp-heat accumulation.

* 茵陈 ** 半枝莲

茵芪肝复颗粒

【处方】茵陈、栀子、大黄、白花蛇舌草、猪苓、柴胡、当归、黄芪。

【功能主治】清热解毒利湿，疏肝补脾。用于慢性乙肝病毒性肝炎，肝胆湿热兼脾虚肝郁证。症见右胁胀满，恶心厌油，纳差食少，口淡乏味。

Virgate Wormwood* and Milkvetch** Liver-soothing Granules

Name of Chinese Phonetic Alphabet Yin Qi Gan Fu Ke Li

Formula Artemisiae Scopariae Herba, Gardeniae Fructus, Rhei Radix et Rhizoma, Hedyotis Diffusae Herba, Polyporus, Bupleuri Radix, Angelicae Sinensis Radix and Astragali Radix.

Actions and Indications Clearing heat, detoxicating and draining dampness, soothing the liver and tonifying the spleen. It is indicated for chronic viral hepatitis B, damp-heat syndrome of the liver and gallbladder associated with syndrome of spleen deficiency and liver depression, manifested as right hypochondriac fullness, nausea, disgusted with oil and fat, poor appetite, anorexia and tastelessness in the mouth.

* 茵陈 ** 黄芪

茵陈五苓丸

【处方】茵陈、泽泻、茯苓、猪苓、白术（炒）、肉桂。

【功能主治】清湿热，利小便。用于肝胆湿热引起的湿热黄疸，脘腹胀满，小便不利。

Virgate Wormwood* Pill for Relieving Jaundice

Name of Chinese Phonetic Alphabet Yin Chen Wu Ling Wan

Formula Artemisiae Scopariae Herba, Alismatis Rhizoma, Poria, Polyporus, Atractylodis Macrocephalae Rhizoma (fried) and Cinnamomi Cortex.

Actions and Indications Clearing damp-heat and inducing diuresis. It is indicated for jaundice of damp-heat, abdominal distention and fullness and difficult urination due to damp-heat of the liver and gallbladder.

* 茵陈

茵栀黄口服液

【处方】茵陈提取物、栀子提取物、黄芩苷、金银花提取物。

【功能主治】清热解毒，利湿退黄。有退黄疸和降低谷丙转氨酶的作用。用于湿热毒邪内蕴所致急性、迁延性、慢性肝炎和重症肝炎（Ⅰ型）。也可用于其他型重症肝炎的综合治疗。

Virgate Wormwood* Jasmine** and Baicalin*** Oral Liquid

Name of Chinese Phonetic Alphabet Yin Zhi Huang Kou Fu Ye

Formula Artemisiae Scopariae Extractum, Gardeniae Extractum, Baicalin and Lonicerae Japonicae Extractum.

Actions and Indications Clearing heat and detoxicating, draining dampness and relieving jaundice. It possesses the effect of relieving jaundice and decreasing glutamic pyruvic transaminase. It is indicated for acute, persisting, chronic and severe hepatitis (Ⅰ type) due to damp-heat and toxin accumulated interiorly, also indicated for comprehensive treatment to other types of severe hepatitides.

* 茵陈 ** 栀子 *** 黄芩苷

茵胆平肝胶囊

【处方】茵陈、龙胆、黄芩、猪胆膏、栀子、白芍（炒）、当归、甘草。

【功能主治】清热利湿，消黄。用于急性黄疸型肝炎，亦可用于慢性肝炎。

【注意】胆道完全阻塞者忌服。

Virgate Wormwood* and Scabrous Gentian** Capsule for Pacifying Liver

Name of Chinese Phonetic Alphabet Yin Dan Ping Gan Jiao Nang

Formula Artemisiae Scopariae Herba, Gentianae Radix et Rhizoma, Scutellariae Radix, Suillus Fel Extractum, Gardeniae Fructus, Paeoniae Radix Alba (fried), Angelicae Sinensis Radix and Glycyrrhizae Radix et Rhizoma.

Actions and Indications Clearing heat and draining dampness, relieving jaundice. It is indicated for acute icterohepatitis, and also for chronic hepatitis.

Warning It is contraindicated for cases with bile tract obstructed completely.

* 茵陈 ** 龙胆

茵莲清肝合剂

【处方】茵陈、板蓝根、绵马贯众、茯苓、郁金、当归、红花、琥珀、白芍（炒）、白花蛇舌草、半枝莲、广藿香、佩兰、砂仁、虎杖、丹参、泽兰、柴胡、重楼。

【功能主治】清热解毒，化湿，舒肝利胆，健脾和胃，养血活血。用于病毒性肝炎，肝炎病毒携带者及肝功能异常患者。

【注意】忌食辛辣油腻食物。

Virgate Wormwood* and Barbed Skullcap** Mixture for Relieving Viral Hepatitis

Name of Chinese Phonetic Alphabet Yin Lian Qing Gan He Ji

Formula Artemisiae Scopariae Herba, Isatidis Radix, Dryopteridis Crassirhizomatis Rhizoma, Poria, Curcumae Radix, Angelicae Sinensis Radix, Carthami Flos, Succinum, Paeoniae Radix Alba (fried), Hedyotis Diffusae Herba, Scutellariae Barbatae Herba, Pogostemonis Herba, Eupatorii Herba, Amomi Fructus, Polygoni Cuspidati Radix et Rhizoma, Salviae Miltiorrhizae Radix et Rhizoma, Lycopi Herba, Bupleuri Radix and Paridis Rhizoma.

Actions and Indications Clearing heat and detoxicating, draining dampness, soothing the liver and draining bile, fortifying the spleen and harmonizing the stomach, nourishing and activating blood. It is indicated for viral hepatitis, cases with viral carrier and hepatic dysfunction.

Warning Pungent and oily foods are prohibited.

* 茵陈 ** 半枝莲

茴香橘核丸

【处方】小茴香（盐炒）、八角茴香、橘核（盐炒）、荔枝核、补骨脂（盐炒）、肉桂、川楝子、延胡索（醋制）、莪术（醋制）、木香、香附（醋制）、青皮（醋炒）、昆布、槟榔、乳香（制）、桃仁、穿山甲（制）。

【功能主治】散寒行气，消肿止痛。用于寒疝，睾丸肿痛。

Fennel* and Satsuma Orange Seed** Pill

Name of Chinese Phonetic Alphabet Hui Xiang Ju He Wan

Formula Foeniculi Fructus (fried with salt), Anisi Stellati Fructus, Semen Citri Reticulatae (prepared with salt), Litchi Semen, Psoraleae Fructus (fried with salt), Cinnamomi Cortex, Toosendan Fructus, Corydalis Rhizoma (prepared with vinegar), Curcumae Rhizoma (prepared with vinegar), Aucklandiae Radix, Cyperi Rhizoma (prepared with vinegar), Citri Reticulatae Pericarpium Viride (fried with vinegar), Laminariae et Eckloniae Thallus, Arecea Semen, Olibanum (prepared), Persicae Semen and Manis Squama (prepared).

Actions and Indications Dissipating cold, moving *qi*, dispersing swelling, alleviating pain. It is indicated for cold abdominal colic, swelling and pain of testes.

* 小茴香 ** 橘核

药制龟苓膏

【处方】龟甲、土茯苓、广金钱草、地黄、防风、川木通、金银花、槐花、茵陈、甘草。

【功能主治】滋阴降火，清热解毒。用于湿热下注引起的湿疹，皮肤瘙痒，便血，尿痛及妇女黄带。

Soft Extract of Tortoise's Shell and Plastron* and Glabrous Greenbrier**

Name of Chinese Phonetic Alphabet Yao Zhi Gui Ling Gao

Formula Testudinis Carapax et Plastrum, Smilacis Glabrae Rhizoma, Desmodii Styracifolii Herba, Rehmanniae Radix, Saposhnikoviae Radix, Clematidis Armandii Caulis, Lonicerae Japonicae Flos, Sophorae Flos, Artemisiae Scopariae Herba and Glycyrrhizae Radix et Rhizoma.

Actions and Indications Enriching *yin* and downbearing fire, clearing heat and detoxicating. It is indicated for eczema, cutaneous pruritus, bloody stool, urodynia, and yellow vaginal discharge due to downward attack of damp-heat.

* 龟甲 ** 土茯苓

按摩乳

【处方】芸香浸膏、乳香、没药、颠茄流浸膏、乌药、川芎、郁金、水杨酸甲酯、薄荷油、桂皮油、丁香油、樟脑、硬脂酸、单硬脂酸甘油酯。

【功能主治】活血化瘀，和络止痛。用于运动劳损，肌肉酸痛，跌打损伤，无名肿毒。

【注意】切勿内服，皮肤破伤者及孕妇忌用。

Massage Emulsion

Name of Chinese Phonetic Alphabet An Mo Ru

Formula Cymbopogonis Distantis Extractum, Olibanum, Myrrha, Belladonnae Extractum, Linderae Radix, Chuanxiong Rhizoma, Curcumae Radix, Methyl Salicylate, Menthae Haplocalycis Oleum, Cinnamomi Oleum, Caryophylli Oleum, Camphora, Stearic Acid and Glyceryl Monostearate.

Actions and Indications Activating blood, resolving stasis, harmonizing collaterals, alleviating pain. It is used for sport strain, mascular soreness and pain, traumatic injury, sprain, swelling and pain of unknown origin.

Warning It is for external use only. The preparation is contraindicated for pregnant women and cases with wound of skin.

鸦胆子油乳注射液

【处方】精制鸦胆子油、精制豆磷脂、甘油。

【功能主治】抗癌药。用于肺癌、肺癌脑转移及消化道肿瘤。

【注意】本品无明显毒副作用，但有少数患者服后有恶心，厌食症状。

Injection of Java Brucea Oil*

Name of Chinese Phonetic Alphabet Ya Dan Zi You Ru Zhu She Ye

Formula Bruceae Fructus Oleum, Purified Soybean Phospholipid and Glycerin.

Actions and Indications Anticarcinogen. It is indicated for cancer of the lung, lung cancer with brain metastaticum and tumor of the digestive tract.

Warning It has not obvious toxic and side effects, but some patients may suffer from nausea, anorexia.

*鸦胆子油

咽速康气雾剂

【处方】人工牛黄、珍珠、雄黄、蟾酥、冰片、麝香等。

【功能主治】解毒、消肿、止痛。用于咽喉肿痛、单双乳蛾的肺胃实热证。

【注意】孕妇禁用。不宜长期使用。

Aerosol for Sore-throat

Name of Chinese Phonetic Alphabet Yan Su Kang Qi Wu Ji

Formula Bovis Calculus Artifactus, Margarita, Realgar, Bufonis Venenum, Borneolum Syntheticum, Moschus, etc.

Actions and Indications Detoxicating, reducing swelling, relieving pain. It is used for sore-throat, unilateral or bilateral tonsillitis due to excess heat in the lung and stomach.

Warning It is contraindicated for pregnant women. Long-term application is prohibited.

咽喉消炎丸

【处方】牛黄、蟾酥（制）、七叶莲、珍珠、冰片、雄黄、百草霜、穿心莲总内酯。

【功能主治】清热解毒，消肿，止痛。用于咽喉肿痛（食管炎，咽喉炎，急、慢性扁桃体炎）。

【注意】忌酒和辛辣食物。

Sore-throat-relieving Pill

Name of Chinese Phonetic Alphabet Yan Hou Xiao Yan Wan

Formula Bovis Calculus, Bufonis Venenum (prepared), Schefflerae Arboricolae Radix, Margarita, Borneolum Syntheticum, Realgar, Gramen Fumi Carbonisatus Pulvis and Andrographolide.

Actions and Indications Clearing heat and detoxicating, dispersing swelling and relieving pain. It is indicated for sore-throat (esophagitis, laryngopharyngitis, acute, chronic tonsillitis).

Warning Wine and pungent foods are prohibited.

咽喉清口服液

【处方】土牛膝、马兰草、车前草、天名精。

【功能主治】清热解毒，利咽止痛。主治肺胃实热所致的咽部肿痛、发热、口渴、便秘，以及急性扁桃体炎、急性咽炎见于上述症状者。

Relieving Sore-throat Oral Liquid

Name of Chinese Phonetic Alphabet Yan Hou Qing Kou Fu Ye

Formula Achyranthis Bidentatae Radix, Wedeliae Chinensis Herba seu Radix, Plantaginis Herba and Carpesii Abrotanoidis Radix et Folium.

Actions and Indications Clearing heat and detoxicating, soothing the throat and relieving pain. It is indicated for sore-throat, fever, thirst, constipation and acute tonsillitis due to excess heat in the lung and stomach, and also used for acute pharyngitis with the above mentioned symptoms.

咳宁糖浆

【处方】松塔、棉花根、枇杷叶。

【功能主治】镇咳祛痰，平喘，扶正固本。用于反复咳嗽，咯痰历年不愈，胸满；慢性支气管炎，感冒。

Syrup for Alleviating Cough

Name of Chinese Phonetic Alphabet Ke Ning Tang Jiang

Formula Pini Strobilus, Gossypii Radix and Eriobotryae Folium.

Actions and Indications Alleviating cough and dispelling phlegm, calming dyspnea, reinforcing and securing healthy *qi*. It is indicated for repeated cough, uncurable spitting phlegm, chest distress, chronic bronchitis and common cold.

咳喘宁片

【处方】桔梗、石膏、罂粟壳、甘草、麻黄、百部、苦杏仁。

【功能主治】宣通肺气，止咳平喘。用于支气管哮喘，咳嗽，老年痰喘。

【注意】高血压及冠状动脉病患者忌服。

Suppressing Bronchial Asthma and Cough Tablet

Name of Chinese Phonetic Alphabet Ke Chuan Ning Pian

Formula Platycodonis Radix, Gypsum Fibrosum, Papaveris Pericarpium, Glycyrrhizae Radix et Rhizoma, Ephedrae Herba, Stemonae Radix and Armeniacae Semen Amarum.

Actions and Indications Diffusing lung-*qi*, suppressing cough and asthma. It is indicated for bronchial asthma, cough, phlegm dyspnea of aged.

Warning It is contraindicated for cases with hypertension and coronary artery diseases.

咳喘顺丸

【处方】半夏、陈皮、瓜蒌子、紫菀、款冬花、桑白皮、前胡、紫苏子、苦杏仁、鱼腥草、茯苓、甘草。

【功能主治】健脾燥湿，宣肺平喘，化痰止咳。用于慢性支气管炎、肺气肿所致的气喘、胸闷、咳嗽痰多。

Relieving Cough and Dyspnea Pill

Name of Chinese Phonetic Alphabet Ke Chuan Shun Wan

Formula Pinelliae Rhizoma, Citri Reticulatae Pericarpium, Trichosanthis Semen, Asteris Radix et Rhizoma, Farfarae Flos, Mori Cortex, Peucedani Radix, Perillae Fructus, Armeniacae Semen Amarum, Houttuyniae Herba, Poria and Glycyrrhizae Radix et Rhizoma.

Actions and Indications Fortifying the spleen and drying dampness, diffusing the lung and calming dyspnea, resolving phlegm and relieving cough. It is indicated for dyspnea, chest distress, cough with profuse phlegm due to chronic bronchitis, pulmonary emphysema.

胃乃安胶囊

【处方】黄芪、三七、人参粉、珍珠层粉、人工牛黄。

【功能主治】补气健脾，宁心安神，行气活血，消炎生肌。用于胃及十二指肠溃疡，慢性胃炎。

Peaceful Stomach Capsule

Name of Chinese Phonetic Alphabet Wei Nai An Jiao Nang

Formula Astragali Radix, Notoginseng Radix et Rhizoma, Ginseng Pulvis, Margaritae Concha Strati Pulvis and Bovis Calculus Artifactus.

Actions and Indications Tonifying *qi* and fortifying the spleen, tranquilizing the mind, moving *qi* and activating blood, counteracting inflammation and promoting tissue regeneration. It is used for gastric and duodenal ulcer and chronic gastritis.

胃力康颗粒

【处方】柴胡、赤芍、枳壳等。

【功能主治】行气活血，泄热和胃。用于胃脘痛气滞血瘀兼肝胃郁热症，症见胃脘疼痛，胀闷，灼热，嗳气，反酸，烦躁易怒，口干口苦；以及慢性浅表性胃炎及消化性溃疡见上述症候者。

Stomachache and Gastritis Relieving Soluble Granules

Name of Chinese Phonetic Alphabet Wei Li Kang Ke Li

Formula Bupleuri Radix, Paeoniae Radix Rubra, Aurantii Fructus, etc.

Actions and Indications Moving *qi*, activating blood, discharging heat, harmonizing the stomach. It is used for epigastric pain of *qi*-stagnation, blood-stasis and accumulation of heat in the liver and stomach type, manifested as pain in stomach duct, abdominal fullness, scorching hot, eructation, acid regurgitation, vexation, dry mouth and bitter taste in the mouth. Also used for chronic superficial gastritis and peptic ulcer with the above mentioned symptoms.

胃乐宁片

【处方】本品为猴头菌菌丝体经加工制成的片。

【功能主治】养阴和胃。用于胃脘疼痛，痞满，腹胀及胃、十二指肠溃疡，慢性萎缩性胃炎。

Mycelium Hedgehog* Tablet for Chronic Atrophic Gastritis

Name of Chinese Phonetic Alphabet Wei Le Ning Pian

Formula Hedgehog Hericii Mycelium.

Actions and Indications Nourishing *yin*, harmonizing the stomach. It is used for stomach duct pain and stuffiness and fullness, abdominal fullness, gastroduodenal ulcer and chronic atrophic gastritis.

* 猴头菌菌丝体

胃安胶囊

【处方】石斛、黄柏、南沙参、山楂、枳壳（炒）、黄精、甘草、白芍。

【功能主治】养阴益胃，补脾消炎，行气止痛。用于萎缩性胃炎，出现胃脘嘈杂、上腹隐痛、咽干口燥、舌红少津、脉细数等胃阴虚证者。

Atrophic Gastritis-relieving Capsule

Name of Chinese Phonetic Alphabet Wei An Jiao Nang

Formula Dendrobii Caulis, Phellodendri Chinensis Cortex, Adenophorae Radix, Crataegi Fructus, Aurantii Fructus (fried), Polygonati Rhizoma, Glycyrrhizae Radix et Rhizoma and Paeoniae Radix Alba.

Actions and Indications Nourishing *yin*, tonifying the stomach and spleen, anti-inflammation, moving *qi* and alleviating pain. It is indicated for atrophic gastritis manifested as gastric upset, upper abdominal dull pain, dry mouth and throat, red tongue and lack of fluid, fine and rapid pulse attributed to syndrome of stomach *yin*-deficiency.

胃苏冲剂

【处方】本品为紫苏梗、香附、陈皮、香橼、佛手、枳壳等药经加工制成的颗粒冲剂。

【功能主治】理气消胀，和胃止痛。主治气滞型胃脘痛，症见胃脘胀痛，窜及两肋，得嗳气或矢气则舒，情绪郁怒则发作加重。胸闷食少，舌苔薄白，脉弦。用于慢性胃炎及消化性溃疡见上述症候者。

Purple Perilla Stem* Soluble Granules

Name of Chinese Phonetic Alphabet Wei Su Chong Ji

Formula Perillae Caulis, Cyperi Rhizoma, Citri Reticulatae Pericarpium, Citri Fructus, Citri Sarcodactylis Fructus, Aurantii Fructus, etc.

Actions and Indications Regulating *qi*, dispersing fullness, harmonizing the stomach, alleviating pain. It is used for pain in stomach duct radiating to hypochondrium, and relieved by eructation and fecal *qi* and severe during mental depression; also for chest distress, anorexia, thin and white tongue fur and string-like pulse due to stagnation of *qi*. It also used for chronic gastritis and peptic ulcer with the above mentioned symptoms.

* 紫苏梗

胃肠宁片

【处方】布渣叶、辣蓼、番石榴叶、火炭母、功劳木。

【功能主治】清热祛湿，健胃止泻。用于急性胃肠炎，小儿消化不良。

Gastroenteritis-relieving Tablet

Name of Chinese Phonetic Alphabet Wei Chang Ning Pian

Formula Microctis Folium, Polygoni Flaccidi Herba, Psidii Guajavae Folium, Polygoni Chinensis Herba and Mahoniae Caulis.

Actions and Indications Clearing heat and draining dampness, fortifying the stomach and relieving diarrhea. It is indicated for acute gastroenteritis and infantile dyspepsia.

胃肠安丸

【处方】本品为木香、沉香、枳壳（麸炒）、檀香、大黄、厚朴（姜制）、朱砂、麝香、巴豆霜、大枣（去核）、川芎等药经加工制成的丸剂。

【功能主治】芳香化浊，理气止痛，健胃导滞。用于消化不良引起的腹泻，肠炎，菌痢，脘腹胀满，腹痛，食积乳积。

Dyspepsia-relieving Pill

Name of Chinese Phonetic Alphabet Wei Chang An Wan

Formula Aucklandiae Radix, Aquilariae Lignum Resinatum, Aurantii Fructus (fried with bran), Santali Albi Lignum, Rhei Radix et Rhizoma, Magnoliae Officinalis Cortex (prepared with ginger), Cinnabaris, Moschus, Crotonis Semen Pulveratum, Jujubae Fructus (removed nucleus), Chuanxiong Rhizoma, etc.

Actions and Indications Resolving turbidity, regulating *qi*, alleviating pain, fortifying the stomach. It is used for diarrhea, enteritis, bacillary dysentery, abdominal fullness and pain and accumulation of milk due to dyspepsia.

胃肠复原膏

【处方】枳壳（麸炒）、太子参、大黄、蒲公英、木香、莱菔子（炒）、赤芍 、紫苏梗、黄芪、桃仁。

【功能主治】益气保元，化瘀去毒，理气通下。用于胃肠手术后腹胀，胃肠活动减弱，老年性慢性便秘，气虚腹胀。

Gastrointestinal-restoration Soft Extract

Name of Chinese Phonetic Alphabet Wei Chang Fu Yuan Gao

Formula Aurantii Fructus (fried with bran), Pseudostellariae Radix, Rhei Radix et Rhizoma, Taraxaci Herba, Aucklandiae Radix, Raphani Semen (fried), Paeoniae Radix Rubra, Perillae Caulis, Astragali Radix and Persicae Semen.

Actions and Indications Tonifying *qi* and protecting original *qi*, resolving stasis and detoxicating, regulating *qi*. It is used for abdominal distention after gastrointestinal surgery, decreasement of gastrointestinal activity, senile chronic constipation and abdominal distention due to *qi* deficiency.

胃复春片

【处方】红参、香茶菜、枳壳（炒）。

【功能主治】健脾益气，活血解毒。用于治疗胃癌癌前期病变及胃癌手术后辅助治疗。

Stomach-restoration Tablet

Name of Chinese Phonetic Alphabet Wei Fu Chun Pian

Formula Ginseng Radix et Rhizoma Rubra, Rabdosiae Glaucocalycis Herba and Aurantii Fructus (fried).

Actions and Indications Fortifying the spleen and tonifying *qi*, activating blood and detoxicating. It is used for precancerous pathological changes of stomach cancer and adjuvant treatment after gastric carcinoma operation.

胃逆康胶囊

【处方】柴胡、白芍、枳实、清半夏等。

【功能主治】疏肝泄热，和胃降逆，制酸止痛。用于肝胃不和郁热症引起的胸脘胁痛，嗳气呃逆，吐酸嘈杂，脘胀纳呆，口干口苦，舌红苔黄等，以及反流性食管炎，功能性消化不良见上述证候者。

Stomach-harmonizing Capsule

Name of Chinese Phonetic Alphabet Wei Ni Kang Jiao Nang

Formula Bupleuri Radix, Paeoniae Radix Alba, Aurantii Fructus Immaturus, Pinelliae Rhizoma Praeparatum cum Alumine, etc.

Actions and Indications Soothing the liver, discharging heat, harmonizing the stomach, directing *qi* downward, inhibiting acidity, alleviating pain. It is used for hypochondriac pain, eructation, hiccup, acid vomiting, gastric upset, anorexia, dry mouth, bitter taste in the mouth, red tongue with yellow fur. It is also used for reflux esophagitis and functional dyspepsia with the above montioned symptoms.

胃益胶囊

【处方】佛手、砂仁、黄柏、川楝子、延胡索、山楂。

【功能主治】疏肝理气，和胃止痛，健脾消食。用于肝胃气滞，脘肋胀痛，食欲不振，嗳气呃逆，以及萎缩性胃炎见上述表现者。

Stomach-benefiting Capsule

Name of Chinese Phonetic Alphabet Wei Yi Jiao Nang

Formula Citri Sarcodactylis Fructus, Amomi Fructus, Phellodendri Chinensis Cortex, Toosendan Fructus, Corydalis Rhizoma and Crataegi Fructus.

Actions and Indications Soothing the liver, regulating *qi*, harmonizing the stomach, alleviating pain, fortifying the spleen and promoting digestion. It is used for fullness and pain of hypochondrium, poor appetite, eructation and hiccup due to stagnation of stomach *qi*, and also used for atrophic gastritis with the above mentioned manifestations.

胃祥宁颗粒

【处方】本品为女贞子经加工组成的颗粒。

【功能主治】舒肝止痛，养阴润肠。用于消化性溃疡，慢性胃炎所致的胃脘痛腹胀，嗳气，口渴，便秘。

Chinese Privet* Soluble Granules

Name of Chinese Phonetic Alphabet Wei Xiang Ning Ke Li

Formula Ligustri Lucidi Fructus (prepared).

Actions and Indications Soothing the liver, alleviating pain, nourishing *yin* and moistening the intestine. It is indicated for peptic ulcer, stomach duct pain, abdominal fullness, belching, thirst and constipation due to chronic gastritis.

* 女贞子

胃福冲剂

【处方】白及、黄芪、蚕砂、延胡索（制）、沉香、威灵仙、地榆、没药、陈皮、马兜铃、木香、马齿苋。

【功能主治】理气和胃，利膈开郁。用于治疗慢性胃炎，胃及十二指肠溃疡。

Harmonizing Stomach Soluble Granules

Name of Chinese Phonetic Alphabet Wei Fu Chong Ji

Formula Bletillae Rhizoma, Astragali Radix,

Bombycis Feculae, Corydalis Rhizoma (prepared), Aquilariae Lignum Resinatum, Clematidis Radix et Rhizoma, Sanguisorbae Radix, Myrrha, Citri Reticulatae Pericarpium, Aristolochiae Fructus, Aucklandiae Radix and Portulacae Herba.

Actions and Indications Regulating *qi*, harmonizing the stomach, relieving deperssion. It is indicated for chronic gastritis, gastroduodenal ulcer.

骨友灵擦剂

【处方】红花、续断、威灵仙、延胡索、防风、蝉蜕、鸡血藤、川乌（制）、制何首乌等。

【功能主治】活血化瘀，消肿止痛。用于骨质增生引起的功能性障碍，软组织损伤及大关节病引的肿胀，疼痛。

【注意】个别患者用药后出现皮肤发痒、发热及潮红，切勿手挠，停药后症状即可消失。

Gu You Ling Liniment

Name of Chinese Phonetic Alphabet Gu You Ling Ca Ji

Formula Carthami Flos, Dipsaci Radix, Clematidis Radix et Rhizoma, Corydalis Rhizoma, Saposhnikoviae Radix, Cicadae Periostracum, Spatholobi Caulis, Aconiti Radix Cocta, Polygoni Multiflori Radix Praeparata, etc.

Actions and Indications Activating blood, resolving stasis, reducing swelling, alleviating pain. It is used for functional disorder and injury of soft tissue due to hyperosteogeny; swelling and pain due to osteoarthrosis deformans.

Warning Itching of skin, fever and tidal flushed complexion occur occasionally. Patient should not scratch the itch, the symptoms will disappear when medication is suspended.

骨龙胶囊

【处方】狗腿骨、穿山龙。

【功能主治】散寒镇痛，活血祛风，强筋壮骨。用于慢性风湿及类风湿性关节炎。

Dog Bone Capsule for Relieving Rheumatism

Name of Chinese Phonetic Alphabet Gu Long Jiao Nang

Formula Canis Os, Dioscoreae Nipponicae Rhizoma.

Actions and Indications Dissipating cold and settling pain, activating blood and dispelling wind, strengthening the sinews and bone. It is indicated for chronic rheumatism and rheumatoid arthritis.

骨仙片

【处方】骨碎补、熟地黄、黑豆、女贞子、牛膝、仙茅、菟丝子、广防己、枸杞子。

【功能主治】填精益髓，壮腰健肾，强壮筋骨，舒筋活络，养血止痛。用于因骨质增生引起的疾患。

【注意】感冒发热勿服。

Relieving Hyperosteogeny Tablet

Name of Chinese Phonetic Alphabet Gu Xian Pian

Formula Drynariae Rhizoma, Rehmanniae Radix Praeparata, Sojae Semen Nigrum, Ligustri Lucidi Fructus, Achyranthis Bidentatae Radix, Curculiginis Rhizoma, Cuscutae Semen, Aristolochiae Fangchi Radix and Lycii Fructus.

Actions and Indications Tonifying vital essence and marrow, fortifying the loin and kidney, strengthening sinews and bone, relaxing sinews and activating collaterals, nourishing blood and alleviating pain. It is used for those diseases due to hyperosteogeny.

Warning It is contraindicated for cases with common cold, fever.

骨折挫伤胶囊

【处方】猪骨（制）、黄瓜子（制）、自然铜（煅）、红花、大黄、当归、乳香（炒）、没药（制）、血竭、土鳖虫。

【功能主治】舒筋活络，接骨止痛。用于跌打损伤，消肿散瘀，扭腰岔气。

【注意】孕妇忌服。

Fracture and Contusion Relieving Capsule

Name of Chinese Phonetic Alphabet Gu Zhe Cuo Shang Jiao Nang

Formula Suillus Os (prepared), Cucumidis Sativi Semen (prepared), Pyritum (calcined), Carthami Flos, Rhei Radix et Rhizoma, Angelicae Sinensis Radix, Olibanum (fried), Myrrha (prepared), Draconis Sanguis and Eupolyphaga seu Steleophaga.

Actions and Indications Relaxing sinews, activating collaterals, bone-knitting, alleviating pain. It is used for sudden lumbar sprain, traumatic injury marked by swelling and blood-stasis.

Warning It is contraindicated for pregnant women.

骨松宝颗粒

【处方】淫羊藿、续断、赤芍、川芎、知母、莪术、三棱、地黄、牡蛎（煅）。

【功能主治】补肾活血，强筋壮骨。用于骨痿（骨质疏松）引起的骨折、骨痛、骨关节炎，以及预防更年期骨质疏松。

Relieving Osteoporosis Soluble Granules

Name of Chinese Phonetic Alphabet Gu Song Bao Ke Li

Formula Epimedii Folium, Dipsaci Radix, Paeoniae Radix Rubra, Chuanxiong Rhizoma, Anemarrhenae Rhizoma, Curcumae Rhizoma, Sparganii Rhizoma, Rehmanniae Radix and Ostreae Concha (calcined).

Actions and Indications Tonifying the kidney, activating blood, strengthening the sinews and bone. It is indicated for fracture, ostealgia and osteoarthritis due to bone wilting disease (osteoporosis), and also for preventing climacteric osteoporosis.

骨刺丸

【处方】制川乌、制草乌、天南星（制）、秦艽、白芷、当归、甘草、薏苡仁（炒）、穿山龙、绵萆薢、红花、徐长卿。

【功能主治】祛风止痛。用于骨质增生，风湿性关节炎，风湿痛。

【注意】肾病患者慎用。

Relieving Bony Spur Bolus

Name of Chinese Phonetic Alphabet Gu Ci Wan

Formula Aconiti Radix Cocta, Aconiti Kusnezoffii Radix Cocta, Arisaematis Rhizoma (prepared), Gentianae Macrophyllae Radix, Angelicae Dahuricae Radix, Angelicae Sinensis Radix, Glycyrrhizae Radix et Rhizoma, Coicis Semen (fried), Dioscoreae Nipponicae Rhizoma, Dioscoreae Spongiosae Rhizoma, Carthami Flos and Cynanchi Paniculati Radix et Rhizoma.

Actions and Indications Dispelling wind and alleviating pain. It is indicated for hyperosteogeny, rheumatic arthritis, rheumatalgia.

Warning It should be used carefully for cases with nephrosis.

骨刺平片

【处方】黄精、独活、威灵仙、鸡血藤 、骨碎补、熟地黄、两面针、川乌（制）、锁阳、狗脊、枸杞子、莱菔子。

【功能主治】补精壮髓，壮筋健骨，通络止痛。用于骨质增生（包括肥大性腰椎炎，颈椎综合征，四肢骨节增生）。

Relieving Bony Spur Tablet

Name of Chinese Phonetic Alphabet Gu Ci Ping Pian

Formula Polygonati Rhizoma, Angelicae Pubescentis Radix, Clematidis Radix et Rhizoma, Spatholobi Caulis, Drynariae Rhizoma, Rehmanniae

Radix Praeparata, Zanthoxyli Radix, Aconiti Radix (prepared), Cynomorii Caulis Carnosus, Cibotii Rhizoma, Lycii Fructus and Raphani Semen.

Actions and Indications Tonifying vital essence and marrow, strengthening the sinews and bone, activating collaterals and alleviating pain. It is indicated for hyperosteogeny (including hypertrophic lumbar vertebrae, cervical syndrome and joints hyperosteogeny of limbs).

骨刺宁胶囊

【处方】威灵仙、急性子、山楂、砂仁、白芷、红花、乌梅。

【功能主治】活血通络，消瘀定痛。用于骨刺，风寒湿痹所引起的疼痛及四肢麻木。

【注意】孕妇慎用。

Relieving Bony Spur Capsule

Name of Chinese Phonetic Alphabet Gu Ci Ning Jiao Nang

Formula Clematidis Radix et Rhizoma, Impatientis Semen, Crataegi Fructus, Amomi Fructus, Angelicae Dahuricae Radix, Carthami Flos and Mume Fructus.

Actions and Indications Activating blood and collaterals, eliminating static blood and alleviating pain. It is indicated for bony spur, pain and numbness of the limbs due to wind-cold-damp impediment.

Warning It should be used carefully for pregnant women.

骨刺消痛涂膜液

【处方】本品为制川乌、威灵仙、乌梅、桂枝、木瓜、牛膝等药经加工制成的涂膜剂。

【功能主治】祛风通络，活血止痛。用于颈椎、腰椎、四肢关节骨质增生引起的肿胀、麻木、疼痛、活动受限。

Relieving Bony Spur Pigment

Name of Chinese Phonetic Alphabet Gu Ci Xiao Tong Tu Mo Ye

Formula Aconiti Radix Cocta, Clematidis Radix et Rhizoma, Mume Fructus, Cinnamomi Ramulus, Chaenomelis Fructus, Achyranthis Bidentatae Radix, etc.

Actions and Indications Dispelling wind and dredging collaterals, activating blood and alleviating pain. It is indicated for swelling, numbness, pain and immobility due to hyperosteogeny of the cervical vertebrae, lumbar vertebrae, joints of limbs.

骨增生镇痛膏

【处方】红花、骨碎补、川芎、当归尾、细辛、猪牙皂、羌活、生川乌、栀子、生草乌、独活、生天南星、姜黄、芥子、干姜、生半夏、樟脑、桉油、雄黄。

【功能主治】温经通络，祛风除湿，消瘀止痛。用于各种骨增生性关节炎，亦可用于风湿性关节炎。

【注意】若出现皮疹等过敏反应则暂停使用。

Analgesic Plaster for Arthritis of Hyperosteogeny

Name of Chinese Phonetic Alphabet Gu Zeng Sheng Zhen Tong Gao

Formula Carthami Flos, Drynariae Rhizoma, Chuanxiong Rhizoma. Angelicae Sinensis Radix (tail part), Asari Radix et Rhizoma, Gleditsiae Fructus Abnormalis, Notopterygii Rhizoma et Radix, Aconiti Radix (fresh), Gardeniae Fructus, Aconiti Kusnezoffii Radix (fresh), Angelicae Pubescentis Radix, Arisaematis Rhizoma (fresh), Curcumae Rhizoma Longae, Sinapis Semen, Zingiberis Rhizoma, Pinelliae Rhizoma (fresh), Camphora, Eucalypti Oleum and Realgar.

Actions and Indications Warming meridians, dredging collaterals, dispelling wind and dampness, dispersing stasis, alleviating pain. It is used for arthritis of hyperosteogeny, rheumatic arthritis.

Warning In case of allergy with erythra, suspend the medication.

秋燥感冒冲剂

【处方】桑叶、北沙参、竹叶、前胡、桔梗、伊贝母、麦冬、苦杏仁（炒）、甘草、山豆根、菊花。

【功能主治】清燥退热，润肺止咳。用于感冒病秋燥证症见恶寒发热，鼻咽口唇干燥，干咳少痰，舌边尖红，苔薄白而干或薄黄少津。

【注意】忌食辛辣厚味。

Autumn Common Cold Soluble Granules

Name of Chinese Phonetic Alphabet Qiu Zao Gan Mao Chong Ji

Formula Mori Folium, Glehniae Radix, Phyllostachydis Henonis Folium, Peucedani Radix, Platycodonis Radix, Fritillariae Pallidiflorae Bulbus, Ophiopogonis Radix, Armeniacae Semen Amarum (fried), Glycyrrhizae Radix et Rhizoma, Sophorae Tonkinensis Radix et Rhizoma and Chrysanthemi Flos.

Actions and Indications Clearing dryness, abatement of fever, moistening the lung to relieve cough. It is indicated for common cold of autumn-dryness syndrome manifested as aversion to cold, fever, dry lips, mouth and throat, dry cough, few productive, red tip and margin of tongue, dry tongue with thin and white tongue fur or thin and yellow tongue fur and few fluid of tongue.

Warning Pungent foods and greasy diet should be avoided.

复方三七口服液

【处方】三七（鲜）、黄芪、人参、葛根。

【功能主治】抗衰，扶正培本，益气强心，健脾固本，滋阴润燥，生津止渴；并有提高机体免疫力，升高白细胞和血红蛋白的作用。用于神倦乏力，气短心悸，阴虚津少，口干舌燥；也用于肿瘤病人虚衰及放疗、化疗手术后出现的一切虚证。

Compound *Sanchi** Oral Liquid for Reinforcing *Qi*

Name of Chinese Phonetic Alphabet Fu Fang San Qi Kou Fu Ye

Formula Notoginseng Radix et Rhizoma (fresh), Astragali Radix, Ginseng Radix et Rhizoma and Puerariae Lobatae Radix.

Actions and Indications Counteracting debility, reinforcing the healthy *qi* and securing body resistence, tonifying *qi* and strengthening the heart, fortifying the spleen, nourishing *yin* and moistening dryness, engendering fluid and quenching thirst, enhancing the immunity, increasing leukocyte and hemoglobin. It is used for fatigue, shortness of breath and palpitation, shortage of fluid, dry mouth and tongue. And also used for deficient patients after radiotherapy, chemotherapy and operation treatments.

*三七

复方大青叶合剂

【处方】大青叶、金银花、羌活、拳参、大黄。

【功能主治】疏风清热，解毒消肿，凉血利胆。用于感冒发热头痛，咽喉红肿，耳下肿痛，胁痛黄疸及流感、腮腺炎，急性病毒性肝炎见上述症状者。

Compound Woad* Mixture for Clearing Heat

Name of Chinese Phonetic Alphabet Fu Fang Da Qing Ye He Ji

Formula Isatidis Folium, Lonicerae Japonicae Flos, Notopterygii Rhizoma et Radix, Bistortae Rhizoma and Rhei Radix et Rhizoma.

Actions and Indications Dispersing wind and clearing heat, detoxicating and dispersing swelling, cooling blood and soothing the gallbladder. It is indicated for common cold, fever, headache, sore-throat, ear pain, hypochondriac pain, jaundice and influenza, parotitis acute viral hepatitis.

*大青叶

复方川贝精片

【处方】麻黄浸膏、五味子（醋炙）、川贝母、远志（去心，甘草炙）、陈皮、法半夏、桔梗、甘草浸膏。

【功能主治】化痰止咳，宣肺平喘。用于痰涎阻肺，肺失宣降所致的急、慢性支气管炎，支气管扩张，咳嗽，痰喘。

【注意】高血压症、心脏病、冠状动脉硬化患者忌服；孕妇慎用。

Compound Sichuan Fritillary* Tablet for Alleviating Bronchitis

Name of Chinese Phonetic Alphabet Fu Fang Chuan Bei Jing Pian

Formula Ephedrae Extractum, Schisandrae Chinensis Fructus (prepared with vinegar), Fritillariae Cirrhosae Bulbus, Polygalae Radix (removed core and prepared with licorice root), Citri Reticulatae Pericarpium, Pinelliae Rhizoma Praeparatum, Platycodonis Radix and Glycyrrhizae Extractum.

Actions and Indications Resolving phlegm and alleviating cough, diffusing the lung and calming dyspnea. It is indicated for acute, chronic bronchitis, bronchiectasis, cough and phlegm dyspnea due to stagnation of phlegm in the lung, and the lung failing in purification.

Warning It is contraindicated for cases with hypertension, heart diseases, coronary arteriosclerosis, and should be used carefully for pregnant women.

* 川贝母

复方天仙胶囊

【处方】天花粉、威灵仙、白花蛇舌草、人工牛黄、龙葵、胆南星、乳香（制）、没药、人参、黄芪、珍珠（制）、猪苓、蛇蜕、冰片、麝香等。

【功能主治】清热解毒，活血化瘀，散结止痛。对食道癌、胃癌有一定的抑制作用。

【注意】孕妇忌服；忌凉、硬、腥、辣食物；不宜与洋地黄类药物同用。

Compound Trichosanthes Root* and Chinese Clematis** Capsule

Name of Chinese Phonetic Alphabet Fu Fang Tian Xian Jiao Nang

Formula Trichosanthis Radix, Clematidis Radix et Rhizoma, Hedyotis Diffusae Herba, Bovis Calculus Artifactus, Solani Nigri Herba, Arisaema cum Bile, Olibanum (prepared), Myrrha, Ginseng Radix et Rhizoma, Astragali Radix, Margarita (prepared), Polyporus, Serpentis Periostracum, Borneolum Syntheticum, Moschus, etc.

Actions and Indications Clearing heat, detoxifying, activating blood, resolving stasis, dissipating mass, alleviating pain. It is used as a supplemental treatment for inhibiting carcinoma of esophagus and gastric carcinoma.

Warning It is contraindicated for pregnant women; incompatible with digitalis preparation; the cool, hard, pungent and fishy foods should be avoided.

* 天花粉 ** 威灵仙

复方木鸡冲剂

【处方】云芝提取物、山豆根、菟丝子、核桃、楸皮。

【功能主治】具有抑制甲胎蛋白升高的作用。用于肝炎，肝硬化，肝癌。

Compound *Muji* Soluble Granules

Name of Chinese Phonetic Alphabet Fu Fang Mu Ji Chong Ji

Formula Corioli Extractum, Sophorae Tonkinensis Radix et Rhizoma, Cuscutae Semen and Juglandis Mandshuricae Cortex.

Actions and Indications The preparation can inhibit the raise of alpha-fetoprotein. It is used for hepatitis, cirrhosis and liver cancer.

复方牛黄清胃丸

【处方】大黄、牵牛子（炒）、栀子（姜炙）、石膏、芒硝、黄芩、黄连、连翘、山楂（炒）、陈皮、厚朴（姜炙）、枳实、香附、猪牙皂、荆芥穗、薄荷、防风、菊花、白芷、桔梗、玄参、甘草、牛黄、冰片。

【功能主治】清热通便。用于胃肠实热引起的口舌生疮，牙龈肿痛，大便秘结，小便短赤。

Compond Bezoar* Pill for Clearing Stomach-fire

Name of Chinese Phonetic Alphabet Fu Fang Niu Huang Qing Wei Wan

Formula Rhei Radix et Rhizoma, Pharbitidis Semen (fried), Gardeniae Fructus (prepared with ginger), Gypsum Fibrosum, Natrii Sulfas, Scutellariae Radix, Coptidis Rhizoma, Forsythiae Fructus, Crataegi Fructus (fried), Citri Reticulatae Pericarpium, Magnoliae Officinalis Cortex (prepared with ginger), Aurantii Fructus Immaturus, Cyperi Rhizoma, Gleditsiae Fructus Abnormalis, Schizonepetae Spica, Menthae Haplocalycis Herba, Saposhnikoviae Radix, Chrysanthemi Flos, Angelicae Dahuricae Radix, Platycodonis Radix, Scrophulariae Radix, Glycyrrhizae Radix et Rhizoma, Bovis Calculus and Borneolum Syntheticum.

Actions and Indications Clearing heat and relaxing the bowels. It is used for aphthae, gingivitis, constipation, scanty dark urine due to excess heat of the stomach and intestine.

*牛黄

复方片仔癀软膏

【处方】片仔癀粉等。

【功能主治】清热，解毒，止痛。用于病毒性、细菌性皮肤病，如带状疱疹、单纯疱疹、脓疱疮、毛囊炎、痤疮。

Compound *Pian Zai Huang** Ointment

Name of Chinese Phonetic Alphabet Fu Fang Pian Zai Huang Ruan Gao

Formula Pian Zai Huang Pulvis, etc.

Actions and Indications Clearing heat and detoxicating, relieving pain. It is used for viral and bacterial dermatosis, such as herpes zoster, herpes simplex, impetigo, folliculitis and acne.

*片仔癀

复方乌鸡口服液

【处方】乌鸡、黄芪（蜜炙）、山药、党参、白术、川芎、茯苓、当归、熟地黄、白芍（酒炒）、牡丹皮、五味子（酒制）、苯甲酸钠、蜂蜜（炼）等。

【功能主治】补气血，益肝肾。主治妇女病：气血两虚或肝肾两虚的月经不调；脾虚或肾虚带下。症见：面色皖白、五心烦热、腰酸膝软、舌红苔白或淡有齿痕、脉细缓或数者。

【注意】服药期间应少食辛辣生冷食物。属湿热等实证者慎用。

Compound Silky Chicken* Oral Liquid

Name of Chinese Phonetic Alphabet Fu Fang Wu Ji Kou Fu Ye

Formula Galli Caro cum Osse Nigro, Astragali Radix (prepared with honey), Dioscoreae Rhizoma, Codonopsis Radix, Atractylodis Macrocephalae Rhizoma, Chuanxiong Rhizoma, Poria, Angelicae Sinensis Radix, Rehmanniae Radix Praeparata, Paeoniae Radix Alba (fried with wine), Moutan Cortex, Schisandrae Chinensis Fructus (prepared with wine), Sodium Benzoate, Mel (refined), etc.

Actions and Indications Tonifying *qi* and blood, invigorating the liver and kidney. It is mainly indicated for gynecopathy such as irregular menstruation due to dual deficiency of *qi* and blood or dual deficiency of liver and kidney; white vaginal discharge due to spleen-deficiency or kidney-deficiency, and manifested as bright pale complexion, vexing heat of the chest, palms and soles, soreness of waist and weakness of kness, red tongue with white or pale and teeth-marked tongue fur, fine and moderate or rapid pulse.

Warning During medication, the pungent and uncooked foods should be limited the amount. It is carefully used for cases attributed to damp-heat syndrome.

*乌鸡

复方丹参片

【处方】丹参浸膏、三七、冰片。

【功能主治】活血化瘀，理气止痛。用于胸中憋闷，心绞痛。

Compound Redroot Sage* Tablet

Name of Chinese Phonetic Alphabet Fu Fang Dan Shen Pian

Formula Salviae Miltiorrhizae Extractum, Notoginseng Radix et Rhizoma and Borneolum Syntheticum.

Actions and Indications Activating blood and resolving stasis, regulating *qi* to alleviate pain. It is used for chest distress and angina pectoris.

*丹参

复方双花口服液

【处方】金银花、连翘、穿心莲、板蓝根。

【功能主治】清热解毒，利咽消肿。用于风热外感、风热乳蛾。症见发热，微恶风，头痛，鼻塞流涕，咽红而痛或咽喉干燥灼痛，舌边尖红苔薄黄或舌红苔黄，脉浮数或数。

【注意】忌食厚味、油腻。

Compound Honeysuckle Flower* Oral Liquid for Relieving Tonsillitis

Name of Chinese Phonetic Alphabet Fu Fang Shuang Hua Kou Fu Ye

Formula Lonicerae Japonicae Flos, Forsythiae Fructus, Andrographis Herba and Isatidis Radix.

Actions and Indications Clearing heat and detoxicating, soothing the throat and dispersing swelling. It is indicated for tonsillitis, manifested as fever, slight aversion to cold, headache, stuffy nose, rhinorrhea, sore-throat, dry throat, red in the tip and margin of the tongue, thin yellow or yellow fur, floating and rapid or rapid pulse.

Warning Pungent and oily foods are prohibited.

*金银花

复方石韦片

【处方】石韦、黄芪、苦参、萹蓄。

【功能主治】清热燥湿，利尿通淋。用于小便不利，尿频，尿急，尿痛，下肢浮肿；也可用于急、慢性肾小球肾炎、肾盂肾炎、膀胱炎、尿道炎见有上述症状者。

Compound Pyrrosia* Tablet for Relieving Strangury

Name of Chinese Phonetic Alphabet Fu Fang Shi Wei Pian

Formula Pyrrosiae Folium, Astragali Radix, Sophorae Flavescentis Radix and Polygoni Avicularis Herba.

Actions and Indications Clearing heat and drying dampness, inducing urine and relieving strangury. It is indicated for difficult urination, frequent urination, urgent urination, urodynia, edema of the lower limbs; also for acute, chronic glomerulonephritis, pyelonephritis, cystitis and urethritis with the above mentioned symptoms.

*石韦

复方田七胃痛胶囊

【处方】三七、延胡索、香附、吴茱萸、瓦楞子、枯矾、甘草、白芍、白及、川楝子、氧化镁、碳酸氢钠、颠茄流浸膏。

【功能主治】制酸止痛，理气化瘀，温中健脾，收敛止血。用于胃酸过多，胃脘痛，胃溃疡，十二指肠球部溃疡及慢性胃炎。

Compound *Sanchi** Capsule for Stomach Pain

Name of Chinese Phonetic Alphabet Fu Fang Tian Qi Wei Tong Jiao Nang

Formula Notoginseng Radix et Rhizoma, Corydalis Rhizoma, Cyperi Rhizoma, Fructus Euodiae, Arcae Concha, Alumen Usta, Glycyrrhizae Radix et Rhizoma, Paeoniae Radix Alba, Bletillae

Rhizoma, Toosendan Fructus, Magnesium Oxide, Sodium Hydrogen Carbonate and Belladonnae Extractum.

Actions and Indications Inhibiting acidity, alleviating pain, regulating *qi*, resolving blood-stasis, warming the middle, fortifying the spleen, relieving bleeding. It is indicated for gastroxia, pain of stomach duct, gastric ulcer, duodenal bulbar ulcer and chronic gastritis.

*三七

复方百部止咳糖浆

【处方】百部(蜜炙)、苦杏仁、桔梗、桑白皮、麦冬、知母、黄芩、陈皮、甘草、天南星(制)、枳壳(炒)。

【功能主治】清肺止咳。用于肺热咳嗽,痰黄黏稠,百日咳。

Compound Sessile Stemona* Syrup for Alleviating Cough

Name of Chinese Phonetic Alphabet Fu Fang Bai Bu Zhi Ke Tang Jiang

Formula Stemonae Radix (prepared with honey), Armeniacae Semen Amarum, Platycodonis Radix, Mori Cortex, Ophiopogonis Radix, Anemarrhenae Rhizoma, Scutellariae Radix, Citri Reticulatae Pericarpium, Glycyrrhizae Radix et Rhizoma, Arisaematis Rhizoma (prepared) and Aurantii Fructus (fried).

Actions and Indications Clearing lung-heat and alleviating cough. It is indicated for cough due to lung-heat; yellow, sticky and thick phlegm and pertussis.

*百部

复方羊角片

【处方】羊角、川芎、白芷、制川乌。

【功能主治】平肝,镇痛。用于偏头痛,血管性头痛,紧张性头痛及神经性头痛。

【注意】忌饮酒及辛辣食品。

Compound Goat Horn* Tablet

Name of Chinese Phonetic Alphabet Fu Fang Yang Jiao Pian

Formula Caprinus Cornu, Chuanxiong Rhizoma, Angelicae Dahuricae Radix and Aconiti Radix Cocta.

Actions and Indications Pacifying the liver, alleviating pain. It is indicated for migraine, vascular headache, tension headache and nervous headache.

Warning Wine and pungent foods should be avoided.

*羊角

复方红根草片

【处方】红根草、鱼腥草、金银花、野菊花、穿心莲。

【功能主治】清热解毒。用于急性咽喉炎、扁桃体炎、肠炎、痢疾。

Compound Clethra Loosetrife* Tablet

Name of Chinese Phonetic Alphabet Fu Fang Hong Gen Cao Pian

Formula Lysimachiae Clethroidis Radix seu Herba, Houttuyniae Herba, Lonicerae Japonicae Flos, Chrysanthemi Indici Flos and Andrographis Herba.

Actions and Indications Clearing heat and detoxicating. It is indicated for acute laryngopharyngitis, tonsillitis, enteritis, dysentery.

*红根草

复方芦荟胶囊

【处方】芦荟、青黛、朱砂、琥珀。

【功能主治】调肝益肾,清热润肠,宁心安神。用于习惯性便秘,大便燥结或因大便数日不通引起的腹胀、腹痛。

【注意】肾功能不全者慎用。

Compound Cape Aloe* Capsule for

Constipation

Name of Chinese Phonetic Alphabet Fu Fang Lu Hui Jiao Nang

Formula Aloe, Indigo Naturalis, Cinnabaris and Succinum.

Actions and Indications Regulating the liver and tonifying the kidney, clearing heat and moistening the intestine, tranquilizing the mind. It is indicated for habitual constipation, dry stools or abdominal distention and pain due to constipation.

Warning It should be used carefully for cases with renal insufficiency.

* 芦荟

复方扶芳藤合剂

【处方】扶芳藤、黄芪、人参。

【功能主治】益气补血，健脾养心。用于气血不足，心脾两虚，症见气短胸闷，少气懒言，神疲乏力，自汗，心悸健忘，失眠多梦，面色不华，脘腹胀满，大便溏软，舌淡胖或有齿痕，脉细弱，以及神经衰弱、白细胞减少症见上述证候者。

【注意】周岁以内婴儿禁服。外感发热病人忌服。

Compound Mixture of Climbing Euonymus*

Name of Chinese Phonetic Alphabet Fu Fang Fu Fang Teng He Ji

Formula Euonymi Fortunei Caulis seu Folium, Astragali Radix and Ginseng Radix et Rhizoma.

Actions and Indications Tonifying *qi* and blood, fortifying the spleen and nourishing the heart blood. It is indicated for insufficiency of *qi* and blood, and dual deficiency of the heart and spleen marked by shortness of breath, oppression in the chest, shortage of *qi* with indolent speaking, lassitude of spirit, fatigue, spontaneous sweating, palpitation, amnesia, insomnia, profuse dreaming, pale complexion, abdominal fullness and distention, sloppy stool, pale and enlarged tongue or tooth-marks tongue, fine and weak pulse. And also used for neurasthenia and leukopenia with above mentioned symptoms.

Warning It is contraindicated for children under one year of age and cases with fever due to external contraction.

* 扶芳藤

复方皂矾丸

【处方】皂矾、西洋参、海马、肉桂 、大枣、核桃仁。

【功能主治】温肾健髓，益气养阴，生血止血。用于再生障碍性贫血症，白细胞减少症、血小板减少症，骨髓增生异常综合征及放疗和化疗引起的骨髓损伤、血细胞减少，属肾阳不足，气血两虚证者。

【注意】忌茶水。

Compound Melanterite* Pill

Name of Chinese Phonetic Alphabet Fu Fang Zao Fan Wan

Formula Malanteritum, Panacis Quinquefolii Radix, Hyppocampus, Cinnamomi Cortex, Jujubae Fructus and Juglandis Semen .

Actions and Indications Warming the kidney and invigorating the marrow, tonifying *qi* and nourishing *yin*, engendering blood and relieving bleeding. It is indicated for aplastic anemia, leukopenia, thrombopenia, myelodysplastic syndrome and marrow injury and cytopenia due to radiotherapy and chemotherapy attributed to insufficiency of kidney-*yang* and dual deficiency of *qi* and blood.

Warning During medication, drinking tea is prohibited.

* 皂矾

复方阿胶浆

【处方】阿胶、人参 、熟地黄、党参、山楂。

【功能主治】补气养血。用于气血两虚，头晕目眩，心悸失眠，食欲不振及白细胞减少症和贫血。

Compound Syrup of Ass-hide Gelatin*

Name of Chinese Phonetic Alphabet Fu Fang E Jiao Jiang

Formula Asini Corii Colla, Ginseng Radix et Rhizoma, Rehmanniae Radix Praeparata, Codonopsis Radix and Crataegi Fructus.

Actions and Indications Tonifying *qi* and blood. It is indicated for dual deficiency of *qi* and blood manifested as dizziness, dizzy vision, palpitation, insomnia, poor appetite, leukopenia and anemia.

* 阿胶

复方陈香胃片

【处方】陈皮、木香、石菖蒲、大黄、碳酸氢钠、重质碳酸镁、氢氧化铝。

【功能主治】行气和胃，制酸止痛。用于气滞型胃脘疼痛、脘腹痞满、嗳气吞酸，胃及十二指肠溃疡、慢性胃炎见上述症状属气滞证者。

Compound Tablet of Mandarin Orange Peel* and Common Aucklandia**

Name of Chinese Phonetic Alphabet Fu Fang Chen Xiang Wei Pian

Formula Citri Reticulatae Pericarpium, Aucklandiae Radix, Acori Tatarinowii Rhizoma, Rhei Radix et Rhizoma, Sodium Hydrogen Carbonate, Magnesium Bicarbonate and Aluminum Hydroxide.

Actions and Indications Moving *qi*, harmonizing the stomach, inhibiting acidity to alleviate pain. It is used for pain in stomach duct, abdominal fullness, eructation and acid regurgitation due to stagnation of *qi*. It also used for gastroduodenal ulcer and chronic gastritis attributed to *qi*-stagnation syndrome.

* 陈皮 ** 木香

复方青黛丸

【处方】青黛、乌梅、蒲公英、紫草、白芷、丹参、白鲜皮、绵马贯众、土茯苓、马齿苋、绵萆薢、山楂（焦）、五味子（酒）等。

【功能主治】清热解毒，消斑化瘀，祛风止痒。用于进行期银屑病，玫瑰糠疹，药疹。

Compound Indigo* Pill for Eliminating Rash

Name of Chinese Phonetic Alphabet Fu Fang Qing Dai Wan

Formula Indigo Naturalis, Mume Fructus, Taraxaci Herba, Arnebiae Radix, Angelicae Dahuricae Radix, Salviae Miltiorrhizae Radix et Rhizoma, Dictamni Cortex, Dryopteridis Crassirhizomatis Rhizoma, Smilacis Glabrae Rhizoma, Portulacae Herba, Dioscoreae Spongiosae Rhizoma, Crataegi Fructus (charred), Schisandrae Chinensis Fructus (prepared with wine), etc.

Actions and Indications Clearing heat and detoxicating, eliminating macula, resolving stasis, dispelling wind and relieving itching. It is indicated for active stage of psoriasis, pityriasis rosea and drug rashcs.

* 青黛

复方苦参肠炎康片

【处方】苦参、黄连、白芍等。

【功能主治】清热燥湿止泻。用于泄泻。症见泄泻急迫、肛门灼热感、腹痛、小便短赤，以及急性肠炎见于以上症候者。

Compound Shrubby Sophora* Tablet for Relieving Enteritis

Name of Chinese Phonetic Alphabet Fu Fang Ku Shen Chang Yan Kang Pian

Formula Sophorae Flavescentis Radix, Coptidis Rhizoma, Paeoniae Radix Alba, etc.

Actions and Indications Clearing heat, drying dampness and relieving diarrhea. It is indicated for diarrhea manifested as urgent diarrhea, scorching heat of the anus, abdominal pain, scanty dark urine and acute enteritis with the above mentioned symptoms.

＊苦参

复方苦参注射液

【处方】苦参、白土苓。

【功能主治】清热利湿，凉血解毒，散结止痛。用于癌性疼痛的出血。

Injection of Compound Shrubby Sophora★

Name of Chinese Phonetic Alphabet Fu Fang Ku Shen Zhu She Ye

Formula Sophorae Flavescentis Radix and Smilacis Opacae Rhizoma.

Actions and Indications Clearing heat and draining dampness, cooling blood and detoxicating, dispersing mass and alleviating pain. It is indicated for bleeding of carcinomatous pain.

＊苦参

复方虎杖烧伤油

【处方】虎杖、冰片。

【功能主治】清热解毒、敛疮止痛。用于各种热源及化学物质所致的体表皮肤有红肿热痛表现的I度烧烫伤。

【注意】忌食辛辣食物。

Compound Bushy Knotweed★ Oils for Burn

Name of Chinese Phonetic Alphabet Fu Fang Hu Zhang Shao Shang You

Formula Polygoni Cuspidati Rhizoma et Radix and Borneolum Syntheticum.

Actions and Indications Clearing heat and detoxicating, astringing sore and relieving pain. It is used for first-degree burn or scald with swelling and pain due to various dermal damages by heat origins and chemical substances.

Warning Pungent foods should be avoided.

＊虎杖

复方罗布麻冲剂

【处方】罗布麻叶、菊花、山楂。

【功能主治】清热，平肝，安神。用于高血压、神经衰弱引起的头晕，心悸，失眠。

Compound Dogbane★ Soluble Granules

Name of Chinese Phonetic Alphabet Fu Fang Luo Bu Ma Chong Ji

Formula Apocyni Veneti Folium, Chrysanthemi Flos and Crataegi Fructus.

Actions and Indications Clearing heat, pacifying the liver, tranquilizing the mind. It is used for hypertension, dizziness, palpitation and insomnia due to neurasthenia.

＊罗布麻

复方金钱草冲剂

【处方】广金钱草、车前草、石韦、玉米须。

【功能主治】清热祛湿，利尿排石，消炎止痛。用于泌尿系结石、尿路感染属湿热下注证者。

Compound Snowbellleaf Tickclover★ Soluble Granules

Name of Chinese Phonetic Alphabet Fu Fang Jin Qian Cao Chong Ji

Formula Desmodii Styracifolii Herba, Plantaginis Herba, Pyrrosiae Folium and Zeae Maydis Stylus.

Actions and Indications Clearing heat and dispelling dampness, inducing diuresis and removing stone, antiphlogistic and alleviating pain. It is indicated for stone of the urinary system, urinary tract infection attributive to downward attack of damp-heat.

＊广金钱草

复方鱼腥草片

【处方】鱼腥草、黄芩、板蓝根、连翘、金银花。

【功能主治】清热解毒。用于风热引起咽喉疼痛，扁桃体炎。

Compound Fishword* Tablet for Tonsillitis

Name of Chinese Phonetic Alphabet Fu Fang Yu Xing Cao Pian

Formula Houttuyniae Herba, Scutellariae Radix, Isatidis Radix, Forsythiae Fructus and Lonicerae Japonicae Flos.

Actions and Indications Clearing heat and detoxicating. It is used for sore-throat, tonsillitis due to exogenous wind-heat.

* 鱼腥草

复方炉甘石外用散

【处方】炉甘石、血竭、铜绿、乳香、自然铜、紫草、朱砂、冰片等。

【功能主治】有消炎止痛、收敛止痒、促进伤口愈合的作用。用于皮肤及伤口感染，渗出型湿疹，体表慢性顽固性溃疡及烧伤、烫伤。

【注意】外用，不能用在毛发处。

Compound Smithsonite* Powder

Name of Chinese Phonetic Alphabet Fu Fang Lu Gan Shi Wai Yong San

Formula Calamina, Draconis Sanguis, Aeruginosum, Olibanum, Pyritum, Arnebiae Radix, Cinnabaris, Borneolum Syntheticum, etc.

Actions and Indications Counteracting inflammation and relieving pain, astringing and relieving itching, promoting wound healing. It is used for skin and wound infection, exudative eczema, chronic and obstinate ulcer of the body surface, burn and scald.

Warning The preparation is for external use only and should not be used on hair region.

* 炉甘石

复方珍珠暗疮片

【处方】珍珠层粉、羚羊角粉、北沙参、赤芍、黄芩、水牛角浓缩粉等。

【功能主治】清热解毒，凉血。用于消除青年脸部痤疮（俗称暗疮）及皮肤湿疹、皮炎。

Compound Pearl* Tablet for Eliminating Acne

Name of Chinese Phonetic Alphabet Fu Fang Zhen Zhu An Chuang Pian

Formula Margaritae Concha Strati Pulvis, Saigae Tataricae Corun Pulvis, Glehniae Radix, Paeoniae Radix Rubra, Scutellariae Radix, Bubali Cornu Pulvis Concentratio, etc.

Actions and Indications Clearing heat and detoxicating, cooling blood. It is used for eliminating acne, eczema and dermatitis.

* 珍珠

复方春砂冲剂

【处方】砂仁叶油、化橘红、白术、枳壳。

【功能主治】行气温中，健脾开胃，止痛消胀。用于脾胃虚寒引起的胃脘痛和消化不良。

Compound Villous Amomum Leaf* Soluble Granules for Promoting Digestion

Name of Chinese Phonetic Alphabet Fu Fang Chun Sha Chong Ji

Formula Amomi Folium Oleum , Citri Grandis Exocarpium, Atractylodis Macrocephalae Rhizoma and Aurantii Fructus.

Actions and Indications Moving *qi* and warming the middle, fortifying the spleen and improving appetite, relieving pain and dispersing distention. It is indicated for stomach duct pain and indigestion due to dual deficiency-cold of the spleen and stomach.

* 砂仁叶

复方荆芥熏洗剂

【处方】荆芥、防风、透骨草、生川乌、虾蟆草、生草乌、苦参。

【功能主治】祛风燥湿，消肿止痛。用于外痔，混合痔，内痔脱垂嵌顿，肛裂，肛周脓肿，肛瘘急性发作。

Compound Fineleaf Schizonepeta* Fumigant for Hemorrhoid

Name of Chinese Phonetic Alphabet Fu Fang Jing Jie Xun Xi Ji

Formula Schizonepetae Herba, Saposhnikoviae Radix, Speranskiae Tuberculatae Herba, Aconiti Radix (raw), Plantaginis Herba, Aconiti Kusnezoffii Radix (raw) and Sophorae Flavescentis Radix.

Actions and Indications Dispelling wind and drying dampness, dispersing swelling and alleviating pain. It is indicated for external hemorrhoid, mixed hemorrhoid, collapsed and incarceration of internal hemorrhoid, anal fissure, perianal abscess and acute attack of anal fistula.

* 荆芥

复方南板蓝根冲剂

【处方】南板蓝根、紫花地丁、蒲公英。

【功能主治】消炎解毒。用于腮腺炎、咽炎、乳腺炎、疮疖肿痛。

Compound Soluble Granules of Common Baphicacanthus*

Name of Chinese Phonetic Alphabet Fu Fang Nan Ban Lan Gen Chong Ji

Formula Baphicacanthis Cusiae Rhizoma et Radix, Violae Herba and Taraxaci Herba.

Actions and Indications Counteracting inflammation and detoxicating. It is indicated for parotitis, pharyngitis, mastitis, abscess and deep-rooted boil.

* 南板蓝根

复方南星止痛膏

【处方】生天南星、生首乌、丁香、肉桂、白芷、细辛、川芎、徐长卿等。

【功能主治】散寒除湿、活血止痛。用于骨性关节炎属寒湿瘀阻证，症见关节疼痛、肿胀、功能障碍，遇寒加重，舌质暗淡或瘀斑。

【注意】本品为外用药品，不宜长期使用。

Compound Jackinthepulpit* Plaster for Relieving Osteoarthritis

Name of Chinese Phonetic Alphabet Fu Fang Nan Xing Zhi Tong Gao

Formula Arisaematis Rhizoma (raw), Polygoni Multiflori Radix (raw), Caryophylli Flos, Cinnamomi Cortex, Angelicae Dahuricae Radix, Asari Radix et Rhizoma, Chuanxiong Rhizoma, Cynanchi Paniculati Radix et Rhizoma, etc.

Actions and Indications Dissipating cold and dampness, activating blood and alleviating pain. It is indicated for osteoarthritis attributive to cold-damp stasis syndrome, manifested as pain, swelling and dysfunction, aggravation when cold, dark or ecchymoses on the tongue.

Warning It is only for external use, and long-term use is prohibited.

* 天南星

复方草珊瑚含片

【处方】草珊瑚浸膏、薄荷脑、薄荷油。

【功能主治】疏风清热，消肿止痛，清利咽喉。用于治疗外感风热所致的风热型急性咽喉炎。

Compound Glabrous Sarcandra* Sucked Tablet

Name of Chinese Phonetic Alphabet Fu Fang Cao Shan Hu Han Pian

Formula Sarcandrae Extractum, Menthol and Menthae Haplocalycis Oleum.

Actions and Indications Dispersing wind and clearing heat, dispersing swelling and relieving pain, soothing the throat. It is indicated for acute laryngopharyngitis due to exogenous wind-heat.

* 草珊瑚

复方胆通片

【处方】溪黄草、茵陈、穿心莲、大黄等。

【功能主治】清热利胆，解痉止痛。用于急、慢性胆囊炎，胆管炎，胆囊、胆道结石并感染，胆囊术后综合征，胆道功能性疾患。

Compound Tablet for Relieving Cholecystitis

Name of Chinese Phonetic Alphabet Fu Fang Dan Tong Pian

Formula Rabdosiae Serrae Herba, Artemisiae Scopariae Herba, Andrographis Herba, Rhei Radix et Rhizoma, etc.

Actions and Indications Clearing heat and draining bile, relieving spasm to alleviate pain. It is indicated for acute, chronic cholecystitis, cholangitis, cholelithiasis and biliary calculi accompanied with infection, syndrome after operation of the gallbladder, functional diseases on biliary tract.

复方夏天无片

【处方】夏天无、夏天无总碱、制草乌、豨莶草、鸡血藤、鸡矢藤、威灵仙、广防己、五加皮、羌活、独活、秦艽、蕲蛇、麻黄、防风、全蝎、僵蚕、马钱子（制）、苍术、乳香（制）、没药（制）、木香、川芎、丹参、当归、三七、骨碎补、赤芍、山楂叶、麝香、冰片、牛膝等。

【功能主治】驱风逐湿，舒筋活络，行血止痛。用于风湿性关节肿痛，坐骨神经痛，脑血栓形成，肢体麻木，屈伸不灵，步履艰难及小儿麻痹后遗症。

【注意】感冒发热者勿服。

Compound Bending Corydalis* Tablet for Rheumatic Arthralgia

Name of Chinese Phonetic Alphabet Fu Fang Xia Tian Wu Pian

Formula Corydalis Decumbentis Rhizoma, Total Decumbensine Alkaloids, Aconiti Kusnezoffii Radix Cocta, Siegesbeckiae Herba, Spatholobi Caulis, Paederiae Scandentis Herba et Radix, Clematidis Radix et Rhizoma, Aristolochiae Fangchi Radix, Acanthopanacis Cortex, Notopterygii Rhizoma et Radix, Angelicae Pubescentis Radix, Gentianae Macrophyllae Radix, Agkistrodon, Ephedrae Herba, Saposhnikoviae Radix, Scorpio, Bombyx Batryticatus, Strychni Semen (prepared), Atractylodis Rhizoma, Olibanum (prepared), Myrrha (prepared), Aucklandiae Radix, Chuanxiong Rhizoma, Salviae Miltiorrhizae Radix et Rhizoma, Angelicae Sinensis Radix, Notoginseng Radix et Rhizoma, Drynariae Rhizoma, Paeoniae Radix Rubra, Crataegi Folium, Moschus, Borneolum Syntheticum, Achyranthis Bidentatae Radix, etc.

Actions and Indications Dispelling wind and dampness, relaxing sinews and activating collaterals, moving blood and alleviating pain. It is indicated for rheumatic arthralgia, sciatica, cerebral thrombosis, numbness of the limbs, immobility of the limbs, difficulty for walk and sequelae of poliomyelitis.

Warning It is contraindicated for cases with common cold and fever.

* 夏天无

复方益母口服液

【处方】益母草、当归、川芎、木香。

【功能主治】活血行气，化瘀止痛。用于气滞血瘀所致的痛经。症见月经期小腹胀痛拒按，经血不畅，血色紫黯成块，乳房胀痛，腰部酸痛。

【注意】孕妇及月经过多者忌服。

Compound Chinese Motherwort* Oral Liquid

Name of Chinese Phonetic Alphabet Fu Fang Yi Mu Kou Fu Ye

Formula Leonuri Herba, Angelicae Sinensis Radix, Chuanxiong Rhizoma and Aucklandiae Radix.

Actions and Indications Activating blood, promoting *qi* moving, resolving stasis, alleviating pain. It is indicated for dysmenorrhea manifested as fullness, pain and tenderness in lower abdomen, purple, dark and clotted menstrual blood, distending pain in breast, soreness and pain of waist due to *qi*-stagnation and blood-stasis.

Warning It is contraindicated for pregnant women and hypermenorrhea.

*益母草

复方益母草膏

【处方】鲜益母草、当归、川芎、红花、白芍、地黄。

【功能主治】调经活血，散瘀止痛。用于经血不调，经闭经少，腰酸腹痛，产后血晕，胞衣不下。

【注意】孕妇忌服。

Compound Chinese Motherwort* Liquid Extract

Name of Chinese Phonetic Alphabet Fu Fang Yi Mu Cao Gao

Formula Leonuri Herba (fresh sample), Angelicae Sinensis Radix, Chuanxiong Rhizoma, Carthami Flos, Paeoniae Radix Alba and Rehmanniae Radix.

Actions and Indications Regulating menstruation, activating blood, dissipating stasis, alleviating pain. It is indicated for irregular menstruation, amenorrhea, soreness of waist, abdominal pain, puerperal faint, retention of placenta.

Warning It is contraindicated for pregnant women.

*益母草

复方消食冲剂

【处方】苍术、白术、神曲茶、山楂、薏苡仁、饿蚂蝗。

【功能主治】健脾利湿，开胃导滞。用于食积不化，食欲不振，便溏消瘦。

Compound Soluble Granules for Promoting Digestion

Name of Chinese Phonetic Alphabet Fu Fang Xiao Shi Chong Ji

Formula Atractylodis Rhizoma, Atractylodis Macrocephalae Rhizoma, Medicata Massa Fermentata, Crataegi Fructus, Coicis Semen and Rhynchosiae Volubilis Herba.

Actions and Indications Fortifying the spleen and draining dampness, promoting digestion. It is used for cases with indigestion, poor appetite, sloppy stool and emaciation.

复方益肝丸

【处方】茵陈、板蓝根、龙胆、野菊花、蒲公英、山豆根、垂盆草、蝉蜕、苦杏仁、人工牛黄、夏枯草、车前子、土茯苓、胡黄连、牡丹皮、丹参、红花、大黄、香附、青皮、枳壳、槟榔、鸡内金、人参、桂枝、五味子、柴胡、炙甘草。

【功能主治】清热利湿，疏肝理脾，化瘀散结。用于慢性肝炎及急性肝炎胁肋胀痛，口干口苦，黄疸，苔黄脉弦。

【注意】勿空腹服用，孕妇禁用。

Relieving Chronic and Acute Hepatitis Pill

Name of Chinese Phonetic Alphabet Fu Fang Yi Gan Wan

Formula Artemisiae Scopariae Herba, Isatidis Radix, Gentianae Radix et Rhizoma, Chrysanthemi Indici Flos, Taraxaci Herba, Sophorae Tonkinensis Radix et Rhizoma, Herba Sedi, Cicadae Periostracum, Armeniacae Semen Amarum, Bovis Calculus Artifactus, Prunellae Spica, Plantaginis Semen, Smilacis Glabrae Rhizoma, Picrorhizae Rhizoma, Moutan Cortex, Salviae Miltiorrhizae Radix et Rhizoma, Carthami Flos, Rhei Radix et Rhizoma, Cyperi Rhizoma, Citri Reticulatae Pericarpium Viride, Aurantii Fructus, Arecae Semen, Galli Gigerii Endothelium Corneum, Ginseng Radix et Rhizoma, Cinnamomi Ramulus, Schisandrae Chinensis Fructus, Bupleuri Radix and Glycyrrhizae Radix et Rhizoma Praeparata cum Melle.

Actions and Indications Clearing heat, draining dampness, soothing the liver, regulating the spleen, resolving stasis, dissipating mass. It is indicated for chronic and acute hepatitis marked by hypochondriac fullness and pain, dry mouth, bitter taste in the mouth, jaundice, yellow tongue fur, string-like pulse.

Warning Fasting medication is prohibited. It is contraindicated for pregnant women.

复方黄芩片

【处方】黄芩、虎杖、穿心莲、十大功劳叶。

【功能主治】清热解毒，凉血消肿。用于咽喉肿痛，口舌生疮，感冒发热，大肠湿热泄泻、热淋涩痛，痈肿疮疡。

Compound Baical Skullcap* Tablet for Relieving Sore-throat

Name of Chinese Phonetic Alphabet Fu Fang Huang Qin Pian

Formula Scutellariae Radix, Polygoni Cuspidati Rhizoma et Radix, Andrographis Herba and Mahoniae Foliom.

Actions and Indications Clearing heat and detoxicating, cooling blood and dispersing swelling. It is used for sore-throat, aphthae, common cold, fever, diarrhea due to damp-heat of the large intestine; heat strangury; abscess and deep-rooted boil.

* 黄芩

复方黄连素片

【处方】盐酸小檗碱、木香、白芍、吴茱萸。

【功能主治】清热燥湿，行气，止痛，止痢止泻。用于大肠湿热，赤白下痢，里急后重或暴注下泻，肛门灼热。

Compound Tablet of Berberine

Name of Chinese Phonetic Alphabet Fu Fang Huang Lian Su Pian

Formula Berberine hydrochloride, Aucklandiae Radix, Paeoniae Radix Alba and Euodiae Fructus.

Actions and Indications Clearing heat and drying dampness, moving *qi* to alleviate pain, relieving dysentery and diarrhea. It is indicated for dysentery with bloody stool, tenesmus or sudden onset of diarrhea, scorching heat in the anus due to damp-heat in the large intestine.

复方雪莲胶囊

【处方】雪莲、延胡索(醋制)、羌活、川乌(制)、独活、草乌(制)、木瓜、香加皮。

【功能主治】温经散寒，祛风逐湿，化瘀消肿，舒筋活络。用于风寒湿邪所致类风湿性关节炎，风湿性关节炎，强直性脊柱炎和各类退行性骨关节病。

【注意】孕妇忌服。

Compound Medusa Saussurea* Capsule for Rheumatoid Arthritis

Name of Chinese Phonetic Alphabet Fu Fang Xue Lian Jiao Nang

Formula Saussureae Herba, Corydalis Rhizoma (prepared with vinegar), Notopterygii Rhizoma et Radix, Aconiti Radix (prepared), Angelicae Pubescentis Radix, Aconiti Kusnezoffii Radix (prepared), Chaenomelis Fructus and Periplocae Cortex.

Actions and Indications Warming the meridians and dissipating cold, dispelling wind and dampness, resolving stasis and dispersing swelling, relaxing sinews and activating collaterals. It is indicated for rheumatoid and rheumatic arthritis, ankylosing spondylitis and various retrograde osteoarticular disease due to wind-cold-damp.

Warning It is contraindicated for pregnant women.

* 雪莲

复方蛇胆陈皮末

【处方】蛇胆汁、朱砂、地龙、僵蚕(制)、陈皮、琥珀。

【功能主治】祛风除痰，镇惊。用于痰多咳嗽，惊风抽搐。

Compound Forest Cobra Bile* and Mandarin Orange Peel** Powder

Name of Chinese Phonetic Alphabet Fu Fang She Dan Chen Pi Mo

Formula Naja Bilis, Cinnabaris, Pheretima, Bombyx Batryticatus (prepared), Citri Reticulatae Pericarpium and Succinum.

Actions and Indications Dispelling wind and eliminating phlegm, settling fright. It is indicated for cough with profuse phlegm, convulsion and spasm.

*蛇胆 **陈皮

复方羚角降压片

【处方】羚羊角、夏枯草、黄芩、槲寄生。

【功能主治】降低血压，预防中风。用于高血压，头晕胀痛。

Compound Antelope Horn* Tablet

Name of Chinese Phonetic Alphabet Fu Fang Ling Jiao Jiang Ya Pian

Formula Saigae Tataricae Cornu, Prunellae Spica, Scutellariae Radix and Visci Herba.

Actions and Indications Lowering blood pressure, preventing apoplexy. It is indicated for hypertension and distending pain of head.

*羚羊角

复方斑蝥胶囊

【处方】斑蝥、人参、黄芪、刺五加、三棱、半枝莲、莪术、山茱萸、女贞子、熊胆粉、甘草。

【功能主治】破血消瘀，攻毒蚀疮。用于原发性肝癌，肺癌，直肠癌，恶性淋巴瘤，妇科恶性肿瘤。

Compound Large Blister Beetle* Capsule

Name of Chinese Phonetic Alphabet Fu Fang Ban Mao Jiao Nang

Formula Mylabris, Ginseng Radix et Rhizoma, Astragali Radix, Acanthopanacis Senticosi Radix et Rhizoma seu Caulis, Sparganii Rhizoma, Scutellariae Barbatae Herba, Curcumae Rhizoma, Corni Fructus, Ligustri Lucidi Fructus, Ursi Fel Pulvis and Glycyrrhizae Radix et Rhizoma.

Actions and Indications Breaking blood, dispersing stasis, detoxifying, necrosing mass. It is used for primary liver cancer, lung cancer, rectal cancer, malignant lymphoma and gynecological malignant tumor.

*斑蝥

复方满山红糖浆

【处方】满山红、百部、罂粟壳、桔梗、远志。

【功能主治】止咳，祛痰，平喘。用于支气管炎及咳嗽、哮喘。

Compound Daurian Rhododendron* Syrup for Relieving Bronchitis

Name of Chinese Phonetic Alphabet Fu Fang Man Shan Hong Tang Jiang

Formula Rhododendri Daurici Folium, Stemonae Radix, Papaveris Pericarpium, Platycodonis Radix and Polygalae Radix.

Actions and Indications Relieving cough, dispelling phlegm and calming dyspnea. It is indicated for bronchitis, cough and asthma.

*满山红

复方鲜竹沥液

【处方】鲜竹沥、鱼腥草、生半夏、生姜、枇杷叶、桔梗、薄荷油。

【功能主治】清热，化痰，止咳。用于痰热咳嗽。

Compound Honon Bamboo Juice* Oral Liquid for Relieving Cough

Name of Chinese Phonetic Alphabet Fu Fang Xian Zhu Li Ye

Formula Phyllostachydis Henonis Succus, Houttuyniae Herba, Pinelliae Rhizoma(raw), Zingiberis Rhizoma Recens, Eriobotryae Folium, Platycodonis Radix and Menthae Haplocalycis Oleum.

Actions and Indications Clearing heat, resolving phlegm and relieving cough. It is indicated for cough due to phlegm-heat.

* 竹沥

复方熊胆乙肝胶囊

【处方】熊胆粉、龙胆、丹参、柴胡、虎杖、板蓝根等。

【功能主治】清热利湿，用于慢性乙型肝炎。症见胸胁胀闷，口黏口苦，恶心厌油，纳呆，倦怠乏力，身自发黄。

Compound Bear Gall★ Capsule for Hepatitis B

Name of Chinese Phonetic Alphabet Fu Fang Xiong Dan Yi Gan Jiao Nang

Formula Ursi Fel Pulvis, Gentianae Radix et Rhizoma, Salviae Miltiorrhizae Radix et Rhizoma, Bupleuri Radix, Polygoni Cuspidati Rhizoma et Radix, Isatidis Radix, etc.

Actions and Indications Clearing heat and draining dampness. It is indicated for chronic hepatitis B, manifested as distention and oppression in hypochondrium, sticky and bitter taste in the mouth, nausea, disgust at oily foods, poor appetite, tiredness, fatigue, yellow appearance of the skin.

* 熊胆

复方熊胆滴眼液

【处方】熊胆粉、冰片。

【功能主治】清热降火，明目退翳。用于肝火上炎之急性细菌性结膜炎，流行性角膜炎。

Compound Bear Gall★ Eye Drops

Name of Chinese Phonetic Alphabet Fu Fang Xiong Dan Di Yan Ye

Formula Ursi Fel Pulvis and Borneolum Syntheticum.

Actions and Indications Clearing heat and downbearing fire, removing nebula to improve vision. It is indicated for acute bacterial keratitis and acute conjunctivitis due to liver-fire flaming upward.

* 熊胆

复方鳖甲软肝片

【处方】鳖甲、赤芍、黄芪、三七等。

【功能主治】软坚散结，化瘀解毒，益气养血。用于慢性肝炎肝纤维化，以及早期肝硬化，症见胁肋隐痛或肋下痞块，面色晦黯，脘腹胀满，纳差便溏，神疲乏力，口干口苦。

Compound Turtle Carapace★ Tablet for Soothing Liver

Name of Chinese Phonetic Alphabet Fu Fang Bie Jia Ruan Gan Pian

Formula Trionycis Carapax, Paeoniae Radix Rubra, Astragali Radix, Notoginseng Radix et Rhizoma, etc.

Actions and Indications Softening hardness and dissipating binds, resolving stasis, detoxifying, tonifying *qi* and nourishing blood. It is indicated for chronic hepatitis, hepatic fibrosis and early stage of cirrhosis manifested as dull pain in hypochondrium, subcostal stuffy lump, gloomy complexion, abdominal fullness, poor appetite, sloppy stools, lassitude of spirit, fatigue, dry mouth, bitter taste in the mouth.

* 鳖甲

复心片

【处方】本品为山楂叶制成的浸膏片。

【功能主治】具有减少左心室做功，降低心肌耗氧量，维持氧代谢平衡，促进微动脉血流及恢复血管径的作用。用于胸闷心痛，心悸气短，冠心病，心绞痛，心律失常。

Chinese Hawthorn* Tablet for Heart Disease

Name of Chinese Phonetic Alphabet Fu Xin Pian

Formula Crataegi Folium Extractum.

Actions and Indications Reducing the work of left ventricle, decreasing the oxygen consumption of myocardium, maintaining the balance of oxygen metabolism, promoting the blood flow of arteriole and recovering the diameter of blood vessel. It is indicated for chest distress, cardialgia, palpitation, shortness of breath, coronary heart disease, angina pectoris and arrhythmia.

* 山楂

复明片

【处方】羚羊角、蒺藜、木贼、菊花、车前子、夏枯草、决明子、人参、山茱萸（制）、石斛、枸杞子、菟丝子、女贞子、石决明、黄连、谷精草、关木通、熟地黄、山药、泽泻、茯苓、牡丹皮、地黄、槟榔。

【功能主治】滋补肝肾，养阴生津，清肝明目。用于肝肾阴虚引起的羞明畏光、视物模糊，及青光眼，初、中期白内障等见有上述症状者。

【注意】禁忌辛辣刺激。

Improving Vision Tablet

Name of Chinese Phonetic Alphabet Fu Ming Pian

Formula Saigae Tataricae Cornu, Tribuli Fructus, Equiseti Hiemalis Herba, Chrysanthemi Flos, Plantaginis Semen, Prunellae Spica, Cassiae Semen, Ginseng Radix et Rhizoma, Corni Fructus (prepared), Dendrobii Caulis, Lycii Fructus, Cuscutae Semen, Ligustri Lucidi Fructus, Haliotidis Concha, Coptidis Rhizoma, Eriocauli Flos, Aristolochiae Manshuriensis Caulis, Rehmanniae Radix Praeparata, Dioscoreae Rhizoma, Alismatis Rhizoma, Poria, Moutan Cortex, Rehmanniae Radix and Arecae Semen.

Actions and Indications Enriching the liver and kidney, tonifying *yin*, engendering fluid and clearing liver-fire to improve vision. It is indicated for photophobia, blurred vision, glaucoma and initial or middle stage of cataract with the above mentioned symptoms due to dual deficiency of liver-*yin* and kidney-*yin* .

Warning Pungent and irritant foods are prohibited.

复胃散胶囊

【处方】黄芪（制）、白芷、白及、延胡索（醋制）、白芍、海螵蛸、甘草（蜜制）。

【功能主治】补气健脾，制酸止痛，止血生肌。用于胃酸过多，吐血便血，食减形瘦，胃及十二指肠溃疡。

Compound Capsule for Stomach-restoration

Name of Chinese Phonetic Alphabet Fu Wei San Jiao Nang

Formula Astragali Radix (prepared), Angelicae Dahuricae Radix, Bletillae Rhizoma, Corydalis Rhizoma (prepared with vinegar), Paeoniae Radix Alba, Sepiae Endoconcha and Glycyrrhizae Radix et Rhizoma (prepared with honey).

Actions and Indications Tonifying *qi* and fortifying the spleen, antiacid and relieving pain, stopping bleeding and promoting tissue regeneration. It is indicated for gastroxia, spitting blood and hematochezia, poor appetite, emaciation, gastric and duodenal ulcer.

香苏正胃丸

【处方】广藿香、紫苏叶、香薷、陈皮、厚朴（姜制）、枳壳（炒）、砂仁、白扁豆（炒）、山楂（炒）、六神曲（炒）、麦芽（炒）、茯苓、甘草、滑石、朱砂。

【功能主治】解表和中，消食行滞。用于小儿暑热感冒，停食停乳，头痛发热，呕吐泄泻，腹痛胀满，小便不利。

Cablin Potchouli* and Purple Perilla Leaf** Pill for Harmonizing Stomach

Name of Chinese Phonetic Alphabet Xiang Su Zheng Wei Wan

Formula Pogostemonis Herba, Perillae Folium, Moslae Herba, Citri Reticulatae Pericarpium, Magnoliae Officinalis Cortex (prepared with ginger), Aurantii Fructus (fried), Amomi Fructus, Lablab Semen Album (fried), Crataegi Fructus (fried), Medicata Massa Fermentata (fried), Hordei Fructus Germinatus (fried), Poria, Glycyrrhizae Radix et Rhizoma, Talcum and Cinnabaris.

Actions and Indications Releasing the exterior and harmonizing the middle, promoting digestion. It is used for children common cold due to summer-heat; stagnant food or milk, headache, fever, vomiting, diarrhea, abdominal fullness and pain, difficulty in urination.

* 广藿香 ** 紫苏叶

香苏调胃片

【处方】广藿香、香薷、木香、紫苏叶、厚朴（姜制）、砂仁、枳壳（去瓤麸炒）、陈皮、茯苓、山楂（炒）、麦芽（炒）、白扁豆（去皮）、葛根、甘草、六神曲（麸炒）、生姜。

【功能主治】解表和中、健胃化滞。用于胃肠积滞，外感时邪引起的身热体倦，饮食少进，呕吐乳食，腹胀便泻，小便不利。

Cablin Potchouli* and Purple Perilla Leaf** Tablet for Regulating Stomach

Name of Chinese Phonetic Alphabet Xiang Su Tiao Wei Pian

Formula Pogostemonis Herba, Moslae Herba, Aucklandiae Radix, Perillae Folium, Magnoliae Officinalis Cortex (prepared with ginger), Amomi Fructus, Aurantii Fructus (removed pulp and fried with bran), Citri Reticulatae Pericarpium, Poria, Crataegi Fructus (fried), Hordei Fructus Germinatus (fried), Lablab Semen Album (removed seed coat), Puerariae Lobatae Radix, Glycyrrhizae Radix et Rhizoma, Medicata Massa Fermentata (fried with bran) and Zingiberis Rhizoma Recens.

Actions and Indications Releasing the exterior and harmonizing the middle, fortifying the stomach and resolving stagnation. It is used for generalized fever, fatigue, poor appetite, vomiting of milk, abdominal distention, diarrhea and oliguria, due to food stagnation in the stomach and intestines, invasion of exogenous seasonal pathogens.

* 广藿香 ** 紫苏叶

香连化滞丸

【处方】黄连、木香、黄芩、枳实（麸炒）、陈皮、青皮（醋炙）、甘草、滑石、厚朴（姜炙）、槟榔（炒）、白术（炒）、当归。

【功能主治】清热利湿，行血化滞。用于湿热凝滞引起的里急后重，腹痛下痢。

【注意】孕妇忌服。

Common Aucklandia* and Golden Thread** Bolus for Dysentery

Name of Chinese Phonetic Alphabet Xiang Lian Hua Zhi Wan

Formula Coptidis Rhizoma, Aucklandiae Radix, Scutellariae Radix, Aurantii Fructus Immaturus (fried with bran), Citri Reticulatae Pericarpium, Citri Reticulatae Pericarpium Viride (prepared with vinegar), Glycyrrhizae Radix et Rhizoma, Talcum, Magnoliae Officinalis Cortex (prepared with vinegar), Arecae Semen (fried), Atractylodis Macrocephalae Rhizoma (fried) and Angelicae Sinensis Radix.

Actions and Indications Clearing heat and draining dampness, moving blood to resolve stagnation. It is indicated for tenesmus, abdominal pain and dysentery due to stagnation of damp-heat.

Warning It is contraindicated for pregnant women.

* 木香 ** 黄连

香连浓缩丸

【处方】黄连（吴茱萸制）、木香。

【功能主治】清热化湿，行气止痛。用于痢疾，里急后重，腹痛泄泻。

Condensed Pill of Common Aucklandia* and Golden Thread**

Name of Chinese Phonetic Alphabet Xiang Lian Nong Suo Wan

Formula Coptidis Rhizoma (prepared with Euodiae Fructus) and Aucklandiae Radix.

Actions and Indications Clearing heat and draining dampness, moving *qi* to relieve pain. It is indicated for dysentery, tenesmus, abdominal pain and diarrhea.

* 木香 ** 黄连

香附丸

【处方】香附（醋制）、当归、川芎、白芍（炒）、熟地黄、白术（炒）、砂仁、陈皮、黄芩。

【功能主治】理气养血。用于气滞血虚，胸闷胁痛，经期腹痛，月经不调。

Nut-grass* Pill for Irregular Menstruation

Name of Chinese Phonetic Alphabet Xiang Fu Wan

Formula Cyperi Rhizoma (prepared with vinegar), Angelicae Sinensis Radix, Chuanxiong Rhizoma, Paeoniae Radix Alba (fried), Rehmanniae Radix Praeparata, Atractylodis Macrocephalae Rhizoma (fried), Amomi Fructus, Citri Reticulatae Pericarpium and Scutellariae Radix.

Actions and Indications Regulating *qi* and nourishing blood. It is used for chest distress, hypochondriac pain, dysmenorrheal and menstrual irregularities due to *qi*-stagnation and blood deficiency.

* 香附

香果健消片

【处方】珍珠香（炒焦）、草果（去壳、炒焦）、糯米。

【功能主治】健胃消食。用于消化不良，气胀饱闷，食积腹痛，胸满腹胀。

Common Aucklandia* and Tsaoko Amomum** Tablet for Promoting Digestion

Name of Chinese Phonetic Alphabet Xiang Guo Jian Xiao Pian

Formula Aucklandiae Radix (charred), Tsaoko Fructus (removed seed coat and charred) and Oryzae Glutinosae Fructus.

Actions and Indications Fortifying the stomach and promoting digestion. It is used for dyspepsia, *qi* distention, food accumulation, abdominal pain, chest distress and abdominal fullness.

* 珍珠香 ** 草果

香砂六君丸

【处方】木香、砂仁、党参、白术（炒）、茯苓、甘草（蜜炙）、陈皮、半夏（制）。

【功能主治】益气健脾，和胃。用于脾虚气滞，消化不良，嗳气食少，脘腹胀满，大便溏泄。

Common Aucklandia* and Villous Amomum** Pill for Fortifying Spleen

Name of Chinese Phonetic Alphabet Xiang Sha Liu Jun Wan

Formula Aucklandiae Radix, Amomi Fructus, Codonopsis Radix, Atractylodis Macrocephalae Rhizoma (fried), Poria, Glycyrrhizae Radix et Rhizoma (prepared with honey), Citri Reticulatae Pericarpium and Pinelliae Rhizoma (prepared).

Actions and Indications Tonifying *qi* and fortifying the spleen, harmonizing the stomach. It is used for dyspepsia, belching, poor appetite, abdominal fullness and sloppy stool due to deficiency of the spleen and *qi* stagnation.

* 木香 ** 砂仁

香砂平胃丸

【处方】苍术、陈皮、厚朴（姜制）、木香、砂仁、甘草。

【功能主治】健胃，舒气，止痛。用于胃肠衰弱，消化不良，胸膈满闷，胃痛呕吐。

Common Aucklandia* and Villous Amomum** Pill for Pacifying Stomach

Name of Chinese Phonetic Alphabet Xiang Sha Ping Wei Wan

Formula Atractylodis Rhizoma, Citri Reticulatae Pericarpium, Magnoliae Officinalis Cortex (prepared with ginger), Aucklandiae Radix, Amomi Fructus and Glycyrrhizae Radix et Rhizoma.

Actions and Indications Fortifying the stomach, soothing *qi*, relieving pain. It is used for dyspepsia, chest distress, stomachache and vomiting due to hypofunction of the stomach and intestines.

* 木香 * 砂仁

香砂枳术丸

【处方】木香、枳实（麸炒）、砂仁、白术（麸炒）。

【功能主治】健脾开胃，行气消痞。用于脾虚气滞，脘腹痞闷，食欲不振，大便溏软。

【注意】忌食生冷食物。

Common Aucklandia* and Villous Amomum** Pill

Name of Chinese Phonetic Alphabet Xiang Sha Zhi Shu Wan

Formula Aucklandiae Radix, Aurantii Fructus Immaturus (fried with bran), Amomi Fructus and Atractylodis Macrocephalae Rhizoma (fried with bran).

Actions and Indications Fortifying the spleen, improving appetite, moving *qi*, relieving distention. It is used for abdominal stuffiness and oppression, poor appetite and sloppy stool due to deficiency of the spleen and stagnation of *qi*.

Warning Uncooked and cold foods should be avoided.

* 木香 ** 砂仁

香砂养胃丸

【处方】木香、砂仁、白术、陈皮、茯苓、半夏（制）、香附（醋制）、枳实（炒）、豆蔻（去壳）、厚朴（姜制）、广藿香、甘草。

【功能主治】温中和胃。用于不思饮食，呕吐酸水，胃脘满闷，四肢倦怠。

Concentrative Pill of Common Aucklandia* and Villous Amomum**

Name of Chinese Phonetic Alphabet Xiang Sha Yang Wei Wan

Formula Aucklandiae Radix, Amomi Fructus, Atractylodis Macrocephalae Rhizoma, Citri Reticulatae Pericarpium, Poria, Pinelliae Rhizoma (prepared), Cyperi Rhizoma (prepared with vinegar), Aurantii Fructus Immaturus (fried), Amomi Fructus Rotundus (removed shell), Magnoliae Officinalis Cortex (prepared with ginger), Pogostemonis Herba and Glycyrrhizae Radix et Rhizoma.

Actions and Indications Warming and harmonizing the stomach. It is used for anorexia, acid vomiting, fullness in stomach duct, tiredness of extremities.

* 木香 ** 砂仁

香菊胶囊

【处方】化香树果序、夏枯草、野菊花、防风、辛夷等。

【功能主治】辛散祛风，清热通窍。用于急、慢性鼻窦炎、鼻炎。

Dyetree* and Wild Chrysanthemum** Capsule for Sinusitis

Name of Chinese Phonetic Alphabet Xiang Ju Jiao Nang

Formula Platycaryae Strobilaceae Infructescentia, Prunellae Spica, Chrysanthemi Indici Flos, Saposhnikoviae Radix, Magnoliae Flos, etc.

Actions and Indications Dispersing wind, clearing heat and dredging the orifices. It is indicated for acute, chronic sinusitis, rhinitis.

* 化香树 ** 野菊花

香菇多糖注射液

【处方】香菇多糖、苯甲醇、氯化钠、注射用水（适量）。

【功能主治】益气健脾，补虚扶正。用于慢性乙型迁延性肝炎及消化道肿瘤的放、化疗辅助药。

【注意】本品为淡黄色、黄色微显乳光的液体，不应有摇不匀的沉淀物。

Lentinan* Injection

Name of Chinese Phonetic Alphabet Xiang Gu Duo Tang Zhu She Ye

Formula Lentinan, Benzyl Alcohol, Sodium Chloride and Injection Water.

Actions and Indications Tonifying *qi* and fortifying the spleen, reinforcing the healthy *qi*. It is used for chronic persistent hepatitis B and auxiliary medicine to radiotherapy and chemotherapy for gastrointestinal tumor.

Warning The product is pale yellow, yellow micro-opalescence liquid and should not contain heterogeneous precipitates while being shaken.

* 香菇多糖

便秘通

【处方】白术、肉苁蓉、枳壳。

【功能主治】健脾益气，润肠通便，适用于虚性便秘，尤其是脾虚及脾肾两虚型便秘患者，症见大便秘结，面色无华，腹胀，神疲气短，头晕耳鸣，腰膝酸软。

【注意】个别患者服用后有口干现象。

Constipation-relieving Extract

Name of Chinese Phonetic Alphabet Bian Mi Tong

Formula Atractylodis Macrocephalae Rhizoma, Cistanches Caulis Carnosus and Aurantii Fructus.

Actions and Indications Fortifying the spleen, tonifying *qi*, moistening the intestines to relax the bowels. It is indicated for constipation due to deficiency, especially spleen deficiency and dual deficiency of the spleen and kidney, manifested as constipation, pale complexion, abdominal distention, lassitude of spirit, shortness of breath, dizziness, tinnitus, soreness and weakness of the waist and knees.

Warning After medication, dry mouth occurs occasionally.

保心包

【处方】苏合香、川芎、丹参、三七、冰片、菊花、葛根、安息香、檀香、丁香、青木香、当归、郁金、沉香、黄芪、赤芍、香附、白芷、薤白、延胡索、决明子、降香、首乌藤、石菖蒲、乳香、没药。

【功能主治】芳香开窍，活血化瘀，通痹止痛。适用于胸痹心痛属于气滞血瘀或痰瘀交阻证型者，并可防治冠心病心绞痛。

Cardialgia-relieving Powder

Name of Chinese Phonetic Alphabet Bao Xin Bao

Formula Styrax, Chuanxiong Rhizoma, Salviae Miltiorrhizae Radix et Rhizoma, Notoginseng Radix et Rhizoma, Borneolum Syntheticum, Chrysanthemi Flos, Puerariae Lobatae Radix, Benzoinum, Santali Albi Lignum, Caryophylli Flos, Aristolochiae Radix, Angelicae Sinensis Radix, Curcumae Radix, Aquilariae Lignum Resinatum, Astragali Radix, Paeoniae Radix Rubra, Cyperi Rhizoma, Angelicae Dahuricae Radix, Allii Macrostemonis Bulbus, Corydalis Rhizoma, Cassiae Semen, Dalbergiae Odoriferae Lignum, Polygoni Multiflori Caulis, Acori Tatarinowii Rhizoma, Olibanum and Myrrha.

Actions and Indications Inducing resuscitation,

activating blood, resolving stasis, alleviating pain. It is used for cardialgia attributed to *qi*-stagnation and blood-stasis or stagnation of phlegm with blood-stasis. It is also used for preventing coronary heart disease, angina pectoris.

保妇康栓

【处方】莪术油、冰片。

【功能主治】行气破瘀，生肌，止痛。用于霉菌性阴道炎，宫颈糜烂。

Suppository for Leukorrheal Disease

Name of Chinese Phonetic Alphabet Bao Fu Kang Shuan

Formula Curcumae Rhizoma Oleum and Borneolum Syntheticum.

Actions and Indications Moving *qi*, breaking stasis, promoting tissue regeneration and alleviating pain. It is indicated for colpomycosis, erosion of cervix.

保赤散

【处方】六神曲（炒）、巴豆霜、天南星（制）、朱砂。

【功能主治】消食导滞，化痰镇惊。用于小儿停乳停食，大便秘结，腹部胀满，痰多。

【注意】泄泻者忌服。

Digestion-promoting Powder for Infant

Name of Chinese Phonetic Alphabet Bao Chi San

Formula Medicata Massa Fermentata (fried), Crotonis Semen Pulveratum, Arisaematis Rhizoma (prepared) and Cinnabaris.

Actions and Indications Promoting digestion and removing food stagnation, resolving phlegm and settling fright. It is used for infantile stagnant milk and food, constipation, abdominal distention and fullness, profuse phlegm.

Warning It is contraindicated for cases with diarrhea.

保和丸

【处方】山楂（焦）、六神曲（炒）、半夏（制）、茯苓、陈皮、连翘、莱菔子（炒）、麦芽（炒）。

【功能主治】消食导滞，和胃。用于食积停滞，脘腹胀满，嗳腐吞酸，不思饮食。

Bao He Pill Digestion-promoting

Name of Chinese Phonetic Alphabet Bao He Wan

Formula Crataegi Fructus (charred), Medicata Massa Fermentata (fried), Pinelliae Rhizoma (prepared), Poria, Citri Reticulatae Pericarpium, Forsythiae Fructus, Raphani Semen (fried) and Hordei Fructus Germinatus (fried) .

Actions and Indications Promoting digestion and removing food stagnation, harmonizing the stomach. It is used for food stagnation, abdominal distention and fullness, eructation and acid regurgitation, anorexia.

保胎丸

【处方】熟地黄、艾叶（炭）、荆芥穗、贝母、槲寄生、菟丝子（酒制）、黄芪、白术（炒）、枳壳（炒）、砂仁、黄芩、厚朴（姜制）、甘草、川芎、白芍、羌活、当归。

【功能主治】补气养血，保产安胎。用于妊娠气虚，腰酸腿痛，胎动不安，屡经流产。

Relieving Excessive Fetal Movement Bolus

Name of Chinese Phonetic Alphabet Bao Tai Wan

Formula Rehmanniae Radix Praeparata, Artemisiae Argyi Folium (carbonated), Schizonepetae Spica, Fritillariae Cirrhosae Bulbus, Visci Herba, Cuscutae Semen (prepared with wine), Astragali Radix, Atractylodis Macrocephalae Rhizoma (fried), Aurantii

Fructus (fried), Amomi Fructus, Scutellariae Radix, Magnoliae Officinalis Cortex (prepared with ginger), Glycyrrhizae Radix et Rhizoma, Chuanxiong Rhizoma, Paeoniae Radix Alba, Notopterygii Rhizoma et Radix and Angelice Sinensis Radix.

Actions and Indications Tonifying *qi* and blood, keeping normal fetal movement. It is used for soreness of waist and pain of legs, excessive fetal movement and abortion due to *qi*-deficiency during pregnancy.

保济丸

【处方】钩藤、菊花、蒺藜、厚朴、木香、苍术、天花粉、广藿香、葛根、茯苓、薄荷、化橘红、白芷、薏苡仁、神曲、稻芽。

【功能主治】解表，祛湿，和中。用于腹痛腹泻，噎食嗳酸，恶心呕吐，肠胃不适，消化不良，舟车晕浪。

【注意】外感燥热者不宜服用。

Bao Ji Pill

Name of Chinese Phonetic Alphabet Bao Ji Wan

Formula Uncariae Ramulus cum Uncis, Chrysanthemi Flos, Tribuli Fructus, Magnoliae Officinalis Cortex, Aucklandiae Radix, Atractylodis Rhizoma, Trichosanthis Radix, Pogostemonis Herba, Puerariae Lobatae Radix, Poria, Menthae Haplocalycis Herba, Citri Grandis Exocarpium, Angelicae Dahuricae Radix, Euryales Semen, Medicata Massa Fermentata and Oryzae Fructus Germinatus.

Actions and Indications Releasing the exterior, dispelling dampness, harmonizing the middle energizer. It is used for abdominal pain and diarrhea, acid regurgitation, nausea and vomiting, gastrointestinal disturbance, indigestion, naupathia and car sickness.

Warning It is contraindicated for cases with exogenous dryness-heat.

保童化痰丸

【处方】黄芩、黄连、胆南星（酒炙）、天竺黄、前胡、浙贝母、桔梗、苦杏仁（炒）、陈皮、化橘红、法半夏、茯苓、甘草、紫苏叶、木香、枳壳（麸炒）、葛根、羌活、党参、朱砂、冰片。

【功能主治】清热化痰，止咳定喘。用于小儿肺胃痰热，感受风寒引起的头痛身热，咳嗽痰盛，气促喘急，烦躁不安。

Resolving Infantile Fever and Cough Pill

Name of Chinese Phonetic Alphabet Bao Tong Hua Tan Wan

Formula Scutellariae Radix, Coptidis Rhizoma, Arisaema cum Bile (prepared with wine), Bambusae Concretio Silicea, Peucedani Radix, Fritillariae Thunbergii Bulbus, Platycodonis Radix, Armeniacae Semen Amarum (fried), Citri Reticulatae Pericarpium, Citri Grandis Exocarpium, Pinelliae Rhizoma Praeparatum, Poria, Glycyrrhizae Radix et Rhizoma, Perillae Folium, Aucklandiae Radix, Aurantii Fructus (fried with bran), Puerariae Lobatae Radix, Notopterygii Rhizoma et Radix, Codonopsis Radix, Cinnabaris and Borneolum Syntheticum.

Actions and Indications Clearing heat and resolving phlegm, relieving cough and panting. It is indicated for infantile headache, fever, cough with excessive phlegm, panting, and irritability due to phlegm-heat of the lung and stomach and attack of exogenous wind-cold.

追风壮骨膏

【处方】川芎、大黄、天麻、地黄、栀子、生川乌、熟地黄、薄荷、白芷、关木通、威灵仙、当归、玄参、香加皮、白术、杜仲、青风藤、五味子、陈皮、山药、乌药、猪苓、甘草、生半夏、青皮、前胡、麻黄、细辛、藁本、连翘、知母、牛膝、苍术、防风、续断、赤石脂、浙贝母、泽泻、何首乌、羌活、黄芩、独活、黄连、金银花、黄柏、僵蚕、楮实子、川楝子、桑枝、荆芥、蒺藜、苦参、地榆、大枫子（打碎）、赤芍、桃枝、榆枝、苦杏仁、槐枝、茵陈、白蔹、柳枝、桃仁、桔梗、苍耳子、生草乌、豹骨、蜈蚣、麝香、肉桂、木香、龙骨、没药、乳香、血竭。

【功能主治】追风散寒，活血止痛。用于风寒湿痹，肩背疼痛，腰酸腿软，筋脉拘挛，四肢麻木，关节酸痛，筋骨无力，行步艰难。

Strengthening Bone Plaster

Name of Chinese Phonetic Alphabet Zhui Feng Zhuang Gu Gao

Formula Chuanxiong Rhizoma, Rhei Radix et Rhizoma, Gastrodiae Rhizoma, Rehmanniae Radix, Gardeniae Fructus, Aconiti Radix (raw), Rehmanniae Radix Praeparata, Menthae Haplocalycis Herba, Angelicae Dahuricae Radix, Aristolochiae Manshuriensis Caulis, Clematidis Radix et Rhizoma, Angelicae Sinensis Radix, Scrophulariae Radix, Periplocae Cortex, Atractylodis Macrocephalae Rhizoma, Eucommiae Cortex, Sinomenii Caulis, Schisandrae Chinensis Fructus, Citri Reticulatae Pericarpium, Dioscoreae Rhizoma, Linderae Radix, Polyporus, Glycyrrhizae Radix et Rhizoma, Pinelliae Rhizoma (raw), Citri Reticularae Pericarpium Viride, Peucedani Radix, Ephedrae Herba, Asari Radix et Rhizoma, Ligustici Rhizoma et Radix, Forsythiae Fructus, Anemarrhenae Rhizoma, Achyranthis Bidentatae Radix, Atractylodis Rhizoma, Saposhnikoviae Radix, Dipsaci Radix, Halloysitum Rubrum, Fritillariae Thunbergii Bulbus, Alismatis Rhizoma, Polygoni Multiflori Radix, Notopterygii Rhizoma et Radix, Scutellariae Radix, Angelicae Pubescentis Radix, Coptidis Rhizoma, Lonicerae Japonicae Flos, Phellodendri Chinensis Cortex, Bombyx Batryticatus, Broussonetiae Fructus, Toosendan Fructus, Mori Ramulus, Schizonepetae Herba, Tribuli Fructus, Sophorae Flavescentis Radix, Sanguisorbae Radix, Hydnocarpi Anthelmintici Semen (shattered), Paeoniae Radix Rubra, Persicae Ramulus, Ulmi Pumilae Ramulus, Armeniacae Semen Amarum, Sophorae Ramulus, Artemisiae Scopariae Herba, Ampelopsis Radix, Salicis Babylonicae Ramulus, Persicae Semen, Platycodonis Radix, Xanthii Fructus, Aconiti Kusnezoffii Radix (raw), Pardi Os, Scolopendra, Moschus, Cinnamomi Cortex, Aucklandiae Radix, Draconis Os, Myrrha, Olibanum and Draconis Sanguis.

Actions and Indications Dispelling wind and dissipating cold, activating blood and alleviating pain. It is indicated for wind-cold-damp impediment syndrome, marked by pain of the shoulder and back, aching and wilting of the waist and legs, spasm, numbness of the limbs, soreness and pain of the joints, weakness and difficulty for walk.

追风透骨丸

【处方】制川乌、白芷、制草乌、香附（制）、甘草、白术（炒）、川芎、没药（制）、乳香（制）、秦艽、地龙、当归、茯苓、赤小豆、羌活、天麻、赤芍、天南星（制）、桂枝、甘松、朱砂。

【功能主治】祛风除湿，通经活络，散寒止痛。用于风寒湿痹，肢节疼痛，肢体麻木。

【注意】不宜久服，属热痹者及孕妇忌服。

Dispelling Wind and Dampness Pill

Name of Chinese Phonetic Alphabet Zhui Feng Tou Gu Wan

Formula Aconiti Radix Cocta, Angelicae Dahuricae Radix, Aconiti Kusnezoffii Radix Cocta, Cyperi Rhizoma (prepared), Glycyrrhizae Radix et Rhizoma, Atractylodis Macrocephalae Rhizoma (fried), Chuanxiong Rhrizoma, Myrrha (prepared), Olibanum (prepared), Gentianae Macrophyllae Radix, Pheretima, Angelicae Sinensis Radix, Poria, Vignae Semen, Notopterygii Rhizoma et Radix, Gastrodiae Rhizoma, Paeoniae Radix Rubra, Arisaematis Rhizoma (prepared), Cinnamomi Ramulus, Nardostachyos Radix et Rhizoma and Cinnabaris.

Actions and Indications Dispelling wind and dampness, dredging meridians and collaterals, dissipating cold and alleviating pain. It is indicated for wind-cold-damp impediment syndrome, marked by pain and numbness of the limbs and joints.

Warning It can't be taken for a long time and is contraindicated for cases with heat impediment and pregnant women.

追风透骨片

【处方】制川乌、香附（制）、川芎、麻黄、制草乌、秦艽、当归、赤小豆、羌活、赤芍细辛、甘草、制天南星、白芷、白术（炒）、没药（制）、乳香（制）、地龙、茯苓、桂枝、天麻、甘松、防风、朱砂。

【功能主治】通经络，祛风湿，镇痛祛寒。用于风寒湿痹，四肢痹痛，神经麻痹。

【注意】孕妇忌服。

Dispelling Wind and Dampness Tablet

Name of Chinese Phonetic Alphabet Zhui Feng Tou Gu Pian

Formula Aconiti Radix Cocta Cyperi Rhizoma (prepared), Chuanxiong Rhizoma, Ephedrae Herba, Aconiti Kusnezoffii Radix Cocta, Gentianae Macrophyllae Radix, Angelicae Sinensis Radix, Vignae Semen, Notopterygii Rhizoma et Radix, Paeoniae Radix Rubra, Asari Radix et Rhizoma, Glycyrrhizae Radix et Rhizoma, Arisaematis Rhizoma Praeparata, Angelicae Dahuricae Radix, Atractylodis Macrocephalae Rhizoma (fried), Myrrha (prepared), Olibanum (prepared), Pheretima, Poria, Cinnamomi Ramulus, Gastrodiae Rhizoma, Nardostachyos Radix et Rhizoma, Saposhnikoviae Radix and Cinnabaris.

Actions and Indications Dredging meridians and collaterals, dispelling wind and dampness, settling pain and dispelling cold. It is used for wind-cold-damp impediment syndrome, marked by pain and numbness of the limbs, neuroparalysis.

Warning It is contraindicated for pregnant women.

独一味片

【处方】本品为独一味经加工制成的片剂。

【功能主治】活血止痛。用于跌打损伤，筋骨扭伤，风湿痹痛；软组织、关节及腰挫伤，骨折，外伤，风湿性关节炎引起的疼痛。

Common Lamiophlomis* Tablet for Traumatic Injury

Name of Chinese Phonetic Alphabet Du Yi Wei Pian

Formula Lamiophlomidis Herba.

Actions and Indications Activating blood, alleviating pain. It is used for traumatic injury, sprain, rheumatic impediment syndrome, pain induced by injury of soft tissue, joint, lumbar sprain, fracture, external injury and rheumatic arthritis.

* 独一味

独圣活血片

【处方】三七、香附（炙）、当归、大黄、延胡索（醋炙）、鸡血藤、甘草。

【功能主治】活血化瘀，消肿止痛，理气解郁。用于跌打损伤，瘀血肿胀及气滞血瘀所致的痛经。

【注意】孕妇慎服。

Blood-activating Tablet for Relieving Traumatic Injury

Name of Chinese Phonetic Alphabet Du Sheng Huo Xue Pian

Formula Notoginseng Radix et Rhizoma, Cyperi Rhizoma (prepared), Angelicae Sinensis Radix, Rhei Radix et Rhizoma, Corydalis Rhizoma (prepared with vinegar), Spatholobi Caulis and Glycyrrhizae Radix et Rhizoma.

Actions and Indications Activating blood, resolving stasis, reducing swelling, alleviating pain, regulating *qi*. It is used for traumatic injury with swelling, dysmenorrhea due to *qi*-stagnation and blood-stasis.

Warning It should be used carefully for pregnant women.

独活寄生合剂

【处方】独活、桑寄生、秦艽、防风、细辛、当归、白芍、川芎、熟地黄、杜仲（盐制）、川牛膝、党参、茯苓、甘草、桂枝。

【功能主治】养血舒筋，祛风除湿。用于风寒湿痹，腰膝冷痛，屈伸不利。

Doubleteeth Pubescent Angelica* and Chinese Taxillus** Mixture

Name of Chinese Phonetic Alphabet Du Huo Ji

Sheng He Ji

Formula Angelicae Pubescentis Radix, Taxilli Herba, Gentianae Macrophyllae Radix, Saposhnikoviae Radix, Asari Radix et Rhizoma, Angelicae Sinensis Radix, Paeoniae Radix Alba, Chuanxiong Rhizoma, Rehmanniae Radix Praeparata, Eucommiae Cortex (prepared with salt), Cyathulae Radix Codonopsis Radix, Poria, Glycyrrhizae Radix et Rhizoma and Cinnamomi Ramulus.

Actions and Indications Nourishing blood and relaxing sinews, dispelling wind and dampness. It is indicated for wind-cold-damp impediment syndrome, marked by cold and pain of the waist and knee, immobility of the limbs.

* 独活 ** 桑寄生

胆石利通片

【处方】硝石、白矾、郁金、三棱、金钱草、大黄等。

【功能主治】理气解郁，化瘀散结，利胆排石。用于胆石病气滞证。症见：右上腹胀满疼痛，痛引肩背，胃脘痞满，厌食油腻。

Relieving Cholelithiasis Tablet

Name of Chinese Phonetic Alphabet Dan Shi Li Tong Pian

Formula Nitrum, Alumen, Curcumae Radix, Sparganii Rhizoma, Lysimachiae Herba, Rhei Radix et Rhizoma, etc.

Actions and Indications Regulating *qi* and relieving depression, resolving stasis and dissipating mass, draining bile and eliminating stone. It is indicated for cholelithiasis, manifested as upper-right abdominal distention and pain, and referring to the shoulder and back, stomach fullness, disgusted for oily diet.

胆石通胶囊

【处方】蒲公英、水线草、茵陈、广金钱草、溪黄草、枳壳、柴胡、大黄、黄芩、鹅胆干膏粉。

【功能主治】清热利湿，利胆排石。用于肝胆湿热，右胁疼痛，口渴呕恶，黄疸口苦，以及胆石症、胆囊炎、胆道炎属肝胆湿热证者。

【注意】孕妇禁服。严重消化道溃疡、心脏病及重症肌无力者忌服。

Removing Gallbladder Stone Capsule

Name of Chinese Phonetic Alphabet Dan Shi Tong Jiao Nang

Formula Taraxaci Herba, Hedyotis Corymbosae Herba, Artemisiae Scopariae Herba, Desmodii Styracifolii Herba, Rabdosiae Serrae Herba, Aurantii Fructus, Bupleuri Radix, Rhei Radix et Rhizoma, Scutellariae Radix, Anserinus Fel Pulvis.

Actions and Indications Clearing heat and draining dampness, draining bile and removing stone. It is indicated for right hypochondriac pain, thirst and vomiting, nausea, jaundice and bitter taste in the mouth due to damp-heat of the liver and gallbladder, and cholelithiasis, cholecystitis, inflammation of biliary tract attributive to damp-heat of the liver and gallbladder.

Warning It is contraindicated for pregnant women and cases with severe peptic ulcer, heart disease and myasthenia gravis.

胆石清片

【处方】硝石、皂矾、羊胆汁、大黄、芒硝、威灵仙、鸡内金、郁金、山楂。

【功能主治】消食化积，清热利胆，行气止痛。用于胆囊结石。

Cholelithiasis-relieving Tablet

Name of Chinese Phonetic Alphabet Dan Shi Qing Pian

Formula Nitrum, Melanteritum, Bilis Caprinus, Rhei Radix et Rhizoma, Natrii Sulfas, Clematidis Radix et Rhizoma, Galli Gigerii Endothelium Corneum , Curcumae Radix and Crataegi Fructus.

Actions and Indications Promoting digestion,

clearing heat and draining bile, moving *qi* to alleviate pain. It is indicated for calculus of the gallbladder.

胆乐片

【处方】柴胡、蒲公英、大黄、茵陈、牛黄、栀子、郁金、薄荷油。

【功能主治】舒肝利胆，清热解毒，消炎止痛。用于急、慢性胆囊炎，胆道结石等胆道疾患。

Relieving Cholecystitis Tablet

Name of Chinese Phonetic Alphabet Dan Le Pian

Formula Bupleuri Radix, Taraxaci Herba, Rhei Radix et Rhizoma, Artemisiae Scopariae Herba, Bovis Calculus, Gardeniae Fructus, Curcumae Radix and Menthae Haplocalycis Oleum.

Actions and Indications Soothing the liver and draining bile, clearing heat and detoxicating, antiphlogistic to alleviate pain. It is indicated for acute or chronic cholecystitis, biliary calculi.

胆宁片

【处方】人工牛黄、水飞蓟素、盐酸小檗碱、延胡索、大黄、蒲公英、金钱草、薄荷油。

【功能主治】清热化湿，疏肝利胆。用于急、慢性胆囊炎，胆道感染，胆结石。

Cholecystitis-relieving Tablet

Name of Chinese Phonetic Alphabet Dan Ning Pian

Formula Bovis Calculus Artifactus, Silybin, Berberine hydrochloride, Corydalis Rhizoma, Rhei Radix et Rhizoma, Taraxaci Herba, Lysimachiae Herba and Menthae Haplocalycis Oleum.

Actions and Indications Clearing heat and draining dampness, soothing the liver and draining bile. It is indicated for acute, chronic cholecystitis, infection of biliary tract, cholelithes.

胆酸止咳片

【处方】粗胆酸、前胡、陈皮、甘草。

【功能主治】止咳化痰。用于支气管炎和感冒引起之咳嗽。

Cholic Acid* Tablet for Relieving Cough

Name of Chinese Phonetic Alphabet Dan Suan Zhi Ke Pian

Formula Crude Cholic Acid, Peucedani Radix, Citri Reticulatae Pericarpium and Glycyrrhizae Radix et Rhizoma.

Actions and Indications Relieving cough and resolving phlegm. It is indicated for cough due to bronchitis and common cold.

* 胆酸

脉君安片

【处方】钩藤、氢氯噻嗪、葛根。

【功能主治】平肝息风，解肌止痛。用于高血压症，头痛眩晕，颈项强痛，失眠心悸，冠心病。

Mai Jun An Tablet

Name of Chinese Phonetic Alphabet Mai Jun An Pian

Formula Uncariae Ramulus cum Uncis, Hydrochlorothiazide and Puerariae Lobatae Radix.

Actions and Indications Pacifying the liver, extinguishing wind, releasing the muscle, alleviating pain. It is used for hypertension, headache, vertigo, rigid and painful nape, insomnia, palpitation, coronary heart disease.

脉络宁注射液

【处方】牛膝、玄参、石斛、金银花。

【功能主治】清热养阴，活血化瘀。用于血栓闭塞性脉管炎，静脉血栓形成，动脉硬化性闭塞症，脑血栓形成及后遗症。

Relieving Cerebral Thrombosis Injection

Name of Chinese Phonetic Alphabet Mai Luo Ning Zhu She Ye

Formula Achyranthis Bidentatae Radix, Scrophulariae Radix, Dendrobii Caulis and Lonicerae Japonicae Flos.

Actions and Indications Clearing heat, nourishing *yin*, activating blood and resolving stasis. It is indicated for thromboangiitis obliterans, phlebothrombosis, arteriosclerotic obliteration, cerebral thrombosis and its sequela.

脉络通片

【处方】郁金、人参、黄连、三七、安息香、檀香、琥珀、降香、甘松、木香、石菖蒲、丹参、麦冬、钩藤、黄芩、夏枯草、槐角、甘草、珍珠、冰片、朱砂、牛黄。

【功能主治】通脉活络，行气化瘀。用于冠状动脉性心脏病引起的心绞痛，防治高血压及脑血管意外。

【注意】孕妇忌服。

Vessel-dredging Tablet

Name of Chinese Phonetic Alphabet Mai Luo Tong Pian

Formula Curcumae Radix, Ginseng Radix et Rhizoma, Coptidis Rhizoma, Notoginseng Radix et Rhizoma, Benzoinum, Santali Albi Lignum, Succinum, Dalbergiae Odoriferae Lignum, Nardostachyos Radix et Rhizoma, Aucklandiae Radix, Acori Tatarinowii Rhizoma, Salviae Miltiorrhizae Radix et Rhizoma, Ophiopogonis Radix, Uncariae Ramulus cum Uncis, Scutellariae Radix, Prunellae Spica, Sophorae Fructus, Glycyrrhizae Radix et Rhizoma, Margarita, Borneolum Syntheticum , Cinnabaris and Bovis Calculus.

Actions and Indications Dredging the vessels, activating collaterals, moving *qi* and resolving stasis. It is indicated for angina pectoris due to coronary cardiopathy, and used for preventing hypertension and cerebrovascular accident.

脉管复康片

【处方】丹参、鸡血藤、郁金、乳香、没药。

【功能主治】活血化瘀，通经活络。用于瘀血阻滞，脉管不通引起的脉管炎、硬皮病、动脉硬化性下肢血管闭塞症，对冠心病、脑血栓后遗症也有一定治疗作用。

【注意】经期减量，孕妇及肺结核患者遵医嘱服用。

Angiitis-relieving Tablet

Name of Chinese Phonetic Alphabet Mai Guan Fu Kang Pian

Formula Salviae Miltiorrhizae Radix et Rhizoma, Spatholobi Caulis, Curcumae Radix, Olibanum and Myrrha.

Actions and Indications Activating blood, resolving stasis, dredging meridians and collaterals. It is indicated for angiitis, scleroderma and arteriosclerotic obliteration of lower limbs due to blood-stasis; and also used for coronary heart disease and sequela of cerebral thrombosis.

Warning Decrement during menstrual period; pregnant women and patients with pulmonary tuberculosis should follow the physician's advice.

胎产金丸

【处方】紫河车、五味子（醋炙）、人参、茯苓、甘草、当归、鳖甲（沙烫醋淬）、香附（醋炙）、延胡索（醋炙）、没药（醋炙）、赤石脂（煅）、黄柏、白薇、艾叶炭、白术（麸炒）、藁本、沉香、肉桂、川芎、牡丹皮、益母草、地黄、青蒿。

【功能主治】补气，养血，调经。用于产后失血过多引起的恶露不净，腰酸腹痛，足膝浮肿，倦怠无力。

Puerperal Precious Bolus

Name of Chinese Phonetic Alphabet Tai Chan Jin Wan

Formula Hominis Placenta, Schisandrae Chinensis Fructus (prepared with vinegar), Ginseng Radix et Rhizoma, Poria, Glycyrrhizae Radix et Rhizoma, Angelicae Sinensis Radix, Trionycis Carapax (scalded in heated soil and quenched by vinegar), Cyperi Rhizoma (prepared with vinegar), Corydalis Rhizoma (prepared with vinegar), Myrrha (prepared with vinegar), Halloysitum Rubrum (calcined), Phellodendri Chinensis Cortex, Cynanchi Atrati Radix et Rhizoma, Artemisiae Argyi Folium (carbonated), Atractylodis Macrocephalae Rhizoma (fried with bran), Ligustici Rhizoma et Radix, Aquilariae Lignum Resinatum, Cinnamomi Cortex, Chuanxiong Rhizoma, Moutan Cortex, Leonuri Herba, Rehmanniae Radix and Artemisiae Annuae Herba.

Actions and Indications Tonifying *qi* and blood, regulating menstruation. It is indicated for puerperal lochiorrhagia, soreness of waist, abdominal pain, edema of feet and tiredness due to puerperal excessive bleeding.

急支糖浆

【处方】本品为鱼腥草、金荞麦、四季青和麻黄等药经加工制成的糖浆剂。

【功能主治】清热化痰，宣肺止咳。用于治疗急性支气管炎、感冒后咳嗽、慢性支气管炎急性发作。

Relieving Acute Bronchitis Syrup

Name of Chinese Phonetic Alphabet Ji Zhi Tang Jiang

Formula Houttuyniae Herba, Fagopyri Dibotryis Rhizoma, Ilicis Chinensis Folium, Ephedrae Herba, etc.

Actions and Indications Clearing heat and resolving phlegm, diffusing the lung and relieving cough. It is indicated for acute bronchitis, cough after common cold, acute attack of chronic bronchitis.

疮疡膏

【处方】白芷、血竭、川芎、红花、当归、大黄、升麻、土鳖虫。

【功能主治】消肿散结，活血化瘀，拔脓生肌。用于慢性下肢溃疡，乳腺炎及疖痛。

Relieving Sore Ointment

Name of Chinese Phonetic Alphabet Chuang Yang Gao

Formula Angelicae Dahuricae Radix, Draconis Sanguis, Chuanxiong Rhizoma, Carthami Flos, Angelicae Sinensis Radix, Rhei Radix et Rhizoma, Cimicifugae Rhizoma and Eupolyphaga seu Steleophaga.

Actions and Indications Dispersing swelling and dissipating mass, activating blood and resolving stasis, discharging pus, promoting tissue regeneration. It is used for chronic ulcer of the lower limb, mastitis and furuncle.

恒制咳喘胶囊

【处方】法半夏、红花、生姜、白及、佛手、甘草、紫苏叶、薄荷、香橼、陈皮、红参、西洋参、砂仁、沉香、丁香、豆蔻、肉桂、赭石（煅）。

【功能主治】益气养阴，温阳化饮，止咳平喘。用于气阴两虚，阳虚痰阻所致的咳嗽痰喘，胸脘满闷，倦怠乏力。

Heng Zhi Capsule for Relieving Cough and Dyspnea

Name of Chinese Phonetic Alphabet Heng Zhi Ke Chuan Jiao Nang

Formula Pinelliae Rhizoma Praeparatum, Carthami Flos, Zingiberis Rhizoma Recens, Bletillae Rhizoma, Citri Sarcodactylis Fructus, Glycyrrhizae Radix et Rhizoma, Perillae Folium, Menthae Haplocalycis Herba, Citri Fructus, Citri Reticulatae Pericarpium, Ginseng Radix et Rhizoma Rubra, Panacis Quinquefolii Radix, Amomi Fructus,

Aquilariae Lignum Resinatum, Caryophylli Flos, Amomi Fructus Rotundus, Cinnamomi Cortex and Haematitum (calcined).

Actions and Indications Replenishing *qi* and nourishing *yin*, warming *yang* and resolving retained fluid, relieving cough and calming dyspnea. It is indicated for cough and dyspnea, chest distress, tiredness and fatigue due to dual deficiency of *qi* and *yin*, *yang*-deficiency and stagnation of phlegm.

烂积丸

【处方】三棱（麸炒）、莪术（醋炙）、山楂（炒）、青皮（醋炙）、陈皮、枳实、槟榔、牵牛子（炒）、大黄。

【功能主治】消积，驱虫。用于脾胃不和引起的食滞积聚，胸满，痞闷，腹胀坚硬，嘈杂吐酸，虫积腹痛，大便秘结。

【注意】孕妇忌服。

Lan Ji Pill

Name of Chinese Phonetic Alphabet Lan Ji Wan

Formula Sparganii Rhizoma (fried with bran), Curcumae Rhizoma (prepared with vinegar), Crataegi Fructus (fried), Citri Reticulatae Pericarpium Viride (prepared with vinegar), Citri Reticulatae Pericarpium, Aurantii Fructus Immaturus, Arecae Semen, Pharbitidis Semen (fried) and Rhei Radix et Rhizoma.

Actions and Indications Removing food stagnation, expelling intestinal worms. It is used for disharmony of the spleen and stomach marked by food stagnation, chest fullness and oppression, abdominal distention, gastric upset, acid vomiting, abdominal pain due to intestinal worms; and constipation.

Warning It is contraindicated for pregnant women.

洁尔阴洗液

【处方】蛇床子、艾叶、独活、石菖蒲、苍术、薄荷、黄柏、黄芩、苦参、地肤子、茵陈、土荆皮、栀子、金银花。

【功能主治】清热燥湿，杀虫止痒。主治妇女湿热带下。症见阴部瘙痒红肿，带下量多，色黄，口苦口干，尿黄便结，舌红苔黄腻，脉弦数。适用于霉菌性、滴虫性及非特异性阴道炎。

【注意事项】本品系外用药。

Jie Er Yin Washings for Cleaning Vagina

Name of Chinese Phonetic Alphabet Jie Er Yin Xi Ye

Formula Cnidii Fructus, Artemisiae Argyi Folium, Angelicae Pubescentis Radix, Acori Tatarinowii Rhizoma, Atractylodis Rhizoma, Menthae Haplocalycis Herba, Phellodendri Chinensis Cortex, Scutellariae Radix, Sophorae Flavescentis Radix, Kochiae Fructus, Artemisiae Scopariae Herba, Pseudolaricis Cortex, Gardeniae Fructus and Lonicerae Japonicae Flos.

Actions and Indications Clearing heat and drying dampness, killing worms and relieving itching. It is indicated for vaginal discharge due to damp-heat, manifested as itching, red and swelling pudendum, profuse yellow vaginal discharge, bitter taste in the mouth and dry mouth, yellow urine and dry stools, red tongue with yellow slimy fur, string-like and rapid pulse, and also used for colpomycosis, trichomonal and nonspecific vaginitis.

Warning Only for external use.

洁白胶囊

【处方】诃子（煨）、肉豆蔻、草果、草豆蔻、沉香、丁香、五灵脂膏、红花、石榴子、木瓜、土木香、寒水石、翼首草等。

【功能主治】健脾和胃，止痛止吐。用于胸腹胀满，胃脘疼痛，消化不良，呕逆泄泻，小便不利。

Jie Bai Capsule for Fortifying Stomach

Name of Chinese Phonetic Alphabet Jie Bai Jiao Nang

Formula Chebulae Fructus (roasted), Myristicae Semen, Tsaoko Fructus, Alpiniae Katsumadai Semen,

Aquilariae Lignum Resinatum, Caryophylli Flos, Trogopterori Extractum, Carthami Flos, Granati Fructus, Chaenomelis Fructus, Inulae Radix, Gypsum Rubrum, Pterocephali Herba, etc.

Actions and Indications Fortifying the spleen and harmonizing the stomach, relieving pain and vomiting. It is indicated for distention and fullness of the chest and abdomen, stomach duct pain, indigestion, vomiting, diarrhea, oliguria.

活力苏口服液

【处方】制何首乌、淫羊藿、黄精（制）、枸杞子、黄芪、丹参。

【功能主治】益气补血，滋养肝肾。用于年老体弱，精神萎靡，失眠健忘，眼花耳聋，脱发或头发早白属气血不足、肝肾亏虚者。

Improving Senile Constitution Oral Liquid

Name of Chinese Phonetic Alphabet Huo Li Su Kou Fu Ye

Formula Polygoni Multiflori Radix Praeparata, Epemedii Folium, Polygonati Rhizoma (prepared), Lycii Fructus, Astragali Radix and Salviae Miltiorrhizae Radix et Rhizoma.

Actions and Indications Tonifying *qi* and blood, nourishing the liver and kidney. It is used for senile debility, listlessness, insomnia, amnesia, dim eyesight, deafness, alopecia or premature graying of hair due to insufficiency of *qi* and blood, and dual deficiency of the liver and kidney.

活心丸

【处方】灵芝、麝香、熊胆、红花、牛黄、珍珠、人参、蟾酥、附子、冰片。

【功能主治】益气活血，温经通脉。主治胸痹，心痛，用于冠心病、心绞痛。

【注意】本品可引起子宫平滑肌收缩，妇女经期及孕妇慎用。

Heart-activating Pill

Name of Chinese Phonetic Alphabet Huo Xin Wan

Formula Ganoderma, Moschus, Ursi Fel, Carthami Flos, Bovis Calculus, Margarita, Ginseng Radix et Rhizoma, Bufonis Venenum, Aconiti Lateralis Radix Praeparata and Borneolum Syntheticum.

Actions and Indications Tonifying *qi*, activating blood, warming meridians and dredging vessels. It is used for chest impediment syndrome, cardialgia, coronary heart disease and angina pectoris.

Warning The preparation can induce the contraction of uterine smooth muscle, and should be used cautiously for cases during menstrual period and for pregnant women.

活血止痛散

【处方】当归、冰片、土鳖虫、自然铜（煅）、乳香（制）、三七。

【功能主治】活血散瘀，消肿止痛。用于跌打损伤，瘀血肿痛。

【注意】孕妇禁用。

Pain-relieving Powder for Traumatic Injury

Name of Chinese Phonetic Alphabet Huo Xue Zhi Tong San

Formula Angelicae Sinensis Radix, Borneolum Syntheticum, Eupolyphaga seu Steleophaga, Pyritum (calcined), Olibanum (prepared) and Notoginseng Radix et Rhizoma.

Actions and Indications Activating blood, dissipating stasis, reducing swelling, alleviating pain. It is used for traumatic injury marked by swelling, pain and blood-stasis.

Warning It is contraindicated for pregnant women.

活血消炎丸

【处方】乳香（醋炙）、没药（醋炙）、石菖蒲浸膏、黄米（蒸熟）、牛黄。

【功能主治】活血解毒，消肿止痛。用于毒热结于脏腑经络引起的痈疽初起，乳痈，红肿作痛。

【注意】孕妇慎服。

Activating Blood and Anti-inflammatory Pill

Name of Chinese Phonetic Alphabet Huo Xue Xiao Yan Wan

Formula Olibanum (prepared with vinegar), Myrrha (prepared with vinegar), Acori Tatarinowii Extractum, Panici Miliacei Fructus (steamed) and Bovis Calculus.

Actions and Indications Activating blood and detoxicating, dispersing swelling and relieving pain. It is used for initial stage of abscess, acute mastitis with swelling and pain due to toxic-heat accumulation in the viscera and meridians.

Warning It should be used carefully for pregnant women.

活血通脉胶囊

【处方】鸡血藤、桃仁、丹参、三七、赤芍、红花、降香、黄精（酒炙）、郁金、川芎、石菖蒲、冰片、陈皮、木香、人参、麦冬、枸杞子。

【功能主治】活血通脉，强心镇痛。用于冠状动脉硬化引起的心绞痛，胸闷气短，心气不足，瘀血作痛。

【注意】孕妇慎用。

Relieving Angina Pectoris Capsule

Name of Chinese Phonetic Alphabet Huo Xue Tong Mai Jiao Nang

Formula Spatholobi Caulis, Persicae Semen, Salviae Miltiorrhizae Radix et Rhizoma, Notoginseng Radix et Rhizoma, Paeoniae Radix Rubra, Carthami Flos, Dalbergiae Odoriferae Lignum, Polygonati Rhizoma (prepared with wine), Curcumae Radix, Chuanxiong Rhizoma, Acori Tatarinowii Rhizoma, Borneolum Syntheticum, Citri Reticulatae Pericarpium, Aucklandiae Radix, Ginseng Radix et Rhizoma, Ophiopogonis Radix and Lycii Fructus.

Actions and Indications Activating blood, dredging vessels, strengthening the heart, settling pain. It is used for angina pectoris, chest distress, shortness of breath due to insufficiency of heart-*qi* and coronary arterioclerosis.

Warning It should be used carefully for pregnant women.

活血解毒丸

【处方】乳香（醋炙）、没药（醋炙）、蜈蚣、黄米（蒸熟）、石菖蒲清膏、雄黄粉。

【功能主治】解毒消肿，活血止痛。用于肺腑毒热，气血凝结引起的痈毒初起，乳痈乳炎，红肿高大，坚硬疼痛，结核，疔毒恶疮，无名肿毒。

【注意】孕妇忌服，忌食辛辣厚味。

Blood-activating Pill for Relieving Abscess

Name of Chinese Phonetic Alphabet Huo Xue Jie Du Wan

Formula Olibanum (prepared with vinegar), Myrrha (prepared with vinegar), Scolopendra, Panici Miliacei Fructus (steamed), Acori Tatarinowii Extractum and Realgar Pulvis.

Actions and Indications Detoxicating and dispersing swelling, activating blood and relieving pain. It is used for initial stage of abscess, acute mastitis with swelling, mass and pain, subcutaneous node, deep-rooted boil, inflammatory swelling of unknown origin due to heat-toxin in the lung, stagnation of *qi* and blood.

Warning It is contraindicated for pregnant women. Pungent foods and greasy diet should be avoided.

活络丸

【处方】蕲蛇（酒制）、麻黄、羌活、竹节香附、天麻、乌梢蛇（酒炙）、细辛、虎骨（油炙）、僵蚕（麸炒）、威灵仙（酒炙）、防风、乳香（醋炙）、肉桂（去粗皮）、附子（炙）、全蝎、地龙、没药（醋炙）、丁香、赤芍、血竭、何首乌（酒炙）、玄参、甘草、熟地黄、白术（麸炒）、茯苓、人参、龟甲（沙烫醋淬）、骨碎补、当归、广藿香、大黄、白芷、川芎、草豆蔻、黄芩、沉香、黄连、青皮（醋炙）、香附（醋炙）、天竺黄、木香、乌药、松香、葛根、豆蔻、麝香、水牛角浓缩粉、冰片、人工牛黄、朱砂、安息香。

【功能主治】祛风，舒筋，活络，除湿。用于风寒湿痹引起的肢体疼痛，手足麻木，筋脉拘挛，中风瘫痪，口眼歪斜，半身不遂，言语不清。

【注意】孕妇忌服。

Collateral-activating Pill

Name of Chinese Phonetic Alphabet Huo Luo Wan

Formula Agkistrodon (prepared with wine), Ephedrae Herba, Notopterygii Rhizoma et Radix, Anemones Raddeanae Rhizoma, Gastrodiae Rhizoma, Zaocys (prepared with wine), Asari Radix et Rhizoma, Tigris Os (prepared with oil), Bombyx Batryticatus (fried with bran), Clematidis Radix et Rhizoma (prepared with wine), Saposhnikoviae Radix, Olibanum (prepared with vinegar), Cinnamomi Cortex (removed rough bark), Aconiti Lateralis Radix Praeparata, Scorpio, Pheretima, Myrrha (prepared with vinegar), Caryophylli Flos, Paeoniae Radix Rubra, Draconis Sanguis, Polygoni Multiflori Radix (prepared with wine), Scrophulariae Radix, Glycyrrhizae Radix et Rhizoma, Rehmanniae Radix Praeparata, Atractylodis Macrocephalae Rhizoma (fried with bran), Poria, Ginseng Radix et Rhizoma, Testudinis Carapax et Plastrum (scalded by sand and quenched by vinegar), Fructus Drynariae, Angelicae Sinensis Radix, Pogostemonis Herba, Rhei Radix et Rhizoma, Angelicae Dahuricae Radix, Chuanxiong Rhizoma, Alpiniae Katsumadai Semen, Scutellariae Radix, Aquilariae Lignum Resinatum, Coptidis Rhizoma, Citri Reticulatae Pericarpium Viride (prepared with vinegar), Cyperi Rhizoma (prepared with vinegar), Bambusae Concretio Silicea, Aucklandiae Radix, Linderae Radix, Pini Resina, Puerariae Lobatae Radix, Amomi Fructus Rotundus, Moschus, Bubali Cornu Puvlis Concentratio, Borneolum Syntheticum, Bovis Calculus Artifactus, Cinnabaris and Benzoinum.

Actions and Indications Dispelling wind, relaxing sinews, activating collaterals, eliminating dampness. It is used for generalized pain, numbness of extremities, muscular spasm, paralysis, deviated eyes and mouth, hemiparalysis and alalia due to wind-cold-damp impediment.

Warning It is contraindicated for pregnant women.

洛布桑胶囊

【处方】红景天、冬虫夏草、手参。

【功能主治】益气养阴，活血通脉。用于胸痹心痛，气阴两虚，心血瘀阻证所致的胸闷，刺痛或隐痛，心悸气短，倦怠懒言，头晕目眩，面色少华等证。冠心病心绞痛见以上表现者。

Luobusang Capsule

Name of Chinese Phonetic Alphabet Luo Bu Sang Jiao Nang

Formula Rhodiolae Crenulatae Radix et Rhizoma, Cordyceps and Gymnadeniae Tuber.

Actions and Indications Tonifying *qi* and nourishing *yin*, activating blood and strengthening pulse beat. It is indicated for chest impediment syndrome, heart pain, chest distress, stabbing pain and dull pain, palpitation, shortness of breath, tiredness, indolent speaking, dizziness, dizzy vision and pale complexion due to dual deficiency of *qi* and *yin*, also used for coronary heart disease, angina pectoris with the above mentioned symptoms.

洋参保肺口服液

【处方】本品为罂粟壳、五味子 (醋炙) 、川贝母、陈皮、麻黄、西洋参等药经加工制成的口服液。

【功能主治】滋阴补肺，止咳定喘。用于阴虚肺弱引起的久嗽咳喘，干咳少痰及口燥咽干，睡卧不安。

American Ginseng★ Oral Liquid

Name of Chinese Phonetic Alphabet Yang Shen

Bao Fei Kou Fu Ye

Formula Papaveris Pericarpium, Schisandrae Chinensis Fructus (prepared with vinegar), Fritillariae Cirrhosae Bulbus, Citri Reticulatae Pericarpium, Ephedrae Herba and Panacis Quinquefolii Radix.

Actions and Indications Enriching lung-*yin*, relieving cough and dyspnea. It is indicated for cough, dyspnea, dry cough, dry mouth and throat and sleep disturbance due to *yin*-deficiency of the lung.

* 西洋参

前列安栓

【处方】黄柏、虎杖、栀子、大黄、泽兰、毛冬青、吴茱萸、威灵仙、石菖蒲、荔枝核。

【功能主治】清热利湿通淋，化瘀散结止痛。主治湿热壅阻症所引起的少腹痛、会阴痛、睾丸疼痛、排尿不利、尿频、尿痛。可用于白浊、劳淋（慢性前列腺炎）等病见以上证候者。

【注意】药物塞入肛门后，如有便意感，腹痛，腹泻等不适症状，可改进使用方法，如将栓剂外涂植物油或将栓剂置入更深些，待直肠适应后，自觉症状可减轻或消失。

Relieving Strangury Suppository

Name of Chinese Phonetic Alphabet Qian Lie An Shuan

Formula Phellodendri Chinensis Cortex, Polygoni Cuspidati Rhizoma et Radix , Gardeniae Fructus, Rhei Radix et Rhizoma, Lycopi Herba, Ilecis Pubescentis Radix, Euodiae Fructus, Clematidis Radix et Rhizoma, Acori Tatarinowii Rhizoma and Litchi Semen.

Actions and Indications Clearing heat, draining dampness and relieving strangury, resolving stasis, dissipating mass, alleviating pain. It is indicated for syndrome of damp-heat obstruction, manifested as lower abdominal pain, perineal pain, pain of the testis, dysuria, frequency of micturition, urodynia; also for whitish turbid urine, stranguria by overstrain (chronic prostatitis) with the above mentioned symptoms.

Warning After inserting the drug to the anus, some patients may feel uncomfortable, such as feeling of defecating, abdominal pain and diarrhea, then the administration method may be improved, for example, smearing plant oil outside of the suppository or pushing it deeper, when the rectum adapts it, the symptoms may be alleviated or disappear.

前列欣胶囊

【处方】桃仁（炒）、没药（炒）、丹参、红花、泽兰、王不留行（炒）、皂角刺、败酱草、蒲公英、川楝子、白芷、石韦、枸杞子、赤芍。

【功能主治】活血化瘀，清热利湿。用于治疗瘀血凝聚，湿热下注所致慢性前列腺炎及前列腺增生的症状改善。症见尿急、尿痛、排尿不畅、滴沥。

【不良反应】偶见胃脘不适者，一般不影响继续治疗。

Relieving Prostatitis Capsule

Name of Chinese Phonetic Alphabet Qian Lie Xin Jiao Nang

Formula Persicae Semen (fried), Myrrha (fried), Salviae Miltiorrhizae Radix et Rhizoma, Carthami Flos, Lycopi Herba, Vaccariae Semen (fried), Gleditsiae Spina, Patriniae Herba, Taraxaci Herba, Toosendan Fructus, Angelicae Dahuricae Radix, Pyrrosiae Folium, Lycii Fructus and Paeoniae Radix Rubra.

Actions and Indications Activating blood and resolving stasis, clearing heat and draining dampness. It is indicated for chronic prostatitis and hyperplasia of prostate due to stagnation of blood-stasis and downward attack of damp-heat, manifested as urgency of urination, urodynia, dysuria and dribbling urine.

Warning Patient may feel uncomfortable in the stomach occasionally which will not affect subsequent treatment.

前列桂黄片

【处方】大黄、猪牙皂、肉桂等。

【功能主治】祛瘀散结，利尿。用于Ⅰ、Ⅱ期前列腺增生，尿路瘀阻证；症见小便频数，尿后余沥，舌紫瘀点，脉涩或弦。

【注意】有胃溃疡病史者，出血性疾病，脾胃虚弱及大便溏稀者慎用。

Cassia Bark* and Rhubarb** Tablet for Relieving Hyperplasia of Prostate

Name of Chinese Phonetic Alphabet Qian Lie Gui Huang Pian

Formula Rhei Radix et Rhizoma, Gleditsiae Fructus Abnormalis, Cinnamomi Cortex, etc.

Actions and Indications Dispelling stasis and mass, inducing diuresis. It is indicated for the first or second stage of hyperplasia of prostate, obstructed urinary tract syndrome, manifested as frequency of micturition, dribbling urine, purple spot on the tongue, rough or string-like pulse.

Warning It should be used carefully for cases with history of gastric ulcer, hemorrhagic diseases, for cases with deficiency of the spleen and stomach and sloppy stool.

* 肉桂 ** 大黄

前列通片

【处方】车前子、黄柏、蒲公英、泽兰、两头尖、黄芪等干浸膏，八角茴香油，肉桂油，琥珀。

【功能主治】清热解毒，清利湿浊，理气活血，消炎止痛，祛瘀通淋。用于急性前列腺炎、前列腺增生。

Relieving Prostatitis Tablet

Name of Chinese Phonetic Alphabet Qian Lie Tong Pian

Formula Plantaginis, Phellodendri Chinensis, Taraxaci, Lycopi, Anemones Raddeanae et Astragali Extractum, etc. Anisi Stellati Oleum, Cinnamomi Oleum and Succinum.

Actions and Indications Clearing heat and detoxicating, clearing and relieving dampness turbid, regulating *qi* and activating blood, antiphlogistic and alleviating pain, removing stasis and relieving strangury. It is indicated for acute prostatitis, hyperplasia of prostate.

前列通胶囊

【处方】桃仁、丹参、红花等。

【功能主治】活血化瘀，清热利湿。用于治疗瘀血凝聚，湿热下注所致的慢性前列腺炎及前列腺增生的症状改善。症见尿急、尿痛、排尿不畅、滴沥不净。

Capsule for Prostatitis

Name of Chinese Phonetic Alphabet Qian Lie Tong Jiao Nang

Formula Persicae Semen, Salviae Miltiorrhizae Radix et Rhizoma, Carthami Flos, etc.

Actions and Indications Activating blood and resolving stasis, clearing heat and draining dampness. It is indicated for chronic prostatitis and hyperplasia of prostate due to stagnation of blood-stasis and downward attack of damp-heat, manifested as urgency of urination, urodynia, dysuria and dribbling urine.

首乌丸

【处方】何首乌（制）、地黄、牛膝（酒制）、桑椹清膏、女贞子（酒制）、桑叶（制）、黑芝麻、墨旱莲清膏、菟丝子（酒蒸）、金樱子清膏、补骨脂（盐炒）、豨莶草（制）、金银花（制）。

【功能主治】补肝肾，强筋骨，乌须发。用于肝肾两虚，头晕目花，耳鸣，腰酸肢麻，须发早白，高血脂症。

Chinese Knotweed* Pill

Name of Chinese Phonetic Alphabet Shou Wu Wan

Formula Polygoni Multiflori Radix (prepared), Rehmanniae Radix, Achyranthis Bidentatae Radix (prepared with wine), Mori Fructus Extractum, Ligustri Lucidi Fructus (prepared with wine), Mori Folium (prepared), Sesami Semen Nigrum, Ecliptae Extractum, Cuscutae Semen (steamed by wine), Rosae Laevigatae Extractum, Psoraleae Fructus (fried with salt),

Siegesbeckiae Herba (prepared) and Lonicerae Japonicae Flos (prepared).

Actions and Indications Tonifying the liver and kidney, strengthening the sinews and bone, and blackening the beard and hair. It is indicated for dizziness, dizzy vision, tinnitus, soreness of waist, numbness of limbs, premature graying of beard and hair, and also for hyperlipemia.

*何首乌

养心芪片

【处方】黄芪、党参、丹参、葛根、淫羊藿、山楂、地黄、当归、黄连、延胡索（炙）、灵芝、人参甘草（炙）。

【功能主治】扶正固本，益气活血，止痛。用于气虚血瘀性冠心病、心绞痛，心肌梗死及合并高血脂、高血糖等症见有上述证候者。

Milkvetch* Tablet for Heart-nourishing

Name of Chinese Phonetic Alphabet Yang Xin Qi Pian

Formula Astragali Radix, Codonopsis Radix, Salviae Miltiorrhizae Radix et Rhizoma, Puerariae Lobatae Radix, Epimedii Folium, Crataegi Fructus, Rehmanniae Radix, Angelicae Sinensis Radix, Coptidis Rhizoma, Corydalis Rhizoma (prepared), Ganoderma, Ginseng Radix et Rhizoma and Glycyrrhizae Radix et Rhizoma (prepared).

Actions and Indications Reinforcing the healthy *qi*, securing the body resistence, tonifying *qi*, activating blood, alleviating pain. It is indicated for coronary heart diseases, angina pectoris and myocardial infarction due to *qi*-deficiency and blood-stasis; and complicated with hyperlipemia and hyperglycemia.

*黄芪

养心定悸颗粒

【处方】地黄、麦冬、红参、大枣、阿胶、黑芝麻、桂枝、生姜、甘草（蜜炙）。

【功能主治】养血益气，复脉定悸。用于气虚血少，心悸气短，心律不齐，盗汗失眠，咽干舌燥，大便干结。

【注意】腹胀便溏、食少苔腻者忌服。

Heart-nourishing Soluble Granules

Name of Chinese Phonetic Alphabet Yang Xin Ding Ji Ke Li

Formula Rehmanniae Radix, Ophiopogonis Radix, Ginseng Radix et Rhizoma Rubra, Jujubae Fructus, Asini Corii Colla, Sesami Semen Nigrum, Cinnamomi Ramulus, Zingiberis Rhizoma Recens and Glycyrrhizae Radix et Rhizoma (prepared with honey).

Actions and Indications Nourishing blood, tonifying *qi*, restoring normal pulse beat and relieving palpitation. It is used for palpitation, shortness of breath, arrhythmia, night sweating, insomnia, dry throat and tongue and hard bound stool due to deficiency of *qi* and insufficiency of blood.

Warning It is contraindicated for cases with abdominal fullness, sloppy stool, poor appetite and greasy tongue fur.

养血生发胶囊

【处方】本品为何首乌、当归、熟地黄、天麻、川芎、木瓜等经加工制成的胶囊剂。

【功能主治】养血补肾，祛风生发。用于斑秃，全秃，脂溢性脱发，头皮发痒，头屑多，油脂多与病后、产后脱发属血虚肾亏者。

Engendering Hair Capsule

Name of Chinese Phonetic Alphabet Yang Xue Sheng Fa Jiao Nang

Formula Polygoni Multiflori Radix, Angelicae Sinensis Radix, Rehmanniae Radix Praeparata, Gastrodiae Rhizoma, Chuanxiong Rhizoma, Chaenomelis Fructus, etc.

Actions and Indications Nourishing blood and tonifying the kidney, dispelling wind, promoting hair-engendering. It is used for alopecia areata, total alopecia,

alopecia seborrhoeica, itching of scalp, much dandruff, alopecia after illness and puerperal alopecia attributed to blood-deficiency and depletion of the kidney.

养血当归糖浆

【处方】当归、白芍、熟地黄、茯苓、甘草（蜜炙）、党参、黄芪、川芎。

【功能主治】补气血，调经。用于贫血虚弱，产后体虚，萎黄肌瘦，月经不调，行经腹痛。

Chinese Angelica* Syrup for Enriching Blood

Name of Chinese Phonetic Alphabet Yang Xue Dang Gui Tang Jiang

Formula Angelicae Sinensis Radix, Paeoniae Radix Alba, Rehmanniae Radix Praeparata, Poria, Glycyrrhizae Radix et Rhizoma (prepared with honey), Codonopsis Radix, Astragali Radix and Chuanxiong Rhizoma.

Actions and Indications Tonifying *qi* and blood, regulating menstruation. It is used for anemia, puerperal debility, sallow complexion, emaciation, irregular menstruation, dysmenorrhea.

* 当归

养血安神糖浆

【处方】仙鹤草、墨旱莲、鸡血藤、熟地黄、地黄、合欢皮、首乌藤。

【功能主治】滋阴养血，宁心安神。用于阴虚血少，头眩心悸，失眠健忘。

Tranquility Syrup

Name of Chinese Phonetic Alphabet Yang Xue An Shen Tang Jiang

Formula Agrimoniae Herba, Ecliptae Herba, Spatholobi Caulis, Rehmanniae Radix Praeparata, Rehmanniae Radix, Albiziae Cortex and Polygoni Multiflori Caulis.

Actions and Indications Enriching *yin*, nourishing blood, tranquilizing the mind. It is used for vertigo, palpitation, insomnia and amnesia due to *yin*-deficiency and insufficiency of blood.

养血饮口服液

【处方】当归、黄芪、鹿角胶、阿胶、大枣。

【功能主治】补气养血，益肾助脾。用于气血两亏，崩漏下血，体虚羸弱，血小板减少及贫血，对放疗和化疗后引起的白细胞减少症有一定的治疗作用

Tonifying Blood Oral Liquid

Name of Chinese Phonetic Alphabet Yang Xue Yin Kou Fu Ye

Formula Angelicae Sinensis Radix, Astragali Radix, Cervi Cornus Colla, Asini Corii Colla and Jujubae Fructus.

Actions and Indications Tonifying *qi* and blood, fortifying the kidney and spleen. It is indicated for metrorrhagia and general debility due to dual deficiency of *qi* and blood; thrombopenia and anemia. The preparation possesses certain curative effect for the treatment of leukopenia due to radiotherapy and chemotherapy.

养血荣筋丸

【处方】当归、鸡血藤、赤芍、何首乌（酒炙）、续断、桑寄生、木香、威灵仙（酒炙）、伸筋草、透骨草、陈皮、补骨脂（盐炒）、油松节、赤小豆、党参、白术（麸炒）。

【功能主治】养血荣筋，祛风通络。用于跌打损伤日久引起的筋骨疼痛，肢体麻木，肌肉萎缩，关节不利，肿胀等陈旧性疾患。

【注意】孕妇忌用。

Sinew-luxuriating Bolus

Name of Chinese Phonetic Alphabet Yang Xue Rong Jin Wan

Formula Angelicae Sinensis Radix, Spatholobi

Caulis, Paeoniae Radix Rubra, Polygoni Multiflori Radix (prepared with wine), Dipsaci Radix, Taxilli Herba, Aucklandiae Radix, Clematidis Radix et Rhizoma (prepared with wine), Lycopodii Herba, Speranskiae Tuberculatae Herba, Citri Reticulatae Pericarpium, Psoraleae Fructus (fried with salt), Pini Lignum Nodi, Vignae Semen, Codonopsis Radix and Atractylodis Macrocephalae Rhizoma (fried with bran).

Actions and Indications Nourishing blood, luxuriating the sinews, dispelling wind, dredging collaterals. It is used for pain of sinews and bone, numbness of extremities, myoatrophy and difficult mobility of joints due to old traumatic injury.

Warning It is contraindicated for pregnant women.

养血清脑颗粒

【处方】当归、川芎、熟地黄、白芍、钩藤、鸡血藤、夏枯草、决明子、珍珠母、延胡索、细辛。

【功能主治】养血平肝，活血通络。用于血虚肝亢所致头痛，眩晕眼花，心烦易怒，失眠多梦。

【注意】低血压者慎用。孕妇忌用。

Nourishing Blood Granules

Name of Chinese Phonetic Alphabet Yang Xue Qing Nao Ke Li

Formula Angelicae Sinensis Radix, Chuanxiong Rhizoma, Rehmanniae Radix Praeparata, Paeoniae Radix Alba, Uncariae Ramulus cum Uncis, Spatholobi Caulis, Prunellae Spica, Cassiae Semen, Margaritifera Concha, Corydalis Rhizoma and Asari Radix et Rhizoma.

Actions and Indications Nourishing blood, pacifying the liver, activating blood, dredging collaterals. It is used for headache, vertigo, blurred vision, vexation, insomnia and profuse dreaming due to deficiency of blood and hyperactivity of the liver.

Warning It should be used cautiously for cases with hypotension and is contraindicated for pregnant women.

养阴降糖片

【处方】黄芪、党参、葛根、枸杞子、玄参、玉竹、地黄、知母、牡丹皮、川芎、虎杖、五味子。

【功能主治】养阴益气，清热活血。用于糖尿病。

Hypoglycemic Tablet of Nourishing *Yin*

Name of Chinese Phonetic Alphabet Yang Yin Jiang Tang Pian

Formula Astragali Radix, Codonopsis Radix, Puerariae Lobatae Radix, Lycii Fructus, Scrophulariae Radix, Polygonati Odorati Rhizoma, Rehmanniae Radix, Anemarrhenae Rhizoma, Moutan Cortex, Chuanxiong Rhizoma, Polygoni Cuspidati Rhizoma et Radix and Schisandrae Chinensis Fructus.

Actions and Indications Tonifying *qi* and nourishing *yin*, clearing heat and activating blood. It is indicated for diabetes.

养阴清肺糖浆

【处方】地黄、玄参、麦冬、川贝母、白芍、薄荷、甘草、牡丹皮。

【功能主治】养阴清肺，清热利咽。用于咽喉干燥疼痛，干咳少痰，痰中带血。

Yin-nourishing and Lung-moistening Syrup

Name of Chinese Phonetic Alphabet Yang Yin Qing Fei Tang Jiang

Formula Rehmanniae Radix, Scrophulariae Radix, Ophiopogonis Radix, Fritillariae Cirrhosae Bulbus, Paeoniae Radix Alba, Menthae Haplocalycis Herba, Glycyrrhizae Radix et Rhizoma and Moutan Cortex.

Actions and Indications Nourishing *yin*, clearing lung-heat, soothing the throat. It is used for dry throat, sore-throat, dry cough with few productive, blood-stained phlegm.

养阴清胃颗粒

【处方】石斛、知母、黄连、苦参、茯苓、白术、黄芪等。

【功能主治】养阴清胃，健脾和中。用于慢性萎缩性胃炎郁热蕴胃、伤及气阴证，症见胃脘痞满或疼痛，胃中灼热，恶心呕吐，反酸呕苦，口臭不爽，大便干。

【注意】忌食辛辣。

Relieving Atrophic Gastritis Soluble Granules

Name of Chinese Phonetic Alphabet Yang Yin Qing Wei Ke Li

Formula Dendrobii Caulis, Anemarrhenae Rhizoma, Coptidis Rhizoma, Sophorae Flavescentis Radix, Poria, Atractylodis Macrocephalae Rhizoma, Astragali Radix, etc.

Actions and Indications Nourishing *yin*, clearing stomach-heat, fortifying the spleen and harmonizing the middle energizer. It is indicated for chronic atrophic gastritis due to heat accumulated in the stomach and manifested as epigastric fullness or pain, scorching stomach, nausea, vomiting, acid regurgitation, bilious vomiting, fetid mouth, dry stool.

Warning Pungent foods are prohibited.

养胃冲剂

【处方】黄芪（炙）、党参、白芍、甘草、陈皮、香附、乌梅、山药。

【功能主治】养胃健脾，理气和中。用于脾虚气滞所致的慢性萎缩性胃炎。

Nourishing Stomach Soluble Granules

Name of Chinese Phonetic Alphabet Yang Wei Chong Ji

Formula Astragali Radix (prepared), Codonopsis Radix, Paeoniae Radix Alba, Glycyrrhizae Radix et Rhizoma, Citri Reticulatae Pericarpium, Cyperi Rhizoma, Mume Fructus and Dioscoreae Rhizoma.

Actions and Indications Nourishing the stomach and fortifying the spleen, regulating *qi* and harmonizing the middle. It is used for chronic atrophic gastritis due to deficiency of the spleen and *qi* stagnation.

养胃舒胶囊

【处方】党参、陈皮、黄精（蒸）、山药、干姜、菟丝子、白术（炒）、玄参、乌梅、山楂、北沙参。

【功能主治】扶正固本，滋阴养胃，调理中焦，行气消导。用于气阴两虚所致的胃脘热胀痛，手足心热，口干、口苦，纳差，消瘦，以及慢性萎缩性胃炎、慢性胃炎属气阴两虚而见有上述症状者。

Nourishing Stomach Capsule

Name of Chinese Phonetic Alphabet Yang Wei Shu Jiao Nang

Formula Codonopsis Radix, Citri Reticulatae Pericarpium, Polygonati Rhizoma (steamed), Dioscoreae Rhizoma, Zingiberis Rhizoma, Cuscutae Semen, Atractylodis Macrocephalae Rhizoma (fried), Scrophulariae Radix, Mume Fructus, Crataegi Fructus and Glehniae Radix.

Actions and Indications Supporting healthy *qi* and strengthening body resistance, enriching *yin* and nourishing the stomach, harmonizing the middle energizer, moving *qi* to improve food retention. It is indicated for epigastric fullness and pain, vexing heat in the palms and soles, dry mouth, bitter taste in the mouth, poor appetite and emaciation due to dual deficiency of *qi* and *yin*. Also used for chronic atrophic gastritis and chronic gastritis with the above mentioned symptoms.

养胃舒颗粒

【处方】党参、白术（炒）、黄精（蒸）、山药、干姜、菟丝子、陈皮、玄参。

【功能主治】益气固本，滋阴养胃，调理中焦，行气消导。用于气阴两虚引起的胃脘灼热胀痛，手足心热，口干，口苦，纳差，及慢性萎缩性胃炎、慢性胃炎有上述证候者。

Nourishing Stomach Granules

Name of Chinese Phonetic Alphabet Yang Wei Shu Ke Li

Formula Codonopsis Radix, Atractylodis Macrocephalae Rhizoma (fried), Polygonati Rhizoma (steamed), Dioscoreae Rhizoma, Zingiberis Rhizoma, Cuscutae Semen, Citri Reticulatae Pericarpium and Scrophulariae Radix.

Actions and Indications Tonifying *qi* and nourishing *yin*, strengthening body resistance, nourishing the stomach, harmonizing the middle energizer, moving *qi* to improve food retention. It is indicated for epigastric fullness and pain, vexing heat in the palms and soles, dry mouth, bitter taste in the mouth and poor appetite due to dual deficiency of *qi* and *yin*. Also used for chronic atrophic gastritis and chronic gastritis with the above mentioned symptoms.

宫血宁胶囊

【处方】重楼。

【功能主治】凉血，收涩止血。用于崩漏下血，月经过多，产后或流产后宫缩不良出血及子宫功能性出血属血热妄行证者。

Metrorrhagia-relieving Capsule

Name of Chinese Phonetic Alphabet Gong Xue Ning Jiao Nang

Formula Paridis Rhizoma.

Actions and Indications Cooling blood, relieving bleeding. It is used for metrorrhagia, profuse menstruation, puerperal or postabortal uterine atony and uterine dysfunctional bleeding attributed to frenetic movement due to heat.

宫瘤清胶囊

【处方】大黄 土鳖虫 水蛭等。

【功能主治】活血逐瘀、消瘤破积、养血清热。用于瘀血内停所致的小腹胀痛，经色紫暗有块，以及子宫浆膜下肌瘤。

【注意】经期停服。

Hysteromyoma-relieving Capsule

Name of Chinese Phonetic Alphabet Gong Liu Qing Jiao Nang

Formula Rhei Radix et Rhizoma, Eupolyphaga seu Steleophaga, Hirudo, etc.

Actions and Indications Activating blood, expelling stasis, reducing mass, nourishing blood, clearing heat. It is used for fullness and pain in lower abdomen, purple and dark menses with blood clot and subserous myoma of uterus.

Warning It should be suspended during menstrual period.

穿龙骨刺片

【处方】穿山龙、淫羊藿、狗脊、川牛膝、熟地黄、枸杞子。

【功能主治】补肾，健骨，活血，止痛。用于骨质增生，骨刺疼痛。

【注意】服药期间遇有感冒发热、腹泻应暂停服用。

Nippon Yam★ Tablet for Relieving Bony Spur

Name of Chinese Phonetic Alphabet Chuan Long Gu Ci Pian

Formula Dioscoreae Nipponicae Rhizoma, Epimedii Folium, Cibotii Rhizoma, Cyathulae Radix, Rehmanniae Radix Praeparata and Lycii Fructus.

Actions and Indications Tonifying the kidney, strengthening the bone, activating blood and alleviating pain. It is indicated for hyperosteogeny, pain due to bony spur.

Warning In cases with common cold, fever and diarrhea, suspend the medicine.

*穿山龙

祛伤消肿酊

【处方】连钱草、生草乌、冰片、莪术、红花、血竭、川芎、桂枝、威灵仙、茅膏菜、了哥王、海风藤、野木瓜、两面针、天南星、白芷、栀子、酢浆草、樟脑、薄荷脑。

【功能主治】活血化瘀，消肿止痛。用于跌打损伤，急性扭挫伤见有皮肤青紫瘀斑，肿胀疼痛。

【注意】外用药。

Removing Stasis Tincture for Traumatic Injury

Name of Chinese Phonetic Alphabet Qu Shang Xiao Zhong Ding

Formula Glechomae Herba, Aconit Kusnezoffii Radix (raw), Borneolum Syntheticum, Curcumae Rhizoma, Carthami Flos, Draconis Sanguis, Chuanxiong Rhizoma, Cinnamomi Ramulus, Clematidis Radix et Rhizoma, Droserae Peltatae Herba, Wikstroemiae Indicae Caulis et Folium, Piperis Kadsurae Caulis, Stauntoniae Chinensis Caulis et Folium, Zanthoxyli Radix, Arisaematis Rhizoma, Angelicae Dahuricae Radix, Gardeniae Fructus, Oxalidis Corniulatae Herba, Camphora and Menthol.

Actions and Indications Activating blood, resolving stasis, reducing swelling, alleviating pain. It is used for traumatic injury, acute sprain and contusion marked by purple ecchymosis of skin, swelling and pain.

Warning It is for external use only.

祛痰灵口服液

【处方】鲜竹沥、鱼腥草。

【功能主治】清热，化痰，解毒。用于肺热痰喘，咳嗽痰多。

【注意】便溏者忌用。

Dispelling Phlegm Oral Liquid

Name of Chinese Phonetic Alphabet Qu Tan Ling Kou Fu Ye

Formula Phyllostachydis Henonis Succus and Houttuyniae Herba.

Actions and Indications Clearing heat, resolving phlegm and detoxicating. It is used for phlegm dyspnea due to lung-heat; cough with profuse phlegm.

Warning It is contraindicated for cases with sloppy stool.

祖师麻片

【处方】本品为祖师麻浸膏粉经加工制成的片剂。

【功能主治】祛风除湿，活血止痛。用于风湿痹症，关节炎，类风湿性关节炎。

Girald Daphne* Tablet for Relieving Rheumatoid Arthritis

Name of Chinese Phonetic Alphabet Zu Shi Ma Pian

Formula Daphnes Giraldii Extractum.

Actions and Indications Dispelling wind and dampness, activating blood and alleviating pain. It is indicated for wind-damp impediment syndrome, arthritis and rheumatoid arthritis.

*祖师麻

祖师麻关节止痛膏

【处方】祖师麻、樟脑、冰片、薄荷脑、水杨酸甲酯、苯海拉明、二甲苯、麝香。

【功能主治】祛风除湿，活血止痛。用于风寒湿痹、瘀血痹阻经脉。症见肢体关节肿痛、畏寒肢冷、局部肿胀有硬结或瘀斑。

【注意】忌贴于创伤处，孕妇慎用。

Plaster of Girald Daphne* for Relieving Arthralgia

Name of Chinese Phonetic Alphabet Zu Shi Ma Guan Jie Zhi Tong Gao

Formula Daphnes Giraldii Cortex, Camphora , Borneolum Syntheticum, Menthol, Methyl Salicylate, Diphenhydramine, Xylene and Moschus.

Actions and Indications Dispelling wind and dampness, activating blood and alleviating pain. It is indicated for swelling and pain of the joints, fear of cold and cold limbs, local swelling with mass or ecchymosis due to wind-cold-damp impediment and blood-stasis.

Warning It is prohibited to be plastered on the injury area and should be used carefully for pregnant women.

*祖师麻

神农镇痛膏

【处方】三七、胆南星、白芷、狗脊、羌活、石菖蒲、防风、升麻、红花、土鳖虫、川芎、当归、血竭、马钱子、没药、樟脑、重楼、薄荷脑、乳香、水杨酸甲酯、冰片、丁香罗勒油、麝香、颠茄流浸膏、熊胆粉。

【功能主治】活血散瘀，消肿止痛。用于跌打损伤，风湿关节痛，腰背酸痛。

【注意】孕妇慎用。

Shen Nong Plaster for Pain-relieving

Name of Chinese Phonetic Alphabet Shen Nong Zhen Tong Gao

Formula Notoginseng Radix et Rhizoma, Arisaema cum Bile, Angelicae Dahuricae Radix, Cibotii Rhizoma, Notopterygii Rhizoma et Radix, Acori Tatarinowii Rhizoma, Saposhnikoviae Radix, Cimicifugae Rhizoma, Carthami Flos, Eupolyphaga seu Steleophaga, Chuanxiong Rhizoma, Angelicae Sinensis Radix, Draconis Sanguis, Strychni Semen, Myrrha, Camphora, Paridis Rhizoma, Menthol, Olibanum, Methyl Salicylate, Borneolum Syntheticum, Ocimi Basilici Oleum, Moschus, Belladonnae Extractum and Ursi Fel Pulvis.

Actions and Indications Activating blood, dissipating stasis, reducing swelling, alleviating pain. It is used for traumatic injury, rheumatic arthralgia, soreness and pain of waist and back.

Warning It should be used cautiously for pregnant women.

神香苏合丸

【处方】麝香、冰片、水牛角浓缩粉、乳香(制)、安息香、白术、香附、木香、沉香、丁香、苏合香。

【功能主治】温通宣痹，行气化浊。用于胸闷、气憋、心绞痛以及气厥、心腹疼痛等及冠心病具有上述证候者。

【注意】孕妇忌服。

Miraculous Storax* Pill

Name of Chinese Phonetic Alphabet Shen Xiang Su He Wan

Formula Moschus, Borneolum Syntheticum, Bubali Cornu Pulvis Concentratio, Olibanum (prepared), Benzoinum, Atractylodis Macrocephalae Rhizoma, Cyperi Rhizoma, Aucklandiae Radix, Aquilariae Lignum Resinatum, Caryophylli Flos and Styrax.

Actions and Indications Diffusing impediment, moving *qi*, resolving turbidity. It is used for chest distress, angina pectoris and syncope due to *qi* disorder; cardioabdominal pain and coronary heart disease with the above mentioned symptoms.

Warning It is contraindicated for pregnant women.

*苏合香

神衰康胶囊

【处方】本品为倒卵叶五加经加工制成的胶囊。

【功能主治】扶正固本，益智安神，补肾健脾。用于脾肾阳虚，腰膝酸软，体虚乏力，失眠，多梦，食欲不振。

Strengthening Body Resistance Capsule

Name of Chinese Phonetic Alphabet Shen Shuai Kang Jiao Nang

Formula Acanthopanacis Obovati Cortex.

Actions and Indications Supporting healthy *qi* to strengthen body resistance, tranquilize the mind, tonify the kidney and fortify the spleen. It is indicated for soreness and weakness of waist and knees, general debility, fatigue, insomnia, profuse dreaming and poor appetite due to dual *yang*-deficiency of the spleen and kidney.

冠心丹参片

【处方】丹参、三七、降香油。

【功能主治】活血化瘀，理气止痛。用于气滞血瘀、冠心病所致的胸闷，胸痹，心悸气短。

Relieving Coronary Heart Disease Tablet of Redroot Sage*

Name of Chinese Phonetic Alphabet Guan Xin Dan Shen Pian

Formula Salviae Miltiorrhizae Radix et Rhizoma, Notoginseng Radix er Rhizoma and Dalbergiae Odoriferae Oleum.

Actions and Indications Activating blood, resolving stasis, regulating *qi* to alleviate pain. It is indicated for chest distress, chest impediment syndrome, palpitation and shortness of breath due to *qi* stagnation, blood-stasis and coronary heart disease.

* 丹参

冠心生脉口服液

【处方】人参、麦冬、五味子（醋炙）、丹参、赤芍、郁金、三七。

【功能主治】益气生津，活血通脉。用于心气不足，心阴虚引起的心悸气短，胸闷作痛，自汗乏力，脉微结代。

【注意】节房事，切忌气恼、劳累过度。

Heart-*qi*-tonifying Oral Liquid

Name of Chinese Phonetic Alphabet Guan Xin Sheng Mai Kou Fu Ye

Formula Ginseng Radix et Rhizoma, Ophiopogonis Radix, Schisandrae Chinensis Fructus (prepared with vinegar), Salviae Miltiorrhizae Radix et Rhizoma, Paeoniae Radix Rubra, Curcumae Radix and Notoginseng Radix et Rhizoma.

Actions and Indications Tonifying *qi*, engendering fluid, activating blood, dredging vessels. It is used for palpitation, shortness of breath, chest distress and pain, spontaneous sweating, fatigue, faint and intermittent pulse due to insufficiency of heart-*qi* and deficiency of heart-*yin*.

Warning Sexual intercourse should be controlled, anger and overstrain should be avoided.

冠心安口服液

【处方】野菊花、川芎、延胡索（醋炙）、珍珠母、茯苓、桂枝、首乌藤、牛膝、降香、三七、半夏（炙）、大枣、甘草（蜜炙）、柴胡、冰片。

【功能主治】宽胸散结，活血行气。用于气滞血瘀型冠心病、心绞痛引起的胸痛，憋气，心悸，气短，乏力，心衰等症。

【注意】孕妇及心气虚、心血瘀阻性冠心病患者慎用。

Relieving Coronary Heart Disease Oral Liquid

Name of Chinese Phonetic Alphabet Guan Xin An Kou Fu Ye

Formula Chrysanthemi Indici Flos, Chuanxiong Rhizoma, Corydalis Rhizoma (prepared with vinegar), Margaritifera Concha, Poria, Cinnamomi Ramulus, Polygoni Multiflori Caulis, Achyranthis Bidentatae Raidx, Dalbergiae Odoriferae Lignum, Notoginseng Radix et Rhizoma, Pinelliae Rhizoma (prepared), Jujubae Fructus, Glycyrrhizae Radix et Rhizoma (prepared with honey), Bupleuri Radix and Borneolum

Syntheticum.

Actions and Indications Soothing the chest, dissipating stagnation, activating blood, moving *qi*. It is used for chest distress and pain, palpitation, shortness of breath, fatigue and heart failure due to *qi*-stagnation and blood-stasis, coronary heart disease and angina pectoris.

Warning It should be used cautiously for pregnant women and cases of coronary heart diasease due to deficiency of heart-*qi* and stagnation of heart-blood.

冠心苏合丸

【处方】苏合香、冰片、乳香（炒）、檀香、青木香。

【功能主治】理气宽胸，止痛。用于心绞痛，胸闷憋气。

【注意】孕妇禁用。

Storax* Pill for Coronary Heart Disease

Name of Chinese Phonetic Alphabet Guan Xin Su He Wan

Formula Styrax, Borneolum Syntheticum, Olibanum (fried), Santali Albi Lignum and Aristolochiae Radix.

Actions and Indications Regulating *qi*, soothing the chest, alleviating pain. It is indicated for angina pectoris and chest distress.

Warning It is contraindicated for pregnant women.

*苏合香

冠心静片

【处方】丹参、赤芍、川芎、红花、玉竹、三七、人参、苏合香。

【功能主治】活血化瘀，益气通脉，宣痹止痛。用于气虚血瘀，胸痹心痛，气短，心悸，冠心病，心绞痛，陈旧性心肌梗死属上述证候者。

【注意】患出血性疾病者慎用。

Relieving Coronary Heart Disease Tablet

Name of Chinese Phonetic Alphabet Guan Xin Jing Pian

Formula Salviae Miltiorrhizae Radix et Rhizoma, Paeoniae Radix Rubra, Chuanxiong Rhizoma, Carthami Flos, Polygonati Odorati Rhizoma, Notoginseng Radix et Rhizoma, Ginseng Radix et Rhizoma and Styrax.

Actions and Indications Activating blood, resolving stasis, tonifying *qi*, dredging vessels, diffusing impediment, alleviating pain. It is used for chest impediment syndrome, cardialgia, shortness of breath, palpitation, coronary heart disease, angina pectoris due to *qi* deficiency and blood-stasis; and old myocardial infarction with the above mentioned symptoms.

Warning It should be used cautiously for cases with hemorrhagic disease.

冠脉宁片

【处方】丹参、没药（炒）、鸡血藤、当归、血竭、延胡索（醋制）、制何首乌、郁金、桃仁（炒）、乳香（炒）、黄精（蒸）、红花、冰片、葛根。

【功能主治】活血化瘀，行气止痛。用于以胸部刺痛、固定不移、入夜更甚，心悸不宁，舌质紫暗，脉沉弦为主症的冠心病，心绞痛，冠状动脉供血不足。

【注意】孕妇忌服。

Alleviating Coronary Heart Disease Tablet

Name of Chinese Phonetic Alphabet Guan Mai Ning Pian

Formula Salviae Miltiorrhizae Radix et Rhizoma, Myrrha (fried), Spatholobi Caulis, Angelicae Sinensis Radix, Draconis Sanguis, Corydalis Rhizoma (prepared with vinegar), Polygoni Multiflori Radix Praeparata, Curcumae Radix, Persicae Semen (fried), Olibanum (fried), Polygonati Rhizoma (steamed), Carthami Flos, Borneolum Syntheticum and Puerariae Lobatae Radix.

Actions and Indications Activating blood, resolving stasis, moving *qi* to alleviate pain. It is indicated for coronary heart disease, angina pectoris and coronary insufficiency marked by fixed stabbing pain in chest which is ever more serious at night, palpitation, purple-dark tongue body, sunken and string-like pulse.

Warning It is contraindicated for pregnant women.

除湿白带丸

【处方】党参、白术（麸炒）、山药、白芍、芡实、车前子（炒）、白果、苍术、陈皮、当归、荆芥（炭）、柴胡、黄柏（炭）、茜草、海螵蛸、牡蛎（煅）。

【功能主治】除湿健脾。用于脾虚湿盛白带。

Relieving Vaginal Discharge Pill

Name of Chinese Phonetic Alphabet Chu Shi Bai Dai Wan

Formula Codonopsis Radix, Atractylodis Macrocephalae Rhizoma (fried with bran), Dioscoreae Rhizoma, Paeoniae Radix Alba, Euryales Semen, Plantaginis Semen (fried), Ginkgo Semen, Atractylodis Rhizoma, Citri Reticulatae Pericarpium, Angelicae Sinensis Radix, Schizonepetae Herba (carbonated), Bupleuri Radix, Phellodendri Chinensis Cortex (carbonated), Rubiae Radix et Rhizoma, Sepiae Endoconcha, Ostreae Concha (calcined).

Actions and Indications Eliminating dampness and fortifying the spleen. It is indicated for vaginal discharge due to prevailing dampness and spleen-deficiency.

除痰止嗽丸

【处方】枳实、白术（麸炒）、陈皮、法半夏、桔梗、浮海石（煅）、前胡、六神曲（麸炒）、防风、黄芩、栀子（姜炙）、黄柏、大黄、知母、天花粉、甘草、冰片、薄荷脑

【功能主治】清肺降火，除痰止嗽。用于肺热痰盛引起的咳嗽气逆，痰黄黏稠，咽喉疼痛，大便干燥。

Dispelling Phlegm and Suppressing Cough Bolus

Name of Chinese Phonetic Alphabet Chu Tan Zhi Sou Wan

Formula Aurantii Fructus Immaturus, Atractylodis Macrocephalae Rhizoma (fried with bran), Citri Reticulatae Pericarpium, Pinelliae Rhizoma Praeparatum, Platycodonis Radix, Pumex (calcined), Peucedani Radix, Medicata Massa Fermentata (fried with bran), Saposhnikoviae Radix, Scutellariae Radix, Gardeniae Fructus (prepared with ginger), Phellodendri Chinensis Cortex, Rhei Radix et Rhizoma, Anemarrhenae Rhizoma, Trichosanthis Radix, Glycyrrhizae Radix et Rhizoma, Borneolum Syntheticum and Menthol.

Actions and Indications Clearing lung-heat and downbearing fire, dispelling phlegm and suppressing cough. It is indicated for cough, *qi* counterflow, yellow, thick and sticky phlegm, sore-throat and dry stool due to lung-heat and excessive phlegm.

结石通片

【处方】金钱草、玉米须、石韦、鸡骨草、茯苓、车前草、海金沙藤、白茅根。

【功能主治】清热利湿，通淋排石，镇痛止血。用于泌尿系统感染，膀胱炎，肾炎水肿，尿路结石，血尿，淋沥混浊，尿道灼痛。

【注意】孕妇忌服。忌食辛、燥、酸、辣食物。

Relieving Lithangiuria Tablet

Name of Chinese Phonetic Alphabet Jie Shi Tong Pian

Formula Lysimachiae Herba, Zeae Maydis Stylus, Pyrrosiae Folium, Abri Herba, Poria, Plantaginis Herba, Lygodii Caulis and Imperatae Rhizoma.

Actions and Indications Clearing heat and draining dampness, relieving strangury and removing stone, alleviating pain and relieving bleeding. It is indicated for urinary system infection, cystitis, nephritic edema, lithangiuria, hematuria, dribbling and turbid urine, scorching pain in urethra.

Warning It is contraindicated for pregnant women. Pungent, dry, and sour foods are prohibited.

结肠宁（灌肠剂）

【处方】蒲黄、丁香蓼。

【功能主治】活血化瘀，清肠止泻。用于慢性结肠炎性腹泻（慢性菌痢、溃疡性结肠炎）。

Enema for Colitis

Name of Chinese Phonetic Alphabet Jie Chang Ning (Guan Chang Ji)

Formula Typhae Pollen and Ludwigiae Prostratae Herba.

Actions and Indications Activating blood and resolving stasis, clearing the intestine and relieving diarrhea. It is indicated for diarrhea due to chronic colitis, chronic bacillary dysentery and ulcerative colitis.

绞股蓝总苷片

【处方】本品为绞股蓝总苷经加工制成的片剂。

【功能主治】养心健脾，益气和血，除痰化瘀，降血脂。用于高血脂症，见有心悸气短，胸闷肢麻，眩晕。

Gypenosides* Tablet for Relieving Hyperlipemia

Name of Chinese Phonetic Alphabet Jiao Gu Lan Zong Gan Pian

Formula Gypenosides.

Actions and Indications Nourishing the heart and fortifying the spleen, tonifying *qi* and harmonizing blood, dispelling phlegm and resolving stasis, decreasing blood lipid. It is indicated for hyperlipemia, manifested as palpitation, shortness of breath, chest distress, numbness of the limbs and vertigo.

* 绞股蓝总苷

十画

珠贝定喘丸

【处方】珍珠、川贝母、琥珀、人工牛黄、细辛、葶苈子、肉桂油、陈皮、紫苏叶油、麻黄、五味子、猪胆粉、人参、氨茶碱、盐酸异丙嗪。

【功能主治】理气化痰，镇咳平喘，补气温肾。用于治疗支气管哮喘、慢性支气管炎等久病喘咳，痰涎壅盛。

【注意】孕妇及妇女月经期慎用。

Pill of Pearl* and Sichuan Fritillary** for Relieving Dyspnea

Name of Chinese Phonetic Alphabet Zhu Bei Ding Chuan Wan

Formula Margarita, Fritillariae Cirrhosae Bulbus, Succinum, Bovis Calculus Artifactus, Asari Radix et Rhizoma, Lepidii Semen, Cinnamomi Oleum, Citri Reticulatae Pericarpium, Perillae Folium Oleum, Ephedrae Herba, Schisandrae Chinensis Fructus, Suillus Bilis Pulvis, Ginseng Radix et Rhizoma, Aminophylline and Promethazine Hydrochloride.

Actions and Indications Regulating *qi* and resolving phlegm, settling cough and calming dyspnea, tonifying *qi* and warming the kidney. It is indicated for bronchial asthma, chronic bronchitis, productive cough and dyspnea.

Warning It should be used carefully for pregnant women and women during menstrual period.

* 珍珠 ** 川贝母

珠珀安神丹

【处方】珍珠、白芍、红参、川芎、茯苓、黄芪、陈皮、甘草、琥珀、丹参、当归、远志、白术、地黄、六神曲、牡蛎、朱砂。

【功能主治】宁心安神，益气养血。用于气血两亏所致的夜不安睡，精神不振，心跳气短。

Pearl* and Amber** Pill for Tranquilization

Name of Chinese Phonetic Alphabet Zhu Po An Shen Dan

Formula Margarita, Paeoniae Radix Alba, Ginseng Radix et Rhizoma Rubra, Chuanxiong Rhizoma, Poria, Astragali Radix, Citri Reticulatae Pericarpium, Glycyrrhizae Radix et Rhizoma, Succinum, Salviae Miltiorrhizae Radix et Rhizoma, Angelicae Sinensis Radix, Polygalae Radix, Atractylodis Macrocephalae Rhizoma, Rehmanniae Radix, Medicata Massa Fermentata, Ostreae Concha and Cinnabaris.

Actions and Indications Tranquilizing the mind, tonifying *qi*, nourishing blood. It is used for disturbed sleep, lassitude of spirit, palpitation and shortness of breath due to dual depletion of *qi* and blood.

*珍珠 **琥珀

珠黄散

【处方】珍珠、牛黄。

【功能主治】清热解毒，去腐生肌。用于咽喉肿痛糜烂，口腔溃疡久不收敛。

Pearl* and Bezoar** Powder

Name of Chinese Phonetic Alphabet Zhu Huang San

Formula Margarita and Bovis Calculus.

Actions and Indications Clearing heat and detoxicating, removing necrosis and promoting tissue regeneration. It is used for sore-throat with erosion and prolonged stomatocace.

*珍珠 **牛黄

桂龙咳喘宁胶囊

【处方】本品为桂枝、龙骨、法半夏、黄连等加工制成的胶囊。

【功能主治】止咳化痰，降气平喘。用于风寒或痰湿阻肺引起的咳嗽，气喘，痰涎壅盛，以及急、慢性支气管炎。

【注意】服药期间忌烟、酒、猪肉、生冷食物。

Dragon's Bone* and Cassia Twig** Capsule for Relieving Cough and Dyspnea

Name of Chinese Phonetic Alphabet Gui Long Ke Chuan Ning Jiao Nang

Formula Cinnamomi Ramulus, Draconis Os, Pinelliae Rhizoma Praeparatum, Coptidis Rhizoma, etc.

Actions and Indications Relieving cough and resolving phlegm, directing *qi* downward and calming dyspnea. It is indicated for cough, dyspnea and profuse phlegm due to stagnation of wind-cold or phlegm-damp in the lung, and also for acute, chronic bronchitis.

Warning Smoke, wine, pork, uncooked and cold foods are prohibited during medication.

*龙骨 **桂枝

桂芍镇痫片

【处方】桂枝、白芍、党参、半夏（制）、柴胡、黄芩、甘草、生姜、大枣。

【功能主治】和营卫，清肝胆。用于治疗各种发作类型的癫痫。

Cassia Twig* White Peony ** Tablet for Epilepsy-relieving

Name of Chinese Phonetic Alphabet Gui Shao Zhen Xian Pian

Formula Cinnamomi Ramulus, Paeoniae Radix Alba, Codonopsis Radix, Pinelliae Rhizoma (prepared), Bupleuri Radix, Scutellariae Radix, Glycyrrhizae Radix et Rhizoma, Zingiberis Rhizoma Recens and Jujubae Fructus.

Actions and Indications Harmonizing nutrient and defense aspects, clearing liver-fire and gallbladder-fire. It is applied for the treatment of various types of epilepsy.

*桂枝 **白芍

桂附地黄丸

【处方】肉桂、附子(制)、熟地黄、山茱萸(制)、牡丹皮、山药、茯苓、泽泻。

【功能主治】温补肾阳。用于肾阳不足，腰膝酸冷，肢体浮肿，小便不利或反多，痰饮喘咳，消渴。

Cassia Bark* Szechuan Aconite** and Chinese Fox-glove*** Bolus

Name of Chinese Phonetic Alphabet Gui Fu Di Huang Wan

Formula Cinnamomi Cortex, Aconiti Lateralis Radix (prepared), Rehmanniae Radix Praeparata, Corni Fructus (prepared), Moutan Cortex, Dioscoreae Rhizoma, Poria and Alismatis Rhizoma.

Actions and Indications Warming and tonifying kidney-*yang*. It is used for soreness and cold of waist and knees, edema, oliguria or profuse urination, phlegm-fluid retention, dyspnea, cough and wasting-thirst due to insufficiency of kidney-*yang*.

* 肉桂 ** 附子 *** 地黄

桂附理中丸

【处方】肉桂、附片、党参、白术(炒)、炮姜、甘草(蜜炙)。

【功能主治】补肾助阳，温中健脾。用于肾阳虚衰，脾胃虚寒，脘腹冷痛，呕吐泄泻，四肢厥冷。

【注意】孕妇慎用。

Cassia Bark* and Szechuan Aconite** Bolus for Warming Middle Energizer

Name of Chinese Phonetic Alphabet Gui Fu Li Zhong Wan

Formula Cinnamomi Cortex, Aconiti Lateralis Radix Praeparata (sliced), Codonopsis Radix, Atractylodis Macrocephalae Rhizoma (fried), Zingiberis Rhizoma Praeparatum and Glycyrrhizae Radix et Rhizoma (prepared with honey).

Actions and Indications Tonifying kidney-*yang*, warming the middle energizer and fortifying the spleen. It is indicated for abdominal cold and pain, vomiting, diarrhea and cold limbs due to declination of kidney-*yang* and deficiency-cold of the spleen and stomach.

Warning It should be used carefully for pregnant women.

* 肉桂 ** 附子

桂林西瓜霜片

【处方】西瓜霜、硼砂(煅)、黄柏、黄连、黄芩、山豆根、射干、浙贝母、青黛、冰片、大黄、甘草、薄荷脑等。

【功能主治】清热解毒，消肿止痛。用于咽喉肿痛，口舌生疮，牙龈肿痛或出血，急、慢性咽喉炎，扁桃体炎，口腔炎，口腔溃疡，小儿鹅口疮及轻度烫火伤与创伤出血。

Gui Lin Watermelon Mirabilite* Tablet for Throat-soothing

Name of Chinese Phonetic Alphabet Gui Lin Xi Gua Shuang Pian

Formula Marabilitum Praeparatum, Borax (calcined), Phellodendri Chinensis Cortex, Coptidis Rhizoma, Scutellariae Radix, Sophorae Tonkinensis Radix et Rhizoma, Belamcandae Rhizoma, Fritillariae Thunbergii Bulbus, Indigo Naturalis, Borneolum Syntheticum, Rhei Radix et Rhizoma, Glycyrrhizae Radix et Rhizoma, Menthol, etc.

Actions and Indications Clearing heat and detoxicating, dispersing swelling and relieving pain. It is used for sore-throat, aphthae, gingivitis, acute and chronic laryngopharyngitis, tonsillitis, stomatitis, stomatocace, children thrush, mild burn and scald and traumatic bleeding.

* 西瓜霜

桂枝茯苓胶囊

【处方】桂枝、茯苓、牡丹皮等。

【功能主治】活血化瘀，缓消癥块。用于妇女血瘀所致下腹宿有癥块，月经量多或漏下不止，血色暗紫，多血块，小腹隐痛或腹痛拒按，舌暗有瘀斑，脉涩或细。

【注意】妊娠者忌服。

Cassia Twig* and Indian Bread** Capsule

Name of Chinese Phonetic Alphabet Gui Zhi Fu Ling Jiao Nang

Formula Cinnamomi Ramulus, Poria, Moutan Cortex, etc.

Actions and Indications Activating blood, resolving stasis, dispersing mass. It is used for mass in the lower abdomen of women, hypermenorrhea or metrorrhagia with dark and clotted blood, dull pain in the lower abdomen or abdominal pain, tenderness, dark tongue with ecchymosis, rough or fine pulse.

Warning It is contraindicated for pregnant women.

* 桂枝 ** 茯苓

桔梗冬花片

【处方】桔梗、款冬花、远志（制）、甘草。

【功能主治】镇咳祛痰。用于咳嗽痰多，支气管炎。

【注意】本品宣散之力较强，对暴咳、咯血等证不宜。

Balloon Flower* and Common Coltsfoot** Tablet

Name of Chinese Phonetic Alphabet Jie Geng Dong Hua Pian

Formula Platycodonis Radix, Farfarae Flos, Polygalae Radix (prepared) and Glycyrrhizae Radix et Rhizoma.

Actions and Indications Settling cough and dispelling phlegm. It is indicated for cough with profuse phlegm and bronchitis.

Warning It has powerful effect of diffusing, and is not suitable for cases with sudden cough and hemoptysis.

* 桔梗 ** 款冬花

根痛平冲剂

【处方】白芍、葛根、桃仁（去皮）、红花、续断、乳香（醋炙）、没药（醋炙）、牛膝、狗脊（砂烫去毛）、伸筋草、地黄、甘草。

【功能主治】活血，通络，止痛。用于风寒阻络所致颈腰椎病，症见肩颈疼痛，活动受限，上肢麻木。

【注意】孕妇忌用。

Alleviating Pain Soluble Granules

Name of Chinese Phonetic Alphabet Gen Tong Ping Chong Ji

Formula Paeoniae Radix Alba, Puerariae Lobatae Radix, Persicae Semen (removed seed coat), Carthami Flos, Dipsaci Radix, Olibanum (prepared with vinegar), Myrrha (prepared with vinegar), Achyranthis Bidentatae Radix, Cibotii Rhizoma(scalded by sand to remove hair), Lycopodii Herba, Rehmanniae Radix and Glycyrrhizae Radix et Rhizoma.

Actions and Indications Activating blood, dredging collaterals, alleviating pain. It is used for cervical spondylopathy or lumbar vertebral disease due to wind-cold obstructing the collaterals marked by pain in shoulder and neck, immobility, numbness of upper limbs.

Warning It is contraindicated for pregnant women.

真菌竹黄胶囊

【处方】本品为肉座菌科植物的子座经提取加工制成的胶囊。

【功能主治】祛风通络，散寒理湿。用于风寒湿痹。

Shiraia Bambusicola Stroma* Capsule for Relieving Impediment Syndrome

Name of Chinese Phonetic Alphabet Zhen Jun Zhu Huang Jiao Nang

Formula Shiraiae Bambusicolae Stroma (fungus) Extract.

Actions and Indications Dispelling wind and dredging collaterals, dissipating cold and regulating damp. It is used for wind-cold-damp impediment syndrome.

＊肉座菌科植物（真菌）子座

莱阳梨止咳口服液

【处方】莱阳梨清膏、麻黄提取液、杏仁水、北沙参流浸膏、百合流浸膏、远志流浸膏、桔梗流浸膏、薄荷脑。

【功能主治】镇咳祛痰。用于伤风感冒引起的咳嗽多痰，急、慢性气管炎。

Lai Yang Pear* Oral Liquid for Relieving Cough

Name of Chinese Phonetic Alphabet Lai Yang Li Zhi Ke Kou Fu Ye

Formula Lai Yang Pyri Fructus (liquid extract), Ephedrae Extractum, Armeniacae Semen Amarum (water solution), Glehniae Radix (liquid extract), Lilii Bulbus (liquid extract), Polygalae Extractum, Platycodonis Extractum and menthod.

Actions and Indications Relieving cough, dispelling phlegm. It is used for cough with profuse phlegm, acute or chronic trachitis induced by common cold.

＊莱阳梨

莲花峰茶

【处方】枳实、川木通、甘草、紫苏、桔梗、天花粉、滑石、小茴香、茯苓、广藿香、槟榔、香薷、木瓜、前胡、桑叶、桑白皮、柴胡、青皮、豆蔻、鬼针草、木香、丁香、山楂、茵陈、泽泻、半夏（制）、防风、九层塔、白术、白扁豆、苍术、陈皮（制）、大腹皮、铁苋菜、水龙、车前子、砂仁、丁癸草、厚朴、麦芽（炒）、桂枝、稻芽（炒）、荆芥、爵床、茶叶。

【功能主治】疏风散寒，清热解暑，祛痰利湿，健脾开胃，理气和中。用于四时感冒，伤暑夹湿，脘腹胀满，呕吐泄泻。

Lian Hua Feng Tea

Name of Chinese Phonetic Alphabet Lian Hua Feng Cha

Formula Aurantii Fructus Immaturus, Clematidis Armandii Caulis, Glycyrrhizae Radix et Rhizoma, Perillae Folium, Platycodonis Radix, Trichosanthis Radix, Talcum, Foeniculi Fructus, Poria, Pogostemonis Herba, Arecae Semen, Moslae Herba, Chaenomelis Fructus, Peucedani Radix, Mori Folium, Mori Cortex, Bupleuri Radix, Citri Reticulatae Pericarpium Viride, Amomi Fructus Rotundus, Bidentis Bipinnatae Herba, Aucklandiae Radix, Caryophylli Flos, Crataegi Fructus, Artemisiae Scopariae Herba, Alismatis Rhizoma, Pinelliae Rhizoma (prepared), Saposhnikoviae Radix, Ocimi Basilici Herba, Atractylodis Macrocephalae Rhizoma, Lablab Semen Album, Atractylodis Rhizoma, Citri Reticulatae Pericarpium (prepared), Arecae Pericarpium, Acalyphae Australis Herba, Jussiaeae Repentis Herba, Plantaginis Semen, Amomi Fructus, Zorniae Diphyllae Herba, Magnoliae Officinalis Cortex, Hordei Fructus Germinatus (fried), Cinnamomi Ramulus, Oryzae Fructus Germinatus (fried), Schizonepetae Herba, Rostellulariae Procumbenstis Herba and Camelliae Sinensis Folium Gemmae.

Actions and Indications Dispersing wind and dissipating cold, clearing heat and releasing summer-heat, dispelling phlegm and draining dampness, fortifying the spleen and improving appetite, regulating-*qi* and harmonizing the middle. It is indicated for seasonal common cold, summer-heat with dampness, abdominal distention and fullness, vomiting and diarrhea.

莲芝消炎胶囊

【处方】穿心莲内酯、山芝麻干浸膏。

【功能主治】清热，解毒，消炎。用于肠胃炎，扁桃体炎，咽喉炎，肺炎。

Antiphlogistic Capsule of Common Andrographis* and Narrowleaf Screwtree**

Name of Chinese Phonetic Alphabet Lian Zhi

Xiao Yan Jiao Nang

Formula Andrographolide and Helicteris Angustifoliae Extractum.

Actions and Indications Clearing heat and detoxicating, antiphlogistic. It is indicated for enterogastritis, tonsillitis, laryngopharyngitis, pneumonia.

*穿心莲 **山芝麻

莲胆消炎片

【处方】穿心莲、苦木。

【功能主治】清热解毒，制菌消炎。用于细菌性痢疾，急性胃肠炎及各种急性感染性疾患。

Anti-inflammation Tablet of Common Andrographis*

Name of Chinese Phonetic Alphabet Lian Dan Xiao Yan Pian

Formula Andrographis Herba and Picrasmae Ramulus et Folium.

Actions and Indications Clearing heat and detoxicating, antibacterial and antiphlogistic. It is indicated for bacillary dysentery, acute gastroenteritis and various infective diseases.

*穿心莲

荷丹片

【处方】荷叶、丹参等。

【功能主治】化痰降浊，活血化瘀。用于高脂血症属痰浊夹瘀证候者。

【注意】孕妇忌用。

Tablet of Lotus Leaf* and Redroot Sage**

Name of Chinese Phonetic Alphabet He Dan Pian

Formula Nelumbinis Folium, Salviae Miltiorrhizae Radix et Rhizoma, etc.

Actions and Indications Resolving phlegm and downbearing turbidity, activating blood and resolving stasis. It is indicated for hyperlipemia attributive to phlegm turbiding mixed up with blood-stasis.

Warning It is contraindicated for pregnant women.

*荷叶 **丹参

荷叶丸

【处方】荷叶、藕节、香墨、小蓟（炭）、知母、当归、白芍、地黄（炭）、玄参、栀子（焦）、白茅根（炭）、大蓟（炭）、黄芩（炭）、棕榈（炭）。

【功能主治】凉血止血。用于咯血，衄血，尿血，便血，崩漏。

Lotus Leaf* Bolus

Name of Chinese Phonetic Alphabet He Ye Wan

Formula Nelumbinis Folium, Nelumbinis Rhizomatic Nodus, Chinese Ink, Cirsii Herba (carbonated), Anemarrhenae Rhizoma, Angelicae Sinensis Radix, Paeoniae Radix Alba, Rehmanniae Radix (carbonated), Scrophulariae Radix, Gardeniae Fructus (charred), Imperatae Rhizoma (carbonated), Cirsii Herba Japonici (carbonated), Scutellariae Radix (carbonated) and Trachycarpi Petiolus Carbonisatus.

Actions and Indications Cooling blood, relieving bleeding. It is indicated for hemoptysis, epistaxis, hematuria, hematochezia, metrorrhagia.

*荷叶

速效救心丸

【处方】川芎、冰片。

【功能主治】行气活血，祛瘀止痛，增加冠脉血流量，缓解心绞痛。用于气滞血瘀型冠心病，心绞痛。

Quick-acting Pill for Coronary Heart Disease

Name of Chinese Phonetic Alphabet Su Xiao

Jiu Xin Wan

Formula Chuanxiong Rhizoma and Borneolum Syntheticum.

Actions and Indications Moving *qi*, activating blood, dispelling stasis, alleviating pain, increasing coronary blood flow, relieving angina pectoris. It is indicated for coronary heart disease and angina pectoris due to *qi*- stagnation and blood-stasis.

速溶阿胶冲剂

【处方】本品为驴皮经煎煮，浓缩、喷雾干燥制成的冲剂。

【功能主治】补血滋阴，润燥，止血。用于血虚萎黄，眩晕心悸，肌痿无力，心烦不眠，肺燥咳嗽，劳嗽咯血，吐血尿血，便血崩漏，妊娠胎漏。

Instant Soluble Granules of Ass-hide Gelatin*

Name of Chinese Phonetic Alphabet Su Rong E Jiao Chong Ji

Formula Asini Corii Colla.

Actions and Indications Tonifying blood and enriching *yin*, moistening dryness, relieving bleeding. It is used for sallow complexion, vertigo, palpitation, myoatrophy, vexation, insomnia, cough due to lung dryness, hemoptysis, hematemesis and hematuria, hematochezia, metrorrhagia, vaginal bleeding during pregnancy.

* 阿胶

夏天无片

【处方】夏天无等。

【功能主治】通络、活血、止痛，用于高血压偏瘫，小儿麻痹后遗症，坐骨神经痛，风湿性关节痛，跌打损伤。

Bending Corydalis* Tablet

Name of Chinese Phonetic Alphabet Xia Tian Wu Pian

Formula Corydalis Decumbentis Rhizoma, etc.

Actions and Indications Dredging collaterals, activating blood, alleviating pain. It is indicated for hemiparalysis due to hypertension; sequela of poliomyelitis, sciatica, rheumatic arthralgia and injury due to fall and strike.

* 夏天无

夏枯草膏

【处方】本品为夏枯草制成的煎膏。

【功能主治】清火，明目，散结，消肿。用于头痛眩晕，瘰疬，瘿瘤，乳痈肿痛，甲状腺肿大，乳腺增生症，高血压症。

【注意】体虚慎用；忌食辛辣油腻及刺激性食物。

Selfheal Fruit-spike* Extract

Name of Chinese Phonetic Alphabet Xia Ku Cao Gao

Formula Prunellae Spica (extract).

Actions and Indications Clearing heat, improving vision, dispersing swelling and mass. It is indicated for headache, vertigo, scrofula, goiter, acute mastitis, thyroid enlargement, hyperplasia of mammary glands and hypertension.

Warning It should be used carefully for cases with debility of constitution. Pungent and irritant foods are prohibited.

* 夏枯草

振源胶囊

【处方】本品为人参果实提取的总皂苷制成的胶囊剂。

【功能主治】滋补强壮，安神益智，增强免疫功能，调节内分泌和自主神经功能紊乱，增强心肌收缩力，提高心脏功能，保肝和抗肿瘤作用。主要用于治疗冠心病，更年期综合征，久病体弱，神经衰弱，隐性糖尿病，亦可用于慢性肝炎和肿瘤的辅助治疗。

【注意】忌与五灵脂、藜芦同服。

Crasis-strengthening Capsule

Name of Chinese Phonetic Alphabet Zhen Yuan Jiao Nang

Formula Ginseng Fructus (total saponin).

Actions and Indications Tonifying and strengthening crasis, tranquilizing the mind, enhancing immunologic function, regulating endocrine and dysautonomia, enhancing myocardial contractive power and cardial function, protecting the liver and antineoplastic effect. It is applied for coronary heart disease, menopausal syndrome, physical debility, prolonged illness, neurasthenia, latent diabetes, and also applied as accessory treatment for chronic hepatitis and tumour.

Warning The preparation cannot be used with Trogopterus Dung* and False hellebore** simultaneously.

* 五灵脂 ** 藜芦

损伤速效止痛气雾剂

【处方】血竭、红花、乳香（醋炙）、冰片、麝香、樟脑。

【功能主治】消肿止痛，活血化瘀，消炎生肌，舒筋活络。用于跌打损伤，扭拉伤，挫撞伤，摈擦伤，骨折脱臼疼痛等急性运动创伤。

Quick-acting Spray for Pain-relieving

Name of Chinese Phonetic Alphabet Sun Shang Su Xiao Zhi Tong Qi Wu Ji

Formula Draconis Sanguis, Carthami Flos, Olibanum (prepared with vinegar), Borneolum Syntheticum, Moschus and Camphora.

Actions and Indications Reducing swelling, alleviating pain, activating blood, resolving stasis, anti-inflammatory, promoting tissue regeneration, relaxing sinews, activating collaterals. It is used for pain due to traumatic injury, sprain, contusion, fracture, dislocation and acute sport injury.

换骨丸

【处方】麻黄、威灵仙（酒炙）、防风、白芷、苍术（米泔炙）、蔓荆子（微炒）、川芎、桑白皮（蜜炙）、苦参、槐角（蜜炙）、人参、何首乌（酒炙）、五味子（醋炙）、木香。

【功能主治】散风祛湿，活络止痛。用于风湿阻络，四肢麻木，周身疼痛，筋骨无力，行步艰难。

Activating Collateral and Alleviating Pain Bolus

Name of Chinese Phonetic Alphabet Huan Gu Wan

Formula Ephedrae Herba, Clematidis Radix et Rhizoma (prepared with wine), Saposhnikoviae Radix, Angelicae Dahuricae Radix, Atractylodis Rhizoma (prepared with rice swilled water), Viticis Fructus (fried), Chuanxiong Rhizoma, Mori Cortex (prepared with honey), Sophorae Flavescentis Radix, Sophorae Fructus (prepared with honey), Ginseng Radix et Rhizoma, Polygoni Multiflori Radix (prepared with wine), Schisandrae Chinensis Fructus (prepared with vinegar) and Aucklandiae Radix.

Actions and Indications Dissipating wind and dampness, activating collaterals and alleviating pain. It is indicated for numbness of the limbs, general pain, weakness of sinews and bone and difficulty for walk due to stagnation of wind-damp in collaterals.

热毒清片

【处方】重楼、南板蓝根、冰片、蒲公英、甘草。

【功能主治】清热解毒，消肿散结。用于热毒内盛所致的腮腺炎、扁桃体炎、喉炎、上呼吸道感染。

Clearing Heat Tablet for Relieving Parotitis

Name of Chinese Phonetic Alphabet Re Du Qing Pian

Formula Paridis Rhizoma, Baphicacanthis Cusiae

Rhizoma et Radix, Borneolum Syntheticum, Taraxaci Herba and Glycyrrhizae Radix et Rhizoma.

Actions and Indications Clearing heat and detoxicating, dispersing swelling and dissipating mass. It is indicated for parotitis, tonsillitis, pharyngitis, upper respiratory tract infection due to excessive heat-toxin.

柴连口服液

【处方】麻黄、柴胡、广藿香、肉桂等。

【功能主治】解表宣肺，化湿和中。用于感冒属风寒、风寒夹湿者，症见恶寒、发热、头痛、鼻塞、咳嗽、咽干或兼脘闷、恶心。

Chinese Hare's Ear* and Chinese Ephedra ** Oral Liquid

Name of Chinese Phonetic Alphabet Chai Lian Kou Fu Ye

Formula Ephedrae Herba, Bupleuri Radix, Pogostemonis Herba, Cinnamomi Cortex, etc.

Actions and Indications Releasing the exterior and diffusing the lung, resolving dampness and harmonizing the middle energizer. It is indicated for common cold attributed to wind-cold type, or wind-cold accompanied with dampness type, manifested as aversion to cold, fever, headache, nasal congestion, cough, dry throat or accompanied with abdominal oppression, nausea.

* 柴胡 ** 麻黄

柴胡口服液

【处方】柴胡。

【功能主治】退热解表。用于外感发热。

Chinese Hare's Ear* Oral Liquid

Name of Chinese Phonetic Alphabet Chai Hu Kou Fu Ye

Formula Bupleuri Radix.

Actions and Indications Defervescence and releasing the exterior. It is indicated for fever due to external contraction.

* 柴胡

柴黄片

【处方】柴胡、黄芩。

【功能主治】清热解表，用于轻、中型风热感冒引起的发热，周身不适，头痛目眩，咽喉肿痛，并主治乙型肝炎。

Chinese Hare's Ear* and Baical Skullcap** Tablet

Name of Chinese Phonetic Alphabet Chai Huang Pian

Formula Bupleuri Radix and Scutellariae Radix.

Actions and Indications Clearing heat and releasing the exterior. It is indicated for common cold, marked by fever, general discomfort, headache and dizzy vision, sore-throat, and also used for hepatitis B.

* 柴胡 ** 黄芩

逍遥丸

【处方】柴胡、当归、白芍、白术（炒）、茯苓、甘草（蜜炙）、薄荷。

【功能主治】疏肝健脾，养血调经。用于肝气不舒，胸胁胀痛，头晕目眩，食欲减退，月经不调。

Xiao Yao Pill

Name of Chinese Phonetic Alphabet XiaoYao Wan

Formula Bupleuri Radix, Angelicae Sinensis Radix, Paeoniae Radix Alba, Atractylodis Macrocephalae Rhizoma (fried), Poria, Glycyrrhizae Radix et Rhizoma (prepared with honey) and Menthae Haplocalycis Herba.

Actions and Indications Soothing the liver and fortifying the spleen, nourishing blood and regulating menstruation. It is indicated for depression of liver-*qi*, hypochondriac distention and pain, dizziness, dizzy vision, poor appetite, irregular menstruation.

眩晕宁片

【处方】泽泻、白术、茯苓、陈皮、半夏（制）、女贞子、墨旱莲、菊花、牛膝、甘草。

【功能主治】健脾利湿，益肝补肾。用于痰湿中阻、肝肾不足引起的头晕。

Relieving Vertigo Tablet

Name of Chinese Phonetic Alphabet Xuan Yun Ning Pian

Formula Alismatis Rhizoma, Atractylodis Macrocephalae Rhizoma, Poria, Citri Reticulatae Pericarpium, Pinelliae Rhizoma (prepared), Ligustri Lucidi Fructus, Ecliptae Herba, Chrysanthemi Flos, Achyranthis Bidentatae Radix and Glycyrrhizae Radix et Rhizoma.

Actions and Indications Fortifying the spleen and draining dampness, tonifying the liver and kidney. It is indicated for dizziness due to stagnation of phlegm-damp and insufficiency of the liver and kidney.

晕可平糖浆

【处方】赭石、夏枯草、法半夏、车前草。

【功能主治】潜阳镇肝。用于内耳眩晕症，头晕目眩症。

Dizziness-relieving Syrup

Name of Chinese Phonetic Alphabet Yun Ke Ping Tang Jiang

Formula Haematitum, Prunellae Spica, Pinelliae Rhizoma Praeparatum and Plantaginis Herba.

Actions and Indications Subduing *yang*, calming the liver. It is used for auditory vertigo, dizziness, dizzy vision.

特制狗皮膏

【处方】枳壳、细辛、赤石脂、青风藤、天麻青皮、羌活、乌药、生川乌、甘草、白蔹、黄柏、川芎、木香、远志、桃仁、白术、生草乌、小茴香、穿山甲、菟丝子、川楝子、蛇床子、威灵仙、大枫子、赤芍、牛膝、补骨脂、续断、附子、杜仲、香附、僵蚕、当归、陈皮、肉桂、儿茶、乳香、血竭、没药、丁香、樟脑、水杨酸甲酯、薄荷油、冰片、盐酸苯海拉明、颠茄流浸膏、氮酮。

【功能主治】祛风散寒，舒筋活血，和络止痛。用于风寒湿痹，腰腿痛，肢体麻木，跌打损伤。

Miraculous Plaster for Relieving Rheumatic Artralgia

Name of Chinese Phonetic Alphabet Te Zhi Gou Pi Gao

Formula Aurantii Fructus, Asari Radix et Rhizoma, Halloysitum Rubrum, Sinomenii Caulis, Gastrodiae Rhizoma, Citri Reticularae Pericarpium Viride, Notopterygii Rhizoma et Radix, Linderae Radix, Aconiti Radix, Glycyrrhizae Radix et Rhizoma, Ampelopsis Radix, Phellodendri Chinensis Cortex, Chuanxiong Rhizoma, Aucklandiae Radix, Polygalae Radix, Persicae Semen, Atractylodis Macrocephalae Rhizoma, Aconiti Kusnezoffii Radix, Foeniculi Fructus, Manis Squama, Cuscutae Semen, Toosendan Fructus, Cnidii Fructus, Clematidis Radix et Rhizoma, Hydnocarpi Anthelmintici Semen, Paeoniae Radix Rubra, Achyranthis Bidentatae Radix, Psoraleae Fructus, Dipsaci Radix, Aconiti Lateralis Radix Praeparata, Eucommiae Cortex, Cyperi Rhizoma, Bombyx Batryticatus, Angelicae Sinensis Radix, Citri Reticulatae Pericarpium, Cinnamomi Cortex, Catechu, Olibanum, Draconis Sanguis, Myrrha, Caryophylli Flos, Camphora, Methylsalicylate, Menthae Haplocalycis Oleum, Borneolum Syntheticum, Diphenhydramine Hydrochloride, Belladonnae Extractum and Azone.

Actions and Indications Dispelling wind and cold, relaxing sinews and activating blood, harmonizing collaterals and alleviating pain. It is used for wind-cold-damp impediment syndrome, pain of the waist and legs, numbness of the limbs and traumatic injury.

钻山风糖浆

【处方】钻山风、勾儿茶、四块瓦、威灵仙、千斤拔、鸡血藤、山姜。

【功能主治】祛风除湿，散瘀镇痛，舒筋活络。用于风寒湿痹引起的腰膝冷痛，肢体麻木，伸屈不利。

Oldham Fissistigma* Syrup for Relieving Impediment Syndrome

Name of Chinese Phonetic Alphabet Zuan Shan Feng Tang Jiang

Formula Fissistigmatis Oldhamii Radix, Berchemiae Floribundae Radix, Chloranthi Herba, Clematidis Radix et Rhizoma, Flemingiae Philippinensis Radix, Spatholobi Caulis, Alpiniae Japonicae Rhizoma seu Herba.

Actions and Indications Dispelling wind and dampness, dispersing stasis and alleviating pain, relaxing sinews and activating collaterals. It is indicated for cold-pain of the waist and knees, numbness and immobility of the limbs due to wind-cold-damp impediment syndrome.

* 钻山风

铁笛口服液

【处方】麦冬、玄参、瓜蒌皮、诃子、青果、凤凰衣、桔梗、浙贝母、茯苓、甘草。

【功能主治】润肺利咽，生津止渴。用于阴虚肺热津亏引起的咽干声哑，咽喉疼痛，口渴烦躁。

【注意事项】忌食辛辣食物。

Tie Di Oral Liquid for Sore-throat

Name of Chinese Phonetic Alphabet Tie Di Kou Fu Ye

Formula Ophiopogonis Radix, Scrophulariae Radix, Trichosanthis Pericarpium, Chebulae Fructus, Canarii Fructus, Ovi Follicularis Membrana, Platycodonis Radix, Fritillariae Thunbergii Bulbus, Poria and Glycyrrhizae Radix et Rhizoma.

Actions and Indications Moistening the lung, soothing the throat, engendering fluid, quenching thirst. It is used for dry throat, hoarseness, sore-throat, thirst, vexation.

Warning Pungent foods should be avoided.

秘制舒肝丸

【处方】川楝子、延胡索（醋炙）、木香、陈皮、厚朴（姜炙）、砂仁、豆蔻、枳壳（麸炒）、沉香、茯苓、白芍、片姜黄、朱砂。

【功能主治】舒肝，解郁，止痛。用于气郁不舒引起的两胁胀满，胃脘刺痛，嗳气吞酸，呕吐酸水，四肢抽搐，倒饱嘈杂，不思饮食。

【注意】孕妇禁服。

Liver-soothing Honeyed Pill

Name of Chinese Phonetic Alphabet Mi Zhi Shu Gan Wan

Formula Toosendan Fructus, Corydalis Rhizoma (prepared with vinegar), Aucklandiae Radix, Citri Reticulatae Pericarpium, Magnoliae Officinalis Cortex (prepared with ginger), Amomi Fructus, Amomi Fructus Rotundus, Aurantii Fructus (fried with bran), Aquilariae Lignum Resinatum, Poria, Paeoniae Radix Alba, Wenyujin Rhizoma Concisum and Cinnabaris.

Actions and Indications Soothing the liver, relieving depression and alleviating pain. It is used for hypochondriac fullness, stabbing pain in stomach duct, eructation, acid regurgitation, acid vomiting, spasm of extremities, gastric upset and anorexia due to stagnation of *qi*.

Warning It is contraindicated for pregnant women.

透骨镇风丸

【处方】香加皮、甘松、荆芥、吴茱萸（甘草炙）、关木通、白芷、羌活、白附子（矾炙）、苦杏仁、麻黄、防风、川乌（甘草、银花炙）、海桐皮、苍术、独活、草乌（甘草、银花炙）、高良姜、木贼、细辛、自然铜（煅醋淬）、青风藤、干姜、丁香、肉豆蔻（煨）、红豆蔻、山柰、草果、没药（醋炙）、牡丹皮、豆蔻、赤芍、三棱（麸炒）、菟丝子、川芎、木瓜、青皮（醋炙）、地骨皮、天麻、全蝎、乳香（醋炙）、韭菜子、牛膝、白芍、莪术（醋炙）、石南藤、当归、肉桂、胡芦巴（盐炙）、大青盐、茯苓、砂仁、枳壳（麸炒）、杜仲（炭）、滑石、朱砂、远志（甘草炙）、熟地黄、血竭、鹿茸、小茴香（盐炙）、龙骨（煅）、人参、甘草、虎骨（油炙）、法半夏、连翘、陈皮、巴戟天（甘草炙）、柏子仁、续断、黄芪、五味子（醋炙）、广藿香、乌药、桔梗、肉苁蓉（酒炙）、罂粟壳、麝香、枳实、龟甲（砂烫醋淬）、川楝子、木香、八角茴香、补骨脂（盐炙）、香附（醋炙）、僵蚕（麸炒）、白术（麸炒）、天南星（矾炙）、厚朴（姜炙）、益智（盐炙）。

【功能主治】疏风散寒，温经通络。用于风寒湿邪、痹阻经络引起的腰背疼痛，肢体麻木，筋骨软弱，半身不遂，跌打损伤，瘀血肿痛。

【注意】孕妇忌服。

Bone-strengthening Bolus

Name of Chinese Phonetic Alphabet Tou Gu Zhen Feng Wan

Formula Periplocae Cortex, Nardostachyos Radix et Rhizoma, Schizonepetae Herba, Euodiae Fructus (prepared with licorice root), Aristolochiae Manshuriensis Caulis, Angelicae Dahuricae Radix, Notopterygii Rhizoma et Radix, Typhonii Rhizoma (prepared with alum), Armeniacae Semen Amarum, Ephedrae Herba, Saposhnikoviae Radix, Aconiti Radix (prepared with licorice root and honeysuckle flower), Erythrinae Orientalis Cortex, Atractylodis Rhizoma, Angelicae Pubescentis Radix, Aconiti Kusnezoffii Radix (prepared with licorice root and honeysuckle flower), Alpiniae Officinarum Rhizoma, Equiseti Hiemalis Herba, Asari Radix et Rhizoma, Pyritum (calcined and quenched by vinegar), Sinomenii Caulis, Zingiberis Rhizoma, Caryophylli Flos, Myristicae Semen (stewed), Galangae Fructus, Kaempferiae Rhizoma, Tsaoko Fructus, Myrrha (prepared with vinegar), Moutan Cortex, Amomi Fructus Rotundus, Paeoniae Radix Rubra, Sparganii Rhizoma (fried with bran), Cuscutae Semen, Chuanxiong Rhizoma, Chaenomelis Fructus, Citri Reticulatae Pericarpium Viride (prepared with vinegar), Lycii Cortex, Gastrodiae Rhizoma, Scorpio, Olibanum (prepared with vinegar), Allii Tuberosi Semen, Achyranthis Bidentatae Radix, Paeoniae Radix Alba, Curcumae Rhizoma (prepared with vinegar), Photiniae Serrulatae Herba, Angelicae Sinensis Radix, Cinnamomi Cortex, Trigonellae Semen (prepared with salt), Halitum, Poria, Amomi Fructus, Aurantii Fructus (fried with bran), Eucommiae Cortex (carbonated), Talcum, Cinnabaris, Polygalae Radix (prepared with licorice root), Rehmanniae Radix Praeparata, Draconis Sanguis, Cervi Cornu Pantotrichum, Foeniculi Fructus (prepared with salt), Draconis Os (calcined), Ginseng Radix et Rhizoma, Glycyrrhizae Radix et Rhizoma, Tigris Os (prepared with oil), Pinelliae Rhizoma Praeparatum, Forsythiae Fructus, Citri Reticulatae Pericarpium, Morindae Officinalis Radix (prepared with licorice root), Platycladi Semen, Dipsaci Radix, Astragali Radix, Schisandrae Chinensis Fructus (prepared with vinegar), Pogostemonis Herba, Linderae Radix, Platycodonis Radix, Cistanches Caulis Carnosus (prepared with wine), Papaveris Pericarpium, Moschus, Aurantii Fructus Immaturus, Testudinis Carapax et Plastrum (scalded by sand and quenched by vinegar), Toosendan Fructus, Aucklandiae Radix, Anisi Stellati Fructus, Psoraleae Fructus (prepared with salt), Cyperi Rhizoma (prepared with vinegar), Bombyx Batryticatus (fried with bran), Atractylodis Macrocephalae Rhizoma (fried with bran), Arisaematis Rhizoma (prepared with alum), Magnoliae Officinalis Cortex (prepared with ginger) and Alpiniae Oxyphyllae Fructus (prepared with salt).

Actions and Indications Dispersing wind and cold, warming and dredging meridians and collaterals. It is used for lumbago, backache, numbness of limbs, hemiparalysis, traumatic injury marked by blood-stasis, swelling and pain.

Warning It is contraindicated for pregnant women.

健儿乐冲剂

【处方】山楂、竹叶卷心、钩藤、白芍、甜叶菊、鸡内金。

【功能主治】清热平肝，清心除烦，健脾消食。用于小儿烦躁不安，夜惊夜啼，夜眠不宁，消化不良。

Children Safeness Soluble Granules

Name of Chinese Phonetic Alphabet Jian Er Le

Chong Ji

Formula Crataegi Fructus, Lingnaniae Chungii Folium Involutus Juvenalis, Uncariae Ramulus cum Uncis, Paeoniae Radix Alba, Steviae Rebaudinae Folium, Galli Gigerii Endothelium Corneum.

Actions and Indications Clearing heat and pacifying the liver, clearing heart-fire and relieving vexation, fortifying the spleen and promoting digestion. It is used for vexation, restlessness, fright and crying at night, insomnia, indigestion of children.

健儿药片

【处方】雄黄、甘草、使君子仁、蜂蜡、郁金、苦杏仁（炒）、巴豆霜。

【功能主治】破积驱虫、开胃进食。用于小儿食积，乳积，发热腹胀，呕吐滞下及腹痛。

【注意】忌生冷、腥荤食物。

Promoting Digestion Tablet for Children

Name of Chinese Phonetic Alphabet Jian Er Yao Pian

Formula Realgar, Glycyrrhizae Radix et Rhizoma, Quisqualis Semen, Cera Flava, Curcumae Radix, Armeniacae Semen Amarum (fried) and Crotonis Semen Pulveratum.

Actions and Indications Expelling worms, promoting digestion. It is used for children accumulation of food and milk, fever, abdominal distention, vomiting and abdominal pain.

Warning Uncooked foods and meat or fish should be avoided.

健儿消食口服液

【处方】黄芪、白术（麸炒）、陈皮、麦冬、黄芩、山楂（炒）、莱菔子（炒）。

【功能主治】健脾益胃，理气消食。用于小儿饮食不节损伤脾胃引起的纳呆食少，脘腹胀满，手足心热，自汗乏力，大便不调，以至厌食。

Promoting Digestion Oral Liquid for Children

Name of Chinese Phonetic Alphabet Jian Er Xiao Shi Kou Fu Ye

Formula Astragali Radix, Atractylodis Macrocephalae Rhizoma (fried with bran), Citri Reticulatae Pericarpium, Ophiopogonis Radix, Scutellariae Radix, Crataegi Fructus (fried) and Raphani Semen (fried).

Actions and Indications Fortifying the spleen and invigorating the stomach, regulating *qi* and promoting digestion. It is used for poor appetite, abdominal distention and fullness, vexing heat in the palms and soles, spontaneous sweating, fatigue, irregular bowel movement and anorexia due to improper diet.

健儿清解液

【处方】金银花、菊花、连翘、山楂、苦杏仁、陈皮。

【功能主治】清热解毒，祛痰止咳，消滞和中。用于口腔糜烂，咳嗽咽痛，食欲不振，脘腹胀满。

Children Oral Liquid for Clearing Heat

Name of Chinese Phonetic Alphabet Jian Er Qing Jie Ye

Formula Lonicerae Japonicae Flos, Chrysanthemi Flos, Forsythiae Fructus, Crataegi Fructus, Armeniacae Semen Amarum and Citri Reticulatae Pericarpium.

Actions and Indications Clearing heat and detoxicating, dispelling phlegm and alleviating cough, promoting digestion and harmonizing the stomach. It is indicated for children stomatitis, cough, sore-throat, anorexia, gastric distension.

健儿散

【处方】山药、川明参、薏苡仁（炒）、麦芽、稻芽（炒）、鸡内金（炒）。

【功能主治】调理脾胃，促进食欲。用于厌食，消瘦，消化不良。

Promoting Digestion Powder for Children

Name of Chinese Phonetic Alphabet Jian Er San

Formula Dioscoreae Rhizoma, Changii Radix, Coicis Semen (fried), Hordei Fructus Germinatus, Oryzae Fructus Germinatus (fried) and Galli Gigerii Endothelium Corneum (fried).

Actions and Indications Regulating the spleen and stomach, promoting digestion. It is used for anorexia, emaciation and dyspepsia in children.

健民咽喉片

【处方】玄参、麦冬、蝉蜕、甘草、桔梗、板蓝根、胖大海、地黄、西青果、甜叶菊、薄荷油。

【功能主治】清咽利喉，养阴生津，解毒泻火。用于咽喉肿痛，失声及上呼吸道炎症。

Jian Min Tablet for Relieving Sore-throat

Name of Chinese Phonetic Alphabet Jian Min Yan Hou Pian

Formula Scrophulariae Radix, Ophiopogonis Radix, Cicadae Periostracum, Glycyrrhizae Radix et Rhizoma, Platycodonis Radix, Isatidis Radix, Sterculiae Lychnophorae Semen, Rehmanniae Radix, Chebulae Fructus, Steviae Rebaudinae Folium and Menthae Haplocalycis Oleum.

Actions and Indications Soothing the throat, nourishing *yin*, engendering fluid, detoxifying, purging fire. It is used for sore-throat, hoarseness, inflammation of upper respiratory tract.

健延龄

【处方】熟地黄、制何首乌、黄精、黑豆、黑芝麻、侧柏叶、黄芪、山药、茯苓、芡实、西洋参、天冬、麦冬、紫河车、珍珠、琥珀、龙骨。

【功能主治】填精髓，养气血，调脏腑，固本元。用于精气虚乏，阴血亏损所致的神疲乏力，食欲减退，健忘失眠，头晕耳鸣及放、化疗后白细胞减少症及高脂血症见有上述症候者。

Securing Sourve-*qi* Capsule

Name of Chinese Phonetic Alphabet Jian Yan Ling

Formula Rehmanniae Radix Praeparata, Polygoni Multiflori Radix Praeparata, Polygonati Rhizoma, Sojae Semen Nigrum, Sesami Semen Nigrum, Platycladi Cacumen, Astragali Radix, Dioscoreae Rhizoma, Poria, Euryales Semen, Panacis Quinquefolii Radix, Asparagi Radix, Ophiopogonis Radix, Hominis Placenta, Margarita, Succinum and Draconis Os.

Actions and Indications Invigorating the vital essence and marrow, nourishing *qi* and blood, regulating the viscera and strengthening the body resistance. It is used for cases with lassitude of spirit, fatigue, poor appetite, amnesia, insomnia, dizziness and tinnitus due to deficiency of *qi* and blood. And also used for leukopenia due to radiotherapy and chemotherapy, and hyperlipemia with the above mentioned symptoms.

健阳片

【处方】蜈蚣粉、淫羊藿提取物粉、甘草提取物粉、蜂王浆。

【功能主治】补肾益精，助阳兴痿。用于肾虚阳衰引起的阳痿、早泄等性功能低下症。

【注意】忌房事过度。肝、肾功能不全者慎用。

Tonifying Kidney-*yang* Tablet

Name of Chinese Phonetic Alphabet Jian Yang Pian

Formula Scolopendrae Pulvis, Epimedii Folium Pulvis (extracted), Glycyrrhize Extractum Pulvis and Apis Regis Lac .

Actions and Indications Tonifying the kidney, essence and *yang*. It is used for impotence, ejaculatio praecox and sexual hypofunction due to declination of kidney-*yang*.

Warning Sexual intemperance is prohibited, and

medication should be used carefully for cases with hepatic or renal insufficiency.

健步强身丸

【处方】知母、黄柏、龟甲（醋淬）、熟地黄、白芍、当归、黄芪（蜜炙）。

【功能主治】补肾健骨，宣痹止痛。用于肝肾阴虚、风湿阻络引起的筋骨痿软，腰腿酸痛，足膝无力，行步艰难。

【注意】孕妇忌服。

Vigorous Bolus for Sinews Wilt

Name of Chinese Phonetic Alphabet Jian Bu Qiang Shen Wan

Formula Anemarrhenae Rhizoma, Phellodendri Chinensis Cortex, Testudinis Carapax et Plastrum (quenched by vinegar), Rehmanniae Radix Praeparata, Paeoniae Radix Alba, Angelicae Sinensis Radix and Astragali Radix (prepared with honey).

Actions and Indications Tonifying the kidney and bone, diffusing impediment and alleviating pain. It is indicated for sinews wilt, soreness and pain of the waist and legs and hardness of walk due to dual *yin*-deficiency of the liver and kidney, and stagnation of wind-damp in collaterals.

Warning It is contraindicated for pregnant women.

健肝乐颗粒

【处方】甘草、白芍。

【功能主治】养血护肝，解毒止痛。有降低转氨酶，消褪黄疸以及改善各类肝炎临床症状的作用。用于治疗急慢性病毒性肝炎。

Fortifying Liver Soluble Granules

Name of Chinese Phonetic Alphabet Jian Gan Le Ke Li

Formula Glycyrrhizae Radix et Rhizoma and Paeoniae Radix Alba.

Actions and Indications Nourishing blood and enriching the liver, detoxicating and relieving pain, decreasing the level of aminotransferase, relieving jaundice. It is indicated for acute, chronic viral hepatitis.

健身宁片

【处方】何首乌、黄精（酒炙）、熟地黄、当归党参、女贞子（酒炙）、桑椹、墨旱莲、乌梅、鹿茸（去毛）。

【功能主治】滋补肝肾，养血健身。用于肝肾不足引起的腰膝腿软，神疲体倦，头晕耳鸣，心悸气短，须发早白。

Strengthening Body Tablet

Name of Chinese Phonetic Alphabet Jian Shen Ning Pian

Formula Polygoni Multiflori Radix, Polygonati Rhizoma (prepared with wine), Rehmanniae Radix Praeparata, Angelicae Sinensis Radix, Codonopsis Radix, Ligustri Lucidi Fructus (prepared with wine), Mori Fructus, Ecliptae Herba, Mume Fructus and Cervi Cornu Panthotrichum (removed hair).

Actions and Indications Enriching the liver and kidney, nourishing blood and strengthening the body. It is indicated for soreness of the waist and weakness of legs, lassitude of spirit, tiredness, dizziness, tinnitus, palpitation, shortness of breath and premature graying of hair due to insufficiency of the liver and kidney.

健肾生发丸

【处方】制何首乌、熟地黄、枸杞子、黄精、五味子、大枣、女贞子（酒制）、菟丝子、苣胜子、桑椹、当归、柏子仁、山药、山茱萸（酒蒸）、茯苓、泽泻（盐水炒）、桑叶、地黄、牡丹皮、黄连、黄柏、杜仲（盐水炒）、牛膝、续断、木瓜、羌活、川芎、白芍、甘草。

【功能主治】补肾益肝，健肾生发。用于肾虚脱发，肾虚腰痛，慢性肾炎，神经衰弱。

Engendering Hair Bolus for Alopecia

Name of Chinese Phonetic Alphabet Jian Shen Sheng Fa Wan

Formula Polygoni Multiflori Radix Praeparata, Rehmanniae Radix Praeparata, Lycii Fructus, Polygonati Rhizoma, Schisandrae Chinensis Fructus, Jujubae Fructus, Ligustri Lucidi Fructus (prepared with wine), Cuscutae Semen, Lactucae Sativae Semen, Mori Fructus, Angelicae Sinensis Radix, Platycladi Semen, Dioscoreae Rhizoma, Corni Fructus (steamed by wine), Poria, Alismatis Rhizoma (fried with salt water), Mori Folium, Rehmanniae Radix, Moutan Cortex, Coptidis Rhizoma, Phellodendri Chinensis Cortex, Eucommiae Cortex (fried with salt water), Achyranthis Bidentatae Radix, Dipsaci Radix, Chaenomelis Fructus, Notopterygii Rhizoma et Radix, Chuanxiong Rhizoma, Paeoniae Radix Alba and Glycyrrhizae Radix et Rhizoma.

Actions and Indications Tonifying the kidney and liver to engender the hair. It is used for alopecia, lumbago, chronic nephritis and neurasthenia due to kidney-deficiency.

健胃片

【处方】山楂（炒）、六神曲（炒）、麦芽（炒）、槟榔（炒焦）、鸡内金（醋炒）、苍术（米泔制）、草豆蔻、陈皮、生姜、柴胡、白芍、川楝子、延胡索（醋炙）、甘草浸膏。

【功能主治】健胃止痛。用于胃弱食滞引起的胃脘胀痛，倒饱嘈杂，嗳气食臭，大便不调。

Fortifying Stomach Tablet

Name of Chinese Phonetic Alphabet Jian Wei Pian

Formula Crataegi Fructus (fried), Medicata Massa Fermentata (fried), Hordei Fructus Germinatus (fried), Arecae Semen (charred), Galli Gigerii Endothelium Corneum (fried with vinegar), Atractylodis Rhizoma (prepared with rice swilled water), Alpiniae Katsumadai Semen, Citri Reticulatae Pericarpium, Zingiberis Rhizoma Recens, Bupleuri Radix, Paeoniae Radix Alba, Toosendan Fructus, Corydalis Rhizoma (prepared with vinegar) and Glycyrrhizae Extractum.

Actions and Indications Fortifying the stomach and alleviating pain. It is used for fullness and pain in stomach duct, gastric upset, eructation with foul odor and disorder of bowels movement due to hypofunction of the stomach and food stagnation.

健胃消炎颗粒

【处方】党参、茯苓、白术（麸炒）、大黄、白芍、丹参、赤芍、川楝子、白及、木香、乌梅、青黛。

【功能主治】健脾和胃，理气活血。用于脾胃不和所致的上腹疼痛、痞满纳差以及慢性胃炎见上述证候者。

【注意】脾胃虚寒或寒湿中阻者不宜服用。

Relieving Chronic Gastritis Granules

Name of Chinese Phonetic Alphabet Jian Wei Xiao Yan Ke Li

Formula Codonopsis Radix, Poria, Atractylodis Macrocephalae Rhizoma (fried with bran), Rhei Radix et Rhizoma, Paeoniae Radix Alba, Salviae Miltiorrhizae Radix et Rhizoma, Paeoniae Radix Rubra, Toosendan Fructus, Bletillae Rhizoma, Aucklandiae Radix, Mume Fructus and Indigo Naturalis.

Actions and Indications Fortifying the spleen, harmonizing the stomach, regulating *qi*, activating blood. It is indicated for pain and fullness in the upper abdomen, poor appetite and chronic gastritis due to spleen-stomach disharmony.

Warning It is contraindicated for cases with deficiency-cold of the spleen and stomach or cold-damp stagnated in the middle energizer.

健胃消食片

【处方】太子参、陈皮、山药、山楂、麦芽（炒）。

【功能主治】健胃消食。用于脾胃虚弱，消化不良。

Fortifying Stomach Tablet for

Promoting Digestion

Name of Chinese Phonetic Alphabet Jian Wei Xiao Shi Pian

Formula Pseudostellariae Radix, Citri Reticulatae Pericarpium, Dioscoreae Rhizoma, Crataegi Fructus and Hordei Fructus Germinatus (fried).

Actions and Indications Fortifying the stomach and promoting digestion. It is used for dyspepsia due to hypofunction of the spleen and stomach.

健胃愈疡片

【处方】本品为柴胡、党参、白芍、延胡索、白及、珍珠层粉、青黛、甘草等药经加工制成的片剂。

【功能主治】疏肝健脾、解痉止痛，止血生肌。主治用于肝郁脾虚、肝胃不和型消化性溃疡活动期，症见胃脘胀痛、嗳气吐酸、烦躁不食、腹胀便溏。

Peptic Ulcer Relieving Tablet

Name of Chinese Phonetic Alphabet Jian Wei Yu Yang Pian

Formula Bupleuri Radix, Codonopsis Radix, Paeoniae Radix Alba, Corydalis Rhizoma, Bletillae Rhizoma, Margaritae Concha Strati Pulvis, Indigo Naturalis, Glycyrrhizae Radix et Rhizoma, etc.

Actions and Indications Soothing the liver, fortifying the spleen, relaxing spasm, alleviating pain, relieving bleeding, promoting tissue regeneration. It is indicated for active stage of peptic ulcer manifested as fullness and pain in stomach duct, eructation, acid vomiting, vexation, anorexia, abdominal fullness and sloppy stool due to liver-*qi* depression, deficiency of the spleen and disharmony of the liver and stomach.

健脑安神片

【处方】黄精（蒸）、淫羊藿、枸杞子、鹿茸、鹿角胶、鹿角霜、红参、大枣（去核）、茯苓、麦冬、龟甲、酸枣仁（炒）、五味子、远志（制）、熟地黄、苍耳子。

【功能主治】滋补强壮，镇惊安神。用于神经衰弱，头痛，头晕，健忘失眠，耳鸣。

【注意】高血压患者忌服。

Mind-tranquilizing Tablet for Neurasthenia

Name of Chinese Phonetic Alphabet Jian Nao An Shen Pian

Formula Polygonati Rhizoma (steamed), Epimedii Folium, Lycii Fructus, Cervi Cornu Pantotrichum, Cervi Cornus Colla, Cervi Cornu Degelatinatum, Ginseng Radix et Rhizoma Rubra, Jujubae Fructus (removed nucleus), Poria, Ophiopogonis Radix, Testudinis Carapax et Plastrum, Ziziphi Spinosae Semen (fried), Schisandrae Chinensis Fructus, Polygalae Radix (prepared), Rehmanniae Radix Praeparata and Xanthii Fructus.

Actions and Indications Tonic, settling fright, tranquilizing the mind. It is used for neurasthenia, headache, dizziness, amnesia, insomnia, tinnitus.

Warning It is contraindicated for hypertension.

健脑补肾丸

【处方】人参、鹿茸、狗鞭、肉桂、金牛草、牛蒡子（炒）、金樱子、杜仲（炭）、川牛膝、金银花、连翘、蝉蜕、山药 远志（甘草水制）、酸枣仁（炒）、砂仁、当归、龙骨（煅）、牡蛎（煅）、茯苓、白术（麸炒）、桂枝、甘草、白芍（酒炒）、豆蔻。

【功能主治】健脑补肾，益气健脾，安神定志。用于肾精亏虚引起的健忘失眠，头晕目眩，耳鸣心悸，腰膝酸软，肾亏遗精，神经衰弱和性功能障碍。

【注意】忌食生冷食物。

Fortifying Mind Pill

Name of Chinese Phonetic Alphabet Jian Nao Bu Shen Wan

Formula Ginseng Radix et Rhizoma, Cervi Cornu Pantotrichum, Canis Testis et Penis, Cinnamomi Cortex, Polygalae Telephioidis Herba, Arctii Fructus (fried), Rosae Laevigatae Fructus, Eucommiae Cortex (carbonated), Cyathulae Radix, Lonicerae Japonicae Flos, Forsythiae Fructus, Cicadae Periostracum, Dioscoreae Rhizoma, Polygalae Radix (prepared with licorice root water), Ziziphi Spinosae Semen (fried), Amomi Fructus,

Angelicae Sinensis Radix, Draconis Os (calcined), Ostreae Concha (calcined), Poria, Atractylodis Macrocephalae Rhizoma (fried with bran), Cinnamomi Ramulus, Glycyrrhizae Radix et Rhizoma, Paeoniae Radix Alba (fried with wine) and Amomi Fructus Rotundus.

Actions and Indications Fortifying the mind, tonifying the kidney and *qi*, fortifying the spleen, tranquilizing the mind. It is indicated for amnesia, insomnia, dizziness, dizzy vision, tinnitus, palpitation, soreness and weakness of the waist and knees, nocturnal emission, neurasthenia and sexual disorder due to deficiency of kidney-essence.

Warning Uncooked foods are prohibited.

健脑胶囊

【处方】当归、天竺黄、肉苁蓉（盐制）、龙齿（煅）、山药、琥珀、五味子（酒制）、天麻、柏子仁（炒）、丹参、益智（盐炒）、人参、远志（甘草制）、菊花、九节菖蒲、赭石、胆南星、酸枣仁（炒）、枸杞子。

【功能主治】健脑益智，安眠补身。用于用脑过度，记忆衰退，神经衰弱，头晕目眩，惊悸失眠，心烦易倦，畏寒体虚，身亏腰痛及老年痴呆症。

Brain-strengthening Capsule

Name of Chinese Phonetic Alphabet Jian Nao Jiao Nang

Formula Angelicae Sinensis Radix, Bambusae Concretio Silicea, Cistanches Caulis Carnosus (prepared with salt), Draconis Dens (calcined), Dioscoreae Rhizoma, Succinum, Schisandrae Chinensis Fructus (prepared with wine), Gastrodiae Rhizoma, Platycladi Semen (fried), Salviae Miltiorrhizae Radix et Rhizoma, Alpiniae Oxyphyllae Fructus (fried with salt), Ginseng Radix et Rhizoma, Polygalae Radix (prepared with licorice root), Chrysanthemi Flos, Anemones Altaicae Rhizoma, Haematitum, Arisaema cum Bile, Ziziphi Spinosae Semen (fried) and Lycii Fructus.

Actions and Indications Strengthening the brain, promoting peaceful sleep. It is used for over mental work, hypomnesia, neurasthenia, dizziness, dizzy vision, palpitation, insomnia, vexation, tiredness, fear of cold, general debility, lumbago and senile dementia.

健脾八珍糕

【处方】党参（炒）、白术（炒）、茯苓、白扁豆（炒）、薏苡仁（炒）、山药（炒）、芡实（炒）、莲子、陈皮。

【功能主治】健脾益胃。用于老年、小儿及病后脾胃虚弱，消化不良，面色萎黄，腹胀便溏。

Fortifying Spleen Cake

Name of Chinese Phonetic Alphabet Jian Pi Ba Zhen Gao

Formula Codonopsis Radix (fried), Atractylodis Macrocephalae Rhizoma (fried), Poria, Lablab Semen Album (fried), Coicis Semen (fried), Dioscoreae Rhizoma (fried), Euryales Semen (fried), Nelumbinis Semen and Citri Reticulatae Pericarpium.

Actions and Indications Fortifying the spleen and stomach. It is indicated for hypofuntion of spleen and stomach, indigestion, sallow complexion, abdominal fullness and sloppy stool after illness in aged and children.

健脾止遗片

【处方】本品为鸡肠、鸡内金等药经加工制成的片剂。

【功能主治】健脾和胃，缩尿止遗。用于脾胃不和的小儿遗尿症。

Enuresis-arresting Tablet

Name of Chinese Phonetic Alphabet Jian Pi Zhi Yi Pian

Formula Galli Intestina, Galli Gigerii Endothelium Corneum , etc.

Actions and Indications Fortifying the spleen, harmonizing the stomach, reducing urination and arresting enuresis. It is used for infantile enuresis due to disharmony of the spleen and stomach.

健脾生血片

【处方】党参、茯苓、白术（炒）、甘草、黄芪、山药、鸡内金（炒）、龟甲（醋制）、麦冬、南五味子（醋制）、龙骨、牡蛎（煅）、大枣、硫酸亚铁。

【功能主治】健脾和胃，养血安神。用于小儿脾胃虚弱及心脾两虚型缺铁性贫血；成人气血两虚型缺铁性贫血。症见面色萎黄或㿠白，食少纳呆，腹胀脘闷，大便不调，烦躁多汗，倦怠乏力，苔薄白，脉细弱。

【注意】忌茶，勿与含鞣酸类药物合用。

Fortifying Spleen and Nourishing Blood Tablet

Name of Chinese Phonetic Alphabet Jian Pi Sheng Xue Pian

Formula Codonopsis Radix, Poria, Atractylodis Macrocephalae Rhizoma (fried), Glycyrrhizae Radix et Rhizoma, Astragali Radix, Dioscoreae Rhizoma, Galli Gierii Endothelium Corneum (fried), Testudinis Carapax et Plastrum (prepared with vinegar), Ophiopogonis Radix, Schisandrae Sphenantherae Fructus (prepared with vinegar), Draconis Os, Ostreae Concha (calcined), Jujubae Fructus and Ferrous Sulfate.

Actions and Indications Fortifying the spleen and harmonizing the stomach, nourishing blood and tranquilizing the mind. It is indicated for children iron-deficiency anemia due to dual hypofunction of the spleen and stomach and dual deficiency of the heart and spleen, or adult iron-deficiency anemia due to dual deficiency of *qi* and blood, manifested as sallow or pale complexion, poor appetite, abdominal distention and oppression, disorder of the bowels, vexation and hyperhidrosis, tiredness, fatigue, thin and white tongue fur, fine and weak pulse.

Warning Tea and medicines containing tannic acid are prohibited to be taken simultaneously.

健脾冲剂

【处方】党参、白术（炒）、陈皮、枳实（炒）、山楂（炒）、麦芽（炒）。

【功能主治】健脾开胃。用于脾胃虚弱，脘腹胀满，食少便溏。

Fortifying Spleen Soluble Granules for Improving Appetite

Name of Chinese Phonetic Alphabet Jian Pi Chong Ji

Formula Codonopsis Radix, Atractylodis Macrocephalae Rhizoma (fried), Citri Reticulatae Pericarpium, Aurantii Fructus Immaturus (fried), Crataegi Fructus (fried) and Hordei Fructus Germinatus (fried).

Actions and Indications Fortifying the spleen, improving appetite. It is used for abdominal fullness, poor appetite and sloppy stool due to hypofunction of the spleen and stomach.

健脾消食丸

【处方】白术（炒）、枳实（炒）、木香、草豆蔻、鸡内金（醋炙）、槟榔（炒焦）、荸荠粉。

【功能主治】健脾，消食。用于小儿脾胃不健引起的乳食停滞，脘腹胀满，食欲不振，面黄肌瘦，大便不调。

Fortifying Spleen Pill for Promoting Digestion

Name of Chinese Phonetic Alphabet Jian Pi Xiao Shi Wan

Formula Atractylodis Macrocephalae Rhizoma (fried), Aurantii Fructus Immaturus (fried), Aucklandiae Radix, Alpiniae Katsumadai Semen, Galli Gierii Endothelium Corneum (prepared with vinegar), Arecae Semen (charred) and Eleocharitis Cormus Dulcis Pulvis.

Actions and Indications Fortifying the spleen, promoting digestion. It is used for stagnant milk or food, abdominal distention and fullness, poor appetite, sallow complexion, emaciation and irregular bowel movement due to dysfunction of the spleen and stomach.

健脾益肾冲剂

【处方】党参、枸杞子、女贞子、白术、菟丝子、补骨脂（盐炙）。

【功能主治】健脾益肾。用于减轻肿瘤病人术后放、化疗副反应，提高机体免疫能力。

Fortifying Spleen and Kidney Soluble Granules

Name of Chinese Phonetic Alphabet Jian Pi Yi Shen Chong Ji

Formula Codonopsis Radix, Lycii Fructus, Ligustri Lucidi Fructus, Atractylodis Macrocephalae Rhizoma, Cuscutae Semen and Psoraleae Fructus (prepared with salt).

Actions and Indications Fortifying the spleen and kidney. It is used for reducing the side effects after radiotherapy and chemotherapy, and increasing the immunologic function of organism.

健脾康儿片

【处方】人参、白术（麸炒）、茯苓、甘草、使君子（炒）、鸡内金（醋炙）、山楂（炒）、山药（炒）、陈皮、黄连、木香。

【功能主治】健脾养胃，消食止泻。用于脾虚胃肠不和，饮食不节引起的腹胀便泻，面黄肌瘦，食少倦怠，小便短少。

【注意】忌食生冷油腻。

Fortifying Spleen Tablet for Children

Name of Chinese Phonetic Alphabet Jian Pi Kang Er Pian

Formula Ginseng Radix et Rhizoma, Atractylodis Macrocephalae Rhizoma (fried with bran), Poria, Glycyrrhizae Radix et Rhizoma, Quisqualis Fructus (fried), Galli Gigerii Endothelium Corneum (prepared with vinegar), Crataegi Fructus (fried), Dioscoreae Rhizoma (fried), Citri Reticulatae Pericarpium, Coptidis Rhizoma and Aucklandiae Radix.

Actions and Indications Fortifying the spleen and nourishing the stomach, promoting digestion and relieving diarrhea. It is used for abdominal distention, diarrhea, sallow complexion, emaciation, poor appetite, tiredness and scanty urination due to disharmony of the stomach and intestine and deficiency of the spleen.

Warning Uncooked and oily foods should be avoided.

健脾糕片

【处方】党参、白术（炒）、陈皮、白扁豆（炒）、茯苓、莲子、山药、薏苡仁（炒）、甘草（蜜炙）、冬瓜子（炒）、鸡内金、芡实（炒）。

【功能主治】开胃健脾。用于脾胃虚弱，身体羸瘦，食欲不振，大便稀溏。

Spleen-fortifying Tablet

Name of Chinese Phonetic Alphabet Jian Pi Gao Pian

Formula Codonopsis Radix, Atractylodis Macrocephalae Rhizoma (fried), Citri Reticulatae Pericarpium, Lablab Semen Album (fried), Poria, Nelumbinis Semen, Dioscoreae Rhizoma, Coicis Semen (fried), Glycyrrhizae Radix et Rhizoma (prepared with honey), Benincasae Semen (fried), Galli Gierii Endothelium Corneum and Euryales Semen (fried).

Actions and Indications Promoting appetite and fortifying spleen. It is used for cases with dual deficiency of the spleen and stomach, emaciation, poor appetite and sloppy stool.

息伤乐酊

【处方】草乌（金银花甘草炙）、防风、白芷、三七、肉桂、大黄、血竭、鸡血藤、艾叶、透骨草、地黄、辣椒、红花、冰片、薄荷脑、樟脑、紫草、雄黄。

【功能主治】活血化瘀，消肿止痛。用于急、慢性扭挫，跌扑筋伤引起的皮肤青紫，瘀血不散，红肿疼痛，活动不利，亦可用于风湿痹痛。

【注意】外用药，切勿入口。皮肤破伤、关节炎急性期者禁用。

Relieving Traumatic Injury Tincture

Name of Chinese Phonetic Alphabet Xi Shang Le Ding

Formula Aconiti Kusnezoffii Radix (prepared with honeysuckle flower and licorice root), Saposhnikoviae Radix, Angelicae Dahuricae Radix, Notoginseng Radix et Rhizoma, Cinnamomi Cortex, Rhei Radix et Rhizoma, Draconis Sanguis, Spatholobi Caulis, Artemisiae Argyi Folium, Speranskiae Tuberculatae Herba, Rehmanniae Radix, Capsici Fructus, Carthami Flos, Borrneolum Syntheticum, Menthol, Camphora, Arnebiae Radix and Realgar.

Actions and Indications Activating blood, resolving stasis, reducing swelling, alleviating pain. It is used for acute, chronic sprain and contusion, traumatic injury with purple skin, swelling and pain. It is also used for rheumatalgia.

Warning The tincture is for external use only and is contraindicated for cases with wound of skin, and acute stage of arthritis.

胰胆炎合剂

【处方】柴胡、黄芩、厚朴、大黄、枳实、蒲公英、赤芍、北败酱、法半夏、甘草。

【功能主治】清泻肝胆湿热。用于急性胰腺炎，急性胆囊炎；也可用于慢性胰腺炎，慢性胆囊炎的急性发作。

Relieving Pancreatitis and Cholecystitis Mixture

Name of Chinese Phonetic Alphabet Yi Dan Yan He Ji

Formula Bupleuri Radix, Scutellariae Radix, Magnoliae Officinalis Cortex, Rhei Radix et Rhizoma, Aurantii Fructus Immaturus, Taraxaci Herba, Paeoniae Radix Rubra, Sonchi Arvensis Herba, Pinelliae Rhizoma Praeparatum and Glycyrrhizae Radix et Rhizoma.

Actions and Indications Clearing and purging damp-heat in the liver and gallbladder. It is indicated for acute pancreatitis and acute cholecystitis, also for acute attack of chronic pancreatitis and chronic cholecystitis.

脂必妥胶囊

【处方】山楂、白术、红曲等。

【功能主治】消痰化瘀、健脾和胃。主治痰瘀互结所致的高脂血症。

【注意】服药期间及停药后应尽量避免高脂饮食。

Zhi Bi Tuo Capsule for Decreasing Hyperlipidemia

Name of Chinese Phonetic Alphabet Zhi Bi Tuo Jiao Nang

Formula Crataegi Fructus, Atractylodis Macrocephalae Rhizoma, Oryzae Fructus Monascus, etc.

Actions and Indications Eliminating phlegm and resolving blood-stasis, fortifying the spleen and harmonizing the stomach. It is indicated for hyperlipemia due to accumulation of phlegm and blood-stasis.

Warning High fat diet should be avoid during and after medication.

脏连丸

【处方】黄连、黄芩、地黄、赤芍、当归、槐角、槐花、荆芥穗、地榆（炭）、阿胶。

【功能主治】清肠止血。用于肠热便血，肛门灼热，痔疮肿痛。

Zang Lian Bolus

Name of Chinese Phonetic Alphabet Zang Lian Wan

Formula Coptidis Rhizoma, Scutellariae Radix, Rehmanniae Radix, Paeoniae Radix Rubra, Angelicae Sinensis Radix, Sophorae Fructus, Sophorae Flos, Schizonepetae Spica, Sanguisorbae Radix (carbonated) and Asini Corii Colla.

Actions and Indications Clearing intestinal heat, relieving bleeding. It is used for hematochezia due to intestine-heat, scorching hot of anus, hemorrhoid with swelling and pain.

脑力静糖浆

【处方】大枣、小麦、甘草流浸膏、甘油磷酸钠（50%）、维生素B_1、维生素B_2、维生素B_6。

【功能主治】养心安神，补脾益气。用于心气不足引起的神经衰弱，头昏目眩，身体虚弱，失眠健忘，精神忧郁，烦躁及小儿不安寐。

Tranquilization Syrup

Name of Chinese Phonetic Alphabet Nao Li Jing Tang Jiang

Formula Jujubae Frurtus, Tritici Aestivi Fructus, Glycyrrhizae Extractum, Sodium Glycerophosphate (50%), Vitamin B_1, Vitamin B_2 and Vitamin B_6.

Actions and Indications Nourishing the heart, tranquilizing the mind, tonifying the spleen and *qi*. It is used for neurasthenia, dizziness, dizzy vision, debility of constitution, insomnia, amnesia, depression of spirit, vexation and infant disturbed sleep due to insufficiency of heart-*qi*.

脑乐静

【处方】甘草浸膏、大枣、小麦。

【功能主治】养心，健脑，安神。用于精神忧郁，易惊失眠，烦躁及小儿夜不安寐。

Brain-fortifying Oral Liquid

Name of Chinese Phonetic Alphabet Nao Le Jing

Formula Glycyrrhizae Extractum, Jujubae Fructus and Tritici Aestivi Fructus.

Actions and Indications Nourishing the heart, fortifying the brain and tranquilizing the mind. It is used for depression of spirit, fluster, insomnia, vexation and disturbed sleep of infant.

脑立清丸

【处方】磁石、赭石、珍珠母、清半夏、酒曲、酒曲（炒）、牛膝、薄荷脑、冰片、猪胆汁（或猪胆膏、猪胆汁粉）。

【功能主治】平肝潜阳，醒脑安神。用于肝阳上亢，头晕目眩，耳鸣口苦，心烦难寐及高血压见上述证候者。

【注意】孕妇及体弱虚寒者忌服。

Dizziness-relieving Pill

Name of Chinese Phonetic Alphabet Nao Li Qing Wan

Formula Magnetitum, Haematitum, Margaritifera Concha, Pinelliae Rhizoma Praeparatum cum Alumine, Vini-fermentum, Vini-fermentum (fried), Achyranthis Bidentatae Radix, Menthol, Borneolum Syntheticum and Suillus Bilis seu Suillus Fel Extractum seu Suillus Bilis Pulvis.

Actions and Indications Pacifying the liver, subduing *yang*, inducing resuscitation, tranquilizing the mind. It is used for dizziness, dizzy vision, tinnitus, bitter taste in the mouth, vexation, difficult sleep and hypertension due to ascendant hyperactivity of liver-*yang*.

Warning It is contraindicated for pregnant women and cases with physical debility.

脑血康胶囊

【处方】水蛭。

【功能主治】活血化瘀，破血散结。用于血瘀中风、半身不遂、口眼歪斜、舌强语謇、舌紫暗、有瘀斑及高血压脑出血后的脑血肿、脑血栓见上述证候者。

【注意】出血者及孕妇禁用。

Leech* Capsule for Resolving Thrombosis

Name of Chinese Phonetic Alphabet Nao Xue Kang Jiao Nang

Formula Hirudo.

Actions and Indications Activating blood, resolving and breaking blood-stasis, dissipating mass. It is indicated for apoplexy, hemiparalysis, deviated eyes and mouth, dysphasia due to stiff tongue; dark tongue with ecchymosis, and cerbral hematoma and cerbral thrombosis due to cerebral hemorrhage with the above mentioned symptoms.

Warning It is contraindicated for cases with hemorrhage, and pregnant women.

* 水蛭

脑安胶囊

【处方】川芎、当归、红花、人参、冰片。

【功能主治】活血化瘀，益气通络。适用于脑血栓形成急性期、恢复期属气虚血瘀证候者。症见急性起病，半身不遂，口舌歪斜，舌强语謇，偏身麻木，气短乏力，口角流涎，手足肿胀，舌暗或有瘀斑，苔薄白。

【注意】出血性中风慎用。

Resolving Cerebral Thrombosis Capsule

Name of Chinese Phonetic Alphabet Nao An Jiao Nang

Formula Chuanxiong Rhizoma, Angelicae Sinensis Radix, Carthami Flos, Ginseng Radix et Rhizoma and Borneolum Syntheticum.

Actions and Indications Activating blood, resolving stasis, tonifying *qi*, dredging collaterals. It is used for acute stage and convalescent period of cerebral thrombosis attributed to *qi*-deficiency and blood-stasis syndrome and manifested as hemiparalysis, deviated tongue and mouth, dysphasia due to stiff tongue; hemilateral numbness, shortness of breath, fatigue, salivation, swelling of limbs, dark tongue with ecchymosis, thin and white tongue fur.

Warning It should be used carefully for hemorrhagic apoplexy.

脑灵素胶囊

【处方】黄精（制）、淫羊藿（羊油制）、苍耳子（炒）、五味子、枸杞子、大枣、远志（制）、熟地黄、麦冬、酸枣仁（炒）、茯苓、龟甲、鹿角胶、人参、鹿茸。

【功能主治】补气血，健脑安神。用于神经衰弱，健忘失眠，头昏心悸，身倦无力，体虚自汗，阳痿遗精。

【注意】高血压患者忌服。

Tranquility Capsule

Name of Chinese Phonetic Alphabet Nao Ling Su Jiao Nang

Formula Polygonati Rhizoma (prepared), Epimedii Folium (prepared with sheep suet), Xanthii Fructus (fried), Schisandrae Chinensis Fructus, Lycii Fructus, Jujubae Fructus, Polygalae Radix(prepared), Rehmanniae Radix Praeparata, Ophiopogonis Radix, Ziziphi Spinosae Semen (fried), Poria, Testudinis Carapax et Plastrum, Cervi Cornus Colla, Ginseng Radix et Rhizoma and Cervi Cornu Pantotrichum.

Actions and Indications Tonifying *qi* and blood, tranquilizing the mind. It is used for neurasthenia, amnesia, insomnia, dizziness, palpitation, tiredness, fatigue, spontaneous sweating, impotence and nocturnal emission.

Warning It is contraindicated for cases with hypertension.

脑脉泰胶囊

【处方】红参、三七、当归、丹参、鸡血藤、红花、银杏叶、山楂、菊花、石决明、何首乌（制）、石菖蒲、葛根。

【功能主治】益气活血，息风豁痰。用于缺血性中风（脑梗死）恢复期中经络属于气虚血瘀证、风痰瘀血闭阻经络证者。症见半身不遂，口舌歪斜，头晕目眩，偏身麻木，面色㿠白,气短乏力，口角流涎。

Relieving Ischemic Stroke Capsule

Name of Chinese Phonetic Alphabet Nao Mai Tai Jiao Nang

Formula Ginseng Radix et Rhizoma Rubra,

Notoginseng Radix et Rhizoma, Angelicae Sinensis Radix, Salviae Miltiorrhizae Radix et Rhizoma, Spatholobi Caulis, Carthami Flos, Ginkgo Folium, Crataegi Fructus, Chrysanthemi Flos, Haliotidis Concha, Polygoni Multiflori Radix Praeparata, Acori Tatarinowii Rhizoma and Puerariae Lobatae Radix.

Actions and Indications Tonifying *qi*, activating blood, extinguishing wind, dispelling phlegm. It is indicated for convalescent period of ischemic stroke attributed to *qi* deficiency with blood-stasis syndrome and manifested as hemiparalysis, deviated eyes and mouth, dysphasia, dizziness, dizzy vision, hemilateral numbness, bright pale complexion, shortness of breath, fatigue and salivation.

脑得生丸

【处方】三七、川芎、红花、山楂（去核）、葛根。

【功能主治】活血化瘀，疏通经络，醒脑开窍。用于脑动脉硬化，缺血性脑中风及脑出血后遗症。

Relieving Cerebral Arteriosclerosis Bolus

Name of Chinese Phonetic Alphabet Nao De Sheng Wan

Formula Notoginseng Radix et Rhizoma, Chuanxiong Rhizoma, Carthami Flos, Crataegi Fructus (removed nucleus) and Puerariae Lobatae Radix.

Actions and Indications Activating blood, resolving stasis, dredging meridians and collaterals. It is indicated for cerebral arteriosclerosis, ischemic cerebral apoplexy and sequela of cerebral hemorrhage.

脑震宁颗粒

【处方】当归、地黄、牡丹皮、丹参、川芎、地龙、酸枣仁（炒）、柏子仁、茯苓、陈皮、竹茹。

【功能主治】凉血活血，化瘀通络，益血安神，宁心定智，除烦止呕。用于脑外伤引起的头痛、头晕、烦躁失眠，健忘惊悸，恶心呕吐。

Brain-calming Granules

Name of Chinese Phonetic Alphabet Nao Zhen Ning Ke Li

Formula Angelicae Sinensis Radix, Rehmanniae Radix, Moutan Cortex, Salviae Miltiorrhizae Radix et Rhizoma, Chuanxiong Rhizoma, Pheretima, Ziziphi Spinosae Semen (fried), Platycladi Semen, Poria, Citri Reticulatae Pericarpium and Bambusae Caulis in Taenias.

Actions and Indications Cooling blood, activating blood, resolving stasis, dredging collaterals, tranquilizing the mind, relieving vexation and vomiting. It is used for headache, dizziness, vexation, insomnia, amnesia, fright palpitation, nausea and vomiting due to brain trauma.

高血压速降丸

【处方】茺蔚子、琥珀、蒺藜（盐炙）、赤芍、天竺黄、阿胶、乌梢蛇（酒炙）、白薇、法半夏、菊花、僵蚕（麸炒）、当归、夏枯草、牛膝、大黄（酒炒）、白芍、化橘红、玄参、远志（甘草水炙）、桂枝、西红花、龙胆、九节菖蒲、石膏、牡丹皮、钩藤、川芎（酒炙）、茯神、羚羊角、麦冬、枳实（炒）、黄芩、天麻、沉香、甘草（蜜炙）、黄柏、柴胡、连翘、地黄、桑叶、蒲黄、地龙、芦荟、全蝎、玳瑁、黄连、降香、朱砂。

【功能主治】清热息风，平肝降逆。用于虚火上升引起的目眩头晕的颈项强直，颜面红赤，烦躁不宁，言语不清，知觉减退。

【注意】感冒或泄泻期间停服。孕妇忌服。

Rapid Relieving Hypertension Pill

Name of Chinese Phonetic Alphabet Gao Xue Ya Su Jiang Wan

Formula Leonuri Fructus, Succinum, Tribuli Fructus (prepared with salt), Paeoniae Radix Rubra, Bambusae Concretio Silicea, Asini Corii Colla, Zaocys (prepared with wine), Cynanchi Atrati Radix et Rhizoma, Pinelliae Rhizoma Praeparatum, Chrysanthemi Flos, Bombyx Batryticatus (fried with bran), Angelicae Sinensis Radix, Pinellae Spica,

Achyranthis Bidentatae Radix, Rhei Radix et Rhizoma (fried with wine), Paeoniae Radix Alba, Citri Grandis Exocarpium, Scrophulariae Radix, Polygalae Radix (prepared with licorice root water), Cinnamomi Ramulus, Croci Stigma, Gentianae Radix et Rhizoma, Anemones Altaicae Rhizoma, Gypsum Fibrosum, Moutan Cortex, Uncariae Ramulus cum Uncis, Chuanxiong Rhizoma (prepared with wine), Poria Sclerotiume Circum Pini Radicem, Saigae Tataricae Cornu, Ophiopogonis Radix, Aurantii Fructus Immaturus (fried), Scutellariae Radix, Gastrodiae Rhizoma, Aquilariae Lignum Resinatum, Glycyrrhizae Radix et Rhizoma Praeparata cum Melle, Phellodendri Chinensis Cortex, Bupleuri Radix, Forsythiae Fructus, Rehmanniae Radix, Mori Folium, Typhae Pollen, Pheretima, Aloe, Scorpio, Eretmochelydis Carapax, Coptidis Rhizoma, Dalbergiae Odoriferae Lignum and Cinnabaris.

Actions and Indications Clearing heat, extinguishing wind, pacifying the liver, checking upward adverse flow of *qi*. It is used for hypertension marked by dizzy vision, dizziness, neck rigidity, flushed face, vexation, alalia and reduction of perception due to deficiency fire flaming upward.

Warning It is contraindicated for cases with common cold, diarrhea and pregnant women.

烧伤净喷雾剂

【处方】五倍子、诃子、刘寄奴、苦参、桉叶。

【功能主治】解毒止痛，利湿消肿。用于各种Ⅰ至Ⅱ度的烧伤烫伤。

Aerosol for Burn

Name of Chinese Phonetic Alphabet Shao Shang Jing Pen Wu Ji

Formula Galla Chinensis, Chebulae Fructus, Artemisiae Anomalae Herba, Sophorae Flavescentis Radix and Eucalypti Folium.

Actions and Indications Detoxicating and alleviating pain, draining dampness and dispersing swelling. It is used for I~II degree burn or scald.

消石片

【处方】威灵仙、核桃、穿破石、半边莲、铁线草、猪苓、郁金、琥珀、乌药等。

【功能主治】清热通淋，止痛排石。用于肾结石、尿道结石、输尿管结石属热淋证者。

Relieving Heat-strangury Tablet

Name of Chinese Phonetic Alphabet Xiao Shi Pian

Formula Clematidis Radix et Rhizoma, Juglandis Semen, Cudraniae Radix, Lobeliae Chinensis Herba, Cynodontis Dactyli Herba, Polyporus, Curcumae Radix, Succinum, Linderae Radix, etc.

Actions and Indications Clearing heat and relieving strangury, alleviating pain and lithagogue. It is indicated for kidney stone, urethral stone and ureter stone attributive to heat strangury syndrome.

消肿止痛酊

【处方】木香、防风、荆芥、细辛、五加皮、肉桂、牛膝、川芎、徐长卿、白芷、莪术、红杜仲、大罗伞、小罗伞、两面针、黄藤、栀子、三棱、沉香、樟脑、薄荷脑。

【功能主治】舒筋活络，消肿止痛。用于跌打扭伤，风湿骨痛，无名肿痛，腮腺炎。

【注意】孕妇忌用。只供外用。

Tincture for Relieving Swelling and Pain

Name of Chinese Phonetic Alphabet Xiao Zhong Zhi Tong Ding

Formula Aucklandiae Radix, Saposhnikoviae Radix, Schizonepetae Herba, Asari Radix et Rhizoma, Acanthopanacis Cortex, Cinnamomi Cortex, Achyranthis Bidentatae Radix, Chuangxiong Rhizoma, Cynanchi Paniculati Radix et Rhizoma, Angelicae Dahuricae Radix, Curcumae Rhizoma, Parabarii Micranthi Caulis seu Radix, Clerodendri Serrati Herba, Ardisiae Punctatae Herba, Zanthoxyli Radix, Fibraureae

Caulis, Gardeniae Fructus, Sparganii Rhizoma, Aquilariae Lignum Resinatum, Camphora and Menthol.

Actions and Indications Relaxing the sinews, activating the collaterals, reducing swelling, alleviating pain. It is used for traumatic sprain, rheumatalgia, inflammatory swelling of unknown origin and parotitis.

Warning It is contraindicated for pregnant women, and is for external use only.

消肿片

【处方】枫香脂、马钱子等。

【功能主治】消肿拔毒，用于瘰疬痰核，流注，乳房肿块，阴疽肿毒。

【注意】孕妇忌服。

Dispersing Swelling Tablet

Name of Chinese Phonetic Alphabet Xiao Zhong Pian

Formula Liquidambaris Resina, Strychni Semen, etc.

Actions and Indications Dispersing swelling and discharging pus. It is indicated for scrofula, metastatic abscess, mammary mass and deep-rooted carbuncle.

Warning It is contraindicated for pregnant women.

消炎利胆片

【处方】穿心莲、溪黄草、苦木。

【功能主治】清热，祛湿，利胆。用于急性胆囊炎，胆道炎症。

Relieving Acute Cholecystitis Tablet

Name of Chinese Phonetic Alphabet Xiao Yan Li Dan Pian

Formula Andrographis Herba, Rabdosiae Serrae Herba and Picrasmae Ramulus et Folium.

Actions and Indications Clearing heat, dispelling dampness and draining bile. It is indicated for acute cholecystitis and inflammation of biliary tract.

消炎退热冲剂

【处方】大青叶、蒲公英、紫花地丁、甘草。

【功能主治】清热解毒，凉血消肿。用于感冒发热，上呼吸道感染，咽喉肿痛及各种疮疖肿痛。

Woad* Soluble Granules for Clearing Heat

Name of Chinese Phonetic Alphabet Xiao Yan Tui Re Chong Ji

Formula Isatidis Folium, Taraxaci Herba, Violae Herba and Glycyrrhizae Radix et Rhizoma.

Actions and Indications Clearing heat and detoxicating, cooling blood and dispersing swelling. It is indicated for common cold, fever, upper respiratory tract infection, sore-throat, abscess and deep-rooted boil.

* 大青叶

消咳喘糖浆

【处方】满山红。

【功能主治】止咳，祛痰，平喘。用于寒痰咳嗽，慢性支气管炎。

Syrup for Relieving Cough and Bronchitis

Name of Chinese Phonetic Alphabet Xiao Ke Chuan Tang Jiang

Formula Rhododendri Daurici Folium.

Actions and Indications Relieving cough, dispelling phlegm and calming dyspnea. It is indicated for cough due to cold phlegm; and chronic bronchitis.

消食退热糖浆

【处方】本品为柴胡、黄芩、知母、青蒿、槟榔、厚朴、水牛角浓缩粉、牡丹皮、荆芥穗、大黄等药经加工制成的糖浆剂。

【功能主治】清热解毒，消食通便。用于小儿瘟疫时毒，高热不退，内兼食滞，大便不畅；小儿呼吸道、消化道急性感染。

【注意】泄泻者忌服。

Promoting Digestion and Defervescence Syrup for Infant

Name of Chinese Phonetic Alphabet Xiao Shi Tui Re Tang Jiang

Formula Bupleuri Radix, Scutellariae Radix, Anemarrhenae Rhizoma, Artemisiae Annuae Herba, Arecae Semen, Magnoliae Officinalis Cortex, Bubali Cornu Pulvis Concentratio, Moutan Cortex, Schizonepetae Spica, Rhei Radix et Rhizoma, etc.

Actions and Indications Clearing heat and detoxicating, promoting digestion and bowels. It is used for infantile seasonal pestilence, high fever, food stagnation, difficulty in defecation, and also used for acute infection of the respiratory tract and digestive tract.

Warning It is contraindicated for cases with diarrhea.

消食健儿糖浆

【处方】南沙参、白术、山药、谷芽、麦芽、九香虫。

【功能主治】健脾消食。用于小儿慢性腹泻，食欲不振及营养不良。

Promoting Digestion Syrup for Infant

Name of Chinese Phonetic Alphabet Xiao Shi Jian Er Tang Jiang

Formula Adenophorae Radix, Atractylodis Macrocephalae Rhizoma, Dioscoreae Rhizoma, Setariae Fructus Germinatus, Hordei Fructus Germinatus and Aspongopus.

Actions and Indications Fortifying the spleen and promoting digestion. It is used for infantile chronic diarrhea, poor appetite and dystrophia.

消络痛片

【处方】芫花枝条、绿豆。

【功能主治】散风，祛湿。用于风湿性关节炎及其他风湿性疾病。

【注意】忌食辛辣等刺激性食物；孕妇忌服。

Relieving Rheumatic Disease Tablet

Name of Chinese Phonetic Alphabet Xiao Luo Tong Pian

Formula Genkwa Ramulus and Phaseoli Radiati Semen.

Actions and Indications Dissipating wind and dispelling dampness. It is indicated for rheumatic arthritis and other rheumatic diseases.

Warning Pungent foods are prohibited, and it is contraindicated for pregnant women.

消栓再造丸

【处方】血竭、赤芍、没药（醋炙）、当归、牛膝、丹参、川芎、桂枝、三七、豆蔻、郁金、枳壳（麸炒）、白术（麸炒）、人参、沉香、金钱白花蛇、僵蚕（麸炒）、白附子、天麻、防己、木瓜、全蝎、威灵仙、黄芪、肉桂、泽泻、茯苓、杜仲（炭）、槐角、麦冬、五味子（醋炙）、骨碎补、松香、山楂、冰片、苏合香、安息香、朱砂。

【功能主治】活血化瘀，息风通络，补气养血，消血栓。用于气虚血滞，风痰阻络引起的中风后遗症，半身不遂，口眼歪斜，言语障碍，胸中郁闷。

Thrombosis-dispersing Bolus

Name of Chinese Phonetic Alphabet Xiao Shuan Zai Zao Wan

Formula Draconis Sanguis, Paeoniae Radix Rubra, Myrrha (prepared with vinegar), Angelicae Sinensis Radix, Achyranthis Bidentatae Radix, Salviae Miltiorrhizae Radix et Rhizoma, Chuanxiong Rhizoma, Cinnamomi Ramulus, Notoginseng Radix et Rhizoma, Amomi Fructus Rotundus, Curcumae Radix, Aurantii Fructus (fried with bran), Atractylodis Macrocephalae Rhizoma (fried with bran), Ginseng Radix et Rhizoma, Aquilariae Lignum Resinatum, Bungarus Parvus, Bombyx Batryticatus (fried with bran), Typhonii Rhizoma, Gastrodiae Rhizoma, Stephaniae Tetrandrae

Radix, Chaenomelis Fructus, Scropio, Clematidis Radix et Rhizoma, Astragali Radix, Cinnamomi Cortex, Alismatis Rhizoma, Poria, Eucommiae Cortex (carbonated), Sophorae Fructus, Ophiopogoins Radix, Schisandrae Chinensis Fructus (prepared with vinegar), Drynariae Rhizoma, Pini Resina, Crataegi Fructus, Borneolum Syntheticum, Styrax, Benzoinum and Cinnabaris.

Actions and Indications Activating blood, resolving stasis, extinguishing wind, dredging collaterals, tonifying *qi*, nourishing blood, dispersing thrombosis. It is used for sequela of apoplexy, hemiparalysis, deviated eyes and mouth, lalopathy and chest distress due to *qi*-deficiency and stagnation of wind-phlegm in collaterals.

消栓胶囊

【处方】黄芪、当归、赤芍、川芎、地龙、桃仁、红花。

【功能主治】补气，活血，通络。用于中风引起的半身不遂，口眼歪斜，语言謇涩，口角流涎，下肢痿废，小便频数。

【注意】凡阴虚阳亢、风火上扰、痰浊蒙蔽者禁用。

Hemiparalysis-relieving Capsule

Name of Chinese Phonetic Alphabet Xiao Shuan Jiao Nang

Formula Astragali Radix, Angelicae Sinensis Radix, Paeoniae Radix Rubra, Chuanxiong Rhizoma, Pheretima, Persicae Semen and Carthami Flos.

Actions and Indications Tonifying *qi*, activating blood, dredging collaterals. It is indicated for hemiparalysis, deviated eyes and mouth, dysphasia, salivation, flaccidity of lower limbs and frequent urination due to apoplexy.

Warning It is contraindicated for cases with *yin*-deficiency and *yang* hyperactivity, wind-fire attack upward and turbid phlegm disturbance.

消栓通冲剂

【处方】黄芪、当归、地黄、桃仁、赤芍、川芎、地龙、枳壳（炒）、三七、丹参、甘草、红花、牛膝、冰片。

【功能主治】益气，活血，祛瘀，通络。用于中风瘫痪，半身不遂，口眼歪斜，语言不清及淤血性头痛，胸痛，肋痛，对中风先兆者（脑血栓形成先兆）亦有一定预防作用。

【注意】孕妇忌服。

Prodromal Thrombosis-preventing Soluble Granules

Name of Chinese Phonetic Alphabet Xiao Shuan Tong Chong Ji

Formula Astragali Radix, Angelicae Sinensis Radix, Rehmanniae Radix, Persicae Semen, Paeoniae Radix Rubra, Chuanxiong Rhizoma, Pheretima, Aurantii Fructus (fried), Notoginseng Radix et Rhizoma, Salviae Miltiorrhizae Radix et Rhizoma, Glycyrrhizae Radix et Rhizoma, Carthami Flos, Achyranthis Bidentatae Radix and Borneolum Syntheticum.

Actions and Indications Tonifying *qi*, activating blood, dispelling stasis, dredging collaterals. It is indicated for paralysis, hemiparalysis, deviated eyes and mouth, alalia, headache of blood-stasis type, chest pain, and preventing the prodromal cerebral thrombosis.

Warning It is contraindicated for pregnant women.

消栓通络片

【处方】川芎、丹参、黄芪、泽泻、三七、槐花、桂枝、郁金、木香、冰片、山楂。

【功能主治】活血化瘀，温经通络。用于血脂增高，脑血栓引起的精神呆滞、舌质发硬、言语迟涩、发音不清、手足发凉、活动疼痛。

【注意】禁食生冷、辛辣、动物油脂食物。

Dispersing Cerebral Thrombosis Tablet

Name of Chinese Phonetic Alphabet Xiao Shuan

Tong Luo Pian

Formula Chuanxiong Rhizoma, Salviae Miltiorrhizae Radix et Rhizoma, Astragali Radix, Alismatis Rhizoma, Notoginseng Radix et Rhizoma, Sophorae Flos, Cinnamomi Ramulus, Curcumae Radix, Aucklandiae Radix, Borneolum Syntheticum and Crataegi Fructus.

Actions and Indications Activating blood, resolving stasis, warming meridians and dredging collaterals. It is used for hyperlipemia, sluggishness of spirit due to cerebral thrombosis; stiff tongue, dysphasia, alalia, cold limbs and pain during movement.

Warning Uncooked, pungent and animal suet foods are prohibited.

消核片

【处方】玄参、海藻、丹参、浙贝母、昆布、半枝莲、牡蛎、漏芦、白花蛇舌草、夏枯草、郁金、芥子、金果榄、甘草。

【功能主治】软坚散结，行气活血，化痰通络。用于女性乳腺增生症，尤其适用于中青年妇女的乳痛症，乳腺小叶增生症。

Relieving Hyperplasia of Mammary Gland Tablet

Name of Chinese Phonetic Alphabet Xiao He Pian

Formula Scrophulariae Radix, Sargassum, Salviae Miltiorrhizae Radix et Rhizoma, Fritillariae Thunbergii Bulbus, Laminariae seu Eckloniae Thalluse, Scutellariae Barbatae Herba, Ostreae Concha, Rhapontici Radix, Hedyotis Diffusae Herba, Prunellae Spica, Curcumae Radix, Sinapis Semen, Tinosporae Radix and Glycyrrhizae Radix et Rhizoma.

Actions and Indications Softening and dispersing mass, moving *qi* and activating blood, resolving phlegm and dredging collaterals. It is indicated for hyperplasia of mammary glands, especially for breast pain, hyperplasia of lobule of mammary gland of young and middle-age women.

消银片

【处方】地黄、牡丹皮、赤芍、当归、苦参、金银花、玄参、牛蒡子、蝉蜕、白鲜皮、防风、大青叶、红花等。

【功能主治】清热凉血，养血润燥，祛风止痒。适用于血热白疕和血虚白疕。

Relieving Psoriasis Tablet

Name of Chinese Phonetic Alphabet Xiao Yin Pian

Formula Rehmanniae Radix, Moutan Cortex, Paeoniae Radix Rubra, Angelicae Sinensis Radix, Sophorae Flavescentis Radix, Lonicerae Japonicae Flos, Scrophulariae Radix, Arctii Fructus, Cicadae Periostracum, Dictamni Cortex, Saposhnikoviae Radix, Isatidis Folium, Carthami Flos, etc.

Actions and Indications Clearing heat and cooling blood, nourishing blood and moistening dryness, dispelling wind and relieving itching. It is indicated for psoriasis due to blood-heat and blood-deficiency.

消痔灵注射液

【处方】明矾、鞣酸、三氯叔丁醇、甘油、枸橼酸钠、亚硫酸氢钠、低分子右旋糖酐注射液。

【功能主治】收敛、止血。用于内痔出血，各期内痔，静脉曲张性混合痔。

【注意】内痔嵌顿发炎、皮赘性外痔忌用。

Injection for Relieving Hemorrhoid

Name of Chinese Phonetic Alphabet Xiao Zhi Ling Zhu She Ye

Formula Alumen, Tannic Acid, Chlorbutanol, Glycerol, Sodium Citrate, Sodium Bisulfite and Low Molecular Dextran Injection.

Actions and Indications Astringing and relieving bleeding. It is indicated for bleeding of internal hemorrhoid, various periods of internal hemorrhoid, varicosis mixed hemorrhoid.

Warning It is contraindicated for inflammation

of incarceration and cutaneous tag of external hemorrhoid.

消痔栓

【处方】龙骨（煅）、轻粉、冰片、珍珠（制）。

【功能主治】收敛，消肿，止痛，止血。用于内外痔疮。

【注意】孕妇禁用。

Relieving Hemorrhoid Suppository

Name of Chinese Phonetic Alphabet Xiao Zhi Shuan

Formula Draconis Os (calcined), Calomelas, Borneolum Syntheticum and Margarita (prepared).

Actions and Indications Astringing, dispersing swelling and alleviating pain, relieving bleeding. It is indicated for internal and external hemorrhoids.

Warning It is contraindicated for pregnant women.

消痤丸

【处方】升麻、柴胡、麦冬、野菊花、黄芩、玄参、生石膏、石斛、龙胆、大青叶、金银花、竹茹、蒲公英、淡竹叶、夏枯草、紫草。

【功能主治】清热解毒。用于痤疮。

Eliminating Acne Pill

Name of Chinese Phonetic Alphabet Xiao Cuo Wan

Formula Cimicifugae Rhizoma, Bupleuri Radix, Ophiopogonis Radix, Chrysanthemi Indici Flos, Scutellariae Radix, Scrophulariae Radix, Gypsum Fibrosum, Dendrobii Caulis, Gentianae Radix et Rhizoma, Isatidis Folium, Lonicerae Japonicae Flos, Bambusae Caulis in Taenias, Taraxaci Herba, Lophatheri Herba, Prunellae Spica and Arnebiae Radix.

Actions and Indications Clearing heat and detoxicating. It is used for acne.

消痛贴膏

【处方】独一味、棘豆、姜黄、花椒、水牛角、水柏枝。

【功能主治】活血化瘀，消肿止痛。用于急、慢性扭挫伤，跌打瘀痛，骨质增生，风湿，类风湿疼痛。亦适用于落枕、肩周炎、腰肌劳损和陈旧性伤痛。

Pain-dispersing Adhesive Plaster

Name of Chinese Phonetic Alphabet Xiao Tong Tie Gao

Formula Lamiophlomidis Radix Rhizoma et Herba, Oxytropis Leptophyllae Radix, Curcumae Longae Rhizoma, Zanthoxyli Pericarpium, Bubali Cornu and Myricariae Germanicae Ramulus.

Actions and Indications Activating blood, resolving stasis, reducing swelling, alleviating pain. It is used for acute, chronic traumatic sprain and contusion, hyperosteogeny, rheumatism, rheumatoid pain, and also used for stiff neck, scapulohumeral periarthritis, lumbar muscle strain and old traumatic pain.

消渴丸

【处方】葛根、地黄、黄芪、天花粉、玉米须、五味子、山药、格列本脲。

【功能主治】滋肾养阴，益气生津。用于多饮，多尿，多食，消瘦，体倦无力，眠差腰痛，尿糖及血糖升高之气阴两虚型消渴。

【注意】服用本品时严禁加服降血糖化学类药物。对严重肾功能不全，少年糖尿病，酮体糖尿，妊娠期糖尿病，糖尿性昏迷症患者不宜使用；肝炎患者慎服。

Relieving Wasting-thirst Pill

Name of Chinese Phonetic Alphabet Xiao Ke Wan

Formula Puerariae Lobatae Radix, Rehmanniae Radix, Astragali Radix, Trichosanthis Radix, Zeae Maydis Stylus, Schisandrae Chinensis Fructus,

Dioscoreae Rhizoma and Glybenzcyclamide.

Actions and Indications Enriching kidney-*yin*, tonifying *qi* and engendering fluid. It is indicated for cases with polydipsia, polyuria and polyphagia, emaciation, tiredness, fatigue, disturbed sleep, lumbago and ascending of glucose in urine and blood attributed to dual deficiency of *qi* and *yin*.

Warning Administration of chemical hypoglycemic medicine simultaneously is prohibited. It is contraindicated for cases with renal insufficiency, diabetes in early youth, ketone diabetes, diabetes during pregnant period, diabetic coma, and should be used carefully for hepatitis.

消渴平片

【处方】人参、黄连、天花粉、天冬、黄芪、丹参、枸杞子、沙苑子、葛根、知母、五倍子、五味子。

【功能主治】益气养阴，清热泻火，益肾缩尿。用于糖尿病。

Relieving Wasting-thirst Tablet

Name of Chinese Phonetic Alphabet Xiao Ke Ping Pian

Formula Ginseng Radix et Rhizoma, Coptidis Rhizoma, Trichosanthis Radix, Asparagi Radix, Astragali Radix, Salviae Miltiorrhizae Radix et Rhizoma, Lycii Fructus, Astragali Complanati Semen, Puerariae Lobatae Radix, Anemarrhenae Rhizoma, Galla Chinensis and Schisandrae Chinensis Fructus.

Actions and Indications Tonifying *qi* and nourishing *yin*, clearing heat, purging fire, tonifying the kidney and reducing urination. It is indicated for diabetes.

消渴安胶囊

【处方】地黄、知母、黄连、枸杞子等。

【功能主治】清热生津，益气养阴，活血化瘀。用于消渴病阴虚燥热兼气虚血瘀证。症见口渴多饮，多食易饥，五心烦热，大便秘结，倦怠乏力，自汗。

Relieving Wasting-thirst Capsule

Name of Chinese Phonetic Alphabet Xiao Ke An Jiao Nang

Formula Rehmanniae Radix, Anemarrhenae Rhizoma, Coptidis Rhizoma, Lycii Fructus, etc.

Actions and Indications Clearing heat, promoting fluid-engendering, tonifying *qi* and nourishing *yin*, activating blood and resolving stasis. It is indicated for diabetes attributed to *yin*-deficiency with dryness-heat associated with *qi*-deficiency and blood-stasis syndrome, and manifested as thirst, polydipsia, polyphagia, vexing heat in the chest, palms and soles, constipation, tiredness, fatigue and spontaneous sweating.

消渴降糖片

【处方】蔗鸡、黄精（制）、甜叶菊、桑椹、山药、天花粉、红参。

【功能主治】清热生津，益气养阴。用于糖尿病。

Relieving Wasting-thirst and Glucose-lowering Tablet

Name of Chinese Phonetic Alphabet Xiao Ke Jiang Tang Pian

Formula Sacchari Sinensis Gemma, Polygonati Rhizoma (prepared), Steviae Rebaudinae Folium, Mori Fructus, Dioscoreae Rhizoma, Trichosanthis Radix and Ginseng Radix et Rhizoma Rubra.

Actions and Indications Clearing heat, engendering fluid, tonifying *qi* and nourishing *yin*. It is indicated for diabetes.

消瘿气瘰丸

【处方】夏枯草、海藻、昆布、海螵蛸、蛤壳（煅）、海胆、陈皮、枳壳（去瓤麸炒）、黄芩、玄参。

【功能主治】消瘿化痰。用于肝郁痰结引起的瘿瘤肿胀，瘰疬结核。

Dispersing Goiter and Scrofula Pill

Name of Chinese Phonetic Alphabet Xiao Ying Qi Luo Wan

Formula Prunellae Spica, Sargassum, Laminariae seu Eckloniae Thallus, Sepiae Endoconchae, Meretricis Concha (calcined), Echinoideae Osseus Concha, Citri Reticulatae Pericarpium, Aurantii Fructus (removed pulp and fried), Scutellariae Radix and Scrophulariae Radix.

Actions and Indications Dispersing goiter and resolving phlegm. It is indicated for swelling of goiter and scrofula due to liver depression and stagnation of phlegm.

消癥益肝片

【处方】蜚蠊。

【功能主治】破血化积，消肿止痛。对原发性肝癌的症状有一定的缓解作用。

Prepared Roach* Tablet

Name of Chinese Phonetic Alphabet Xiao Zheng Yi Gan Pian

Formula Blatta (roach).

Actions and Indications Resolving mass, reducing swelling, alleviating pain. The preparation possesses remittent action for primary liver cancer.

*蜚蠊

海马多鞭丸

【处方】海马、蛤蚧、韭菜子、锁阳、鹿茸（去毛）、补骨脂（制）、小茴香（制）、菟丝子（制）、沙苑子（制）、山茱萸（制）、白术（炒）、杜仲（盐制）、红参、母丁香、牛膝、茯苓、山药、黄芪、当归、龙骨（煅）、甘草（制）、肉桂、雀脑、五味子、枸杞子、狗鞭、驴鞭、牛鞭、貂鞭、熟地黄、附子（制）、肉苁蓉、巴戟天、淫羊藿。

【功能主治】补肾壮阳，添精增髓。用于气血两亏引起的面黄肌瘦，梦遗滑精，早泄，阳痿不举，腰腿酸痛。

【注意】高血压患者慎用。

Sea Horse* Pill for Erect Disorder

Name of Chinese Phonetic Alphabet Hai Ma Duo Bian Wan

Formula Hippocampus, Gecko, Allii Tuberosi Semen, Cynomorii Caulis Carnosus, Cervi Cornu Pantotrichum (removed hair), Psoraleae Fructus (prepared), Foeniculi Fructus (prepared), Cuscutae Semen (prepared), Astragali Complanati Semen (prepared), Corni Fructus (prepared), Atractylodis Macrocephalae Rhizoma (fried), Eucommiae Cortex (prepared with salt), Ginseng Radix et Rhizoma Rubra, Caryophylli Fructus, Achyranthis Bidentatae Radix, Poria, Dioscoreae Rhizoma, Astragali Radix, Angelicae Sinensis Radix, Draconis Os (calcined), Glycyrrhizae Radix et Rhizoma (prepared), Cinnamomi Cortex, Passeris Encephalon, Schisandrae Chinensis Fructus, Lycii Fructus, Canis Testis et Penis, Asini Testis et Penis, Bovis Testis et Penis, Martis Zibellinae Testis et Penis, Rehmanniae Radix Praeparata, Aconiti Lateralis Radix Praeparata, Cistanches Caulis Carnosus, Morindae Officinalis Radix and Epimedii Folium.

Actions and Indications Tonifying kidney-*yang*, marrow and essence. It is used for cases with sallow complexion, emaciation, oneirogmus, spermatorrhea, ejaculatio praecox, impotence, erect disorder, soreness and pain of waist and knees due to dual depletion of *qi* and blood.

Warning It should be used carefully for hypertension.

*海马

海马补肾丸

【处方】熟地黄、鲜雀肉（带头去嘴爪）、驴肾、狗肾、鹿筋、附子（制）、肉苁蓉（酒制）、覆盆子、母丁香、淫羊藿（制）、山药、党参、核桃仁、补骨脂（盐制）、茴香（盐制）、菟丝子、沙苑子（盐炒）、当归、山茱萸（酒制）、牛膝、枸杞子、五味子（酒制）、茯苓、人参、鹿茸、黄芪、龙骨（煅）、海马、狗脊、肉桂、甘草、蛤蚧、豹骨（制）、杜仲（炭）等。

【功能主治】滋阴补肾，强壮健脑。用于身体衰弱，气血两亏，肾气不足，面黄肌瘦，心悸气短，腰酸腿疼，健忘虚喘。

Sea Horse* Pill for Tonifying Kidney

Name of Chinese Phonetic Alphabet Hai Ma Bu Shen Wan

Formula Rehmanniae Radix Praeparata, Passeris Caro Dulcis (retained head and removed beak), Asini Ren, Canis Ren, Cervi Tendo, Aconiti Lateralis Radix Praeparata, Cistanches Caulis Carnosus (prepared with wine), Rubi Fructus, Caryophylli Fructus, Epimedii Folium (prepared), Dioscoreae Rhizoma, Codonopsis Radix, Juglandis Semen , Psoraleae Fructus (prepared with salt), Foeniculi Fructus (prepared with salt), Cuscutae Semen, Astragali Complanati Semen (fried with salt), Angelicae Sinensis Radix, Corni Fructus (prepared with wine), Achyranthis Bidentatae Radix, Lycii Fructus, Schisandrae Chinensis Fructus (prepared with wine), Poria, Ginseng Radix et Rhizoma, Cervi Cornu Pantotrichum, Astragali Radix, Draconis Os (calcined), Hippocampus, Cibotii Rhizoma, Cinnamomi Cortex, Glycyrrhizae Radix et Rhizoma, Gecko, Pardi Os (prepared), Eucommiae Cortex (carbonated), etc.

Actions and Indications Enriching *yin*, tonifying the kidney and mind. It is used for general debility, sallow complexion, emaciation, palpitation, shortness of breath, soreness of waist and pain of legs, amnesia and dyspnea due to dual depletion of *qi* and blood and insufficiency of kidney-*qi*.

*海马

海马舒活膏

【处方】海马、三七、血竭、川芎、红花、栀子、官桂、香附、白芷、樟脑、薄荷脑、冰片。

【功能主治】活血化瘀，舒筋活络，消肿止痛。用于跌打损伤，瘀血肿痛，劳伤疼痛，风湿骨痛，闭合性新旧软组织挫伤，肌肉劳损。

【注意】皮肤有溃疡或外伤者勿直接贴用，皮肤过敏者慎用。

Sea Horse* Plaster

Name of Chinese Phonetic Alphabet Hai Ma Shu Huo Gao

Formula Hippocampus, Notoginseng Radix et Rhizoma, Draconis Sanguis, Chuanxiong Rhizoma, Carthami Flos, Gardeniae Fructus, Cinnamomi Cortex, Cyperi Rhizoma, Angelicae Dahuricae Radix, Camphora, Menthol and Borneolum Syntheticum.

Actions and Indications Activating blood, resolving stasis, relaxing sinews, activating collaterals, reducing swelling and alleviating pain. It is used for injury due to fall and strike; swelling and pain, rheumatalgia, closed new or old soft tissue contusion and muscular strain.

Warning This plaster cannot be applied on skin directly for cases with ulcer or trauma, and should be used carefully for cases with skin allergy.

*海马

海龙蛤蚧口服液

【处方】海龙、蛤蚧、人参、羊鞭、黄芩、熟地黄、菟丝子、何首乌、地黄、陈皮、当归、黄芪、阳起石、莲须、甘草、川芎、泽泻、锁阳、豆蔻、沉香、鹿茸、枸杞子、肉苁蓉、淫羊藿(羊油炙)、肉桂、韭菜子、蛇床子、花椒等。

【功能主治】温肾壮阳，补益精血。用于腰足酸软，面色㿠白，阳痿遗精，宫冷不孕，头目眩晕。

【注意】感冒，发热，咽喉痛时忌服。

Pipe Fish* and Giant Gecko** Oral Liquid

Name of Chinese Phonetic Alphabet Hai Long Ge Jie Kou Fu Ye

Formula Syngnathus, Gecko, Ginseng Radix et Rhizoma, Testis et Penis Garprinus, Scutellariae Radix, Rehmanniae Radix Praeparata, Cuscutae Semen, Polygoni Multiflori Radix, Rehmanniae Radix, Citci Reticulatae Pericarpium, Angelicae Sinensis Radix, Astragali Radix, Tremolitum, Nelumbinis Stamen, Glycyrrhizae Radix et Rhizoma, Chuanxiong Rhizoma,

Alismatis Rhizoma, Cynomorii Caulis Carnosus, Amomi Fructus Rotundus, Aquilariae Lignum Resinatum, Cervi Cornu Pantotrichum, Lycii Fructus, Cistanches Caulis Carnosus, Epimedii Folium (prepared with sheep suet), Cinnamomi Cortex, Allii Tuberosi Semen, Cnidii Fructus, Zanthoxyli Pericarpium, etc.

Actions and Indications Warming kidney-*yang*, tonifying essence and blood. It is used for soreness and weakness of waist and legs, bright pale complexion, impotence, nocturnal emission, uterus-coldness, sterility and vertigo.

Warning It is contraindicated for cases with common cold, fever and laryngeal pain.

* 海龙 ** 蛤蚧

海洋胃药片

【处方】海星、陈皮（炭）、牡蛎（煅）、瓦楞子（煅）、黄芪、白术（炒）、枯矾、干姜、胡椒。

【功能主治】益气健脾，温中止痛。用于脾胃虚弱，胃寒作痛，胃酸过多及由胃、十二指肠溃疡所致上述证候。

【注意】忌生冷食物；孕妇忌服。

Oceanic Medicinals Stomachic Tablet

Name of Chinese Phonetic Alphabet Hai Yang Wei Yao Pian

Formula Asterias, Citri Reticulatae Pericarpium (carbonated), Ostreae Concha (calcined), Arcae Concha (calcined), Astragali Radix, Atractylodis Macrocephalae Rhizoma (fried), Alumen Usta, Zingiberis Rhizoma and Piperis Fructus.

Actions and Indications Tonifying *qi* and fortifying the spleen, warming the middle and relieving pain. It is indicated for deficiency of the spleen and stomach, stomach pain, gastroxia, and gastroduodenal ulcer with the above mentioned symptoms.

Warning It is contraindicated for pregnant women, uncooked and cold foods should be avoided.

润肺止嗽丸

【处方】天冬、地黄、天花粉、瓜蒌子（蜜炙）、桑白皮（蜜炙）、紫苏子（炒）、苦杏仁（去皮炒）、紫菀、浙贝母、款冬花、桔梗、五味子（醋炙）、前胡、青皮（醋炙）、陈皮、黄芪（蜜炙）、酸枣仁（炒）、黄芩、知母、淡竹叶、甘草（蜜炙）。

【功能主治】清肺定喘，止嗽化痰。用于肺气虚弱引起的咳嗽喘促，痰涎壅盛，久嗽声哑。

Moistening Lung and Suppressing Cough Bolus

Name of Chinese Phonetic Alphabet Run Fei Zhi Sou Wan

Formula Asparagi Radix, Rehmanniae Radix, Trichosanthis Radix, Trichosanthis Semen (prepared with honey), Mori Cortex (prepared with honey), Perillae Fructus (fried), Armeniacae Semen Amarum (removed seed coat and fried), Asteris Radix et Rhizoma, Fritillariae Thunbergii Bulbus, Farfarae Flos, Platycodonis Radix, Schisandrae Chinensis Fructus (prepared with vinegar), Peucedani Radix, Citri Reticularae Pericarpium Viride (prepared with vinegar), Citri Reticulatae Pericarpium, Astragali Radix (prepared with honey), Ziziphi Spinosae Semen (fried), Scutellariae Radix, Anemarrhenae Rhizoma, Lophatheri Herba and Glycyrrhizae Radix et Rhizoma (prepared with honey).

Actions and Indications Clearing lung-heat and calming panting, suppressing cough and resolving phlegm. It is indicated for cough and panting, excessive phlegm, chronic cough and hoarseness due to deficiency of lung-*qi*.

润肺膏

【处方】莱阳梨清膏、黄芪（蜜炙）、紫菀（蜜炙）、百部（蜜炙）、川贝母、党参。

【功能主治】润肺益气，止咳化痰。用于肺虚气弱、胸闷不畅，久咳痰嗽，气喘自汗，慢性气管炎。

Soft Extract of Moistening Lung

Name of Chinese Phonetic Alphabet Run Fei Gao

Formula Lai Yang Pyri Fructus (liquid extract), Astragali Radix (prepared with honey), Asteris Radix et Rhizoma (prepared with honey), Stemonae Radix (prepared with honey), Fritillariae Cirrhosae Bulbus and Codonopsis Radix.

Actions and Indications Moistening the lung, tonifying *qi*, relieving cough, resolving phlegm. It is used for chest distress, chronic cough, productive cough, dyspnea, spontaneous sweating and chronic trachitis due to deficiency of *qi* and the lung.

益中生血片

【处方】党参、山药、薏苡仁、陈皮等。

【功能主治】健脾和胃，益气生血。用于缺铁性贫血属脾胃虚弱、气血两虚证；症见面色萎黄或苍白，头晕目眩，纳差，心悸气短，食后腹胀，神疲乏力，唇舌色淡，脉细弱。

Engendering Blood Tablet

Name of Chinese Phonetic Alphabet Yi Zhong Sheng Xue Pian

Formula Codonopsis Radix, Dioscoreae Rhizoma, Coicis Semen, Citri Reticulatae Pericarpium, etc.

Actions and Indications Fortifying the spleen, harmonizing the stomach, tonifying *qi* to engender blood. It is indicated for hypoferric anemia attributed to hypofunction of the spleen and stomach, dual deficiency of *qi* and blood, and manifested as sallow or pale complexion, dizziness, dizzy vision, poor appetite, palpitation, shortness of breath, abdominal fullness after meal, lassitude of spirit, fatigue, pale lips and tongue, fine and weak pulse.

益气止血冲剂

【处方】党参、黄芪、白术（炒）、茯苓、白及、功劳叶、地黄、防风。

【功能主治】益气，止血，固表，健脾。用于咯血、吐血，久服可预防感冒。

Soluble Granules of Tonifying *Qi* and Relieving Bleeding

Name of Chinese Phonetic Alphabet Yi Qi Zhi Xue Chong Ji

Formula Codonopsis Radix, Astragali Radix, Atractylodis Macrocephalae Rhizoma (fried), Poria, Bletillae Rhizoma, Mahoniae Folium, Rehmanniae Radix and Saposhnikoviae Radix.

Actions and Indications Tonifying *qi*, relieving bleeding, securing the exterior and fortifying the spleen. It is indicated for hemoptysis, hematemesis, prolonged administration for preventing common cold.

益气复脉胶囊

【处方】红参、麦冬、五味子。

【功能主治】益气复脉，养阴生津。能改善冠状动脉循环，降低心肌耗氧量。用于气阴两亏，心悸气短，脉微自汗，冠心病、心绞痛和衰老。

Restoring Normal Pulse Beat Capsule

Name of Chinese Phonetic Alphabet Yi Qi Fu Mai Jiao Nang

Formula Ginseng Radix et Rhizoma Rubra, Ophiopogonis Radix and Schisandrae Chinensis Fructus.

Actions and Indications Tonifying *qi* to restore normal pulse beat, nourishing *yin* and engendering fluid. It can improve the coronary artery circulation, reduce oxygen consumption of myocardium, and is indicated for palpitation, shortnes of breath, faint pulse, spontaneous sweating, coronary heart disease, angina pectoris and senility due to dual depletion of *qi* and *yin*.

益气维血颗粒

【处方】猪血提取物、黄芪等。

【功能主治】补血益气。用于血虚证、气血两虚证的证候治疗；症见面色萎黄或苍白，头晕目眩，神疲乏力，少气懒言，自汗，唇舌色淡，脉细弱，以及低色素小细胞性贫血见上述诸证候者。

Tonifying Blood Granules

Name of Chinese Phonetic Alphabet Yi Qi Wei Xue Ke Li

Formula Suillus Saguis (extract), Astragali Radix, etc.

Actions and Indications Tonifying *qi* and blood. It is indicated for blood-deficiency syndrome and dual deficiency of *qi* and blood, and manifested as sallow or pale complexion, dizziness, dizzy vision, lassitude of spirit, fatigue, shortness of breath with indolent speaking, spontaneous sweating, pale lips and tongue, fine and weak pulse, and hypochromic microcytic anemia with the above mentioned symptoms.

益心口服液

【处方】麦冬、当归、五味子、知母、人参、石菖蒲。

【功能主治】益气，养阴，通脉。用于心气虚或气阴两虚型的胸痹患者，症见心悸，乏力，胸痛，胸闷，心烦，失眠，汗多，眩晕，口干，面色少华或面色潮红，舌质淡红，胖嫩或有齿痕，脉弦细或沉细、涩、结代等；亦用于冠心病心绞痛见有上述证候者。

Chest-pain-relieving Oral Liquid

Name of Chinese Phonetic Alphabet Yi Xin Kou Fu Ye

Formula Ophiopogonis Radix, Angelicae Sinensis Radix, Schisandrae Chinensis Fructus, Anemarrhenae Rhizoma, Ginseng Radix et Rhizoma and Acori Tatarinowii Rhizoma.

Actions and Indications Tonifying *qi*, nourishing *yin*, dredging vessels. It is used for chest impediment syndrome manifested as palpitation, fatigue, chest pain, chest distress, vexation, insomnia, hyperhidrosis, vertigo, dry mouth, lusterless complexion or flushed complexion, light red or swollen and tender tongue or tooth-marked tongue, string-like and fine pulse or sunken and fine pulse, rough, bound and intermittent pulse due to dual deficiency of *qi* and *yin* or deficiency of heart-*qi*. The preparation is also used for coronary heart disease and angina pectoris with the above mentioned symptoms.

益心宁神片

【处方】人参茎叶总皂苷、合欢藤、五味子、灵芝。

【功能主治】补气生津，养心安神。用于心悸气短，多梦失眠，记忆力减退，神经衰弱。

Heart-nourishing and Mind-tranquilizing Tablet

Name of Chinese Phonetic Alphabet Yi Xin Ning Shen Pian

Formula Total saponin of Ginseng Folium et Caulis, Albiziae Caulis, Schisandrae Chinensis Fructus and Ganoderma.

Actions and Indications Tonifying *qi*, engendering fluid, nourishing the heart and tranquilizing the mind. It is used for palpitation, shortness of breath, profuse dreaming, insomnia, hypomnesia and neurasthenia.

益心复脉冲剂

【处方】生晒参、麦冬、五味子、黄芪、丹参、川芎。

【功能主治】益气养阴，活血复脉。用于气阴两虚，心血内阻，胸痹心痛，胸闷不舒，心悸，脉结代。

【注意】孕妇忌服。

Restoring Normal Pulse Beat Soluble Granules

Name of Chinese Phonetic Alphabet Yi Xin Fu Mai Chong Ji

Formula Ginseng Radix et Rhizoma Exsiccatus, Ophiopogonis Radix, Schisandrae Chinensis Fructus,

Astragali Radix, Salviae Miltiorrhizae Radix et Rhizoma and Chuanxiong Rhizoma.

Actions and Indications Tonifying *qi* and nourishing *yin*, activating blood and restoring normal pulse beat. It is used for internal stagnation of heart-blood, chest impediment disease and heart pain, chest distress, palpitation and bound and intermittent pulse beat due to dual deficiency of *qi* and *yin*.

Warning It is contraindicated for pregnant women.

益心通脉颗粒

【处方】黄芪、人参、北沙参、玄参、丹参、川芎等。

【功能主治】益气养阴，活血化瘀。用于冠心病稳定型心绞痛证属气阴两虚、心脉瘀阻者。症见胸闷心痛，倦怠气短，心悸自汗，咽干口燥，盗汗等。

Relieving Coronary Heart Disease Soluble Granules

Name of Chinese Phonetic Alphabet Yi Xin Tong Mai Ke Li

Formula Astragali Radix, Ginseng Radix et Rhizoma, Glehniae Radix, Scrophulariae Radix, Salviae Miltiorrhizae Radix et Rhizoma, Chuanxiong Rhizoma, etc.

Actions and Indications Tonifying *qi* and nourishing *yin*, activating blood and resolving stasis. It is indicated for coronary heart disease and stable type angina pectoris attributed to dual deficiency of *qi* and *yin* and heart vessel obstruction and manifested as chest distress, heart pain, tiredness, shortness of breath, palpitation, spontaneous sweating, dry mouth and throat, night sweating.

益心舒胶囊

【处方】人参、麦冬、五味子、黄芪、丹参、川芎、山楂。

【功能主治】益气复脉，活血化瘀，养阴生津。用于气阴两虚，心悸脉结代，胸闷不舒、胸痛及冠心病心绞痛见有上述症状者。

Relieving Chest Distress Capsule

Name of Chinese Phonetic Alphabet Yi Xin Shu Jiao Nang

Formula Ginseng Radix et Rhizoma, Ophiopogonis Radix, Schisandrae Chinensis Fructus, Astragali Radix, Salviae Miltiorrhizae Radix et Rhizoma, Chuanxiong Rhizoma and Crataegi Fructus.

Actions and Indications Tonifying *qi* to restore normal pulse beat, activating blood to resolve stasis, nourishing *yin* to engender fluid. It is indicated for palpitation, bound and intermittent pulse, chest distress and chest pain due to dual deficiency of *qi* and *yin*, and also used for coronary heart disease, angina pectoris with the above mentioned symptoms.

益母丸

【处方】益母草、当归、川芎、木香。

【功能主治】调经养血，化瘀生新。用于气逆血滞，血亏血寒引起的经期不准，腹痛白带，腰酸倦怠，血虚头晕，耳鸣，产后败血不净。

【注意】孕妇及月经过多者忌服。

Chinese Motherwort* Bolus

Name of Chinese Phonetic Alphabet Yi Mu Wan

Formula Leonuri Herba, Angelicae Sinensis Radix, Chuanxiong Rhizoma and Aucklandiae Radix.

Actions and Indications Regulating menstruation, nourishing blood, resolving stasis. It is used for irregular menstrual cycle, dysmenorrhea, leukorrhagia, soreness of the waist, tiredness, dizziness, tinnitus and puerperal lochiorrhea due to *qi* counterflow and blood Stagnation.

Warning It is contraindicated for pregnant women and hypermenorrhea.

* 益母草

益母草膏

【处方】益母草。

【功能主治】子宫收缩药。用于调经及产后子宫出血，子宫复原不全。

【注意】孕妇禁用。

Chinese Motherwort* Liquid Extract

Name of Chinese Phonetic Alphabet Yi Mu Cao Gao

Formula Leonuri Extractum.

Actions and Indications It is an uterotonic, and indicated for regulating menstruation, puerperal endometrorrhagia and subinvolution of uterus.

Warning It is contraindicated for pregnant women.

* 益母草

益血生胶囊

【处方】阿胶、龟甲胶、鹿角胶、鹿血、牛髓、紫河车、鹿茸、茯苓、黄芪（蜜制）、白芍、当归、党参、熟地黄、白术（麸炒）、制何首乌、大枣、山楂（炒）、麦芽（炒）、鸡内金（炒）、知母（盐制）、大黄（酒制）、花生衣。

【功能主治】健脾生血，补肾填精。用于脾肾两亏所致的血虚诸症，各种类型贫血及血小板减少症。对慢性再生障碍性贫血也有一定疗效。

【注意】虚热者慎用。

Blood-engendering Capsule

Name of Chinese Phonetic Alphabet Yi Xue Sheng Jiao Nang

Formula Asini Corii Colla, Testudinis Carapacis et Plastri Colla, Cervi Cornus Colla, Cervi Sanguis, Bovis Spinalis Medulla, Hominis Placenta, Cervi Cornu Pantotrichum, Poria, Astragali Radix (prepared with honey), Paeoniae Radix Alba, Angelicae Sinensis Radix, Codonopsis Radix, Rehmanniae Radix Praeparata, Atractylodis Macrocephalae Rhizoma (fried with bran), Polygoni Multiflori Radix Praeparata, Jujubae Fructus, Crataegi Fructus (fried), Hordei Fructus Germinatus (fried), Galli Gigerii Endothelium Corneum (fried), Anemarrhenae Rhizoma (prepared with salt), Rhei Radix et Rhizoma (prepared with wine) and Arachidis Hypogaeae Testa.

Actions and Indications Fortifying the spleen, engendering blood, tonifying the kidney and essence. It is indicated for various types of anemia and thrombopenia due to dual depletion of the spleen and kidney and blood deficiency. It also shows certain curative effect for chronic aplastic anemia.

Warning It should be used carefully for cases with deficiency-heat syndrome.

益肝灵片

【处方】水飞蓟素。

【功能主治】保肝药。具有改善肝功能、保护肝细胞膜的作用，用于急、慢性肝炎及迁延性肝炎。

Nourishing Liver Tablet

Name of Chinese Phonetic Alphabet Yi Gan Ling Pian

Formula Silybin.

Actions and Indications Protecting the liver. It possesses the effect of improving hepatic function and protecting hepatic cell membrane. It is indicated for acute, chronic and persistent hepatitis.

益坤丸

【处方】熟地黄、当归、白芍、阿胶、人参、黄芪（蜜炙）、山药、甘草、益母草膏、血余炭、鸡冠花、延胡索（醋炙）、乳香（醋炙）、没药（醋炙）、小茴香（盐炙）、松香（炙）、鹿角、锁阳、艾叶炭、续断、补骨脂（盐炙）、杜仲炭、菟丝子、白薇、黄柏、茯苓、白术（麸炒）、白芷、陈皮、木香、砂仁、紫苏叶、藁本、川芎、牡丹皮、红花、益母草、赤石脂（煅）、黄芩、青蒿、肉桂。

【功能主治】补气养血，调经散寒。用于气虚血衰引起的月经不调，行经腹痛，宫寒带下，腰酸体倦。

【注意】孕妇忌服。

Menstruation-regulating Bolus

Name of Chinese Phonetic Alphabet Yi Kun Wan

Formula Rehmanniae Radix Praeparata, Angelicae Sinensis Radix, Paeoniae Radix Alba, Asini Corii Colla, Ginseng Radix et Rhizoma, Astragali Radix (prepared with honey), Dioscoreae Rhizoma, Glycyrrhizae Radix et Rhizoma, Leonuri Extractum, Crinis Carbonisatus, Celosiae Cristatae Flos, Corydalis Rhizoma (prepared with vinegar), Olibanum (prepared with vinegar), Myrrha (prepared with vinegar), Foeniculi Fructus (prepared with salt), Pini Resina (prepared), Cervi Cornu, Cynomorii Caulis Carnosus, Artemisiae Argyi Folium Carbonisatus, Dipsaci Radix, Psoraleae Fructus (prepared with salt), Eucommiae Cortex Carbonisatus, Cuscutae Semen, Cynanchi Atrati Radix et Rhizoma, Phellodendri Chinensis Cortex, Poria, Atractylodis Macrocephalae Rhizoma (fried with bran), Angelicae Dahuricae Radix, Citri Reticulatae Pericarpium, Aucklandiae Radix, Amomi Fructus, Perillae Folium, Ligustici Rhizoma et Radix, Chuanxiong Rhizoma, Moutan Cortex, Carthami Flos, Leonuri Herba, Halloysitum Rubrum (calcined), Scutellariae Radix, Artemisiae Annuae Herba and Cinnamomi Cortex.

Actions and Indications Tonifying *qi*, nourishing blood, regulating menstruation, dissipating cold. It is indicated for irregular menstruation, abdominal pain during menstruation, uterus-coldness with vaginal discharge, soreness of waist and tiredness due to dual deficiency of *qi* and blood.

Warning It is contraindicated for pregnant women.

益肾兴阳胶囊

【**处方**】鹿茸、驴肾（酒炙）、狗肾（酒炙）、肉苁蓉（酒炙）、菟丝子、人参、黄芪、淫羊藿干膏粉、蚕蛾（去足翅）。

【**功能主治**】补肾益气，壮阳固精。用于肾阳亏气虚引起的腰腿酸软，精神疲倦，头晕耳鸣，失眠健忘，阳痿，遗精早泄。

【**注意**】实热或湿热者忌用。

Kidney-*yang* Tonifying Capsule

Name of Chinese Phonetic Alphabet Yi Shen Xing Yang Jiao Nang

Formula Cervi Cornu Pantotrichum, Asini Ren (prepared with wine), Canis Ren (prepared with wine), Cistanches Caulis Carnosus (prepared with wine), Cuscutae Semen, Ginseng Radix et Rhizoma, Astragali Radix, Epimedii Extractum Pulvis and Bombycis Imagine Masculi (removed feet and wings).

Actions and Indications Tonifying the kidney and *qi*, strengthening *yang* to arrest essence. It is used for soreness of the waist and weakness of legs, lassitude of spirit, dizziness, tinnitus, insomnia, amnesia, impotence, nocturnal emission and ejaculatio praecox due to depletion of kidney-*yang* and *qi*-deficiency.

Warning It is contraindicated for cases with excess heat and damp-heat.

益肾补骨液

【**处方**】骨碎补、何首乌、茯苓、续断、白芍、当归、党参、熟地黄、黄精、枸杞子、自然铜（煅，醋淬）、陈皮。

【**功能主治**】滋补肝肾，强壮筋骨。用于肝肾不足引起的劳伤腰痛，筋骨折伤。

Tonifying Sinews and Bone Oral Liquid

Name of Chinese Phonetic Alphabet Yi Shen Bu Gu Ye

Formula Psoraleae Fructus, Polygoni Multiflori Radix, Poria, Dipsaci Radix, Paeoniae Radix Alba, Angelicae Sinensis Radix, Codonopsis Radix, Rehmanniae Radix Praeparata, Polygonati Rhizoma, Lycii Fructus, Pyritum (calcined and quenched by vinegar) and Citri Reticulatae Pericarpium.

Actions and Indications Enriching the liver and kidney, strengthening the sinews and bone. It is used for overstrain, lumbago and fracture due to insufficiency of the liver and kidney.

益肾灵冲剂

【**处方**】枸杞子、女贞子、附子（制）、芡实

（炒）、车前子（炒）、补骨脂（炒）、覆盆子、五味子、桑椹、沙苑子、韭菜子（炒）、淫羊藿、金樱子。

【功能主治】益肾壮阳。用于肾亏阳痿，早泄、遗精、少精、死精。

Tonifying Kidney-*yang* Soluble Granules

Name of Chinese Phonetic Alphabet Yi Shen Ling Chong Ji

Formula Lycii Fructus, Ligustri Lucidi Fructus, Aconiti Lateralis Radix Praeparata, Euryales Semen (fried), Plantaginis Semen (fried), Psoraleae Fructus (fried), Rubi Fructus, Schisandrae Chinensis Fructus, Mori Fructus, Astragali Complanati Semen, Allii Tuberosi Semen (fried), Epimedii Folium and Rosae Laevigatae Fructus.

Actions and Indications Tonifying the kidney-*yang*. It is used for impotence, ejaculatio praecox, nocturnal emission, oligospermia and death spermia due to depletion of the kidney.

益肾液

【处方】枸杞子、菟丝子、覆盆子、车前子（盐制）、五味子（酒制）。

【功能主治】填精补髓，益肾扶阳。用于身体虚弱，肾亏阳痿，梦遗滑精，尿液浑浊。

Tonifying Kidney Liquid

Name of Chinese Phonetic Alphabet Yi Shen Ye

Formula Lycii Fructus, Cuscutae Semen, Rubi Fructus, Plantaginis Semen (prepared with salt) and Schisandrae Chinensis Fructus (prepared with wine).

Actions and Indications Tonifying vital essence, marrow and the kidney, reinforcing the *yang-qi*. It is used for general debility, impotence, dream emission, spermatorrhea and turbid urine.

益肾蠲痹丸

【处方】本品为骨碎补、熟地黄、当归、延胡索、寻骨风等经加工制成的丸剂。

【功能主治】温补肾阳，益肾壮督，搜风剔邪，蠲痹通络。用于症见发热，关节疼痛、肿大、红肿热痛、屈伸不利，肌肉疼痛，瘦削或僵硬，畸形的顽痹（类风湿性关节炎）。

【注意】偶有皮肤瘙痒反应；孕妇禁服。

Relieving Rheumatoid Arthritis Pill

Name of Chinese Phonetic Alphabet Yi Shen Juan Bi Wan

Formula Psoraleae Fructus, Rehmanniae Radix Praeparata, Angelicae Sinensis Radix, Corydalis Rhizoma, Aristolochiae Mollissimae Rhizoma seu Herba, etc.

Actions and Indications Warming and tonifying kidney-*yang*, strengthening the governor vessel, expelling wind and pathogen, activating collaterals. It is used for rheumatoid arthritis manifested as pain and swelling of joints, inability of pulling and stretching in limbs, myalgia, emaciation or rigidity.

Warning Cutaneous pruritus occurs occasionally. It is contraindicated for pregnant women.

益肺清化膏

【处方】黄芪、党参、北沙参、麦冬、仙鹤草、川贝母、苦杏仁等。

【功能主治】益气养阴，清热解毒，化痰止咳。用于气阴两虚、阴虚内热型晚期肺癌的辅助治疗。症见：气短、乏力、咳嗽、咯血、胸痛。

Tonifying Lung and Detoxicating Solf Extract

Name of Chinese Phonetic Alphabet Yi Fei Qing Hua Gao

Formula Astragali Radix, Codonopsis Radix, Glehniae Radix, Ophiopogonis Radix, Agrimoniae Herba, Fritillariae Cirrhosae Bulbus, Armeniacae Semen Amarum, etc.

Actions and Indications Tonifying *qi* and nourishing *yin*, clearing heat and detoxicating, resolving phlegm and relieving cough. It is used as an adjunctive treatment for late stage of cancer of pulmonary carcinoma caused by dual deficiency of *qi* and *yin*, *yin*-deficiency and internal heat, manifested as shortness of breath, fatigue, cough, hemoptysis and pectoralgia.

益胆片

【处方】郁金、金银花、白矾、甘草、硝石、滑石粉、玄参。

【功能主治】行气散结，清热通淋。用于胆结石，肾结石，膀胱结石，阻塞性黄疸，胆囊炎等病见湿热蕴结之证者。

Promoting Lithecbole Tablet

Name of Chinese Phonetic Alphabet Yi Dan Pian

Formula Curcumae Radix, Lonicerae Japonicae Flos, Alumen, Glycyrrhizae Radix et Rhizoma, Nitrum, Talci Pulvis and Scrophulariae Radix.

Actions and Indications Moving *qi* to dissipate mass, clearing heat and relieving strangury. It is indicated for calculus of the gallbladder, kidney and vesical calculus, obstructive jaundice, cholecystitis, attributive to accumulation of damp-heat.

益脉康片

【处方】本品为灯盏细辛浸膏片。

【功能主治】活血化瘀，有改善脑血循环，增加脑血流量，增加心肌对缺血、缺氧的耐受性，改善微循环的作用。用于缺血性脑血管及脑出血后遗瘫痪，眼底视网膜静脉阻塞，冠心病，血管炎性皮肤病，风湿病。

Ischemic Cerebrovascular Disease Relieving Tablet

Name of Chinese Phonetic Alphabet Yi Mai Kang Pian

Formula Erigerontis Extractum.

Actions and Indications Activating blood, resolving stasis, improving cerebral blood circulation, increasing cerebral blood flow, increasing the tolerance of ischemia and hypoxia in cardiac muscle, improving microcirculation. It is indicated for ischemic cerebrovascular disease and paralysis due to cerebral hemorrhage; ocular fundus retina vein obstruction, coronary heart disease, vasculitic dermatosis and rheumatism.

益津降糖口服液

【处方】人参、白术、茯苓、仙人掌、甘草。

【功能主治】健脾益气，生津止渴。用于气阴两虚所致的消渴及Ⅱ型糖尿病，症见乏力，自汗，口渴喜饮，多尿，多食善饥，舌苔花剥，少津，脉细少力。

【注意】孕妇慎用。

Hypoglycemic Oral Liquid for Diabetes

Name of Chinese Phonetic Alphabet Yi Jin Jiang Tang Kou Fu Ye

Formula Ginseng Radix et Rhizoma, Atractylodis Macrocephalae Rhizoma, Poria, Opuntiae Dillenii Radix et Caulis and Glycyrrhizae Radix et Rhizoma.

Actions and Indications Fortifying the spleen, tonifying qi, engendering fluid to quench thirst. It is used for type Ⅱ diabetes due to dual deficiency of *qi* and *yin*, and manifested as fatigue, spontaneous sweating, thirst, polydipsia, polyuria and polyphagia, peeling tongue fur, lack of fluid and fine pulse.

Warning It should be used carefully for pregnant women.

益脑胶囊

【处方】龟甲胶、远志、龙骨、灵芝、五味子、麦冬、石菖蒲、党参、人参、茯苓。

【功能主治】补气养阴，滋肾健脑，益智安神。用于神经衰弱，脑动脉硬化引起的体倦头晕，失眠多梦，记忆力减退属于心肝肾不足，气、阴两虚患者。

Brain-tonifying Capsule

Name of Chinese Phonetic Alphabet Yi Nao Jiao Nang

Formula Testudinis Carapacis et Plastri Colla, Polygalae Radix, Draconis Os, Ganoderma, Schisandrae Chinensis Fructus, Ophiopogonis Radix, Acori Tatarinowii Rhizoma, Codonopsis Radix, Ginseng Radix et Rhizoma and Poria.

Actions and Indications Tonifying *qi*, nourishing *yin*, enriching the kidney, tranquilizing the mind. It is used for neurasthenia, tiredness, dizziness, insomnia, profuse dreaming and hypomnesia due to cerebral arteriosclerosis and attributed to insufficiency of the heart, liver and kidney, and dual deficiency of *qi* and *yin*.

益虚宁片

【处方】枸杞子、何首乌（黑豆汁制）、党参、当归、地黄、五味子、菟丝子、女贞子、牛膝、牡丹皮、麦冬、甘草。

【功能主治】养阴益气，补血安神。用于失眠少寝、头发脱落，耳鸣头晕、腰痛腿软。

Tranquilizing Mind Tablet

Name of Chinese Phonetic Alphabet Yi Xu Ning Pian

Formula Lycii Fructus, Polygoni Multiflori Radix (prepared with juice of black soya bean), Codonopsis Radix, Angelicae Sinensis Radix, Rehmanniae Radix, Schisandrae Chinensis Fructus, Cuscutae Semen, Ligustri Lucidi Fructus, Achyranthis Bidentatae Radix, Moutan Cortex, Ophiopogonis Radix and Glycyrrhizae Radix et Rhizoma.

Actions and Indications Nourishing *yin*, tonifying *qi* and blood, tranquilizing the mind. It is indicated for insomnia, alopecia, tinnitus, dizziness, lumbago and weakness of the legs.

益龄精

【处方】制何首乌、金樱子、桑椹、女贞子（酒蒸）、豨莶草（蜜酒蒸）、川牛膝（酒蒸）、菟丝子（酒蒸）。

【功能主治】补肝肾，益精髓。用于肝肾不足引起的头晕目眩，耳鸣心悸，乏力，咽干失眠，及高血压而见有上述症状者。

Oral Liquid of Tonifying Vital Essence

Name of Chinese Phonetic Alphabet Yi Ling Jing

Formula Polygoni Multiflori Radix Praeparata, Rosae Laevigatae Fructus, Mori Fructus, Ligustri Lucidi Fructus (steamed by wine), Siegesbeckiae Herba (steamed by honeyed wine), Cyathulae Radix (steamed by wine) and Cuscutae Semen (steamed by wine).

Actions and Indications Tonifying the liver, kidney and vital essence. It is indicated for dizziness, dizzy vision, tinnitus, palpitation, fatigue, dry throat, insomnia and hypertension with the above mentioned symptoms due to dual insufficiency of the liver and kidney.

宽胸气雾剂

【处方】细辛油、檀香油、高良姜油、荜茇油、冰片。

【功能主治】理气止痛。用于缓解心绞痛。

Relieving Angina Pectoris Aerosol

Name of Chinese Phonetic Alphabet Kuan Xiong Qi Wu Ji

Formula Asari Oleum, Lignum Satali Albi Oleum, Alpiniae Officinarum Oleum, Piperis Longi Fructus Oleum and Borneolum Syntheticum.

Actions and Indications Regulating *qi* and alleviating pain. It is used for relieving angina pectoris.

宽胸舒气化滞丸

【处方】沉香、木香、青皮（醋炙）、陈皮、牵牛子（炒）。

【功能主治】舒气宽中，消积化滞。用于肝胃不和，气郁结滞引起的两肋胀满，呃逆积滞，胃脘刺痛，积聚痞块，大便秘结。

【注意】孕妇忌服。

Soothing Liver and Stomach Bolus

Name of Chinese Phonetic Alphabet Kuan Xiong Shu Qi Hua Zhi Wan

Formula Aquilariae Lignum Resinatum, Aucklandiae Radix, Citri Reticulatae Pericarpium Viride (prepared with vinegar), Citri Reticulatae Pericarpium and Pharbitidis Semen (fried).

Actions and Indications Soothing *qi* movement, resolving stagnation to promote digestion. It is used for hypochondriac fullness, hiccup, food stagnation, stabbing pain in stomach duct, stagnated stuffy lump and constipation due to stagnation of *qi* and disharmony of the liver and stomach.

Warning It is contraindicated for pregnant women.

烫伤油

【处方】马尾连、紫草、黄芩、冰片、地榆、大黄。

【功能主治】消炎，止痛，去腐生肌。用于Ⅰ、Ⅱ度烧烫伤和酸碱灼伤。

Relieving Scalding Oils

Name of Chinese Phonetic Alphabet Tang Shang You

Formula Thalictri Rhizoma et Radix, Arnebiae Radix, Scutellariae Radix, Borneolum Syntheticum, Sanguisorbae Radix and Rhei Radix et Rhizoma.

Actions and Indications Counteracting inflammation and alleviating pain, removing necrosis and promoting tissue regeneration. It is used for Ⅰ ~ Ⅱ degree burn or scald, or burn by acid or base.

诺迪康胶囊

【处方】红景天。

【功能主治】益气活血，通脉止痛。用于胸痹，表现为胸闷，刺痛或隐痛，心悸气短，神疲乏力，少气懒言，头晕目眩，以及冠心病、心绞痛见以上证候者。

Bigflower Rhodiola* Capsule

Name of Chinese Phonetic Alphabet Nuo Di Kang Jiao Nang

Formula Rhodiolae Crenulatae Radix et Rhizoma.

Actions and Indications Tonifying *qi*, activating blood, dredging vessels, alleviating pain. It is used for chest impediment syndrome manifested as chest distress, stabbing or dull pain, palpitation, shortness of breath, lassitude of spirit, fatigue, indolent speaking, dizziness and dizzy vision, and also used for coronary heart disease and angina pectoris with the above mentioned manifestations.

* 红景天

调中四消丸

【处方】牵牛子（炒）、熟大黄、香附（醋炙）、五灵脂（醋炙）、猪牙皂。

【功能主治】消食化滞，利水止痛。用于停食腹胀脘痛，二便不利。

【注意】孕妇忌服。年老体弱者勿服。

Digestion-promoting Pill

Name of Chinese Phonetic Alphabet Tiao Zhong Si Xiao Wan

Formula Pharbitidis Semen (fried), Rehmanniae Radix Praeparata, Cyperi Rhizoma (prepared with vinegar), Trogopterori Faeces (prepared with vinegar) and Gleditsiae Fructus Abnormalis.

Actions and Indications Promoting digestion and improving food stagnation, inducing diuresis and relieving pain. It is indicated for abdominal distention and pain due to indigestion; difficulty in urination and defecation.

Warning It is contraindicated for pregnant women and senile debility.

调经丸

【处方】当归、白芍（酒炒）、川芎、熟地黄、艾叶（炭）、香附（醋制）、陈皮、半夏（制）、茯苓、甘草、白术（炒）、吴茱萸（制）、小茴香（盐炒）、延胡索（醋制）、没药（制）、益母草、牡丹皮、续断、黄芩（酒炒）、麦冬、阿胶。

【功能主治】理气和血，调经止痛。用于气郁血滞，月经不调，经来腹痛，崩漏白带。

Regulating Menstruation Bolus

Name of Chinese Phonetic Alphabet Tiao Jing Wan

Formula Angelicae Sinensis Radix, Paeoniae Radix Alba (fried with wine), Chuanxiong Rhizoma, Rehmanniae Radix Praeparata, Artemisiae Argyi Folium (carbonated), Cyperi Rhizoma (prepared with vinegar), Citri Reticulatae Pericarpium, Pinelliae Rhizoma (prepared), Poria, Glycyrrhizae Radix et Rhizoma, Atractylodis Macrocephalae Rhizoma (fried), Euodiae Fructus (prepared), Foeniculi Fructus (fried with salt), Corydalis Rhizoma (prepared with vinegar), Myrrha (prepared), Leonuri Herba, Moutan Cortex, Dipsaci Radix, Scutellariae Radix (fried with wine), Ophiopogonis Radix and Asini Corii Colla.

Actions and Indications Regulating *qi* and harmonizing blood, regulating menstruation and relieving pain. It is used for irregular menstruation, dysmenorrhea, metrorrhagia and leukorrhagia due to stagnation of *qi* and blood.

调经止痛片

【处方】当归、党参、川芎、香附（醋炙）、益母草、泽兰叶、大红袍。

【功能主治】补气活血，调经止痛。用于月经不调，经期腹痛，产后瘀血不尽。

Regulating Menstruation Tablet

Name of Chinese Phonetic Alphabet Tiao Jing Zhi Tong Pian

Formula Angelicae Sinensis Radix, Codonopsis Radix, Chuanxiong Rhizoma, Cyperi Rhizoma (prepared with vinegar), Leonuri Herba, Lycopi Folium and Myrsines Africanae Herba.

Actions and Indications Tonifying *qi* and activating blood, regulating menstruation and relieving pain. It is used for irregular menstruation, dysmenorrhea, puerperal prolonged blood-stasis.

调经至宝丸

【处方】大黄、木香、牵牛子（炒）、枳实（麸炒）、莪术（醋煮）、五灵脂（醋炒）、陈皮、黄芩、鳖甲（醋制）、香附（醋炒）、三棱（醋炒）、苍术（米泔水炒）、当归、山楂、槟榔。

【功能主治】破瘀，调经。用于妇女血瘀积聚，月经闭止，经期紊乱，行经腹痛。

【注意】体质衰弱、血虚经闭、大便溏薄及孕妇忌服。

Precious Pill for Regulating Menstruation

Name of Chinese Phonetic Alphabet Tiao Jing Zhi Bao Wan

Formula Rhei Radix et Rhizoma, Aucklandiae Radix, Pharbitidis Semen (fried), Aurantii Fructus Immaturus (fried with bran), Curcumae Rhizoma (cooked with vinegar), Trogopterori Faeces (fried with vinegar), Citri Reticulatae Pericarpium, Scutellariae Radix, Trionycis Carapax (prepared with vinegar), Cyperi Rhizoma (fried with vinegar), Sparganii Rhizoma (fried with vinegar), Atractylodis Rhizoma (fried with rice swilled water), Angelicae Sinensis Radix, Crataegi Fructus and Arecae Semen.

Actions and Indications Breaking blood and expelling stasis, regulating menstruation. It is used for amenorrhea, irregular menstruation and abdominal pain during menstruation due to blood-stasis.

Warning It is contraindicated for debility of

crasis, amenorrhea due to blood deficiency; sloppy stools and pregnant women.

调经促孕丸

【处方】鹿茸（去毛）、淫羊藿（羊油炙）、仙茅、续断、桑寄生、菟丝子、枸杞子、覆盆子、山药、莲子（去心）、茯苓、黄芪、白芍、酸枣仁（炒）、钩藤、丹参、赤芍、鸡血藤。

【功能主治】补肾健脾，养血调经。用于脾肾阳虚引起的经血不调，月经过少，久不孕育。

【注意】阴虚火旺、月经量过多者不宜服用。

Menstruation-regulating and Sterility-promoting Pill

Name of Chinese Phonetic Alphabet Tiao Jing Cu Yun Wan

Formula Cervi Cornu Pantotrichum (removed hair), Epimedii Folium (prepared with sheep suet), Curculiginis Rhizoma, Dipsaci Radix, Taxilli Herba, Cuscutae Semen, Lycii Fructus, Rubi Fructus, Dioscoreae Rhizoma, Nelumbinis Semen (removed plumule), Poria, Astragali Radix, Paeoniae Radix Alba, Ziziphi Spinosae Semen (fried), Uncariae Ramulus cum Uncis, Salviae Miltiorrhizae Radix et Rhizoma, Paeoniae Radix Rubra and Spatholobi Caulis.

Actions and Indications Tonifying the kidney and fortifying the spleen, nourishing blood and regulating menstruation. It is indicated for irregular menstruation, hypomenorrhea and sterility in women due to dual *yang*-deficiency of the spleen and kidney.

Warning It is contraindicated for cases with hypermenorrhea and *yin*-deficiency with effulgent fire.

调经活血片

【处方】木香、川芎、赤芍、延胡索（醋制）、当归、熟地黄、丹参、泽兰、红花、乌药、鸡血藤、 白术、香附（制）、菟丝子、吴茱萸（甘草水制）。

【功能主治】调经活血，行气止痛。用于月经不调，行经腹痛。

Menstruation-regulating and Blood-activating Tablet

Name of Chinese Phonetic Alphabet Tiao Jing Huo Xue Pian

Formula Aucklandiae Radix, Chuanxiong Rhizoma, Paeoniae Radix Rubra, Corydalis Rhizoma (prepared with vinegar), Angelicae Sinensis Radix, Rehmanniae Radix Praeparata, Salviae Miltiorrhizae Radix et Rhizoma, Lycopi Herba, Carthami Flos, Linderae Radix, Spatholobi Caulis, Atractylodis Macrocephalae Rhizoma, Cyperi Rhizoma (prepared), Cuscutae Semen and Euodiae Fructus (prepared with licorice root water).

Actions and Indications Regulating menstruation, activating blood, promoting *qi* moving, alleviating pain. It is indicated for irregular menstruation, dysmenorrhea.

调胃丹

【处方】木香、砂仁、甘草、槟榔、枳实（麸炒）、厚朴（姜制）、香附（醋制）、豆蔻、五灵脂（醋制）、高良姜、丁香、肉桂。

【功能主治】健胃宽中，舒肝顺气。用于胃酸胃寒，胸中胀满，倒饱嘈杂。

【注意】孕妇忌服。

Stomach-regulating Pill

Name of Chinese Phonetic Alphabet Tiao Wei Dan

Formula Aucklandiae Radix, Amomi Fructus, Glycyrrhizae Radix et Rhizoma, Arecae Semen, Aurantii Fructus Immaturus (fried with bran), Magnoliae Officinalis Cortex (prepared with ginger), Cyperi Rhizoma (prepared with vinegar), Amomi Fructus Rotundus, Trogopterori Faeces (prepared with vinegar), Alpiniae Officinarum Rhizoma, Caryophylli Flos and Cinnamomi Cortex.

Actions and Indications Fortifying the stomach, soothing the liver, directing *qi* movement. It is used for inhibiting acidity, stomach-cold syndrome, chest fullness and gastric upset.

Warning It is contraindicated for pregnant women.

调胃消滞丸

【处方】厚朴（姜汁制）、羌活、神曲、枳壳、香附（制）、半夏（制）、防风、前胡、川芎（酒蒸）、白芷、薄荷、砂仁、草果、木香、豆蔻、茯苓、苍术、广藿香、乌药（醋制）、甘草、紫苏叶、陈皮（蒸）。

【功能主治】健胃消食，解表化湿。用于感冒风寒，发热头痛，消化不良，腹痛泄泻。

Stomach-regulating and Digestion-promoting Pill

Name of Chinese Phonetic Alphabet Tiao Wei Xiao Zhi Wan

Formula Magnoliae Officinalis Cortex (prepared with ginger juice), Notopterygii Rhizoma et Radix, Medicata Massa Fermentata, Aurantii Fructus, Cyperi Rhizoma (prepared), Pinelliae Rhizoma (prepared), Saposhnikoviae Radix, Peucedani Radix, Chuanxiong Rhizoma (steamed by wine), Angelicae Dahuricae Radix, Menthae Haplocalycis Herba, Amomi Fructus, Tsaoko Fructus, Aucklandiae Radix, Amomi Fructus Rotundus, Poria, Atractylodis Rhizoma, Pogostemonis Herba, Linderae Radix (prepared with vinegar), Glycyrrhizae Radix et Rhizoma, Perillae Folium and Citri Reticulatae Pericarpium (steamed).

Actions and Indications Fortifying the stomach and promoting digestion, releasing the exterior and resolving dampness. It is used for common cold of wind-cold type fever, headache, dyspepsia, abdominal pain and diarrhea.

调胃舒肝丸

【处方】砂仁、厚朴（姜炙）、豆蔻、青皮（醋炙）、枳壳（麸炒）、陈皮、山楂（炒）、柴胡（醋炙）、郁金、香附（醋炙）、木香、片姜黄、甘草。

【功能主治】舒肝和胃，解郁止痛。用于脾胃不和，肝郁不舒引起的胃脘刺痛，两胁胀满，嗳气吞酸，饮食无味。

【注意】孕妇忌服。

Liver-stomach-regulating Bolus

Name of Chinese Phonetic Alphabet Tiao Wei Shu Gan Wan

Formula Amomi Fructus, Magnoliae Officinalis Cortex (prepared with ginger), Amomi Fructus Rotundus, Citri Reticulatae Pericarpium Viride (prepared with vinegar), Aurantii Fructus (fried with bran), Citri Reticulatae Pericarpium, Crataegi Fructus (fried), Bupleuri Radix (prepared with vinegar), Curcumae Radix, Cyperi Rhizoma (prepared with vinegar), Aucklandiae Radix, Wenyujin Rhizoma Concisum and Glycyrrhizae Radix et Rhizoma.

Actions and Indications Soothing the liver, harmonizing the stomach, relieving depression and alleviating pain. It is used for stabbing pain in stomach duct, hypochondriac fullness, eructation, acid regurgitation and poor appetite due to disharmony of the spleen and stomach, and depression of the liver.

Warning It is contraindicated for pregnant women.

桑菊银翘散

【处方】桑叶、菊花、金银花、连翘、川贝母、桔梗、薄荷、淡竹叶、荆芥、芦根、牛蒡子、苦杏仁、蝉蜕、僵蚕、滑石、绿豆、淡豆豉、甘草。

【功能主治】辛凉透表，宣肺止咳，清热解毒。用于外感风热，憎寒壮热，头痛咳嗽，咽喉肿痛。

White Mulberry Leaf* and Chrysanthemum** Powder

Name of Chinese Phonetic Alphabet Sang Ju Yin Qiao San

Formula Mori Folium, Chrysanthemi Flos, Lonicerae Japonicae Flos, Forsythiae Fructus, Fritillariae Cirrhosae Bulbus, Platycodonis Radix, Menthae Haplocalycis Herba, Lophatheri Herba,

Schizonepetae Herba, Phragmitis Rhizoma, Arctii Fructus, Armeniacae Semen Amarum, Cicadae Periostracum, Bombyx Batryticatus, Talcum, Phaseoli Radiati Semen, Sojae Semen Praeparatum and Glycyrrhizae Radix et Rhizoma.

Actions and Indications Outthrusting through the exterior, diffusing the lung and relieving cough, clearing heat and detoxicating. It is used for aversion to cold, high fever, headache, cough and sore-throat due to external contraction of wind-heat.

* 桑叶 ** 菊花

桑菊感冒冲剂

【处方】桑叶、菊花、连翘、薄荷、桔梗、苦杏仁、甘草、芦根。

【功能主治】疏风清热，宣肺止咳。用于风热感冒初起，头痛，咳嗽，口干，咽痛。

White Mulberry Leaf* and Chrysanthemum** Soluble Granules for Common Cold

Name of Chinese Phonetic Alphabet Sang Ju Gan Mao Chong Ji

Formula Mori Folium, Chrysanthemi Flos, Forsythiae Fructus, Menthae Haplocalycis Herba, Platycodonis Radix, Armeniacae Semen Amarum, Glycyrrhizae Radix et Rhizoma and Phragmitis Rhizoma.

Actions and Indications Dispersing wind and clearing heat, diffusing the lung and relieving cough. It is indicated for initial stage of common cold (wind-heat) type, marked by headache, cough, dry mouth, sore-throat.

* 桑叶 ** 菊花

桑麻丸

【处方】桑叶、黑芝麻（炒）。

【功能主治】滋养肝肾，祛风明目。用于肝肾不足，头晕眼花，视物不清，迎风流泪。

White Mulberry* Leaf and Black Sesame** Pill

Name of Chinese Phonetic Alphabet Sang Ma Wan

Formula Mori Folium and Sesami Semen Nigrum (fried).

Actions and Indications Enriching the liver and kidney, dispelling wind to improve vision. It is used for dizziness, poor vision, blurred vision, overflow of tear induced by wind due to insufficiency of the liver and kidney.

* 桑 ** 黑芝麻

通天口服液

【处方】川芎、赤芍、天麻、羌活、白芷、细辛、菊花、薄荷等。

【功能主治】活血化瘀、祛风止痛。用于瘀血阻滞、风邪上扰所致的偏头痛发作期。症见头部胀痛或刺痛，痛有定出，反复发作，头晕目眩或恶心呕吐、恶风。

Migraine-relieving Oral Liquid

Name of Chinese Phonetic Alphabet Tong Tian Kou Fu Ye

Formula Chuanxiong Rhizoma, Paeoniae Radix Rubra, Gastrodiae Rhizoma, Notopterygii Rhizoma et Radix, Angelicae Dahuricae Radix, Asari Radix et Rhizoma, Chrysanthemi Flos, Menthae Haplocalycis Herba, etc.

Actions and Indications Activating blood, resolving stasis, dispelling wind, alleviating pain. It is used for attack stage of migraine due to blood-stasis manifested as fixed distending pain or stabbing pain with repeated attack, dizziness, dizzy vision, nausea, vomiting.

通心络胶囊

【处方】人参、水蛭、全蝎、檀香、土鳖虫、蜈蚣、蝉蜕、降香、赤芍、酸枣仁（炒）、冰片、乳香（制）。

【功能主治】益气活血，通络止痛。用于冠心病心绞痛证属心气虚乏、血瘀络阻者。症见胸部憋闷、刺痛、绞痛、气短乏力、心悸自汗、舌质紫暗或有瘀斑、脉细涩或结代。

【注意】出血性疾患，孕妇及妇女经期禁用。

Improving Coronary Heart Disease Capsule

Name of Chinese Phonetic Alphabet Tong Xin Luo Jiao Nang

Formula Ginseng Radix et Rhizoma, Hirudo, Scorpio, Santali Albi Lignum, Eupolyphaga seu Steleophaga, Scorlopendra, Cicadae Periostracum, Dalbergiae Odoriferae Lignum, Paeoniae Radix Rubra, Ziziphi Spinosae Fructus (fried), Borneolum Syntheticum and Olibanum (prepared).

Actions and Indications Tonifying *qi*, activating blood, dredging collaterals, alleviating pain. It is indicated for coronary heart disease and angina pectoris attributed to deficiency of *qi* and blood-stasis, and manifested as chest distress with stabbing pain or colicky pain, shortness of breath, fatigue, palpitation, spontaneous sweating, purple tongue with ecchymosis, fine and rough or bound and intermittent pulse.

Warning It is contraindicated for women during menstrual period, pregnant women and cases with hemorrhagic disease.

通乳冲剂

【处方】黄芪、熟地黄、通草、瞿麦、天花粉、路路通、漏芦、党参、当归、川芎、白芍（酒炒）、王不留行、柴胡、穿山甲（烫）、鹿角霜。

【功能主治】益气养血，通络下乳。用于产后气血亏损，乳少，无乳，乳汁不通。

Promoting Lactogenesis Soluble Granules

Name of Chinese Phonetic Alphabet Tong Ru Chong Ji

Formula Astragali Radix, Rehmanniae Radix Praeparata, Tetrapanacis Medulla, Dianthi Herba, Trichosanthis Radix, Liquidambaris Fructus, Rhapontici Radix, Codonopsis Radix, Angelicae Sinensis Radix, Chuanxiong Rhizoma, Paeoniae Radix Alba (fried with wine), Vaccariae Semen, Bupleuri Radix, Manis Squma (scalded) and Cervi Cornu Degelatinatum.

Actions and Indications Tonifying *qi* and nourishing blood, dredging the collaterals, promoting lactation. It is indicated for oligogalactia and agalactia due to puerperal depletion of *qi* and blood.

通经甘露丸

【处方】当归、桃仁（去皮）、牡丹皮、三棱（麸炒）、牛膝、大黄（酒炒）、莪术（醋炙）、红花、肉桂（去粗皮）、干漆（煅）。

【功能主治】活血祛瘀，通经止痛。用于血瘀阻滞所致的经闭不通，小腹疼痛，或经血量少，拒按及癥瘕积块。

【注意】孕妇忌服。

Amenorrhea-relieving Pill

Name of Chinese Phonetic Alphabet Tong Jing Gan Lu Wan

Formula Angelicae Sinensis Radix, Persicae Semen (removed seed coat), Moutan Cortex. Sparganii Rhizoma (fried with bran), Achyranthis Bidentatae Radix, Rhei Radix et Rhizoma (fried with wine), Curcumae Rhizoma (prepared with vinegar), Carthami Flos, Cinnamomi Cortex (removed rough bark) and Toxicodendri Resina (calcined).

Actions and Indications Activating blood, dispelling stasis, regulating menstruation, alleviating pain. It is used for amenorrhea, pain in lower abdomen, hypomenorrhea, abdominal mass with tenderness due to blood-stasis.

Warning It is contraindicated for pregnant women.

通幽润燥丸

【处方】枳壳（去瓤麸炒）、木香、厚朴（姜炙）、桃仁（去皮）、红花、当归、苦杏仁（去皮炒）、火麻仁、郁李仁、熟地黄、地黄、黄芩、槟榔、熟大黄、大黄、甘草。

【功能主治】清热导滞，润肠通便。用于胃肠积热，幽门失润引起：脘腹胀痛，大便不通。

【注意】孕妇忌服，年老体弱者慎服。

Moistening Intestines Bolus

Name of Chinese Phonetic Alphabet Tong You Run Zao Wan

Formula Aurantii Fructus (removed pulp and fried with bran), Aucklandiae Radix, Magnoliae Officinalis Cortex (prepared with ginger), Persicae Semen (removed seed coat), Carthami Flos, Angelicae Sinensis Radix, Armeniacae Semen Amarum (removed seed coat and fried), Cannabis Fructus, Pruni Semen, Rehmanniae Radix Praeparata, Rehmanniae Radix, Scutellariae Radix, Arecae Semen, Rhei Radix et Rhizoma Praeparata, Rhei Radix et Rhizoma and Glycyrrhizae Radix et Rhizoma.

Actions and Indications Clearing heat and removing food stagnation, moistening the intestines to promote the bowels. It is indicated for abdominal disention and pain, constipation due to accumulated heat in the stomach and intestines, pyloric loss of moistness.

Warning It is contraindicated for pregnant women and should be used carefully for senile debility.

通便灵胶囊

【处方】番泻叶、当归、肉苁蓉。

【功能主治】泻热导滞、润肠通便。用于热结便秘，长期卧床便秘，一时性腹胀便秘，老年习惯性便秘。

Constipation-relieving Capsule

Name of Chinese Phonetic Alphabet Tong Bian Ling Jiao Nang

Formula Sennae Folium, Angelicae Sinensis Radix and Cistanches Caulis Carnosus.

Actions and Indications Purging heat and removing food stagnation, moistening the intestines to promote the bowels. It is indicated for constipation due to heat retention or lying in bed for a long time, occasional abdominal distention, constipation and senile habitual constipation.

通脉冲剂

【处方】丹参、川芎、葛根。

【功能主治】活血通脉。用于缺血性心脑血管疾病，动脉硬化，脑血栓、脑缺血，冠心病，心绞痛。

Relieving Angiocardiopathy and Cerebrovascular Diseases Soluble Granules

Name of Chinese Phonetic Alphabet Tong Mai Chong Ji

Formula Salviae Miltiorrhizae Radix et Rhizoma, Chuanxiong Rhizoma and Puerariae Lobatae Radix.

Actions and Indications Activating blood, dredging the vessels. It is indicated for ischemic angiocardiopathy and cerebrovascular diseases, arteriosclerosis, cerebral thrombosis, cerebral ischemia, coronary heart disease and angina pectoris.

通脉宝膏

【处方】金银花、天花粉、野菊花、当归、蒲公英、赤芍、天葵子、石斛、鸡血藤、玄参、甘草、牛膝、苦地丁、黄芪、黄芩、白术（麸炒）、延胡索（醋炙）。

【功能主治】清热解毒，益气滋阴，活血通络。用于血栓闭塞性脉管炎证属热毒炽盛，热盛伤阴者，及血栓性静脉炎。

【注意】虚寒型患者慎用。忌食无鳞鱼、螃蟹、猪脂油，忌烟、酒。

Thick Paste for Thromboangiitis Obliterans

Name of Chinese Phonetic Alphabet Tong Mai Bao Gao

Formula Lonicerae Japonicae Flos, Trichosanthis Radix, Chrysanthemi Indici Flos, Angelicae Sinensis Radix, Taraxaci Herba, Paeoniae Radix Rubra, Semiaquilegiae Radix, Dendrobii Caulis, Spatholobi Caulis, Scrophulariae Radix, Glycyrrhizae Radix et Rhizoma, Achyranthis Bidentatae Radix, Corydalis Bungeanae Herba, Astragali Radix, Scutellariae Radix, Atractylodis Macrocephalae Rhizoma (fried with bran) and Corydalis Rhizoma (prepared with vinegar).

Actions and Indications Clearing heat, detoxifying, tonifying *qi*, enriching *yin*, activating blood, dredging collaterals. It is indicated for thromboangiitis obliterans due to exuberant heat-toxin and exuberant damaging *yin*; and also used for thrombotic phlebitis.

Warning It should be used cautiously for cases with deficiency-cold type. Nonscale fishes, crab, smoking, wine and lard are prohibited.

通脉降脂片

【处方】笔管草、川芎、荷叶、三七、花椒。

【功能主治】降脂化浊，活血。用于治疗高脂血症，防治动脉粥样硬化。

Hyperlipemia-relieving Tablet

Name of Chinese Phonetic Alphabet Tong Mai Jiang Zhi Pian

Formula Equiseti Debilis Herba, Chuanxiong Rhizoma, Nelumbinis Folium, Notoginseng Radix et Rhizoma and Zanthoxyli Pericarpium.

Actions and Indications Decreasing blood-lipid and resolving turbidity, activating blood. It is indicated for hyperlipemia and preventing atherosclerosis.

通宣理肺口服液

【处方】紫苏叶、前胡、桔梗、苦杏仁、麻黄、甘草、半夏（炙）、茯苓、枳壳、黄芩、陈皮。

【功能主治】解表散寒，宣肺止嗽。用于感冒咳嗽，发热恶寒，鼻塞流涕，头痛无汗，肢体酸痛。

Cough-alleviating Oral Liquid

Name of Chinese Phonetic Alphabet Tong Xuan Li Fei Kou Fu Ye

Formula Perillae Folium, Peucedani Radix, Platycodonis Radix, Armeniacae Semen Amarum, Ephedrae Herba, Glycyrrhizae Radix et Rhizoma, Pinelliae Rhizoma (prepared), Poria, Aurantii Fructus, Scutellariae Radix and Citri Reticulatae Pericarpium.

Actions and Indications Releasing the exterior and dissipating cold, diffusing the lung and alleviating cough. It is indicated for cough due to common cold, marked by fever, aversion to cold; stuffy nose, rhinorrhea, headache, anhidrosis, aching pain of the limbs and body.

通脉养心口服液

【处方】地黄、鸡血藤、麦冬、甘草、制何首乌、阿胶、五味子、党参、龟甲（醋制）、大枣、桂枝。

【功能主治】养心补血，通脉止痛。用于胸痹心痛，心悸怔忡，心绞痛，心律不齐。

Relieving Heart Pain Oral Liquid

Name of Chinese Phonetic Alphabet Tong Mai Yang Xin Kou Fu Ye

Formula Rehmanniae Radix, Spatholobi Caulis, Ophiopogonis Radix, Glycyrrhizae Radix et Rhizoma, Polygoni Multiflori Radix Praeparata, Asini Corii Colla, Schisandrae Chinensis Fructus, Codonopsis Radix, Testudinis Carapax et Plastrum (prepared with vinegar), Jujubae Fructus and Cinnamomi Ramulus.

Actions and Indications Nourishing the heart, tonifying blood, dredging the vessel to alleviate pain. It is used for chest impediment, heart pain, palpitation, fearful throbbing, angina pectoris and arrhythmia.

通络开痹片

【处方】马钱子粉、川牛膝、当归、全蝎等。

【功能主治】祛风通络，活血散结。用于类风湿性关节炎患者的寒热错杂、瘀血阻络证。

Relieving Rheumatoid Arthritis Tablet

Name of Chinese Phonetic Alphabet Tong Luo Kai Bi Pian

Formula Strychni Semen Pulvis, Cyathulae Radix, Angelicae Sinensis Radix, Scorpio, etc.

Actions and Indications Dispelling wind and dredging the collaterals, activating blood and dispersing mass. It is indicated for rheumatoid arthritis due to cold-heat complex, blood-stasis obstructing the collaterals .

通窍耳聋丸

【处方】柴胡、龙胆、芦荟、大黄、黄芩、青黛、天南星（矾炙）、木香、青皮（醋炙）、陈皮、当归、栀子（姜炙）。

【功能主治】清肝泻火，通窍润便。用于肝经热盛，头目眩晕，耳聋蝉鸣，耳部肿痛，目赤口苦，胸膈满闷，大便燥结。

【注意】忌食辛辣。孕妇忌服。

Improving Audition Pill

Name of Chinese Phonetic Alphabet Tong Qiao Er Long Wan

Formula Bupleuri Radix, Gentianae Radix et Rhizoma, Aloe, Rhei Radix et Rhizoma, Scutellariae Radix, Indigo Naturalis, Arisaematis Rhizoma (prepared with alum), Aucklandiae Radix, Citri Reticulatae Pericarpium Viride (prepared with vinegar), Citri Reticulatae Pericarpium, Angelicae Sinensis Radix and Gardeniae Fructus (prepared with ginger).

Actions and Indications Clearing the liver-fire, dredging the orifices and promoting the bowel movement. It is indicated for vertigo, deafness, otalgia, conjunctival congestion, bitter taste in the mouth, hypochondriac fullness and dry stools due to exuberant heat of liver meridian.

Warning Pungent foods should be avoided. It is contraindicated for pregnant women.

通窍镇痛散

【处方】石菖蒲、郁金、荜茇、香附（醋炙）、木香、丁香、檀香、沉香、苏合香、安息香、冰片、乳香。

【功能主治】行气活血，通窍止痛。用于痰瘀痹阻，心胸憋闷疼痛，或中恶气闭，霍乱吐泻。

【注意】孕妇忌服，忌辛辣食物。

Pain-settling Powder

Name of Chinese Phonetic Alphabet Tong Qiao Zhen Tong San

Formula Acori Tatarinowii Rhizoma, Curcumae Radix, Piperis Longi Fructus, Cyperi Rhizoma (prepared with vinegar), Aucklandiae Radix, Caryophylli Flos, Santali Albi Lignum, Aquilariae Lignum Resinatum, Styrax, Benzoinum, Borneolum Synthcticum and Olibanum.

Actions and Indications Moving *qi*, activating blood, dredging orifices, alleviating pain. It is used for chest distress and pain due to stagnation of phlegm; fright due to blockade of *qi*, cholera morbus marked by vomiting and diarrhea.

Warning It is contraindicated for pregnant women. Pungent foods should be avoided.

通痹片

【处方】本品为制马钱子、白花蛇、人参、当归、蜈蚣、制川乌、天麻、全蝎、地龙等药经加工制成的糖衣片。

【功能主治】调补气血，祛风胜湿，活血通络，消肿止痛。用于寒湿阻络，肝肾两虚症，包括风湿性关节炎，类风湿性关节炎。

【注意】孕妇禁用。肝肾功能损害与高血压患者慎用。

Relieving Rheumatic Arthritis Tablet

Name of Chinese Phonetic Alphabet Tong Bi

Pian

Formula Strychni Semen Praeparata, Agkistrodontis, Ginseng Radix et Rhizoma, Angelicae Sinensis Radix, Scolopendra, Aconiti Radix Cocta, Gastrodiae Rhizoma, Scorpio, Pheretima, etc.

Actions and Indications Regulating and tonifying *qi* and blood, dispelling wind and dampness, activating blood and dredging collaterals, dispersing swelling and alleviating pain. It is indicated for rheumatic arthritis and rheumatoid arthritis due to stagnation of cold-damp and dual deficiency of the liver and kidney.

Warning It is contraindicated for pregnant women and should be used carefully for cases with injury of liver and kidney function and hypertension.

通塞脉片

【处方】当归、金银花、党参、玄参、黄芪、牛膝、石斛、甘草。

【功能主治】培补气血，养阴清热，活血化瘀，通经活络。用于血栓闭塞性脉管炎（脱疽）的毒热证。

【注意】属脉管炎阴寒证者慎用。

Relieving Thromboangiitis Obliterans Tablet

Name of Chinese Phonetic Alphabet Tong Sai Mai Pian

Formula Angelicae Sinensis Radix, Lonicerae Japonicae Flos, Codonopsis Radix, Scrophulariae Radix, Astragali Radix, Achyranthis Bidentatae Radix, Dendrobii Caulis and Glycyrrhizae Radix et Rhizoma.

Actions and Indications Tonifying *qi* and blood, nourishing *yin*, clearing heat, activating blood, resolving stasis, dredging meridians and collaterals. It is indicated for thromboangiitis obliterans (digital gangrene) attributed to heat-toxin syndrome.

Warning It should be used cautiously for thromboangiitis obliterans of *yin*-cold syndrome.

十一画

理中丸

【处方】党参、白术（土炒）、甘草（蜜炙）、炮姜。

【功能主治】温中散寒，健胃。用于脾胃虚寒，呕吐泄泻，胸满腹痛，消化不良。

Li Zhong Bolus for Stomach-regulating Pill

Name of Chinese Phonetic Alphabet Li Zhong Wan

Formula Codonopsis Radix, Atractylodis Macrocephalae Rhizoma (fried with earth), Glycyrrhizae Radix et Rhizoma (prepared with honey) and Zingiberis Rhizoma Praeparatum.

Actions and Indications Warming the middle, dissipating cold, fortifying the stomach. It is used for vomiting, diarrhea, chest distress, abdominal pain and indigestion due to dual deficiency-cold of the spleen and stomach.

理气定喘丸

【处方】紫苏子（炒）、紫苏梗、紫苏叶、陈皮、法半夏、茯苓、芥子（炒）、莱菔子（炒）、苦杏仁（炒）、川贝母、桑白皮（蜜炙）、款冬花、紫菀、黄芪（蜜炙）、白术（麸炒）、百合、麦冬、天冬、知母、地黄、当归、何首乌（酒炙）、阿胶（蛤粉炙）。

【功能主治】祛痰止咳，补肺定喘。用于肺虚痰盛引起的咳嗽痰喘，胸膈满闷，心悸气短，口渴咽干。

Relieving Cough and Dyspnea Honeyed Pill

Name of Chinese Phonetic Alphabet Li Qi Ding Chuan Wan

Formula Perillae Fructus (fried), Perillae Caulis, Perillae Folium, Citri Reticulatae Pericarpium, Pinelliae Rhizoma Praeparatum, Poria, Sinapis Semen (fried), Raphani Semen (fried), Armeniacae Semen Amarum (fried), Fritillariae Cirrhosae Bulbus, Mori Cortex (prepared with honey), Farfarae Flos, Asteris Radix et Rhizoma, Astragali Radix (prepared with honey), Atractylodis Macrocephalae Rhizoma (fried with bran), Lilii Bulbus, Ophiopogonis Radix, Asparagi Radix, Anemarrhenae Rhizoma, Rehmanniae Radix, Angelicae Sinensis Radix, Polygoni Multiflori Radix (prepared with wine) and Asini Corii Colla (prepared with clam powder).

Actions and Indications Dispelling phlegm and relieving cough, tonifying the lung and calming dyspnea. It is indicated for cough and dyspnea marked by chest distress, palpitation, shortness of breath, thirst and dry throat due to lung-deficiency and excessive phlegm.

培坤丸

【处方】黄芪（蜜炙）、陈皮、甘草（蜜炙）、白术（炒）、北沙参、茯苓、当归（酒炒）、麦冬、川芎、酸枣仁（炒）、白芍（酒炒）、砂仁、杜仲（炭）、核桃仁、胡芦巴（盐炒）、艾叶（醋炒）、龙眼肉、山茱萸（制）、远志（制）、熟地黄、五味子（蒸）。

【功能主治】补气血，滋肝肾。用于妇女血亏，消化不良，月经不调，赤白带下，小腹冷痛，久不受孕。

【注意】抑郁气滞，内有湿者忌服。

Bolus of Tonifying Blood in Women

Name of Chinese Phonetic Alphabet Pei Kun Wan

Formula Astragali Radix (prepared with honey), Citri Reticulatae Pericarpium, Glycyrrhizae Radix et Rhizoma (prepared with honey), Atractylodis Macrocephalae Rhizoma (fried), Glehniae Radix, Poria, Angelicae Sinensis Radix (fried with wine), Ophiopogonis Radix, Chuanxiong Rhizoma, Ziziphi Spinosae Semen (fried), Paeoniae Radix Alba (fried with wine), Amomi Fructus, Eucommiae Cortex (carbonated), Juglandis Semen , Trigonellae Semen (fried with salt), Artemisiae Argyi Folium (fried with vinegar), Longan Arillus, Corni Fructus (prepared), Polygalae Radix (prepared), Rehmanniae Radix Praeparata and Schiandrae Chinensis Fructus (steamed).

Actions and Indications Tonifying *qi* and blood, enriching the liver and kidney. It is indicated for blood depletion in women, indigestion, irregular menstruation, red and white vaginal discharge, cold-pain in the lower abdomen and sterility.

Warning It is contraindicated for cases with *qi*-stagnation and internal dampness.

梅花点舌胶囊

【处方】牛黄、珍珠、麝香、蟾酥（制）、熊胆、雄黄、朱砂、硼砂、葶苈子、乳香（制）、没药（制）、血竭、沉香、冰片。

【功能主治】清热解毒，消肿止痛。用于疔疮痈肿初起，咽喉牙龈肿痛，口舌生疮。

【注意】孕妇忌服。

Relieving Abscess and Aphthae Capsule

Name of Chinese Phonetic Alphabet Mei Hua Dian She Jiao Nang

Formula Bovis Calculus, Margarita, Moschus, Bufonis Venenum (prepared), Ursi Fel, Realgar, Cinnabaris, Borax, Lepidii Semen, Olibanum (prepared), Myrrha (prepared), Draconis Sanguis, Aquilariae Lignum Resinatum and Borneolum Syntheticum.

Actions and Indications Clearing heat and detoxicating, dispersing swelling and relieving pain. It is indicated for initial stage of deep-rooted boil and abscess, sore-throat, gingivitis, aphthae.

Warning It is contraindicated for pregnant women.

萃仙丸

【处方】莲须、续断、韭菜子（盐炒）、沙苑子（炒）、五味子、覆盆子（盐炒）、制何首乌、补骨脂（盐炒）、核桃仁、茯苓、鱼鳔（制）、人参、枸杞子、莲子（炒）、牡蛎（煅）、鹿茸、芡实（炒）、山药、金樱子。

【功能主治】补肾固精，益气健脾。用于肾虚精亏，阳痿早泄，体弱乏力，腰膝酸软。

Emission-arresting Pill

Name of Chinese Phonetic Alphabet Cui Xian Wan

Formula Nelumbinis Stamen, Dipsaci Radix, Allii Tuberosi Semen, (fried with salt), Astragali Complanati Semen (fried), Schiandrae Chinensis Fructus, Rubi Fructus (fried with salt), Polygoni Multiflori Radix Praeparata, Psoraleae Fructus (fried with salt), Juglandis Semen, Poria, Piscis Colla (prepared), Ginseng Radix et Rhizoma, Lycii Fructus, Nelumbinis Semen (fried), Ostreae Concha (calcined), Cervi Cornu Pantotrichum, Euryales Semen (fried), Dioscoreae Rhizoma and Rosae Laevigatae Fructus.

Actions and Indications Tonifying the kidney, arresting emission, fortifying the spleen and tonifying *qi*. It is used for impotence, ejaculatio praecox, physical debility, fatigue, soreness and weakness of the waist and knees due to deficiency of the kidney and depletion of essence.

黄氏响声丸

【处方】胖大海、大黄、蝉蜕、川芎、诃子、桔梗、甘草、薄荷、方儿茶、连翘、川贝母、薄荷脑。

【功能主治】利咽开音，清热化痰，消肿止痛。用于喉部急、慢性炎症引起的声音嘶哑，对早期声带小结、缩小声带息肉也有一定疗效。

【注意】胃寒便溏者慎用。外感风寒、风热引起的嘶哑禁用。

Huangshi Xiangsheng Pill for Relieving Hoarseness

Name of Chinese Phonetic Alphabet Huang Shi Xiang Sheng Wan

Formula Sterculiae Lychnophorae Semen, Rhei Radix et Rhizoma, Cicadae Periostracum, Chuanxiong Rhizoma, Chebulae Fructus, Platycodonis Radix, Glycyrrhizae Radix et Rhizoma, Menthae Haplocalycis Herba, Catechu Extractum, Forsythiae Fructus, Fritillaria Cirrhosae Bulbus, and Menthol.

Actions and Indications Soothing the throat and improving hoarseness, clearing heat and resolving phlegm, dispersing swelling, alleviating pain. It is indicated for hoarseness due to acute, chronic inflammation of the throat, It also acts certain curative effect on early stage of vocal nodules, reducing polyp of vocal cord.

Warning It should be used carefully for cases with stomach-cold, sloppy stool. It is contraindicated for cases with hoarseness due to exogenous wind-cold or wind-heat.

黄杨宁片

【处方】本品为黄杨科植物小叶黄杨及其同属植物经提取加工制成的片剂。

【功能主治】行气活血，通络止痛。用于气滞血瘀所致的胸痹心痛，脉象结代及冠心病、心律失常见上述证候者。

【注意】服用初期出现的轻度四肢麻木感，头昏，胃肠道不适，可在短期内自行消失。

Chinese Box* Tablet

Name of Chinese Phonetic Alphabet Huang Yang Ning Pian

Formula Buxi Sinicae Ramulus Extractum or the plants of same genus.

Actions and Indications Moving *qi*, activating blood, dredging collaterals, alleviating pain. It is used for chest impediment, cardialgia, bound and intermittent pulse due to *qi*-stagnation and blood-stasis; coronary heart disease and arrhythmia with the above mentioned symptoms.

Warning Mild numbness of limbs, vertigo, gastrointestinal disturbance occur at the initial stage of medication but the symptoms may disappear in a short period.

* 黄杨

黄芪生脉饮

【处方】黄芪、党参、麦冬、五味子。

【功能主治】益气滋阴，养心补肺。用于气阴两虚，心悸气短的冠心病患者。

Milkvetch* Liquid for Coronary Heart Disease

Name of Chinese Phonetic Alphabet Huang Qi Sheng Mai Yin

Formula Astragali Radix, Codonopsis Radix, Ophiopogonis Radix and Schisandrae Chinensis Fructus.

Actions and Indications Tonifying *qi* and enriching *yin*, tonifying the heart and lung. It is used for coronary heart disease marked by palpitation, shortness of breath due to dual deficiency of *qi* and *yin*.

* 黄芪

黄芪健胃膏

【处方】黄芪、白芍、桂枝、生姜、甘草、大枣。

【功能主治】补气温中，止痛。用于脾胃虚寒，腹痛拘急，心悸自汗，并用于胃、十二指肠溃疡病，胃肠功能紊乱。

【注意】舌红苔黄，消化道出血时忌用。

Milkvetch* Soft Extract for Fortifying Stomach

Name of Chinese Phonetic Alphabet Huang Qi Jian Wei Gao

Formula Astragali Radix, Paeoniae Radix Alba, Cinnamomi Ramulus, Zingiberis Rhizoma Recens, Glycyrrhizae Radix et Rhizoma and Jujubae Fructus.

Actions and Indications Tonifying *qi* and warming the middle, relieving pain. It is indicated for abdominal pain and spasm, palpitation and spontaneous sweating, also for gastric and duodenal ulcer, gastrointestinal disorder due to dual deficiency-cold of the spleen and stomach.

Warning It is contraindicated for hemorrhage of the digestive tract and red tongue with yellow fur.

* 黄芪

黄芪精

【处方】本品为黄芪制成的口服液。

【功能主治】益气补血，固本止汗。用于气虚血亏，表虚自汗，四肢乏力，精神不足或久病衰弱，脾胃不壮。

Oral Liquid of Milkveteh*

Name of Chinese Phonetic Alphabet Huang Qi Jing

Formula Astragali Radix.

Actions and Indications Tonifying *qi* and blood, securing the body resistance to arrest sweating. It is used for spontaneous sweating, weakness of limbs, lassitude of spirit and hypofunction of the spleen and stomach due to dual deficiency of *qi* and blood.

* 黄芪

黄连上清片

【处方】黄连、大黄、连翘、薄荷、旋覆花、黄芩、荆芥穗、栀子、防风、石膏、桔梗、黄柏、蔓荆子（炒）、白芷、甘草、川芎、菊花。

【功能主治】清热通便，散风止痛。用于头晕目眩，暴发火眼，牙齿疼痛，口舌生疮，咽喉肿痛，耳痛耳鸣，大便秘结，小便短赤。

【注意】禁食辛辣物，孕妇忌服。

Golden Thread* Tablet for Clearing Heat

Name of Chinese Phonetic Alphabet Huang Lian Shang Qing Pian

Formula Coptidis Rhizoma, Rhei Radix et Rhizoma, Forsythiae Fructus, Menthae Haplocalycis Herba, Inulae Flos, Scutellariae Radix, Schizonepetae Spica, Gardeniae Fructus, Saposhnikoviae Radix, Gypsum Fibrosum, Platycodonis Radix, Phellodendri Chinensis Cortex, Viticis Fructus (fried), Angelicae

Dahuricae Radix, Glycyrrhizae Radix et Rhizoma, Chuanxiong Rhizoma and Chrysanthemi Flos.

Actions and Indications Clearing heat and relaxing the bowels, dissipating wind and relieving pain. It is used for dizziness, dizzy vision, sudden conjunctivitis, toothache, aphthae, sore-throat, ear pain, tinnitus, constipation, scanty and dark urine.

Warning Pungent foods are prohibited and it is contraindicated for pregnant women.

* 黄连

黄连羊肝丸

【处方】黄连、胡黄连、黄芩、黄柏、龙胆、柴胡、青皮（醋炒）、木贼、密蒙花、茺蔚子、决明子（炒）、石决明（煅）、夜明砂、鲜羊肝。

【功能主治】泻火明目。用于肝火旺盛，目赤肿痛，视物昏暗，羞明流泪，胬肉攀睛。

Golden Thread* and Goat Liver** Bolus

Name of Chinese Phonetic Alphabet Huang Lian Yang Gan Wan

Formula Coptidis Rhizoma, Picrorhizae Rhizoma, Scutellariae Radix, Phellodendri Chinensis Cortex, Gentianae Radix et Rhizoma, Bupleuri Radix, Citri Reticulatae Pericarpium Viride (fried with vinegar), Equiseti Hiemalis Herba, Buddlejae Flos, Leonuri Fructus, Cassiae Semen (fried), Haliotidis Concha (calcined), Vespertilionis Faeces and Caprinus Jecur.

Actions and Indications Purging fire and improving vision. It is indicated for conjunctival congestion, blurred vision, photophobia, lacrimation and pterygium due to intense liver-fire.

* 黄连 ** 羊肝

黄连胶囊

【处方】黄连。

【功能主治】清热燥湿，泻火解毒。用于湿热痞满，呕吐，泻痢，黄疸，高热神昏，心火亢盛，心烦不寐、吐衄，目赤吞酸，牙痛，消渴，痈肿疔疮。

Golden Thread* Capsule for Relieving Dysentery

Name of Chinese Phonetic Alphabet Huang Lian Jiao Nang

Formula Coptidis Rhizoma.

Actions and Indications Clearing heat and drying dampness, purging fire and detoxicating. It is indicated for vomiting, dysentery, jaundice, high fever and loss of consciousness, hyperactive heart-fire, vexation and insomnia, hematemesis, red eye, acid regurgitation, toothache, waisting-thirst, abscess and furuncle.

* 黄连

黄栀花口服液

【处方】黄芩、金银花、大黄、栀子。

【功能主治】清肺泻热。用于小儿外感热证，症见发热、头痛、咽痛、心烦、口渴、大便干结、小便短赤；小儿急性上呼吸道感染见有上述证候者。

Baical Skullcap* Jasmin** and Honeysuckle Flower*** Oral Liquid

Name of Chinese Phonetic Alphabet Huang Zhi Hua Kou Fu Ye

Formula Scutellariae Radix, Lonicerae Japonicae Flos, Rhei Radix et Rhizoma and Gardeniae Fructus.

Actions and Indications Clearing and purging lung-heat. It is used for infantile heat-syndrome with external contraction, manifested as fever, headache, sore-throat, vexation, thirst, hard bound stool, scanty and dark urine, and infantile acute upper respiratory tract infection with the above mentioned symptoms.

* 黄芩 ** 栀子 *** 金银花

黄疸肝炎丸

【处方】竹叶、柴胡、青叶胆、茵陈、白芍（酒炙）、栀子（炒）、郁金（醋炙）、延胡索（醋炙）、枳壳（麸炒）、槟榔、香附（醋炙）、青皮、佛手、甘草。

【功能主治】舒肝利胆，除湿理气。用于湿热熏蒸，皮肤黄染，胸胁胀痛，小便短赤，急性肝炎，胆囊炎。

【注意】肝硬化及虚寒者忌用。

Relieving Icterohepatitis Bolus

Name of Chinese Phonetic Alphabet Huang Dan Gan Yan Wan

Formula Phyllostachydis Henonis Folium, Bupleuri Radix, Swertiae Mileensis Herba, Artemisiae Scopariae Herba, Paeoniae Radix Alba (prepared with wine), Gardeniae Fructus (fried), Curcumae Radix (prepared with vinegar), Corydalis Rhizoma (prepared with vinegar), Aurantii Fructus (fired with bran), Arecae Semen, Cyperi Rhizoma (prepared with vinegar), Citri Reticularae Pericarpium Viride, Citri Sarcodactylis Fructus and Glycyrrhizae Radix et Rhizoma.

Actions and Indications Soothing the liver and draining bile, dispelling dampness and regulating *qi*. It is indicated for yellow skin, chest and hypochondriac distention and pain, scanty dark urine, acute hepatitis and cholecystitis due to damp-heat.

Warning It is contraindicated for cases with cirrhosis and deficiency-cold.

雪山金罗汉止痛涂膜剂

【处方】铁棒锤、麝香、西红花、雪莲花、冰片、五灵脂等。

【功能主治】活血、消肿、止痛。用于急、慢性扭伤挫伤，风湿性关节炎，痛风，肩周炎，骨质增生所致的肢体关节疼痛肿胀，以及神经性疼痛。

Jin Luo Han Pain-alleviating Pigmentum

Name of Chinese Phonetic Alphabet Xue Shan Jin Luo Han Zhi Tong Tu Mo Ji

Formula Aconiti Penduli Radix, Moschus, Croci Stigma, Saussureae Herba cum Flos, Borneolum Syntheticum, Trogopterori Faeces, etc.

Actions and Indications Activating blood, reducing swelling, alleviating pain. It is used for acute, chronic traumatic sprain, contusion, rheumatic arthritis, gout; scapulohumeral periarthritis, arthralgia and neuralgia due to hyperosteogeny.

排石冲剂

【处方】金钱草、车前子（盐水炒）、关木通、徐长卿、石韦、瞿麦、忍冬藤、滑石、苘麻子、甘草。

【功能主治】清热利水，通淋排石。用于输尿管结石，膀胱结石属湿热证者。

Lithagogue Soluble Granules

Name of Chinese Phonetic Alphabet Pai Shi Chong Ji

Formula Lysimachiae Herba, Plantaginis Semen (fried with salt water), Aristolochiae Manshuriensis Caulis, Cynanchi Paniculati Radix et Rhizoma, Pyrrosiae Folium, Dianthi Herba, Lonicerae Japonicae Caulis, Talcum, Abutili Semen and Glycyrrhizae Radix et Rhizoma.

Actions and Indications Clearing heat and inducing diuresis, relieving strangury to remove stone. It is indicated for ureterolith, vesical calculus attributive to damp-heat syndrome.

接骨七厘片

【处方】乳香（炒）、血竭、土鳖虫、硼砂、骨碎补（烫）、没药（炒）、当归、自然铜（煅）、大黄（酒炒）。

【功能主治】活血化瘀，接骨止痛。用于跌打损伤，续筋接骨，血瘀疼痛。

【注意】孕妇忌服。

Qi Li Tablet for Bone-knitting

Name of Chinese Phonetic Alphabet Jie Gu Qi Li Pian

Formula Olibanum (fried), Draconis Sanguis, Eupolyphaga seu Steleophaga, Borax, Drynariae Rhizoma (scalded), Myrrha (fried), Angelicae Sinensis Radix, Pyritum (calcined) and Rhei Radix et Rhizoma (fried with wine).

Actions and Indications Activating blood, resolving stasis, knitting bone, alleviating pain. It is used for traumatic injury, fracture.

Warning It is contraindicated for pregnant women.

接骨丸

【处方】甜瓜子、土鳖虫、马钱子粉、郁金、骨碎补、续断、桂枝（炒）、地龙（广地龙）、自然铜（煅醋淬）。

【功能主治】活血散瘀，消肿止痛。用于跌打损伤，青紫肿痛，闪腰岔气，筋断骨折，瘀血作痛。

【注意】不能多服久服。孕妇忌服。

Bone-knitting Pill

Name of Chinese Phonetic Alphabet Jie Gu Wan

Formula Melo Semen, Eupolyphaga seu Steleophaga, Strychni Semen Pulvis, Curcumae Radix, Drynariae Rhizoma, Dipsaci Radix, Cinnamomi Ramulus (fried), Pheretima and Pyritum (calcined and quenched by vinegar).

Actions and Indications Activating blood, dissipating stasis, reducing swelling, alleviating pain. It is used for traumatic injury, sudden lumbar sprain, fracture with blood-stasis and pain.

Warning It is contraindicated for pregnant women. Long-term medication is prohibited.

救急散

【处方】天南星（矾炙）、僵蚕（麸炒）、白附子（矾炙）、天竺黄、天麻、荆芥穗、薄荷、牛蒡子（炒）、陈皮、木香、黄芩、黄连、大黄、莲子心、玄参、西河柳、滑石、雄黄、麝香、冰片、牛黄、朱砂。

【功能主治】解表清热，镇惊化痰。用于内热食滞，外感风寒引起的身热口渴，咳嗽痰盛，咽喉肿痛，惊风抽搐，夜卧不安，隐疹不出。

Relieving Exogenous Wind-cold Powder

Name of Chinese Phonetic Alphabet Jiu Ji San

Formula Arisaematis Rhizoma (prepared with alum), Bombyx Batryticatus (fried with bran), Typhonii Rhizoma (prepared with alum), Bambusae Concretio Silicea, Gastrodiae Rhizoma, Schizonepetae Spica, Menthae Haplocalycis Herba, Arctii Fructus(fried), Citri Reticulatae Pericarpium, Aucklandiae Radix, Scutellariae Radix, Coptidis Rhizoma,Rhei Radix et Rhizoma, Nelumbinis Plumula,Scrophulariae Radix, Tamaricis Cacumen, Talcum, Realgar, Moschus, Borneolum Synthetcum, Bovis Calculus and Cinnabaris.

Actions and Indications Releasing the exterior, clearing heat, settling fright and resolving phlegm. It is used for dyspepsia due to internal heat; generalized fever, thirst, productive cough, sore-throat, convulsion, spasm, disturbed sleep and latent urticaria due to exogenous wind-cold.

虚寒胃痛冲剂

【处方】黄芪（炙）、甘草（炙）、桂枝、党参、白芍、高良姜、大枣、干姜。

【功能主治】温胃止痛，健脾益气。用于脾虚胃弱，胃脘隐痛，喜温喜按，空腹痛重，十二指肠球部溃疡，慢性萎缩性胃炎。

Relieving Stomachache Soluble Granules

Name of Chinese Phonetic Alphabet Xu Han Wei Tong Chong Ji

Formula Astragali Radix (prepared), Glycyrrhizae Radix et Rhizoma (prepared), Cinnamomi Ramulus, Codonopsis Radix, Paeoniae Radix Alba, Alpiniae Officinarum Rhizoma, Jujubae Fructus and Zingiberis Rhizoma.

Actions and Indications Warming the stomach and relieving pain, fortifying the spleen and enriching *qi*. It is indicated for hypofunction of the spleen and stomach, dull pain of the stomach duct, like of warmth and pressing, severity during fasting, duodenal bulbar ulcer, chronic atrophic gastritis.

蛇胆川贝枇杷膏

【处方】蛇胆汁、川贝母、枇杷叶、桔梗、半夏、薄荷脑。

【功能主治】润肺止咳，祛痰定喘。用于外感风热引起的咳嗽痰多、胸闷、气喘。

Forest Cobra Bile★ Sichuan Fritillary★★ and Loquat Leaf ★★★Soft Extract

Name of Chinese Phonetic Alphabet She Dan Chuan Bei Pi Pa Gao

Formula Naja Bilis, Fritillariae Cirrhosae Bulbus, Eriobotryae Folium, Platycodonis Radix, Pinelliae Rhizoma and Menthol.

Actions and Indications Moistening the lung and relieving cough, dispelling phlegm and calming dyspnea. It is indicated for cough with profuse phlegm, chest distress and dyspnea due to external contraction of wind-heat.

* 蛇胆汁 ** 川贝母 *** 枇杷叶

蛇胆川贝胶囊

【处方】蛇胆汁、川贝母。

【功能主治】清肺，止咳，除痰。用于肺热咳嗽，痰多。

Forest Cobra Bile★ and Sichuan Fritillary★★ Capsule

Name of Chinese Phonetic Alphabet She Dan Chuan Bei Jiao Nang

Formula Naja Bilis and Fritillariae Cirrhosae Bulbus.

Actions and Indications Clearing lung-heat, relieving cough and eliminating phlegm. It is indicated for productive cough due to lung-heat.

* 蛇胆汁 ** 川贝母

蛇胆陈皮散

【处方】蛇胆汁、陈皮（蒸）。

【功能主治】顺气化痰，祛风健胃。用于风寒咳嗽，痰多呕逆。

Powder of Forest Cobra Bile★ and Mandarin Orange Peel★★

Name of Chinese Phonetic Alphabet She Dan Chen Pi San

Formula Naja Bilis and Citri Reticulatae Pericarpium (steamed).

Actions and Indications Directing *qi* downward to resolve phlegm, dispelling wind and fortifying the stomach. It is indicated for cough, hiccup with profuse phlegm due to wind-cold.

* 蛇胆汁 ** 陈皮

蛇胆追风丸

【处方】蛇胆汁、地龙（制）、川芎（酒蒸）、桂枝、白芍、独活、防风、僵蚕、胆南星、当归（酒蒸）、白附子（制）、甘草、姜半夏、荆芥、制草乌、制川乌、化橘红。

【功能主治】舒筋活络，散风化痰。用于筋骨软弱，风湿骨痛，手足麻木。

【注意】孕妇禁服。

Pill of Forest Cobra Bile★ for Relieving Ostealgia

Name of Chinese Phonetic Alphabet She Dan Zhui Feng Wan

Formula Naja Bilis, Pheretima (prepared), Chuanxiong Rhizoma (steamed by wine), Cinnamomi Ramulus, Paeoniae Radix Alba, Angelicae Pubescentis Radix, Saposhnikoviae Radix, Bombyx Batryticatus, Arisaema cum Bile, Angelicae Sinensis Radix (steamed by wine), Typhonii Rhizoma (prepared), Glycyrrhizae Radix et Rhizoma, Pinelliae Rhizoma Praeparatum cum Zingibere et Alumine, Schizonepetae Herba, Aconiti Kusnezoffii Radix Cocta, Aconiti Radix Cocta and Citri

Grandis Exocarpium.

Actions and Indications Relaxing sinews and activating collaterals, dissipating wind and resolving phlegm. It is indicated for wilting of sinews and bone, rheumatic ostealgia and numbness of the hands and feet.

Warning It is contraindicated for pregnant women.

* 蛇胆汁

婴儿素

【处方】白扁豆（炒）、山药、鸡内金（炒）、白术（炒）、川贝母、木香（炒）、碳酸氢钠、牛黄。

【功能主治】健脾，消食，止泻。用于消化不良，乳食不进，腹痛腹泻。

Digestion-relieving Powder for Infant

Name of Chinese Phonetic Alphabet Ying Er Su

Formula Lablab Semen Album (fried), Dioscoreae Rhizoma, Galli Gigerii Endothelium Corneum (fried), Atractylodis Macrocephalae Rhizoma (fried), Fritillariae Cirrhosae Bulbus, Aucklandiae Radix (fried), Sodium Bicarbonate and Bovis Calculus.

Actions and Indications Fortifying the spleen, promoting digestion, relieving diarrhea. It is used for dyspepsia, refusing milk and foods feeding, abdominal pain and diarrhea in infants.

银屑冲剂

【处方】土茯苓、菝葜。

【功能主治】祛风解毒。用于银屑病。

Glabrous Greenbrier* Soluble Granules for Psoriasis

Name of Chinese Phonetic Alphabet Yin Xie Chong Ji

Formula Smilacis Glabrae Rhizoma and Smilacis Chinae Rhizoma.

Actions and Indications Dispelling wind and detoxicating. It is indicated for psoriasis.

* 土茯苓

银屑灵

【处方】苦参、甘草、白鲜皮、防风、土茯苓、蝉蜕、金银花、黄柏、赤芍、连翘、生地黄、当归。

【功能主治】清热解毒，祛风燥湿，活血化瘀。用于银屑病。

【注意】忌食刺激性食物，孕妇慎用。

Relieving Psoriasis Pill

Name of Chinese Phonetic Alphabet Yin Xie Ling

Formula Sophorae Flavescentis Radix, Glycyrrhizae Radix et Rhizoma, Dictamni Cortex, Saposhnikoviae Radix, Smilacis Glabrae Rhizoma, Cicadae Periostracum, Lonicerae Japonicae Flos, Phellodendri Chinensis Cortex, Paeoniae Radix Rubra, Forsythiae Fructus, Rehmanniae Radix and Angelicae Sinensis Radix.

Actions and Indications Clearing heat and detoxicating, dispelling wind and drying dampness, activating blood and resolving stasis. It is indicated for psoriasis.

Warning Irritative foods are prohibited and it should be used carefully for pregnant women.

银杏露

【处方】白果、葶苈。

【功能主治】镇咳、化痰、定喘。用于急慢性支气管炎，排痰不爽，久咳气喘。

Gingkgo* Oral Liquid for Relieving Bronchitis

Name of Chinese Phonetic Alphabet Yin Xing Lu

Formula Ginkgo Semen and Rorippae Indicae Herba seu Flos.

Actions and Indications Settling cough, resolving phlegm and calming dyspnea. It is indicated for acute, chronic bronchitis, difficult expectoration, chronic cough and dyspnea.

* 白果

银黄冲剂

【处方】金银花提取物、黄芩提取物。

【功能主治】清热，解毒，消炎。用于急、慢性扁桃体炎，急慢性咽喉炎，上呼吸道感染。

Honeysuckle Flower* and Baical Skullcap** Soluble Granules

Name of Chinese Phonetic Alphabet Yin Huang Chong Ji

Formula Lonicerae Japonicae Flos (extract) and Scutellariae Radix (extract) .

Actions and Indications Clearing heat, detoxicating, counteracting inflammation. It is indicated for acute and chronic tonsillitis, acute and chronic laryngopharyngitis, upper respiratory tract infection.

* 金银花 ** 黄芩

银翘伤风胶囊

【处方】金银花、连翘、牛蒡子、桔梗、芦根、薄荷、淡豆豉、甘草、淡竹叶、荆芥、牛黄。

【功能主治】辛凉解表，清热解毒。用于外感风热，温病初起，发热恶寒，高热口渴，头痛目赤，咽喉肿痛。

Honeysuckle Flower* and Weeping Forsythia** Capsule for Relieving Common Cold

Name of Chinese Phonetic Alphabet Yin Qiao Shang Feng Jiao Nang

Formula Lonicerae Japonicae Flos, Forsythiae Fructus, Arctii Fructus, Platycodonis Radix, Phragmitis Rhizoma, Menthae Haplocalycis Herba, Sojae Semen Praeparatum, Glycyrrhizae Radix et Rhizoma, Lophatheri Herba, Schizonepetae Herba and Bovis Calculus.

Actions and Indications Releasing the exterior, clearing heat and detoxicating. It is indicated for external contraction of wind-heat and initial stage of warm disease marked by aversion to cold with fever, high fever and thirst, headache and conjunctival congestion, sore-throat.

* 金银花 ** 连翘

银翘解毒片

【处方】金银花、连翘、薄荷、荆芥、淡豆豉、桔梗、牛蒡子（炒）、淡竹叶、甘草。

【功能主治】辛凉解表，清热解毒。用于风热感冒，发热头痛，咳嗽，口干，咽喉疼痛。

Honeysuckle Flower* and Weeping Forsythia** Detoxicating Tablet

Name of Chinese Phonetic Alphabet Yin Qiao Jie Du Pian

Formula Lonicerae Japonicae Flos, Forsythiae Fructus, Menthae Haplocalycis Herba, Schizonepetae Herba, Sojae Semen Praeparatum, Platycodonis Radix, Arctii Fructus (fried), Lophatheri Herba and Glycyrrhizae Radix et Rhizoma.

Actions and Indications Releasing the exterior, clearing heat and detoxicating. It is indicated for wind-heat common cold, marked by fever, headache, cough, dry mouth, sore-throat.

* 金银花 ** 连翘

银蒲解毒片

【处方】金银花、蒲公英、野菊花、紫花地丁、夏枯草。

【功能主治】清热解毒。用于风热型急性咽炎，症见咽痛、充血，咽干或具灼热感，舌苔薄黄；湿热型肾盂肾炎，症见尿频短急，灼热疼痛，头身疼痛，小腹坠胀，肾区叩击痛。

Honeysuckle Flower* and Dandelion** Tablet

Name of Chinese Phonetic Alphabet Yin Pu Jie Du Pian

Formula Lonicerae Japonicae Flos, Taraxaci Herba, Chrysanthemi Indici Flos, Violae Herba and Prunellae Spica.

Actions and Indications Clearing heat and detoxicating. It is indicated for acute pharyngitis of wind-heat type, manifested as sore-throat, congestion, dry throat that may be scorching hot, thin and yellow tongue fur; pyelonephritis of damp-heat type, manifested as urinary frequency, urinary urgency, causalgia, headache and general pain, bearing-down fullness in the lower abdomen, percussion pain in the renal region.

* 金银花 ** 蒲公英

甜梦胶囊

【处方】刺五加、黄精、蚕蛾、桑椹、党参、黄芪、砂仁、枸杞子、山楂、熟地黄、淫羊藿（制）、陈皮、茯苓、马钱子（制）、法半夏、泽泻、山药。

【功能主治】益气补肾，健脾和胃，养心安神。用于肾气不足，气血亏虚引起的头昏耳鸣，视减听衰，失眠健忘，食欲不振，腰膝酸软，心慌气短，中风后遗症；对脑功能减退，冠状血管疾患，脑血管栓塞及脱发也有一定作用。

Sweet Dream Capsule

Name of Chinese Phonetic Alphabet Tian Meng Jiao Nang

Formula Acanthopanacis Senticosi Radix et Rhizoma seu Caulis, Polygonati Rhizoma, Bombycis Imagine Masculi, Mori Fructus, Codonopsis Radix, Astragali Radix, Amomi Fructus, Lycii Fructus, Crataegi Fructus, Rehmanniae Radix Praeparata, Epimedii Folium (prepared), Citri Reticulatae Pericapium, Poria, Strychni Semen (prepared), Pinelliae Rhizoma Praeparatum, Alismatis Rhizoma and Dioscoreae Rhizoma.

Actions and Indications Tonifying *qi* and the kidney, fortifying the spleen, harmonizing the stomach, nourishing the heart and tranquilizing the mind. It is used for dizziness, tinnitus, hypopsia, hypoacusis, insomnia, amnesia, poor appetite,soreness and weakness of the waist and knees, fluster, shortness of breath and sequela of apoplexy due to insufficiency of kidney-*qi* and dual deficiency of *qi* and blood. It also possesses certain curative effect for anencephaloneuria, coronary vessel disease, cerebral embolism and alopecia.

偏瘫复原丸

【处方】黄芪、人参、当归、川芎、赤芍、熟地黄、丹参、三七、牛膝、天麻、僵蚕（炒）、全蝎、钩藤、白附子（矾炙）、秦艽、地龙、威灵仙、防风、杜仲（炭）、补骨脂（盐炙）、骨碎补、香附（醋炙）、沉香、肉桂、豆蔻、茯苓、泽泻、桂枝、白术（炒）、枳壳（炒）、麦冬、法半夏、安息香、甘草、冰片。

【功能主治】补气活血，祛风化痰。用于气虚血瘀，风痰阻络引起的中风瘫痪，半身不遂，口眼歪斜，言语不清，足膝浮肿，行步艰难，筋骨疼痛，手足拘挛。

Hemiparalysis-recovering Bolus

Name of Chinese Phonetic Alphabet Pian Tan Fu Yuan Wan

Formula Astragali Radix, Ginseng Radix et Rhizoma, Angelicae Sinensis Radix, Chuanxiong Rhizoma, Paeoniae Radix Rubra, Rehmanniae Radix Praeparata, Salviae Miltiorrhizae Radix et Rhizoma, Notoginseng Radix et Rhizoma, Achyranthis Bidentatae Radix, Gastrodiae Rhizoma, Bombyx Batryticatus (fried), Scorpio, Uncariae Ramulus cum Uncis, Typhonii Rhizoma (prepared with alum), Gentianae Macrophyllae Radix, Pheretima, Clematidis Radix et Rhizoma, Saposhnikoviae Radix, Eucommiae Cortex (carbonated), Psoraleae Fructus (prepared with salt), Drynariae Rhizoma, Cyperi Rhizoma (prepared with vinegar), Aquilariae Lignum Resinatum, Cinnamomi Cortex, Amomi Fructus Rotundus, Poria, Alismatis

Rhizoma, Cinnamomi Ramulus, Atractylodis Macrocephalae Rhizoma (fried), Aurantii Fructus (fried), Ophiopogonis Radix, Pinelliae Rhizoma Praeparatum, Benzoinum, Glycyrrhizae Radix et Rhizoma and Borneolum Syntheticum.

Actions and Indications Tonifying *qi*, activating blood, dispelling wind, resolving phlegm. It is used for apoplexy, hemiparalysis, deviated eyes and mouth, alalia, edema of feet, difficult walking, pain of sinews and bone and spasm of limbs due to *qi*-deficiency and blood-stasis and stagnation of wind-phlegm in collaterals.

猪苓多糖注射液

【处方】本品为多孔菌科真菌猪苓提取的猪苓多糖，加氯化钠制成的灭菌水溶液。

【功能主治】调节机体免疫功能，对慢性肝炎、肿瘤病有一定疗效。与抗肿瘤化疗药物合用，可增强疗效，减轻毒副作用。

【注意】本品不可供静脉注射。

Polyporus Polysaccharide* Injection

Name of Chinese Phonetic Alphabet Zhu Ling Duo Tang Zhu She Ye

Formula Polyporus Polysaccharide and Sodium Chloride.

Actions and Indications Regulating immune function of organism. It has certain curative effect for chronic hepatitis and tumor. It is used for enhancement effect and reduction of toxic effects in combination with antineoplastic chemotherapy drugs.

Warning The product should not be used as intravenous injection.

* 猪苓多糖

脚气散

【处方】荆芥穗、白芷、枯矾。

【功能主治】祛风燥湿，杀虫止痒。用于脚癣趾间糜烂，刺痒难忍。

Tinea Pedis Relieving Powder

Name of Chinese Phonetic Alphabet Jiao Qi San

Formula Schizonepetae Spica, Angelicae Dahuricae Radix and Alumen Usta.

Actions and Indications Dispelling wind, drying dampness, killing worm, relieving pruritus. It is used for interphalangeal erosion due to tinea pedis with stabbing itching.

康尔心胶囊

【处方】三七、人参、麦冬、丹参、枸杞子、何首乌、山楂。

【功能主治】益气活血，滋阴补肾，增加冠脉血流量，降血脂。用于治疗冠心病，心绞痛，胸闷气短。

Relieving Coronary Heart Disease Capsule

Name of Chinese Phonetic Alphabet Kang Er Xin Jiao Nang

Formula Notoginseng Radix et Rhizoma, Ginseng Radix et Rhizoma, Ophiopogonis Radix, Salviae Miltiorrhizae Radix et Rhizoma, Lycii Fructus, Polygoni Multiflori Radix and Crataegi Fructus.

Actions and Indications Tonifying *qi*, activating blood, nourishing kidney-*yin*, increasing coronary blood flow, lowering blood-lipid. It is indicated for coronary heart disease, angina pectoris, chest distress and shortness of breath.

康妇消炎栓

【处方】苦参、败酱草、紫花地丁、穿心莲、蒲公英、猪胆粉、紫草、芦荟等。

【功能主治】清热解毒，利湿散结，杀虫止痒。用于湿热所致的腰痛，小腹痛，带下病，阴痒，阴蚀。

Relieving Gynecological Inflammation Suppository

Name of Chinese Phonetic Alphabet Kang Fu Xiao Yan Shuan

Formula Sophorae Flavescentis Radix, Patriniae Herba, Violae Heaba, Andrographis Herba, Taraxaci Herba, Suillus Bilis Pulvis, Arnebiae Radix, Aloe, etc.

Actions and Indications Clearing heat and detoxicating, draining dampness and dispersing mass, killing worms and relieving itching. It is indicated for lumbago, lower abdominal pain, leukorrheal disease and prutitus vulvae due to damp-heat.

鹿角胶

【处方】本品为鹿角经水煎熬、浓缩制成的固体胶。

【功能主治】温补肝肾，益精养血。用于阳痿滑精，腰膝酸冷，虚劳羸瘦，崩漏下血，便血尿血，阴疽肿痛。

Solid of Deerhorn Glue*

Name of Chinese Phonetic Alphabet Lu Jiao Jiao

Formula Cervi Cornus Colla.

Actions and Indications Warming and tonifying the liver and kidney, essence and nourishing blood. It is used for impotence, spermatorrhea, soreness and cold of the waist and knees, consumptive disease, emaciation, metrorrhagia and metrostaxis, hematochezia, hematuria and deep-rooted carbuncle.

* 鹿角胶

鹿茸精注射液

【处方】本品为梅花鹿鹿茸经提取加工制成的灭菌水溶液。

【功能主治】增强肌体活力及促进细胞新陈代谢。用于神经衰弱，食欲不振，营养不良，性功能减退及健忘症。

Pilose Deerhorn* Essence Injection

Name of Chinese Phonetic Alphabet Lu Rong Jing Zhu She Ye

Formula Cervi Cornu Pantotrichum.

Actions and Indications Enhancing the body activity, promoting the cellular metabolism. It is indicated for neurasthenia, poor appetite, malnutrition, sexual hypoesthesia and amnesia.

* 鹿茸

鹿筋壮骨酒

【处方】鹿筋、鹿骨、当归、木瓜、党参、玉竹、黄芪、重楼、虎杖、桂枝、续断、肉桂、红花、枸杞子、秦艽、制川乌、制草乌。

【功能主治】祛风除湿，舒筋活血。用于四肢麻木，风湿性关节炎。

【注意】孕妇及高血压者忌服。

Deer Sinew* Wine for Relieving Rheumatic Arthritis

Name of Chinese Phonetic Alphabet Lu Jin Zhuang Gu Jiu

Formula Cervi Tendo, Cervi Os, Angelicae Sinensis Radix, Chaenomelis Fructus, Codonopsis Radix, Polygonati Odorati Rhizoma, Astragali Radix, Paridis Rhizoma, Polygoni Cuspidati Rhizoma et Radix, Cinnamomi Ramulus, Dipsaci Radix, Cinnamomi Cortex, Carthami Flos, Lycii Fructus, Gentianae Macrophyllae Radix, Aconiti Radix Cocta and Aconiti Kusnezoffii Radix Cocta.

Actions and Indications Dispelling wind and dampness, relaxing sinews and activating blood. It is indicated for numbness of the limbs and rheumatic arthritis.

Warning It is contraindicated for pregnant women and cases with hypertension.

* 鹿筋

麻仁丸

【处方】火麻仁、苦杏仁、大黄、枳实（炒）、厚朴（姜制）、白芍（炒）。

【功能主治】润肠通便。用于肠燥便秘。胶囊更适应于老年人无力性便秘，习惯性便秘，痔疮便秘。

【注意】体虚弱、大病初愈者慎用。

Hemp Fimble* Bolus

Name of Chinese Phonetic Alphabet Ma Ren Wan

Formula Cannabis Fructus, Armeniacae Semen Amarum, Rhei Radix et Rhizoma, Aurantii Fructus Immaturus (fried), Magnoliae Officinalis Cortex (prepared with ginger) and Paeoniae Radix Alba (fried).

Actions and Indications Moistening the intestines to relax the bowels. It is indicated for constipation due to intestinal dryness.The capsule is more suitable for senile atonic constipation, habitual constipation and hemorrhoidal constipation.

Warning It should be used carefully for cases with debility and cases who just recovered.

* 火麻仁

麻仁润肠丸

【处方】火麻仁、苦杏仁（去皮炒）、大黄、木香、陈皮、白芍。

【功能主治】润肠通便。用于肠胃积热，胸腹胀满，大便秘结。

【注意】孕妇忌服。

Hemp Fimble* Intestines-moistening Bolus

Name of Chinese Phonetic Alphabet Ma Ren Run Chang Wan

Formula Cannabis Fructus, Armeniacae Semen Amarum (removed seed coat and fried), Rhei Radix et Rhizoma, Aucklandiae Radix, Citri Reticulatae Pericarpium and Paeoniae Radix Alba.

Actions and Indications Moistening the intestines to relax the bowels. It is indicated for accumulated heat in the stomach and intestines, thoracic and abdominal distention, constipation.

Warning It is contraindicated for pregnant women.

* 火麻仁

麻仁滋脾丸

【处方】大黄（制）、火麻仁、当归、厚朴（姜制）、苦杏仁（炒）、枳实（麸炒）、郁李仁、白芍。

【功能主治】润肠通便，健胃消食。用于胸腹胀痛，大便不通，饮食无味，烦躁不宁。

【注意】孕妇遵医嘱服用。

Hemp Fimble* Bolus for Moistening Intestines

Name of Chinese Phonetic Alphabet Ma Ren Zi Pi Wan

Formula Rhei Radix et Rhizoma (prepared), Cannabis Fructus, Angelicae Sinensis Radix, Magnoliae Officinalis Cortex (prepared with ginger), Armeniacae Semen Amarum (fried), Aurantii Fructus Immaturus (fried with bran), Pruni Semen and Paeoniae Radix Alba.

Actions and Indications Moistening the intestines to relax the bowels, invigorating the stomach and promoting digestion. It is indicated for abdominal fullness and pain, constipation, poor appetite, vexation.

Warning Pregnant women should follow the physician's advice.

* 火麻仁

痔宁片

【处方】地榆（炒炭）、侧柏叶（炒炭）、地黄、槐角、白芍（酒制）、荆芥（炒炭）、当归、黄芩、枳壳、刺猬皮（制）、乌梅、甘草。

【功能主治】清热凉血，润燥疏风。用于实热内结或湿热瘀滞所致痔疮出血、肿痛。

【注意】孕妇慎用。

Relieving Hemorrhoidal Bleeding Tablet

Name of Chinese Phonetic Alphabet Zhi Ning Pian

Formula Sanguisorbae Radix (carbonated), Platycladi Cacumen (carbonated), Rehmanniae Radix, Sophorae Fructus, Paeoniae Radix Alba (prepared with wine), Schizonepetae Herba (carbonated), Angelicae Sinensis Radix, Scutellariae Radix, Aurantii Fructus, Erinacei Corium (prepared), Mume Fructus and Glycyrrhizae Radix et Rhizoma.

Actions and Indications Clearing heat and cooling blood, moistening dryness and dispelling wind. It is indicated for bleeding, swelling and pain of hemorrhoid due to excess heat binding interior, or stagnation of damp-heat.

Warning It should be used carefully for pregnant women.

痔疮片

【处方】大黄、蒺藜、功劳木、白芷、冰片、猪胆汁。

【功能主治】清热解毒，凉血止痛，祛风消肿。用于各种痔疮，肛裂，大便秘结。

Relieving Hemorrhoid Tablet

Name of Chinese Phonetic Alphabet Zhi Chuang Pian

Formula Rhei Radix et Rhizoma, Tribuli Fructus, Mahoniae Caulis, Angelicae Dahuricae Radix, Borneolum Syntheticum and Suillus Bilis.

Actions and Indications Clearing heat and detoxicating, cooling blood and alleviating pain, dispelling wind and dispersing swelling. It is indicated for various hemorrhoids, anal fissure and constipation.

痔疮栓

【处方】柿蒂、大黄、冰片、芒硝、田螺壳（炒）、橄榄核（炒炭）。

【功能主治】清热通便，止血，消肿止痛，收敛固脱。用于各期内痔、混合痔之内痔部分，轻度脱垂。

Suppository for Relieving Hemorrhoid

Name of Chinese Phonetic Alphabet Zhi Chuang Shuan

Formula Kaki Calyx, Rhei Radix et Rhizoma, Borneolum Syntheticum, Natrii Sulfas, Cipangopaludinae Concha (fried), Canarii Albi Semen (carbonated).

Actions and Indications Clearing heat and relaxing the bowels, relieving bleeding, dispersing swelling and alleviating pain, astringing and securing collapse. It is indicated for all periods of internal hemorrhoid, internal hemorrhoid part of mixed hemorrhoid with slight prolapse.

痔特佳片

【处方】当归、黄芩、防风、枳壳（炒）、鞣质、阿胶、地榆炭、槐角（炒）。

【功能主治】清热消肿，凉血止血，收敛。用于一、二期内痔，血栓性外痔，肛窦炎、直肠炎。

Hemorrhoid-relieving Tablet

Name of Chinese Phonetic Alphabet Zhi Te Jia Pian

Formula Angelicae Sinensis Radix, Scutellariae Radix, Saposhnikoviae Radix, Aurantii Fructus (fried) Tannin, Asini Corii Colla, Sanguisorbae Radix Carbonisatus and Sophorae Fructus (fried).

Actions and Indications Clearing heat, reducing swelling, cooling blood, relieving bleeding, astringent. It is used for Ⅰ or Ⅱ stage of internal hemorrhoid, thrombosed external hemorrhoid, anal sinusitis and rectitis.

情安喘定片

【处方】榕树叶、鱼腥草、胡颓子叶、五指毛桃、珍珠层粉、冰片等。

【功能主治】平喘，止咳，祛痰，消炎。用于慢性支气管炎，支气管哮喘。

【注意】甲亢、心律不齐或高血压合并症等心血管疾病患者慎用。

Qing An Tablet for Relieving Chronic Bronchitis

Name of Chinese Phonetic Alphabet Qing An Chuan Ding Pian

Formula Fici Microcarpae Folium, Houttuyniae Herba, Elaeagni Pungentis Folium, Fici Simplicissimae Radix, Margaritae Concha Strati Pulvis, Borneolum Syntheticum, etc.

Actions and Indications Calming dyspnea, relieving cough, dispelling phlegm and antiphlegistic. It is indicated for chronic bronchitis, bronchial asthma.

Warning It should be used carefully for cases with hyperthyroidism, arrhythmia or hypertension complicated with angiocardiopathy.

清开灵注射液

【处方】胆酸、水牛角粉、黄芩提取物、珍珠层粉。

【功能主治】清热解毒，镇痛安神。对于温热病引起的高热不退，烦躁不安，咽喉肿痛，舌红或绛，苔黄，脉数者适宜；多用于湿热型肝炎和上呼吸道感染病。

【注意】久病体虚患者出现腹泻的慎用。

Qingkailing Injection

Name of Chinese Phonetic Alphabet Qing Kai Ling Zhu She Ye

Formula Cholic acid, Bubali Cornu Pulvis, Scutellariae Radix (extract) and Margaritae Concha Strati Pulvis.

Actions and Indications Clearing heat and detoxifying, settling pain, tranquilizing the mind. It is indicated for warm-heat disease marked by unabatement of high fever, agitation, sore-throat, red or crimson tongue with yellow fur and rapid pulse, and is most used for hepatitis of damp-heat type and upper respiratory tract infection.

Warning It should be used carefully for cases with physical debility with diarrhea due to prolonged illness.

清气化痰丸

【处方】黄芩（酒炒）、瓜蒌仁霜、半夏（制）、胆南星、陈皮、苦杏仁、枳实、茯苓。

【功能主治】清肺化痰。用于肺热咳嗽，痰多黄稠，胸脘满闷。

Relieving Cough Pill

Name of Chinese Phonetic Alphabet Qing Qi Hua Tan Wan

Formula Scutellariae Radix (fried with wine), Trichosanthis Semen Pulveratum, Pinelliae Rhizoma (prepared), Arisaema cum Bile, Citri Reticulatae Pericarpium, Armeniacae Semen Amarum, Aurantii Fructus Immaturus and Poria.

Actions and Indications Clearing lung-heat and resolving phlegm. It is indicated for cough due to lung-heat; profuse and yellow thick phlegm, and chest upset.

清火片

【处方】大青叶、大黄、石膏、薄荷脑。

【功能主治】清热泻火，通便。用于咽喉肿痛，牙痛，头目眩晕，口鼻生疮，风火目赤，大便不通。

【注意】无实热者及孕妇慎用。

Fire-purging Tablet

Name of Chinese Phonetic Alphabet Qing Huo Pian

Formula Isatidis Folium, Rhei Radix et Rhizoma, Gypsum Fibrosum and Menthol.

Actions and Indications Clearing heat and purging fire, relaxing the bowels. It is indicated for sore-throat, toothache, vertigo, aphthae, conjunctival congestion, difficult bowel movement.

Warning It should be used carefully for cases

without excess heat and pregnant women.

清火栀麦胶囊

【处方】穿心莲、栀子、麦冬。

【功能主治】清热解毒，凉血消肿。用于咽喉肿痛，发热，牙痛，目赤。

Jasmin* and Lily-turf** Capsule for Relieving Sore-throat

Name of Chinese Phonetic Alphabet Qing Huo Zhi Mai Jiao Nang

Formula Andrographis Herba, Gardeniae Fructus and Ophiopogonis Radix.

Actions and Indications Clearing heat and detoxicating, cooling blood and dispersing swelling. It is used for sore-throat, fever, toothache, conjunctival congestion.

* 栀子 ** 麦冬

清心滚痰丸

【处方】金礞石（煅）、大黄、沉香、黄芩、甘遂（醋炙）、牵牛子、猪牙皂、人参、肉桂、金钱白花蛇（去头晒干）、朱砂粉、牛黄、冰片、羚羊角粉、水牛角浓缩粉、珍珠粉等。

【功能主治】清心涤痰，泻火通便。用于顽痰蒙蔽心窍引起的神智错乱，疯狂，羊痫风症。

【注意】孕妇忌服，体弱者慎服。

Phlegm-removing Pill

Name of Chinese Phonetic Alphabet Qing Xin Gun Tan Wan

Formula Micae Lapis Aureus (calcined), Rhei Radix et Rhizoma, Aquilariae Lignum Resinatum, Scutellariae Radix, Kansui Radix (prepared with vinegar), Pharbitidis Semen, Gleditsiae Fructus Abnormalis, Ginseng Radix et Rhizoma, Cinnamomi Cortex, Bungarus Parvus (removed head and dried), Cinnabaris Pulvis, Bovis Calculus, Borneolum Syntheticum, Saigae Tataricae Cornu Pulvis, Bubali Cornu Pulvis Concentratio, Margaritae Pulvis, etc.

Actions and Indications Clearing heart-fire, removing phlegm, purging fire, promoting bowels movement. It is used for mental disorder, mania and epilepsy due to phlegm blocking upper orifices.

Warning It is contraindicated for pregnant women, and should be used cautiously for cases with physical debility.

清宁丸

【处方】大黄、绿豆、车前草、白术（炒）、黑豆、半夏（制）、香附（醋制）、桑叶、桃枝、牛乳、厚朴（姜制）、麦芽、陈皮、侧柏叶。

【功能主治】清热泻火，通便。用于咽喉肿痛，口舌生疮，头晕耳鸣，目赤牙痛，腹中胀满，大便秘结。

【注意】孕妇忌服。

Fire-purging Bolus

Name of Chinese Phonetic Alphabet Qing Ning Wan

Formula Rhei Radix et Rhizoma, Phaseoli Radiati Semen, Plantaginis Herba, Atractylodis Macrocephalae Rhizoma (fried), Sojae Semen Nigrum, Pinelliae Rhizoma (prepared), Cyperi Rhizoma (prepared with vinegar), Mori Folium, Persicae Ramulus, Vaccae Lac, Magnoliae Officinalis Cortex (prepared with ginger), Hordei Fructus Germinatus, Citri Reticulatae Pericarpium and Platycladi Cacumen.

Actions and Indications Clearing heat and purging fire, relaxing the bowels. It is indicated for sore-throat, aphthae, dizziness, tinnitus, conjunctival congestion, toothache, abdominal fullness, constipation.

Warning It is contraindicated for pregnant women.

清血内消丸

【处方】金银花、连翘、拳参、大黄、蒲公英、黄芩、黄柏、关木通、玄明粉、赤芍、桔梗、瞿麦玄参、薄荷、雄黄、甘草、栀子（姜炙）、乳香（醋炙）、没药（醋炙）。

【功能主治】清热祛湿，消肿败毒。用于脏腑积热，风湿毒热引起的疮疡初起，红肿，疮疡，憎寒发热，二便不利。

【注意】孕妇忌服。

Clearing Viscera Heat Pill for Relieving Sore

Name of Chinese Phonetic Alphabet Qing Xue Nei Xiao Wan

Formula Lonicerae Japonicae Flos, Forsythiae Fructus, Bistortae Rhizoma, Rhei Radix et Rhizoma, Taraxaci Herba, Scutellariae Radix, Phellodendri Chinensis Cortex, Aristolochiae Manshuriensis Caulis, Natrii Sulfas Exsiccatus, Paeoniae Radix Rubra, Platycodonis Radix, Dianthi Herba, Scrophulariae Radix, Menthae Haplocalycis Herba, Realgar, Glycyrrhizae Radix et Rhizoma, Gardeniae Fructus (prepared with ginger), Olibanum (prepared with vinegar) and Myrrha (prepared with vinegar).

Actions and Indications Clearing heat and dispelling dampness, dispersing swelling and detoxicating. It is used for initial stage of sore and ulcer with red, swelling, aversion to cold, fever, difficulty in urination and defecation due to accumulated heat in the viscera, invasion of wind-damp and heat toxin.

Warning It is contraindicated for pregnant women.

清肝利胆口服液

【处方】茵陈、金银花、栀子、厚朴、防己等。

【功能主治】清利肝胆湿热。主治纳呆、胁痛、疲倦乏力、尿黄、苔腻、脉弦。

Clearing Liver-heat Oral Liquid

Name of Chinese Phonetic Alphabet Qing Gan Li Dan Kou Fu Ye

Formula Artemisiae Scopariae Herba, Lonicerae Japonicae Flos, Gardeniae Fructus, Magnoliae Officinalis Cortex, Stephaniae Tetrandrae Radix, etc.

Actions and Indications Clearing and draining damp-heat in the liver and gallbladder. It is indicated for loss of appetite, hypochondriac pain, tiredness, fatigue, yellow urine, greasy tongue fur, string-like pulse.

清肝降压胶囊

【处方】夏枯草、何首乌（制）、槐花（炒）、桑寄生、丹参、葛根（煨）、泽泻（盐炒）、小蓟、远志（去心）、川牛膝。

【功能主治】清热平肝，补益肝肾。用于高血压病肝火亢盛、肝肾阴虚证，症见眩晕、头痛、面红目赤、急躁易怒、口干口苦、腰膝酸软、心悸不寐、耳鸣健忘、便秘溲黄。

【注意】孕妇慎服。

Clearing Liver-fire and Lowering Blood Pressure Capsule

Name of Chinese Phonetic Alphabet Qing Gan Jiang Ya Jiao Nang

Formula Prunellae Spica, Polygoni Multiflori Radix Praeparata, Sophorae Flos (fried), Taxilli Herba, Salviae Miltiorrhizae Radix et Rhizoma, Puerariae Lobatae Radix (stewed), Alismatis Rhizoma (prepared with salt), Cirsii Herba, Polygalae Radix (removed core) and Cyathulae Radix.

Actions and Indications Clearing heat, pacifying the liver, tonifying the liver and kidney. It is used for hypertension due to hyperactivity of liver-fire, dual *yin*-deficiency of the liver and kidney, and manifested as vertigo, headache, flushed face, conjunctival congestion, vexation, dry and bitter taste in the mouth, soreness and weakness of the waist and knees, palpitation, insomnia, tinnitus, amnesia, constipation, yellow urine.

Warning It should be used cautiously for pregnant women.

清肺化痰丸

【处方】胆南星（砂炒）、苦杏仁、法半夏（砂炒）、枳壳（炒）、黄芩（酒炙）、川贝母、麻黄（炙）、桔梗、白苏子、瓜蒌子、陈皮、莱菔子（炒）、款冬花（炙）、茯苓、甘草。

【功能主治】降气化痰，止咳平喘。用于肺热咳嗽，痰多作喘，痰涎壅盛，肺气不畅。

Relieving Cough Honeyed Bolus

Name of Chinese Phonetic Alphabet Qing Fei Hua Tan Wan

Formula Arisaema cum Bile (fried with sand), Armeniacae Semen Amarum, Pinelliae Rhizoma Praeparatum (fried with sand), Aurantii Fructus (fried), Scutellariae Radix (prepared with wine), Fritillariae Cirrhosae Bulbus, Ephedrae Herba (prepared), Platycodonis Radix, Perillae Frutescentis Fructus, Trichosanthis Semen, Citri Reticulatae Pericarpium, Raphani Semen (fried), Farfarae Flos (prepared), Poria and Glycyrrhizae Radix et Rhizoma.

Actions and Indications Directing *qi* downward to resolve phlegm, suppressing cough and dyspnea. It is indicated for cough due to lung-heat; dyspnea due to profuse phlegm and lung-*qi* failing to diffuse.

清肺抑火丸

【处方】黄芩、栀子、知母、浙贝母、黄柏、苦参、桔梗、前胡、天花粉、大黄。

【功能主治】清肺止咳，化痰通便。用于肺热咳嗽，痰黄黏稠，口干咽痛，大便干燥。

【注意】孕妇慎用。

Cough-suppressing Pill

Name of Chinese Phonetic Alphabet Qing Fei Yi Huo Wan

Formula Scutellariae Radix, Gardeniae Fructus, Anemarrhenae Rhizoma, Fritillariae Thunbergii Bulbus, Phellodendri Chinensis Cortex, Sophorae Flavescentis Radix, Platycodonis Radix, Peucedani Radix, Trichosanthis Radix and Rhei Radix et Rhizoma.

Actions and Indications Clearing lung-heat and relieving cough, resolving phlegm and promoting bowels movement. It is indicated for cough due to lung-heat, marked by yellow, thick and sticky phlegm, dry mouth and sore-throat, dry stools.

Warning It should be used carefully for pregnant women.

清肺消炎丸

【处方】本品为麻黄、石膏、地龙、牛蒡子、葶苈子、人工牛黄、苦杏仁（炒）、羚羊角等药经加工制成的丸剂。

【功能主治】清肺化痰，止咳平喘。用于上呼吸道感染，急性支气管炎和慢性支气管炎的急性发作，以及肺部感染引起的咳嗽痰稠、喘息气急属热象者。

【注意】心功能不全者慎用。

Relieving Upper Respiratory Tract Infection Pill

Name of Chinese Phonetic Alphabet Qing Fei Xiao Yan Wan

Formula Ephedrae Herba, Gypsum Fibrosum, Pheretima, Arctii Fructus, Lepidii Semen, Bovis Calculus Artifactus, Armeniacae Semen Amarum (fried), Saigae Tataricae Cornu, etc.

Actions and Indications Clearing lung-heat and resolving phlegm, suppressing cough and dyspnea. It is indicated for upper respiratory tract infection, acute bronchitis and acute attack of chronic bronchitis, and cough with thick phlegm and shortness of breath due to lung infection attributive to heat syndrome.

Warning It should be used carefully for cases with cardiac insufficiency.

清泻丸

【处方】大黄、黄芩、枳实、甘草、朱砂。

【功能主治】清热，通便，消滞。用于肠热、积滞、便秘。

Heat-clearing and Purgation Bolus

Name of Chinese Phonetic Alphabet Qing Xie Wan

Formula Rhei Radix et Rhizoma, Scutellariae Radix, Aurantii Fructus Immaturus, Glycyrrhizae Radix et Rhizoma and Cinnabaris.

Actions and Indications Clearing heat, relaxing the bowels, removing food stagnation. It is used for intestinal heat, food stagnation and constipation.

清咽利膈丸

【处方】射干、连翘、栀子、黄芩、大黄、牛蒡子（炒）、薄荷、天花粉、玄参、荆芥穗、防风、桔梗、甘草。

【功能主治】清热利咽，消肿止痛。用于外感时毒，脏腑积热，咽喉肿痛，面赤，痰涎壅盛，口苦舌干，大便秘结，小便黄赤。

【注意】忌食辛辣食物。

Seasonal Toxin Expelling Pill

Name of Chinese Phonetic Alphabet Qing Yan Li Ge Wan

Formula Belamcandae Rhizoma, Forsythiae Fructus, Gardeniae Fructus, Scutellariae Radix, Rhei Radix et Rhizoma, Arctii Fructus (fired), Menthae Haplocalycis Herba, Trichosanthis Radix, Scrophulariae Radix, Schizonepetae Spica, Saposhnikoviae Radix, Platycodonis Radix and Glycyrrhizae Radix et Rhizoma.

Actions and Indications Clearing heat and soothing the throat, dispersing swelling and relieving pain. It is used for sore-throat, flushed complexion, profuse phlegm, bitter taste in the mouth, dry tongue, constipation, yellow and dark urine due to exogenous seasonal toxin and accumulation of heat in the viscera.

Warning Pungent foods should be avoided.

清咽润喉丸

【处方】射干、山豆根、桔梗、僵蚕（麸炒）、栀子（姜炙）、牡丹皮、青果、金果榄、麦冬、玄参、知母、地黄、白芍、浙贝母、甘草、冰片、水牛角、浓缩粉。

【功能主治】清热利咽，消肿止痛。用于风热内壅，肺胃热盛，口渴心烦，咳嗽多痰，咽喉肿痛，失声声哑。

【注意】忌食辛辣食物。

Throat-soothing Honeyed Pill

Name of Chinese Phonetic Alphabet Qing Yan Run Hou Wan

Formula Belamcandae Rhizoma, Sophorae Tonkinensis Radix et Rhizoma, Platycodonis Radix, Bombyx Batryticatus (fried with bran), Gardeniae Fructus (prepared with ginger), Moutan Cortex, Canarii Fructus, Tinosporae Radix, Ophiopogonis Radix, Scrophulariae Radix, Anemarrhenae Rhizoma, Rehmanniae Radix, Paeoniae Radix Alba, Fritillariae Thunbergii Bulbus, Glycyrrhizae Radix et Rhizoma, Borneolum Syntheticum and Bubali Cornu Pulvis Concentratio.

Actions and Indications Clearing heat and soothing the throat, dispersing swelling and relieving pain. It is used for thirst, vexation, productive cough, sore-throat and hoarseness due to wind-heat accumulation and exuberant heat of the lung and stomach.

Warning Pungent foods should be avoided.

清咽滴丸

【处方】青黛、甘草、诃子、薄荷脑、冰片、人工牛黄、聚乙二醇。

【功能主治】疏风清热，解毒利咽。用于风热喉痹，咽痛，咽干、口渴；或微恶风、发热，咽部红肿，舌边尖红，苔薄白或薄黄，脉浮数或滑数，适于急性咽炎见上述证候者。

【注意】孕妇慎用。

Soothing Throat Dripping Pill

Name of Chinese Phonetic Alphabet Qing Yan Di Wan

Formula Indigo Naturalis, Glycyrrhizae Radix et Rhizoma, Chebulae Fructus, Menthol, Borneolum Syntheticum, Bovis Calculus Artifactus and Polyethylene glycol.

Actions and Indications Dispersing wind and clearing heat, detoxicating and soothing the throat. It is used for sore-throat, marked by dry throat, thirst, or slight aversion to cold, fever, pharyngitis, red tip and margin of the tongue, thin and white or thin and yellow tongue fur, floating and rapid pulse or slippery and rapid pulse, also used for acute pharyngitis with the above mentioned symptoms.

Warning It should be used cautiously for pregnant women.

清胃保安丸

【处方】白术（麸炒）、六神曲（麸炒）、陈皮、茯苓、砂仁、青皮（醋炙）、厚朴（姜炙）、麦芽（炒）、甘草、槟榔、枳壳（去瓤麸炒）、枳实、酒曲、山楂（炒）。

【功能主治】消食，和胃止呕。用于小儿停食停乳，肚腹胀满，呕吐，心烦，口渴，不思饮食。

Harmonizing Stomach Pill for Infant

Name of Chinese Phonetic Alphabet Qing Wei Bao An Wan

Formula Atractylodis Macrocephalae Rhizoma (fried with bran), Medicata Massa Fermentata (fried with bran), Citri Reticulatae Pericarpium, Poria, Amomi Fructus, Citri Reticulatae Pericarpium Viride (prepared with vinegar), Magnoliae Officinalis Cortex (prepared with ginger), Hordei Fructus Germinatus (fried), Glycyrrhizae Radix et Rhizoma, Arecae Semen, Aurantii Fructus (removed pulp and fried with bran), Aurantii Fructus Immaturus, Vine-fermentum and Crataegi Fructus (fried).

Actions and Indications Promoting digestion, harmonizing the stomach and relieving vomiting. It is used for stagnant food or milk, abdominal distention and fullness, vomiting, vexation, thirst and anorexia in infant.

清胃黄连丸

【处方】黄连、石膏、桔梗、甘草、知母、玄参、地黄、牡丹皮、天花粉、连翘、栀子、黄柏、黄芩、赤芍。

【功能主治】清胃泻火，解毒消肿。用于口舌生疮，齿龈、咽喉肿痛。

【注意】孕妇慎用。

Golden Thread* Pill for Clearing Stomach-fire

Name of Chinese Phonetic Alphabet Qing Wei Huang Lian Wan

Formula Coptidis Rhizoma, Gypsum Fibrosum, Platycodonis Radix, Glycyrrhizae Radix et Rhizoma, Anemarrhenae Rhizoma, Scrophulariae Radix, Rehmanniae Radix, Moutan Cortex, Trichosanthis Radix, Forsythiae Fructus, Gardeniae Fructus, Phellodendri Chinensis Cortex, Scutellariae Radix and Paeoniae Radix Rubra.

Actions and Indications Clearing stomach-fire, detoxicating and dispersing swelling. It is used for aphthae, gingivitis, sore-throat.

Warning It should be used cautiously for pregnant women.

*黄连

清音丸

【处方】桔梗、寒水石、薄荷、诃子、甘草、乌梅、青黛、硼砂（煅）、冰片。

【功能主治】清音，利咽。用于肺热、胃热，口干舌燥，声哑失声。

【注意】忌烟、酒及辛辣之物。风寒音哑者忌用。

Voice-improving Bolus

Name of Chinese Phonetic Alphabet Qing Yin Wan

Formula Platycodonis Radix, Gypsum Rubrum, Menthae Haplocalycis Herba, Chebulae Fructus, Glycyrrhizae Radix et Rhizoma, Mume Fructus, Indigo Naturalis, Borax (calcined) and Borneolum Syntheticum.

Actions and Indications Improving voice, soothing the throat. It is used for dry mouth and tongue, hoarseness and aphonia due to lung-heat and stomach-heat.

Warning Smoking, drinking and pungent foods should be avoided. It is contraindicated for aphonia of wind-cold type.

清宫寿桃丸

【处方】驴肾、鹿肾、狗肾、枸杞子、人参、天冬、麦冬、地黄、当归。

【功能主治】补肾生精，益元强壮。用于肾虚衰老所致头昏疲倦，记忆力衰退，腰膝酸软，耳鸣，眼花流泪，夜尿多，尿有余沥等症。

【注意】阴虚火旺者不宜服用。

Tonifying Senile Source-*qi* Pill

Name of Chinese Phonetic Alphabet Qing Gong Shou Tao Wan

Formula Asini Ren, Cervi Testis et Penis, Canis Ren, Lycii Fructus, Ginseng Radix et Rhizoma, Asparagi Radix, Ophiopogonis Radix, Rehmanniae Radix and Angelicae Sinensis Radix.

Actions and Indications Tonifying the kidney and essence, enriching source-*qi*. It is used for dizziness, tiredness, hypomnesis, soreness and weakness of the waist and knees, tinnitus, lacrimation and frequent urination at night with dripping urination due to deficiency of the kidney in the aged.

Warning It is contraindicated for cases with *yin*-deficiency with effulgent fire.

清热化湿口服液

【处方】黄芩、法半夏、滑石、青蒿、淡豆豉、射干等。

【功能主治】清热利湿，化痰止咳。用于儿童急性支气管炎。症见发热，咳嗽，痰液黏稠，兼见呕恶纳呆，便溏不爽，溲黄，舌红苔腻。

Alleviating Children Acute Bronchitis Oral Liquid

Name of Chinese Phonetic Alphabet Qing Re Hua Shi Kou Fu Ye

Formula Scutellariae Radix, Pinelliae Rhizoma Praeparatum, Talcum, Artemisiae Annuae Herba, Sojae Semen Praeparatum, Belamcandae Rhizoma, etc.

Actions and Indications Clearing heat and draining dampness, resolving phlegm and relieving cough. It is indicated for children acute bronchitis, manifested as fever, cough, sticky and thick phlegm, accompanied with vomiting, nausea anorexia, sloppy stool, yellow urine, red tongue and greasy fur.

清热灵冲剂

【处方】黄芩、连翘、大青叶、甘草。

【功能主治】清热解毒。用于感冒发热，咽喉肿痛。

Heat-clearing Soluble Granules

Name of Chinese Phonetic Alphabet Qing Re Ling Chong Ji

Formula Scutellariae Radix, Forsythiae Fructus, Isatidis Folium and Glycyrrhizae Radix et Rhizoma.

Actions and Indications Clearing heat and detoxicating. It is used for common cold, fever, sore-throat.

清热明目茶

【处方】决明子（炒）、菊花、甜叶菊。

【功能主治】清热祛风，平肝明目。用于高血压、头眩、头痛、目赤目昏。

Improving Vision Tea

Name of Chinese Phonetic Alphabet Qing Re Ming Mu Cha

Formula Cassiae Semen (fried), Chrysanthemi Flos and Steviae Rebaudinae Folium.

Actions and Indications Clearing heat and dispelling wind, pacifying the liver and improving vision. It is indicated for hypertension, vertigo, headache, conjunctival congestion, blurring of vision.

清热消炎宁胶囊

【处方】本品为九节茶经加工制成的胶囊。

【功能主治】清热解毒，消炎止痛，舒筋活络。用于流行性感冒，咽喉炎，肺炎，菌痢，急性胃肠炎，阑尾炎，烧伤，疮疡脓肿，蜂窝织炎。

Glabrous Sarcandra* Capsule for Clearing Heat

Name of Chinese Phonetic Alphabet Qing Re Xiao Yan Ning Jiao Nang

Formula Sarcandrae Herba.

Actions and Indications Clearing heat and detoxicating, counteracting inflammation, relieving pain, relaxing the sinews and activating the collaterals. It is indicated for influenza, laryngopharyngitis, pneumonia, bacillary dysentery, acute gastroenteritis, appendicitis, burn, sore and abscess, cellulitis.

* 九节茶

清热银花糖浆

【处方】金银花、菊花、白茅根、通草、大枣、甘草、绿茶叶。

【功能主治】清热解毒，通利小便。用于温邪头痛，目赤口渴，湿热郁滞，小便不利。

Syrup of Honeysuckle Flower* for Clearing Heat

Name of Chinese Phonetic Alphabet Qing Re Yin Hua Tang Jiang

Formula Lonicerae Japonicae Flos, Chrysanthemi Flos, Imperatae Rhizoma, Tetrapanacis Medulla, Jujubae Fructus, Glycyrrhizae Radix et Rhizoma and Camelliae Sinensis Folium Gemmae.

Actions and Indications Clearing heat and detoxicating, inducing diuresis. It is used for headache, conjunctival congestion, thirst, and oliguria due to stagnation of damp-heat.

* 金银花

清热散结片

【处方】本品为千里光浸膏片。

【功能主治】清炎解毒，散结止痛。用于急性结膜炎，急性咽喉炎，急性扁桃体炎，急性肠炎，急性菌痢，上呼吸道炎，急性支气管炎，淋巴结炎，疮疖疼痛，中耳炎，皮炎湿疹。

Tablet for Clearing Heat and Dissipating Stasis

Name of Chinese Phonetic Alphabet Qing Re San Jie Pian

Formula Senecionis Scandentis Extractum.

Actions and Indications Antiphlogistic and detoxicating, dissipating mass and relieving pain. It is indicated for acute conjunctivitis, acute laryngopharyngitis, acute tonsillitis, acute enteritis, acute bacillary dysentery, inflammation of upper respiratory tract, acute bronchitis, lymphadenitis, abscess and deep-rooted boil, otitis media, eczematous dermatitis.

清热暗疮片

【处方】金银花、大黄浸膏、穿心莲浸膏、牛黄、栀子浸膏、珍珠层粉、蒲公英浸膏、甘草、山豆根浸膏。

【功能主治】清热解毒，凉血散瘀，泻火通腑。用于治疗痤疮，疖痈。

【注意】孕妇慎用。

Clearing Heat and Acne-eliminating Tablet

Name of Chinese Phonetic Alphabet Qing Re An Chuang Pian

Formula Lonicerae Japonicae Flos, Rhei Extractum, Andrographis Extractum, Bovis Calculus, Gardeniae Extractum, Margaritae Concha Strati Pulvis, Taraxaci Extractum, Glycyrrhizae Radix et Rhizoma and Sophorae Tonkinensis Extractum.

Actions and Indications Clearing heat and detoxicating, cooling blood and removing blood-stasis, purging fire and activating the viscera. It is used for acne, furuncle and carbuncle.

Warning It should be used cautiously for pregnant women.

清热解毒片

【处方】生石膏、金银花、玄参、地黄、连翘、栀子、甜地丁、黄芩、龙胆、板蓝根、知母、麦冬。

【功能主治】清热解毒。用于治疗流感，上呼吸道感染及各种发热性疾病。

Influenza-relieving Tablet

Name of Chinese Phonetic Alphabet Qing Re Jie Du Pian

Formula Gypsum Fibrosum, Lonicerae Japonicae Flos, Scrophulariae Radix, Rehmanniae Radix, Forsythiae Fructus, Gardeniae Fructus, Gueldenstaedtiae Multiflorae Herba, Scutellariae Radix, Gentianae Radix et Rhizoma, Isatidis Radix, Anemarrhenae Rhizoma and Ophiopogonis Radix.

Actions and Indications Clearing heat and detoxicating. It is used for influenza, upper respiratory tract infection and febrile diseases.

清热镇咳糖浆

【处方】葶苈子、矮地茶、鱼腥草、荆芥、知母、前胡、板栗壳、浮海石。

【功能主治】镇咳祛痰。用于感冒咽炎，肺热咳嗽。

Syrup for Settling Cough

Name of Chinese Phonetic Alphabet Qing Re Zhen Ke Tang Jiang

Formula Lepidii Semen, Ardisiae Japonicae Herba, Houttuyniae Herba, Schizonepetae Herba, Anemarrhenae Rhizoma, Peucedani Radix, Cupula Castaneae Mollissimae and Pumex.

Actions and Indications Relieving cough and dispelling phlegm. It is indicated for pharyngitis due to common cold; cough due to lung-heat.

清眩丸

【处方】川芎、白芷、薄荷、荆芥穗、石膏。

【功能主治】散风解热。用于风热头晕目眩，偏正头痛、鼻塞牙痛。

Qing Xuan Bolus

Name of Chinese Phonetic Alphabet Qing Xuan Wan

Formula Chuanxiong Rhizoma, Angelicae Dahuricae Radix, Menthae Haplocalycis Herba, Schizonepetae Spica and Gypsum Fibrosam.

Actions and Indications Dispersing wind, releasing heat. It is used for dizziness and dizzy vision due to wind-heat; migraine and overall headache, nasal congestion, toothache.

清眩治瘫丸

【处方】天麻、蕲蛇（酒炙）、僵蚕、全蝎、地龙、威灵仙、决明子、牛膝、血竭、没药（醋炙）、丹参、川芎、赤芍、香附（醋炙）、桑寄生、玄参、葛根、枳壳（炒）、安息香、郁金、槐角、沉香、人参、骨碎补、茯苓、白术（炒）、麦冬、黄连、黄芩、地黄、法半夏、泽泻、黄芪、水牛角浓缩粉、山楂、冰片、牛黄、白附子（矾炙）、珍珠。

【功能主治】活血降压，化痰息风。用于肝阳上亢，肝火内炽引起的头目眩晕、项强脑胀，胸中闷热，惊恐虚烦，半身不遂，口眼歪斜，痰涎壅盛，言语不清，血压升高。

Hemiparalysis-relieving Bolus

Name of Chinese Phonetic Alphabet Qing Xuan Zhi Tan Wan

Formula Gastrodiae Rhizoma, Agkistrodon (prepared with wine), Bombyx Batryticatus, Scorpio, Pheretima, Clematidis Radix et Rhizoma, Cassiae Semen, Achyranthis Bidentatae Radix, Draconis Sanguis, Myrrha (prepared with vinegar), Salviae

Miltiorrhizae Radix et Rhizoma, Chuanxiong Rhizoma, Paeoniae Radix Rubra, Cyperi Rhizoma (prepared with vinegar), Taxilli Herba, Scrophulariae Radix, Puerariae Lobatae Radix, Aurantii Fructus (fried), Benzoinum, Curcumae Radix, Sophorae Fructus, Aquilariae Lignum Resinatum, Ginseng Radix et Rhizoma, Drynariae Rhizoma, Poria, Atractylodis Macrocephalae Rhizoma (fried), Ophiopogonis Radix, Coptidis Rhizoma, Scutellariae Radix, Rehmanniae Radix, Pinelliae Rhizoma Praeparatum, Alismatis Rhizoma, Astragali Radix, Bubali Cornu Pulvis Concentratio, Crataegi Fructus, Borneolum Syntheticum, Bovis Calculus, Typhonii Rhizoma (prepared with alum) and Margarita.

Actions and Indications Activating blood, lowering blood pressure, resolving phlegm, extinguishing wind. It is used for vertigo, neck rigidity, oppression and feverish sensation in chest, fright, vexation, hemiparalysis, deviated eyes and mouth, alalia, hypertension due to ascendant hyperactivity of liver-*yang* and intense liver fire.

清脑降压胶囊

【处方】黄芩、夏枯草、槐角、磁石（煅）、牛膝、当归、地黄、丹参、水蛭、钩藤、决明子、地龙、珍珠母。

【功能主治】平肝潜阳，清脑降压。用于肝阳上亢，血压偏高，头昏头晕，失眠健忘。

Lowering Blood Pressure Capsule

Name of Chinese Phonetic Alphabet Qing Nao Jiang Ya Jiao Nang

Formula Scutellariae Radix, Prunellae Spica, Sophorae Fructus, Magnetitum (calcined), Achyranthis Bidentatae Radix, Angelicae Sinensis Radix, Rehmanniae Radix, Salviae Miltiorrhizae Radix et Rhizoma, Hirudo, Uncariae Ramulus cum Uncis, Cassiae Semen, Pheretima and Margaritifera Concha.

Actions and Indications Pacifying the liver, subduing *yang*, lowering blood pressure. It is used for high blood pressure tendency, dizziness, insomnia and amnesia due to hyperactivity of liver-*yang*.

清凉眼药膏

【处方】熊胆、冰片、薄荷脑、西瓜霜、硼砂、炉甘石（煅）。

【功能主治】消炎，抑菌，收敛。用于结膜炎，睑缘炎，沙眼，麦粒肿。

Qing Liang Eye Ointment

Name of Chinese Phonetic Alphabet Qing Liang Yan Yao Gao

Formula Ursi Fel, Borneolum Syntheticum, Menthol, Mirabilitum Praeparatum, Borax, and Calamina (calcined).

Actions and Indications Counteracting inflammation, bacteriostasis, astringing. It is indicated for conjunctivitis, blepharitis marginalis, trachoma, hordeolum.

清淋冲剂

【处方】瞿麦、萹蓄、关木通、车前子（盐炒）、滑石、栀子、大黄、甘草（炙）。

【功能主治】清热泻火，利水通淋。用于膀胱湿热，尿频涩痛，淋沥不畅，癃闭不通，小腹胀满，口干咽燥。

【注意】孕妇忌服，体质虚弱者不宜服。

Relieving Strangury Soluble Granules

Name of Chinese Phonetic Alphabet Qing Lin Chong Ji

Formula Dianthi Herba, Polygoni Avicularis Herba, Aristolochiae Manshuriensis Caulis, Plantaginis Semen (fried with salt), Talcum, Gardeniae Fructus, Rhei Radix et Rhizoma and Glycyrrhizae Radix et Rhizoma (prepared).

Actions and Indications Clearing heat and purging fire, inducing diuresis and relieving strangury. It is indicated for frequency of micturition and urodynia, difficult urination, distention and fullness in the lower abdomen, dry mouth and throat due to damp-heat of the bladder.

Warning It is contraindicated for pregnant women and cases with general debility.

清喉利咽颗粒

【处方】黄芩、西青果、桔梗、竹茹、橘红、胖大海、枳壳、桑叶、紫苏子、紫苏梗、沉香、薄荷脑、香附（醋制）。

【功能主治】清热利咽。用于咽喉肿痛，喉核红肿疼痛，咽干口渴，急性咽炎，扁桃体炎及慢性咽炎。

Throat-soothing Granules

Name of Chinese Phonetic Alphabet Qing Hou Li Yan Ke Li

Formula Scutellariae Radix, Chebulae Fructus, Platycodonis Radix, Bambusae Caulis in Taenias, Citri Exocarpium Rubrum, Sterculiae Lychnophorae Semen, Aurantii Fructus, Mori Folium, Perillae Fructus, Perillae Caulis, Aquilariae Lignum Resinatum, Menthol and Cyperi Rhizoma (prepared with vinegar).

Actions and Indications Clearing heat, soothing the throat. It is used for sore-throat, tonsillitis, dry throat, thirst, acute pharyngitis, chronic pharyngitis.

清喉咽合剂

【处方】地黄、麦冬、玄参、连翘、黄芩。

【功能主治】养阴，清咽，解毒。用于局限性的咽白喉，轻度中毒型白喉，急性扁桃体炎，咽峡炎。

Throat-soothing Mixture

Name of Chinese Phonetic Alphabet Qing Hou Yan He Ji

Formula Rehmanniae Radix, Ophiopogonis Radix, Scrophulariae Radix, Forsythiae Fructus and Scutellariae Radix.

Actions and Indications Nourishing *yin*, soothing the throat, detoxifying. It is indicated for localized pharyngeal diphtheria, mild toxic diphtheria, acute tonsillitis and isthmitis.

清暑益气丸

【处方】人参、黄芪（蜜炙）、白术（麸炒）、六神曲（麸炒）、苍术（米泔制）、麦冬、泽泻、五味子（醋炙）、当归、黄柏、葛根、青皮（醋炙）、陈皮、升麻、甘草。

【功能主治】祛暑利湿，补气生津。用于体弱受暑引起的头晕身热，四肢倦怠，自汗心烦，咽干口渴。

Summer-heat-clearing Bolus

Name of Chinese Phonetic Alphabet Qing Shu Yi Qi Wan

Formula Ginseng Radix et Rhizoma, Astragali Radix (prepared with honey), Atractylodis Macrocephalae Rhizoma (fried with bran), Medicata Massa Fermentata (fried with bran), Atractylodis Rhizoma (prepared with rice swilled water), Ophiopogonis Radix, Alismatis Rhizoma, Schisandrae Chinensis Fructus (prepared with vinegar), Angelicae Sinensis Radix, Phellodendri Chinensis Cortex, Puerariae Lobatae Radix, Citri Reticulatae Pericarpium Viride (prepared with vinegar), Citri Reticulatae Pericarpium, Cimicifugae Rhizoma and Glycyrrhizae Radix et Rhizoma.

Actions and Indications Dispelling summer-heat and draining dampness, tonifying *qi* and engendering fluid. It is indicated for dizziness, feverish sensation of the body, tiredness of extremities, spontaneous sweating, vexation, dry throat and thirst due to physical debility and summer-heat stroke.

清暑解毒冲剂

【处方】芦根、薄荷、金银花、甘草、淡竹叶、滑石粉、夏枯草。

【功能主治】清暑解毒，生津止咳，并能防治痱热疖。用于夏季暑热，高温作业。

Relieving Summer-heat Soluble Granules

Name of Chinese Phonetic Alphabet Qing Shu Jie Du Chong Ji

Formula Phragmitis Rhizoma, Menthae Haplocalycis Herba, Lonicerae Japonicae Flos, Glycyrrhizae Radix et Rhizoma, Lophatheri Herba, Talci Pulvis and Prunellae Spica.

Actions and Indications Clearing summer-heat and detoxicating, engendering fluid and relieving cough, preventing miliaria and furuncle. It is used for resisting summer-heat and high temperature operation.

清膈丸

【处方】金银花、连翘、玄参、射干、山豆根、黄连、大黄、龙胆、石膏、玄明粉、桔梗、麦冬、薄荷、地黄、硼砂、甘草、冰片、牛黄、水牛角浓缩粉。

【功能主治】清热利咽，消肿止痛。用于内蕴毒热引起的口渴咽干，咽喉肿痛，声哑失声，面赤，大便燥结。

【注意】孕妇忌服。

Heat-toxin-expelling Bolus

Name of Chinese Phonetic Alphabet Qing Ge Wan

Formula Lonicerae Japonicae Flos, Forsythiae Fructus, Scrophulariae Radix, Belamcandae Rhizoma, Sophorae Tonkinensis Radix et Rhizoma, Coptidis Rhizoma, Rhei Radix et Rhizoma, Gentianae Radix et Rhizoma, Gypsum Fibrosum, Natrii Sulfas Exsiccatus, Platycodonis Radix, Ophiopogonis Radix, Menthae Haplocalycis Herba, Rehmanniae Radix, Borax, Glycyrrhizae Radix et Rhizoma, Borneolum Syntheticum, Bovis Calculus and Bubali Cornu Pulvis Concentratio.

Actions and Indications Clearing heat and soothing the throat, dispersing swelling and relieving pain. It is indicated for thirst, dry throat, sore-throat, hoarseness, flushed complexion and dry stools due to internal accumulation of heat-toxin.

Warning It is contraindicated for pregnant women.

清瘟解毒片

【处方】天花粉、葛根、白芷、桔梗、连翘、玄参、甘草、大青叶、柴胡、羌活、川芎、赤芍、防风、黄芩、牛蒡子、淡竹叶。

【功能主治】清瘟解毒。用于时疫感冒，发热，怕冷，无汗头痛，口渴咽干，四肢酸痛，痄腮。

Clearing Seasonal Pestilence Tablet

Name of Chinese Phonetic Alphabet Qing Wen Jie Du Pian

Formula Trichosanthis Radix, Puerariae Lobatae Radix, Angelicae Dahuricae Radix, Platycodonis Radix, Forsythiae Fructus, Scrophulariae Radix, Glycyrrhizae Radix et Rhizoma, Isatidis Folium, Bupleuri Radix, Notopterygii Rhizoma et Radix, Chuanxiong Rhizoma, Paeoniae Radix Rubra, Saposhnikoviae Radix, Scutellariae Radix, Arctii Fructus and Lophatheri Herba.

Actions and Indications Clearing seasonal pestilence and detoxicating. It is used for seasonal common cold, marked by fever, fear of cold, anhidrosis, headache, thirst, dry throat, aching pain of extremities, mumps.

添精补肾膏

【处方】党参、远志（甘草制）、淫羊藿、黄芪（蜜炙）、茯苓、狗脊、肉苁蓉（酒蒸）、熟地黄、当归、巴戟天（酒制）、杜仲（盐炒）、枸杞子、锁阳（酒蒸）、川牛膝、龟甲胶、鹿角胶。

【功能主治】壮元阳，补精血。用于肾阳亏虚，精血不足引起的腰膝酸软，形寒肢冷，阳痿泄精，神经衰弱。

【注意】伤风感冒忌服。

Oral Thick Paste of Tonifying Kidney

Name of Chinese Phonetic Alphabet Tian Jing Bu Shen Gao

Formula Codonopsis Radix, Polygalae Radix (prepared with licorice root), Epimedii Folium, Astragali Radix (prepared with honey), Poria, Cibotii Rhizoma, Cistanches Caulis Carnosus (steamed by wine), Rehmanniae Radix Praeparata, Angelicae Sinensis Radix, Morindae Officinalis Radix (prepared with wine), Eucommiae Cortex (fried with salt), Lycii Fructus, Cynomorii Caulis Carnosus (steamed by wine), Cyathulae Radix, Testudinis Carapacis et Plastri Colla and Cervi Cornus Colla.

Actions and Indications Strengthening source *yang*, tonifying essence and blood. It is used for soreness and weakness of the waist and knees, cold limbs, impotence, nocturnal emission and neurasthenia due to deficiency of kidney-*yang* and dual deficiency of essence and blood.

Warning It is contraindicated for cases with common cold.

混元丸

【处方】紫河车、人参、黄芪、山药、甘松、益智（盐炒）、远志（甘草炙）、桔梗、茯苓、天竺黄、木香、砂仁、香附（醋炙）、梅花、莪术（醋炙）、牡丹皮、天花粉、滑石、甘草。

【功能主治】健脾，益肾。用于小儿先天不足，后天失调，脾胃虚弱引起的体质软弱，发育不良，面黄肌瘦，饮食少进，遗尿便溏。

Strengthening Children Constitution Pill

Name of Chinese Phonetic Alphabet Hun Yuan Wan

Formula Hominis Placenta, Ginseng Radix et Rhizoma, Astragali Radix, Dioscoreae Rhizoma, Nardostachyos Radix et Rhizoma, Alpineae Oxyphyllae Fructus (fried with salt), Polygalae Radix (prepared with licorice root), Platycodonis Radix, Poria, Bambusae Concretio Silicea, Aucklandiae Radix, Amomi Fructus, Cyperi Rhizoma (prepared with vinegar), Mume Flos, Curcumae Rhizoma (prepared with vinegar), Moutan Cortex, Trichosanthis Radix, Talcum and Glycyrrhizae Radix et Rhizoma.

Actions and Indications Fortifying the spleen and tonifying the kidney. It is used for children debility of constitution, dysplasia, sallow complexion and emaciation, poor appetite, enuresis and sloppy stool due to congenital deficiency, postnatal imbalance and deficiency of the spleen and stomach.

深海龙胶囊

【处方】海龙、海马、鹿茸、羊鞭（砂烫）、蛇床子、淫羊藿、肉苁蓉、五味子、人参、黄芪、大枣、茯苓、砂仁、山药、干姜、附片、当归、熟地黄、天冬、麦冬、枸杞子、桃仁、水蛭、牡丹皮、牛膝、甘草（炙）。

【功能主治】温补肾阳，补髓填精。用于因肾阳不足所致的腰膝酸软、畏寒肢冷、神疲乏力、头晕耳鸣、心悸失眠、小便频数及性功能减退等症。亦能增强心功能、降低血脂，可作为心脏病的辅助治疗药。

Pipe Fish* Capsule

Name of Chinese Phonetic Alphabet Shen Hai Long Jiao Nang

Formula Syngnathus, Hippocampus, Cervi Cornu Pantotrichum, Carprinus Testis et Penis (scalded by sand), Cnidii Fructus, Epimedii Folium, Cistanches Caulis Carnosus, Schisandrae Chinensis Fructus, Ginseng Radix et Rhizoma, Astragali Radix, Jujubae Fructus, Poria, Amomi Fructus, Dioscoreae Rhizoma, Zingiberis Rhizoma, Aconiti Lateralis Radix Praeparata (sliced), Angelicae Sinensis Radix, Rehmanniae Radix Praeparata, Asparagi Radix, Ophiopogoni Radix, Lycii Fructus, Persicae Semen, Hirudo, Moutan Cortex, Achyranthis Bidentatae Radix and Glycyrrhize Radix et Rhizoma (prepared).

Actions and Indications Warming and tonifying kidney-*yang*, marrow and essence. It is used for soreness and weakness of the waist and knees, fear of cold, cold limbs, lassitude of spirit, fatigue, dizziness, tinnitus, palpitation, insomnia, frequent urination and sexual hypoesthesia due to insufficiency of kidney-*yang*. It also acts for enhancing the heart function, decreasing blood-lipid and as an accessory treatment for heart disease.

*海龙

羚贝止咳糖浆

【处方】紫菀（蜜）、茯苓、麻黄、知母、金银花、陈皮、半夏（制）、前胡、远志（制）、平贝母、罂粟壳、山楂、羚羊角。

【功能主治】宣肺化痰，止咳平喘。用于小儿肺热咳嗽及痰湿咳嗽。

Syrup of Antelope Horn* and Ussuri Fritillary** for Relieving Cough

Name of Chinese Phonetic Alphabet Ling Bei Zhi Ke Tang Jiang

Formula Asteris Radix et Rhizoma (prepared with honey), Poria, Ephedrae Herba, Anemarrhenae Rhizoma, Lonicerae Japonicae Flos, Citri Reticulatae Pericarpium, Pinelliae Rhizoma (prepared), Peucedani Radix, Polygalae Radix (prepared), Fritillariae Ussuriensis Bulbus, Papaveris Pericarpium, Crataegi Fructus and Saigae Tataricae Cornu.

Actions and Indications Diffusing lung and resolving phlegm, relieving cough and calming dyspnea. It is indicated for children productive cough due to lung-heat and phlegm-damp.

*羚羊角 **平贝母

羚羊角胶囊

【处方】羚羊角。

【功能主治】平肝息风，清肝明目，散血解毒。用于高热惊痫，神昏痉厥，子痫抽搐，癫痫发狂，头痛眩晕，目赤翳障，温毒发斑，痈肿疮毒。

Antelope Horn* Capsule

Name of Chinese Phonetic Alphabet Ling Yang Jiao Jiao Nang

Formula Saigae Tataricae Cornu.

Actions and Indications Pacifying the liver, extinguishing wind, clearing liver-fire, improving vision and detoxifying. It is used for high fever, convulsion, obnubilation, spasm, eclampsia, epilepsy, headache, vertigo, conjunctival febrile congestion, eruptive disease, carbuncle due to pyogenic toxin.

*羚羊角

羚羊清肺丸

【处方】浙贝母、桑白皮（蜜炙）、前胡、麦冬、天冬、天花粉、地黄、玄参、石斛、桔梗、枇杷叶（蜜炙）、苦杏仁（炒）、金果榄、金银花、大青叶、栀子、黄芩、板蓝根、牡丹皮、薄荷、甘草、大黄、陈皮、羚羊角粉。

【功能主治】清肺利咽，止嗽。用于肺胃热盛，感受时邪，身热头晕，四肢酸懒，咳嗽痰盛，咽喉肿痛，鼻衄咳血，口干舌燥。

Antelope Horn* Bolus for Clearing Lung-heat

Name of Chinese Phonetic Alphabet Ling Yang Qing Fei Wan

Formula Fritillariae Thunbergii Bulbus, Mori Cortex (prepared with honey), Peucedani Radix, Ophiopogonis Radix, Asparagi Radix, Trichosanthis Radix, Rehmanniae Radix, Scrophulariae Radix, Dendrobii Caullis, Platycodonis Radix, Eriobotryae Folium (prepared with honey), Armeniacae Semen Amarum (fried), Tinosporae Radix, Lonicerae Japonicae Flos, Isatidis Folium, Gardeniae Fructus, Scutellariae Radix, Isatidis Radix, Moutan Cortex, Menthae Haplocalycis Herba, Glycyrrhizae Radix et Rhizoma, Rhei Radix et Rhizoma, Citri Reticulatae Pericarpium and Saigae Tataricae Cornu Pulvis.

Actions and Indications Clearing lung-heat and soothing the throat, relieving cough. It is used for feverish sensation of the body, dizziness, soreness of the limbs, productive cough, sore-throat, epistaxis, hemoptysis, dry mouth and tongue due to exuberant heat of the lung and stomach, and invasion of exogenous seasonal pathogens.

*羚羊角

羚羊感冒胶囊

【处方】羚羊角、牛蒡子、淡豆豉、金银花、荆芥、连翘、淡竹叶、桔梗、薄荷脑、甘草。

【功能主治】清热解表。用于流行性感冒，伤风咳嗽，头晕发热，咽喉肿痛。

Antelope Horn* Capsule for Relieving Common Cold

Name of Chinese Phonetic Alphabet Ling Yang Gan Mao Jiao Nang

Formula Saigae Tataricae Cornu, Arctii Fructus, Sojae Semen Praeparatum, Lonicerae Japonicae Flos, Schizonepetae Herba, Forsythiae Fructus, Lophatheri Herba, Platycodonis Radix, Menthol and Glycyrrhizae Radix et Rhizoma.

Actions and Indications Clearing heat and releasing the exterior. It is indicated for influenza, common cold with cough, dizziness, fever, sore-throat.

* 羚羊角

羚珠散

【处方】羚羊角粉、珍珠粉、牛黄、僵蚕、胆南星、朱砂、琥珀、冰片、石菖蒲油。

【功能主治】退热、镇静、定惊。用于小儿外感发热、神态不安，咳嗽有痰；对风热感冒、乳蛾（扁桃体）、风痧、水痘、痄腮等病毒性感染疗效更佳。

Antelope Horn* and Pearl** Powder

Name of Chinese Phonetic Alphabet Ling Zhu San

Formula Saigae Tataricae Cornu Pulvis, Magaritae Pulvis, Bovis Calculus, Bombyx Batryticatus, Arisaema cum Bile, Cinnabaris, Cutis Succinum, Borneolum Syntheticum and Acori Tatarinowii Oleum.

Actions and Indications Antipyretic and tranquilizing. It is used for fever, restlessness, productive cough, common cold, tonsillitis, rubella, chicken pox and mumps in children.

* 羚羊角 ** 珍珠

羚翘解毒丸

【处方】羚羊角、金银花、连翘、牛蒡子（炒）、荆芥穗、淡豆豉、薄荷、桔梗、淡竹叶、甘草。

【功能主治】疏风清热，解毒。用于风热感冒，恶寒发热，头晕目眩，咳嗽，咽痛。

Antelope Horn* and Weeping Forsythia** Detoxicating Bolus

Name of Chinese Phonetic Alphabet Ling Qiao Jie Du Wan

Formula Saigae Tataricae Cornu, Lonicerae Japonicae Flos, Forsythiae Fructus, Arctii Fructus (fried), Schizonepetae Spica, Sojae Semen Praeparatum, Menthae Haplocalycis Herba, Platycodonis Radix, Lophatheri Herba and Glycyrrhizae Radix et Rhizoma.

Actions and Indications Dispersing wind and clearing heat, detoxicating. It is indicated for common cold due to attack of wind-heat, marked by aversion to cold, fever, dizziness, dizzy vision, cough, sore-throat.

* 羚羊角 ** 连翘

断血流胶囊

【处方】断血流。

【功能主治】出血诸证。

Chinese Clinopodium* Capsule

Name of Chinese Phonetic Alphabet Duan Xue Liu Jiao Nang

Formula Clinopodii Herba.

Actions and Indications The preparation is used for various hemorrhagic syndromes.

* 断血流

寄生追风液

【处方】独活、白芍、槲寄生、熟地黄、杜仲（炒）、牛膝、秦艽、桂枝、防风、细辛、党参、甘草、当归、川芎、茯苓。

【功能主治】补肝肾，祛风湿，止痹痛。用于肝肾两亏，风寒湿痹引起的腰膝冷痛，腿足屈伸不利，以及慢性风湿性关节炎，腰肌劳损，跌打损伤后期具有上述症状者。

【注意】舌红口苦，烦热心悸，关节红肿热者痛者禁用。

Colored Mistletoe* Oral Liquid

Name of Chinese Phonetic Alphabet Ji Sheng Zhui Feng Ye

Formula Angelicae Pubescentis Radix, Paeoniae Radix Alba, Visci Herba, Rehmanniae Radix Praeparata, Eucommiae Cortex (fried), Achyranthis Bidentata Radix, Gentianae Macrophyllae Radix, Cinnamomi Ramulus, Saposhnikoviae Radix, Asari Radix et Rhizoma, Codonopsis Radix, Glycyrrhizae Radix et Rhizoma, Angelicae Sinensis Radix, Chuanxiong Rhizoma and Poria.

Actions and Indications Tonifying the liver and kidney, dispelling wind-damp, alleviating pain. It is indicated for cold-pain of the waist and knees, immobility of lower limbs, chronic rheumatic arthritis, lumbar muscle strain due to dual depletion of the liver and kidney, and stagnation of wind-cold-damp. It is also indicated for injury due to fall and strike.

Warning It is contraindicated for cases with red tongue, bitter taste in the mouth, heat vexation, palpitation, red, swelling and pain in the joints.

*槲寄生

颈复康冲剂

【处方】黄芪、党参、丹参、白芍、生地黄、石决明、威灵仙、花蕊石（煅）、葛根、黄柏、秦艽、王不留行（炒）、川芎、苍术、羌活、桃仁（去皮）、乳香（制）、没药（制）、红花、地龙（酒炙）、土鳖虫（酒炙）。

【功能主治】活血通络，散风止痛。用于颈椎病引起的脑供血不足，头晕，颈项僵硬，肩背酸痛，手臂麻木。

【注意】孕妇忌服。消化道溃疡，肾性高血压等患者慎服。

Relieving Cervical Spondylopathy Soluble Granules

Name of Chinese Phonetic Alphabet Jing Fu Kang Chong Ji

Formula Astragali Radix, Codonopsis Radix, Salviae Miltiorrhizae Radix et Rhizoma, Paeoniae Radix Alba, Rehmanniae Radix, Haliotidis Concha, Clematidis Radix et Rhizoma, Ophicalcitum (calcined), Puerariae Lobatae Radix, Phellodendri Chinensis Cortex, Gentianae Macrophyllae Radix, Vaccariae Semen (fried), Chuanxiong Rhizoma, Atractylodis Rhizoma, Notopterygii Rhizoma et Radix, Persicae Semen (removed seed coat), Olibanum (prepared), Myrrha (prepared), Carthami Flos, Pheretima (prepared with wine) and Eupolyphaga seu Steleophaga (prepared with wine).

Actions and Indications Activating blood, dredging collaterals, dissipating wind, alleviating pain. It is indicated for insufficiency of blood supply to brain, marked by dizziness, neck rigidity, soreness and pain of shoulder and back, numbness of arm due to cervical spondylopathy.

Warning It is contraindicated for pregnant women and should be used cautiously for cases with ulcer of digestive tract and renal hypertension.

颈痛灵药酒

【处方】熟地黄、何首乌、黑芝麻、当归、丹参、黄芪、天麻、葛根、千年健、地枫皮、枸杞子、白芍、骨碎补、威灵仙、狗脊、蛇蜕、桂枝、牛膝、木瓜、乳香、没药、山药、槲寄生、甘草、人参、鹿茸、麝香。

【功能主治】滋补肝肾，活络止痛。用于各种颈椎病引起的疼痛。

【注意】孕妇忌服，高血压病人慎服。

Medicated Wine for Cervical Spondylopathy

Name of Chinese Phonetic Alphabet Jing Tong Ling Yao Jiu

Formula Rehmanniae Radix Praeparata, Polygoni Multiflori Radix, Sesami Semen Nigrum, Angelicae Sinensis Radix, Salviae Miltiorrhizae Radix et Rhizoma, Astragali Radix, Gastrodiae Rhizoma, Puerariae Lobatae Radix, Homalomenae Rhizoma, Illicii Cortex, Lycii Fructus, Paeoniae Radix Alba, Psoraleae Fructus, Clematidis Radix et Rhizoma, Cibotii Rhizoma, Serpentis Periostracum, Cinnamomi Ramulus, Achyranthis Bidentatae Radix, Chaenomelis Fructus, Olibanum, Myrrha, Dioscoreae Rhizoma, Visci Herba, Glycyrrhizae Radix et Rhizoma, Ginseng Radix et Rhizoma, Cervi Cornu Pantotrichum and Moschus.

Actions and Indications Enriching and tonifying the liver and kidney, activating collaterals and alleviating pain. It is used for pain due to cervical spondylopathy.

Warning It is contraindicated for pregnant women and should be used carefully for hypertension.

维血宁合剂

【处方】虎杖、太子参、仙鹤草、地黄、鸡血藤、熟地黄、墨旱莲、白芍（炒）。

【功能主治】滋补肝肾，凉血清热。用于血小板减少症及血热所致的出血。

Thrombocytopenia-relieving Mixture

Name of Chinese Phonetic Alphabet Wei Xue Ning He Ji

Formula Polygoni Cuspidati Rhizoma et Radix , Pseudostellariae Radix, Agrimoniae Herba, Rehmanniae Radix, Spatholobi Caulis, Rehmanniae Radix Praeparata, Ecliptae Herba and Paeoniae Radix Alba (fried).

Actions and Indications Enriching and tonifying the liver and kidney, cooling blood, clearing heat. It is indicated for thrombocytopenia, hemorrhage due to blood-heat.

维C银翘片

【处方】金银花、连翘、荆芥、淡豆豉、淡竹叶、牛蒡子、芦根、桔梗、甘草、马来酸氯、苯那敏、对乙酰氨基酚、维生素C、薄荷油。

【功能主治】辛凉解表，清热解毒。用于流行性感冒引起的发热头痛、咳嗽、口干、咽喉疼痛。

Honeysuckle Flower* and Weeping Forsythia** Tablet

Name of Chinese Phonetic Alphabet Wei C Yin Qiao Pian

Formula Lonicerae Japonicae Flos, Forsythiae Fructus, Schizonepetae Herba, Sojae Semen Praeparatum, Lophatheri Herba, Arctii Fructus, Phragmitis Rhizoma, Platycodonis Radix, Glycyrrhizae Radix et Rhizoma, Chlorpheniramine Maleate, Paracetamol, Vitamin C and Menthae Haplocalycis Oleum.

Actions and Indications Releasing the exterior, clearing heat and detoxicating. It is indicated for influenza, marked by fever, headache, cough, dry mouth, sore-throat.

* 金银花 ** 连翘

绿雪胶囊

【处方】寒水石、滑石、磁石、石膏、玄参、升麻、甘草、青木香、丁香、石菖蒲、玄明粉、硝石、水牛角浓缩粉、青黛、朱砂。

【功能主治】清热解毒，镇惊安神。用于外感时邪引起的高热神昏，头痛脑胀，咽痛口渴，面赤腮肿，大便燥结，小儿急热惊风。

【注意】孕妇忌服。

Heat-clearing and Mind-tranquilizing Capsule

Name of Chinese Phonetic Alphabet Lu Xue Jiao Nang

Formula Gypsum Rubrum, Talcum, Magnetitum, Gypsum Fibrosum, Scrophulariae Radix, Cimicifugae Rhizoma, Glycyrrhizae Radix et

Rhizoma, Aristolochiae Radix, Caryophylli Flos, Acori Tatarinowii Rhizoma, Natrii Sulfas Exsiccatus, Nitrum, Bubali Cornu Pulvis Concentratio, Indigo Naturalis and Cinnabaris.

Actions and Indications Clearing heat and detoxifying, settling fright and tranquilizing the mind. It is used for high fever, coma, headache, sore-throat, thirst, flushed face, dry stools and infantile acute convulsion of heat type due to invasion of exogenous seasonal pathogens.

Warning It is contraindicated for pregnant women.

十二画

琥珀还睛丸

【处方】琥珀、菊花、青葙子、黄连、黄柏、知母、石斛、地黄、麦冬、天冬、党参（去芦）、山药、茯苓、甘草（蜜炙）、枳壳（去瓤麸炒）、川芎、当归、熟地黄、枸杞子、沙苑子、菟丝子、肉苁蓉（酒炙）、杜仲（炭）、羚羊角粉、水牛角浓缩粉、苦杏仁（去皮炒）。

【功能主治】补益肝肾，清热明目。用于肝肾两亏，虚火上炎引起的内外翳障，瞳仁散大，视力减退，夜盲昏花，目涩羞明，迎风流泪。

Amber* Bolus for Improving Vision

Name of Chinese Phonetic Alphabet Hu Po Huan Jing Wan

Formula Succinum, Chrysanthemi Flos, Celosiae Semen, Coptidis Rhizoma, Phellodendri Chinensis Cortex, Anemarrhenae Rhizoma, Dendrobii Caulis, Rehmanniae Radix, Ophiopogonis Radix, Asparagi Radix, Codonopsis Radix (removed rhizome), Dioscoreae Rhizoma, Poria, Glycyrrhizae Radix et Rhizoma (prepared with honey), Aurantii Fructus (removed pulp and fried with bran), Chuanxiong Rhizoma, Angelicae Sinensis Radix, Rehmanniae Radix Praeparata, Lycii Fructus, Astragali Complananti Semen, Cuscutae Semen, Cistanches Caulis Carnosus (prepared with wine), Eucommiae Cortex (carbonated), Saigae Tataricae Cornu Pulvis, Bubuli Cornu Pulvis Concentratio and Armeniacae Semen Amarum (removed seed coat and fried).

Actions and Indications Tonifying the liver and kidney, clearing heat, improving vision. It is indicated for internal or external nebula, platycoria, poor vision, night blindness, dry eyes, photophobia and overflow of tear induced by wind due to dual deficiency of the liver and kidney and deficiency-fire flaming upward.

* 琥珀

琥珀抱龙丸

【处方】山药（炒）、朱砂、甘草、琥珀、天竺黄、檀香、枳壳（炒）、茯苓、胆南星、枳实（炒）、红参。

【功能主治】镇惊安神，清热化痰。用于发热抽搐，烦躁不安，痰喘气急，惊痫不安。

【注意】慢惊及久病、气虚者忌服。

Amber* Pill for Tranquilizing

Name of Chinese Phonetic Alphabet Hu Po Bao Long Wan

Formula Dioscoreae Rhizoma (fried), Cinnabaris, Glycyrrhizae Radix et Rhizoma, Succinum, Bambusae Concretio Silicea, Santali Albi Lignum, Aurantii Fructus (fried), Poria, Arisaema cum Bile, Aurantii Fructus Immaturus (fried) and Ginseng Radix et Rhizoma Rubra.

Actions and Indications Tranquilizing the mind, clearing heat and resolving phlegm. It is used for fever, spasm, vexation, restlessness, phlegm dyspnea and fright epilepsy.

Warning It is contraindicated for cases with chronic convulsion, prolonged illness and *qi*-deficiency.

* 琥珀

琥珀消石冲剂

【处方】赤小豆、当归、琥珀、海金沙、金钱草、鸡内金、蒲黄、牛膝、郁金。

【功能主治】清热利湿，通淋消石。用于石淋、血淋，也可用于泌尿系统结石属湿热瘀结证者。

【注意】本品所含沉淀系有效成分，服用时将沉淀物一同服下。素体虚寒者不宜服用。

Amber* Soluble Granules for Relieving Strangury

Name of Chinese Phonetic Alphabet Hu Po Xiao Shi Chong Ji

Formula Vignae Semen, Angelicae Sinensis Radix, Succinum, Lygodii Spora, Lysimachiae Herba, Galli Gigerii Endothelium Corneum , Typhae Pollen, Achyranthis Bidentatae Radix and Curcumae Radix.

Actions and Indications Clearing heat and draining dampness, relieving strangury and removing stone. It is indicated for stone strangury, blood strangury, also for stone of the urinary system attributive to damp-heat binding syndrome.

Warning The deposition in the liquid is effective and it should be taken together with the liquid. It is not suitable for cases with deficiency-cold.

* 琥珀

散风活血膏

【处方】当归、独活、秦艽、血竭、白芷、杜仲、羌活、生川乌、荆芥、防风、干姜、穿山甲、川芎、地黄、玄参、生草乌、甘草、麻黄、没药、高良姜、肉桂、苍术、乳香、龙骨（煅）、麝香、樟脑、海螵蛸。

【功能主治】散风活血，强筋壮骨。用于受风受寒，四肢麻木，腰腿酸痛，跌打损伤，筋骨疼痛。

Relieving Traumatic Injury Plaster

Name of Chinese Phonetic Alphabet San Feng Huo Xue Gao

Formula Angelicae Sinensis Radix, Angelicae Pubescentis Radix, Gentianae Macrophyllae Radix, Draconis Sanguis, Angelicae Dahuricae Radix, Eucommiae Cortex, Notopterygii Rhizoma et Radix, Aconiti Radix (raw), Schizonepetae Herba, Saposhnikoviae Radix, Zingiberis Rhizoma, Manis Squama, Chuanxiong Rhizoma, Rehmanniae Radix, Scrophulariae Radix, Aconiti Kusnezoffii Radix (raw), Glycyrrhizae Radix et Rhizoma, Ephedrae Herba, Myrrha, Alpiniae Officinarum Rhizoma, Cinnamomi Cortex, Atractylodis Rhizoma, Olibanum, Draconis Os (calcined), Moschus, Camphora and Sepiae Endochoncha.

Actions and Indications Dissipating wind, activating blood, strengthening sinews and bone. It is used for numbness of limbs, soreness and pain of the waist and legs due to attack of wind and cold; traumatic injury and ostealgia.

散风活络丸

【处方】乌梢蛇（酒炙）、草乌（甘草、银花炙）、附子（炙）、威灵仙（酒炙）、防风、麻黄、海风藤、细辛、白附子（矾炙）、胆南星（酒炙）、蜈蚣、地龙、乳香（醋炙）、桃仁（去皮）、红花、当归、川芎、赤芍、桂枝、牛膝、骨碎补、熟地黄、党参、白术（麸炒）、茯苓、木香、香附（醋炙）、草豆蔻、石菖蒲、黄芩、大黄、牛黄、冰片。

【功能主治】舒筋活络，祛风除湿。用于风寒湿痹引起的中风瘫痪，口眼歪斜，半身不遂，腰腿疼痛，手足麻木，筋脉拘挛，步行艰难。

【注意】孕妇忌服。

Relieving Apoplexy Pill

Name of Chinese Phonetic Alphabet San Feng Huo Luo Wan

Formula Zaocys (prepared with wine), Aconiti Kusnezoffii Radix (prepared with licorice root and honeysuckle flower), Aconiti Lateralis Radix Praeparata, Clematidis Radix et Rhizoma (prepared with wine), Saposhnikoviae Radix, Ephedrae Herba, Piperis Kadsurae Caulis, Asari Radix et Rhizoma, Typhonii Rhizoma (prepared with alum), Arisaema cum Bile (prepared with wine), Scolopendra, Pheretima, Olibanum (prepared with vinegar),

Persicae Semen (removed seed coat), Carthami Flos, Angelicae Sinensis Radix, Chuanxiong Rhizoma, Paeoniae Radix Rubra, Cinnamomi Ramulus, Achyranthis Bidentatae Radix, Drynariae Rhizoma, Rehmanniae Radix Praeparata, Codonopsis Radix, Atractylodis Macrocephalae Rhizoma (fried with bran), Poria, Aucklandiae Radix, Cyperi Rhizoma (prepared with vinegar), Alpiniae Katsumadai Semen, Acori Tatarinowii Rhizoma, Scutellariae Radix, Rhei Radix et Rhizoma, Bovis Calculus and Borneolum Syntheticum.

Actions and Indications Relaxing sinews and activating collaterals, dispelling wind and dampness. It is indicated for apoplexy, paralysis, deviated eyes and mouth, hemiplegia, pain of the waist and legs, numbness of the limbs, spasm and difficulty for walk due to wind-cold-damp impediment syndrome.

Warning It is contraindicated for pregnant women.

散结灵胶囊

【处方】乳香（醋炙）、木鳖子、当归、没药（醋炙）、地龙、石菖蒲、枫香脂、五灵脂（醋炙）、香墨、草乌（甘草银花炙）。

【功能主治】散结消肿，活血止痛。用于阴疽初起，皮色不变，肿硬作痛，瘰疬。

【注意】孕妇忌服。

Mass-dissipating Capsule

Name of Chinese Phonetic Alphabet San Jie Ling Jiao Nang

Formula Olibanum (prepared with vinegar), Momordicae Semen, Angelicae Sinensis Radix, Myrrha (prepared with vinegar), Pheretima, Acori Tatarinowii Rhizoma, Liquidambaris Resina, Trogopterori Faeces (prepared with vinegar), Chines Ink and Aconiti Kusnezoffii Radix (prepared with licorice root and honeysuckle flower).

Actions and Indications Dissipating mass, reducing swelling, activating blood, alleviating pain. It is used for initial stage of deep-rooted carbuncle with swelling, pain, scrofula.

Warning It is contraindicated for pregnant women.

朝阳丸

【处方】黄芪、鹿茸粉、鹿角霜、大黄、大枣、黄芩、薄荷、冰片、玄参。

【功能主治】温肾健脾，疏肝散郁，化湿解毒。适用于慢性肝炎属于脾肾不足，肝郁血滞，痰湿内阻者。症见面色晦暗或㿠白，神疲乏力，纳呆腹胀，胁肋隐痛，胁下痞块，小便清或淡黄，大便溏或不爽，腰酸腿软，面颈血痣或见肝胀，舌体胖大、舌色暗淡、舌苔白或腻。脉弦而濡或沉弦或弦细等。

【注意】忌食生、冷、酒、蒜及油腻之品。有黄疸者不宜服用或遵医嘱服用。

Chao Yang Pill

Name of Chinese Phonetic Alphabet Chao Yang Wan

Formula Astragali Radix, Cervi Cornu Pantotrichum Pulvis, Cervi Cornu Degelatinatum, Rhei Radix et Rhizoma, Jujubae Fructus, Scutellariae Radix, Menthae Haplocalycis Herba, Borneolum Syntheticum and Scrophulariae Radix.

Actions and Indications Warming the kidney and fortifying the spleen, soothing the liver and relieving depression, resolving dampness and detoxicating. It is indicated for chronic hepatitis due to spleen-kidney insufficiency, liver depression and impeded blood flow, internal retention of phlegm and dampness, manifested as dim or bright pale complexion, lassitude of spirit, fatigue, poor appetite and abdominal distention, hypochondriac and subcostal dull pain, hypochondriac mass, clear or yellowish urination, sloppy stool, soreness of the waist and weakness of the legs, facial and cervical blood nevus or liver palms, enlarged and pale tongue, white or greasy tongue fur, string-like and soggy or sunken and string-like or string-like and fine pulse.

Warning Uncooked and cold foods, wine, garlic

and oily foods should be avoided. It is contraindicated for cases with jaundice, or patient should follow the physician's advice.

葛根芩连微丸

【处方】葛根、黄芩、黄连、甘草（蜜炙）。

【功能主治】解肌，清热，止泻止痢。用于泄泻痢疾、身热烦渴、菌痢、肠炎。

Lobed Kudzuvine* Baikal Skullcap** and Gold Thread *** Mini-pill

Name of Chinese Phonetic Alphabet Ge Gen Qin Lian Wei Wan

Formula Puerariae Lobatae Radix, Scutellariae Radix, Coptidis Rhizoma and Glycyrrhizae Radix et Rhizoma (prepared with honey).

Actions and Indications Releasing the flesh, clearing heat, relieving diarrhea and dysentery. It is used for diarrhea and dysentery, fever and polydipsia, bacillary dysentery and enteritis.

* 葛根 ** 黄芩 *** 黄连

越鞠丸

【处方】香附（醋制）、川芎、栀子（炒）、苍术（炒）、六神曲（炒）。

【功能主治】理气解郁，宽中除满。用于胸脘痞闷，腹中胀满，饮食停滞，嗳气吞酸。

Yueju Pill for Regulating *Qi*

Name of Chinese Phonetic Alphabet Yue Ju Wan

Formula Cyperi Rhizoma (prepared with vinegar), Chuanxiong Rhizoma, Gardeniae Fructus (fried), Atractylodis Rhizoma (fried) and Medicate Massa Fermentata (fried).

Actions and Indications Regulating *qi*, relieving depression, soothing the middle to eliminate oppression in chest. It is used for oppression in chest, abdominal fullness, food stagnation, eructation and acid regurgitation.

越鞠保和丸

【处方】栀子（姜制）、六神曲（麸炒）、香附（醋制）、川芎、苍术、木香、槟榔。

【功能主治】舒肝解郁，开胃消食。用于气郁停滞，倒饱嘈杂，胸腹胀痛，消化不良。

Yueju Baohe Pill for Promoting Digestion

Name of Chinese Phonetic Alphabet Yue Ju Bao He Wan

Formula Gardeniae Fructus (prepared with ginger), Medicata Massa Fermentata (fried with bran), Cyperi Rhizoma (prepared with vinegar), Chuanxiong Rhizoma, Atractylodis Rhizoma, Aucklandiae Radix and Arecae Semen.

Actions and Indications Soothing the liver, relieving depression, improving appetite, promoting digestion. It is used for gastric upset, thoracic and abdominal fullness and pain, and indigestion due to stagnation of *qi*.

紫地宁血散

【处方】大叶紫珠、地菍。

【功能主治】清热凉血，收敛止血。用于治疗胃及十二指肠溃疡或胃炎引起的吐血，便血。

Large-leaved Callicarpa* and Lesser Melastoma** Powder

Name of Chinese Phonetic Alphabet Zi Di Ning Xue San

Formula Callicarpae Macrophyllae Radix et Folium and Melastomatis Dodecandri Herba.

Actions and Indications Clearing heat, cooling blood, relieving bleeding, astringent. It is indicated for hematemesis and hematochezia due to gastric, duodenal ulcer or gastritis.

* 大叶紫珠 ** 地菍

紫金锭

【处方】山慈菇、红大戟、千金子霜、五倍子、麝香、朱砂、雄黄。

【功能主治】辟瘟解毒，消肿止痛。用于中暑，脘腹胀痛，恶心呕吐，痢疾泄泻，小儿痰厥；外治疔疮疖肿，痄腮，丹毒，喉风。

【注意】孕妇忌服。

Zijin Troche

Name of Chinese Phonetic Alphabet Zi Jin Ding

Formula Cremastrae seu Pleiones Psedobulbus, Knoxiae Radix, Euphorbiae Semen Pulveratum, Galla Chinensis, Moschus, Cinnabaris and Realgar.

Actions and Indications Exorcising pestilence, detoxifying, dispersing swelling and alleviating pain. It is indicated for summer-heat stroke, abdominal fullness and pain, nausea, vomiting, dysentery, diarrhea, infantile phlegm syncope. External use for deep-rooted boil, sore, furunculosis, mumps, erysipelas and acute pyogenic infection of pharynx.

Warning It is contraindicated for pregnant women.

紫河车胶囊

【处方】本品为紫河车制成的胶囊。

【功能主治】温肾补精，益气养血。用于虚劳羸瘦，骨蒸盗汗，咳嗽气喘，食少气短，阳痿遗精，不孕少乳。

Human Placenta* Capsule

Name of Chinese Phonetic Alphabet Zi He Che Jiao Nang

Formula Hominis Placenta.

Actions and Indications Warming the kidney, tonifying essence, *qi* and blood. It is indicated for consumptive disease, emaciation, night sweating, cough, dyspnea, poor appetite, shortness of breath, impotence, nocturnal emission, sterility and oligogalactia.

* 紫河车

紫珠止血液

【处方】紫珠叶。

【功能主治】清热解毒，收敛止血。用于胃肠道出血、便血、咯血以及外伤出血。

Taiwan Beautyberry* Oral Liquid for Relieving Bleeding

Name of Chinese Phonetic Alphabet Zi Zhu Zhi Xue Ye

Formula Callicarpae Formosanae Folium.

Actions and Indications Clearing heat, detoxifying, astringent, relieving bleeding. It is used for hemorrhage of gastrointestinal tract, hematochezia, hemoptysis and traumatic bleeding.

* 紫珠

紫雪散

【处方】石膏、寒水石、滑石、磁石、玄参、木香、沉香、升麻、甘草、芒硝（制）、硝石（精制）、丁香、麝香、羚羊角、朱砂、水牛角浓缩粉。

【功能主治】清热解毒，止痉开窍。用于热病，高热烦躁，神昏谵语，惊风抽搐，斑疹吐衄，尿赤便秘。

【注意】孕妇禁用。

Heat-clearing and Convulsion-relieving Powder

Name of Chinese Phonetic Alphabet Zi Xue San

Formula Gypsum Fibrosum, Gypsum Rubrum, Talcum, Magnetitum, Scrophulariae Radix, Aucklandiae Radix, Aquilariae Lignum Resinatum, Cimicifugae Rhizoma, Glycyrrhizae Radix et Rhizoma, Natrii Sulfas (prepared), Nitrum (refined), Caryophylli Flos, Moschus, Saigae Tataricae Cornu, Cinnabaris and Bubali Cornu Pulvis Concentratio.

Actions and Indications Clearing heat and detoxifying, alleviating spasm, inducing resuscitation. It is used for heat disease marked by high fever, vexation coma, delirious speech, convulsion, spasm, macular macula, hemoptysis, epistaxis, deep coloured urine and constipation.

Warning It is contraindicated for pregnant women.

喘息灵胶囊

【处方】何首乌、甘草、马兜铃、五味子、知母等。

【功能主治】平喘，止咳，祛痰。用于急、慢性支气管炎，支气管哮喘。

Relieving Dyspnea and Cough Capsule

Name of Chinese Phonetic Alphabet Chuan Xi Ling Jiao Nang

Formula Polygoni Multiflori Radix, Glycyrrhizae Radix et Rhizoma, Aristolochiae Fructus, Schisandrae Chinensis Fructus, Anemarrhenae Rhizoma, etc.

Actions and Indications Relieving dyspnea and cough, dispelling phlegm. It is indicated for acute, chronic bronchitis, bronchial asthma.

喉炎丸

【处方】硼砂（煅）、黄连、蟾酥、熊胆、牛黄、冰片、珍珠、五倍子、细辛、麝香、人指甲、水牛角浓缩粉。

【功能主治】清热解毒，消肿止痛。用于咽喉肿痛，单双乳蛾，痈疽疮疖肿痛。

【注意】孕妇慎服。

Laryngitis-relieving Pill

Name of Chinese Phonetic Alphabet Hou Yan Wan

Formula Borax (calcined), Coptidis Rhizoma, Bufonis Venenum, Ursi Fel, Bovis Calculus, Borneolum Syntheticum, Margarita, Galla Chinensis, Asari Radix et Rhizoma, Moschus, Unguis Hominis and Bubali Cornu Pulvis Concentratio.

Actions and Indications Clearing heat and detoxicating, dispersing swelling and relieving pain. It is indicated for sore-throat, unilateral or bilateral tonsillitis, abscess and deep-rooted boil.

Warning It should be used carefully for pregnant women.

喉症丸

【处方】板蓝根、牛黄、冰片、猪胆汁、玄明粉、青黛、雄黄、硼砂、百草霜、蟾酥（酒制）。

【功能主治】清热解毒，消肿止痛。用于咽炎、喉炎、扁桃体炎及一般疮疖。

【注意】孕妇忌服。

Laryngopathy-relieving Pill

Name of Chinese Phonetic Alphabet Hou Zheng Wan

Formula Isatidis Radix, Bovis Calculus, Borneolum Syntheticum, Suillus Bilis, Natrii Sulfas Exsiccatus, Indigo Naturalis, Realgar, Borax, Gramen Fumi Carbonisatus and Bufonis Venenum (prepared with wine).

Actions and Indications Clearing heat and detoxicating, dispersing swelling and relieving pain. It is used for pharyngitis, laryngitis, tonsillitis, abscess and deep-rooted boil.

Warning It is contraindicated for pregnant women.

喉疾灵胶囊

【处方】牛黄、板蓝根、诃子、桔梗、猪牙皂、连翘、天花粉、冰片、珍珠粉、山豆根、了哥王、广东土牛膝。

【功能主治】清热解毒，散肿止痛。用于腮腺炎，扁桃体炎，急性咽炎，慢性咽炎急性发作及一般喉痛。

【注意】孕妇忌服。

Laryngopathy-relieving Capsule

Name of Chinese Phonetic Alphabet Hou Ji Ling Jiao Nang

Formula Bovis Calculus, Isatidis Radix, Chebulae Fructus, Platycodonis Radix, Gleditsiae Fructus Abnormalis, Forsythiae Fructus, Trichosanthis Radix, Borneolum Syntheticum, Magaritae Pulvis, Sophorae Tonkinensis Radix et Rhizoma, Wikstroemiae Indicae Caulis et Folium and Eupatorii Chinensis Radix.

Actions and Indications Clearing heat, detoxicating, dispersing swelling and relieving pain. It is indicated for parotitis, tonsillitis, acute pharyngitis, acute attack of chronic pharyngitis and sore-throat.

Warning It is contraindicated for pregnant women.

喉康散

【处方】冰片、珍珠层粉、生晒参、薄荷脑、青黛、玄明粉、硼砂（煅）、天花粉、甘草、穿心莲叶。

【功能主治】清热解毒，消炎止痛。用于各种咽喉疾患，如急性、慢性咽炎，喉炎，扁桃体炎，口腔溃疡。

Relieving Laryngitis Powder

Name of Chinese Phonetic Alphabet Hou Kang San

Formula Borneolum Syntheticum, Margaritae Concha Strati Pulvis, Ginseng Radix et Rhizoma Exsiccatus, Menthol, Indigo Naturalis, Natrii Sulfas Exsiccatus, Borax (calcined), Trichosanthis Radix, Glycyrrhizae Radix et Rhizoma and Andrographis Folium.

Actions and Indications Clearing heat and detoxicating, counteracting inflammation and relieving pain. It is indicated for various throat diseases, such as acute and chronic pharyngitis, laryngitis, tonsillitis, ulcerative stomatitis.

蛤蚧定喘丸

【处方】蛤蚧、瓜蒌子、紫菀、麻黄、鳖甲（醋制）、黄芩、甘草、麦冬、黄连、百合、紫苏子（炒）、石膏、苦杏仁（炒）、石膏（煅）。

【功能主治】滋阴清肺，止咳定喘。用于虚劳久咳，年老哮喘，气短发热，胸满郁闷，自汗盗汗，不思饮食。

Honeyed Bolus of Giant Gecko* for Relieving Asthma

Name of Chinese Phonetic Alphabet Ge Jie Ding Chuan Wan

Formula Gecko, Trichosanthis Semen, Asteris Radix et Rhizoma, Ephedrae Herba, Trionycis Carapax (prepared with vinegar), Scutellariae Radix, Glycyrrhizae Radix et Rhizoma, Ophiopogonis Radix, Coptidis Rhizoma, Lilii Bulbus, Perillae Fructus (fried), Gypsum Fibrosum, Armeniacae Semen Amarum (fried) and Gypsum Fibrosum (calcined).

Actions and Indications Enriching *yin* and clearing lung-heat, relieving cough and calming dyspnea. It is indicated for chronic cough due to consumptive disease; senile asthma, marked by shortness of breath, fever, chest distress, spontaneous and night sweating, anorexia.

* 蛤蚧

跌打万花油

【处方】乌药、大蒜、红花、黑老虎、葛花、大黄、苏木、威灵仙、砂仁、紫草、羌活、蔓荆子、独活、干姜、荜茇、骨碎补、柳枝、栀子、辣蓼、化橘红、青皮、陈皮、白及、草豆蔻、卷柏、皂角刺、白芷、苍耳子、桃仁、黄连、赤芍、野菊花、桉油、冰片、荷叶、肉豆蔻、莪术（制）、大枫子（仁）、金银花叶、牡丹皮、川芎（制）、两面针、泽兰、樟脑油、蓖麻子、三棱（制）、蒲黄、丁香罗勒油、生天南星、紫草茸、白胡椒、香附（制）、马齿苋、葱白、胶香、薄荷油、松节油、水杨酸甲酯、茴香油、桂皮油、水翁花、徐长卿、木棉皮、土细辛、声色草、伸筋藤、蛇床子、铁包金、倒扣草、山白芷、朱砂根、过塘蛇、九节茶、地耳草、一点红、谷精草、土田七、木棉花、鸭脚艾、防风、侧柏叶、马钱子、大风艾、腊梅花、墨旱莲、九层塔。

【功能主治】主治跌打损伤，扭挫撞伤，外伤出血，水火烫伤，局部红肿疼痛。

【注意】外用，擦敷患处。

Multiple Usage Oils for External Injury

Name of Chinese Phonetic Alphabet Die Da Wan Hua You

Formula Linderae Radix, Allii Bulbus, Carthami Flos, Kadsurae Coccineae Radix, Flos Puerariae Lobatae, Rhei Radix et Rhizoma, Sappan Lignum, Clematidis Radix et Rhizoma, Amomi Fructus, Arnebiae Radix, Notopterygii Rhizoma et Radix, Viticis Fructus, Angelicae Pubescentis Radix, Zingiberis Rhizoma, Piperis Longi Fructus, Drynariae Rhizoma, Salicis Babylonicae Ramulus, Gardeniae Fructus, Polygoni Flaccidi Herba, Citri Grandis Exocarpium, Citri Reticulatae Pericarpium Viride, Citri Reticulatae Pericarpium, Bletillae Rhizoma, Alpiniae Katsumadai Semen, Selaginellae Herba, Gleditsiae Spina, Angelicae Dahuricae Radix, Xanthii Fructus, Persicae Semen, Copidis Rhizoma, Paeoniae Radix Rubra, Chrysanthemi Indici Flos, Eucalypti Oleum, Borneolum Syntheticum, Nelumbinis Folium, Myristicae Semen, Curcumae Rhizoma (prepared), Hydnocarpi Anthelmintici Semen, Lonicerae Japonicae Folium, Moutan Cortex, Chuanxiong Rhizoma (prepared), Zanthoxyli Radix, Lycopi Herba, Camphora Oleum, Ricini Semen, Sparganii Rhizoma (prepared), Typhae Pollen, Ocimi Basilici Oleum, Arisaematis Rhizoma (raw), Lacca, Orixae Japonicae Radix, Cyperi Rhizoma (prepared), Portulacae Herba, Allii Bulbus Fistulosi, Liquidambaris Formosanae Resina, Menthae Haplocalycis Oleum, Terebinthinae Oleum, Methyl Salicylate, Foeniculi Oleum, Cinnamomi Oleum, Cleistocalycis Operculati Flos Immaturus, Cynanchi Paniculati Radix et Rhizoma, Gossampini Cortex, Tylophorae Ovatae Radix et Rhizoma, Polycarpaeae Corymbosae Herba, Tinosporae Sinensis Caulis, Cnidii Fructus, Berchemiae Lineatae Radix, Achyranthis Asperae Herba, Inulae Cappae Radix, Ardisiae Crenatae Radix, Jussiaeae Repentis Herba, Sarcandrae Herba, Hyperici Japonici Herba, Duchesneae Indicae Herba, Eriocauli Flos, Stahlianthi Involucrati Rhizoma, Gossampini Flos, Artemisiae Lactiflorae Herba, Saposhnikoviae Radix, Platycladi Cacumen, Strychni Semen, Blumeae Balsamiferae Folium et Ramulus, Chimonanthi Praecocis Flos Immaturus, Ecliptae Herba and Ocimi Basilici Herba.

Actions and Indications The preparation is used for traumatic injury, sprain, contusion, traumatic bleeding, scald and burn with topical swelling and pain.

Warning It is for external use on affected part only.

跌打丸

【处方】三七、当归、白芍、赤芍、桃仁、红花、血竭、刘寄奴、骨碎补（烫）、续断、苏木、牡丹皮、乳香（制）、没药（制）、姜黄、枳实（炒）、三棱（醋制）、防风、甜瓜子、桔梗、甘草、关木通、自然铜（煅）、土鳖虫。

【功能主治】活血散瘀，消肿止痛。用于跌打损伤，筋断骨折，瘀血肿痛，闪腰岔气。

【注意】孕妇禁用。

Traumatic Injury Pill

Name of Chinese Phonetic Alphabet Die Da Wan

Formula Notoginseng Radix et Rhizoma, Angelicae Sinensis Radix, Paeoniae Radix Alba, Paeoniae Radix Rubra, Persicae Semen, Carthami Flos, Draconis Sanguis, Artemisiae Anomalae Herba, Drynariae Rhizoma (scalded), Dipsaci Radix, Sappan Lignum, Moutan Cortex, Olibanum (prepared), Myrrha (prepared), Curcumae Longae Rhizoma, Aurantii Fructus Immaturus (fried), Sparganii Rhizoma (prepared with vinegar), Saposhnikoviae Radix, Melo Semen, Platycodonis Radix, Glycyrrhizae Radix et Rhizoma, Aristolochiae Manshuriensis Caulis, Pyritum (calcined) and Eupolyphaga seu Steleophaga.

Actions and Indications Activating blood, dissipating stasis, reducing swelling, alleviating pain. It is used for traumatic injury and fracture marked by swelling, pain and blood-stasis, sudden lumbar sprain and contusion.

Warning It is contraindicated for pregnant women.

跌打镇痛膏

【处方】土鳖虫、草乌、马钱子、大黄、降香、两面针、黄芩、黄柏、虎杖、冰片、薄荷油、樟脑、水杨酸甲酯、薄荷脑。

【功能主治】活血止痛，散瘀消肿，祛风胜湿。用于急、慢性扭挫伤，慢性腰腿痛，风湿关节痛。

【注意】孕妇及皮肤过敏者慎用。

Plaster for Traumatic Injury

Name of Chinese Phonetic Alphabet Die Da Zhen Tong Gao

Formula Eupolyphaga seu Steleophaga, Aconiti Kusnezoffii Radix, Strychni Semen, Rhei Radix et Rhizoma, Dalbergiae Odoriferae Lignum, Zanthoxyli Radix, Scutellariae Radix, Phellodendri Chinensis Cortex, Polygoni Cuspidati Rhizoma et Radix , Borneolum Syntheticum, Menthae Haplocalycis Oleum, Camphora, Methyl Salicylate and Menthol.

Actions and Indications Activating blood, alleviating pain, dissipating stasis, reducing swelling, dispelling wind and dampness. It is used for acute, chronic sprain, contusion, chronic pain of the waist and legs, rheumatic arthralgia.

Warning It should be used cautiously for pregnant women and cases with skin allergy.

暑热感冒冲剂

【处方】连翘、竹叶、北沙参、竹茹、荷叶、生石膏、知母、佩兰、丝瓜络、香薷、菊花。

【功能主治】祛暑解表，清热，生津。用于感冒病暑热证候；症见发热重，恶寒轻，汗出热不退，心烦口渴，溲赤、苔黄、脉数。

【注意】饮食宜清淡，忌食辛辣物。

Relieving Summer-heat Common Cold Soluble Granules

Name of Chinese Phonetic Alphabet Shu Re Gan Mao Chong Ji

Formula Forsythiae Fructus, Phyllostachydis Henonis Folium, Glehniae Radix, Bambusae Caulis in Taenias, Nelumbinis Folium, Gypsum Fibrosum, Anemarrhenae Rhizoma, Eupatorii Herba, Luffae Fructus Retinervus, Moslae Herba and Chrysanthemi Flos.

Actions and Indications Dispelling summer-heat and releasing the exterior, clearing heat, engendering fluid. It is used for common cold with summer-heat pattern, manifested as fever, aversion to cold, sweating but unabated fever, vexation, thirst, brown urine, yellow tongue fur, rapid pulse.

Warning Bland diet should be taken and pungent foods should be avoided.

暑症片

【处方】猪牙皂、细辛、薄荷、广藿香、木香、白芷、防风、陈皮、半夏（制）、桔梗、甘草、绵马贯众、白矾（煅）、雄黄、朱砂。

【功能主治】祛寒辟瘟，化浊开窍。用于夏令中恶昏厥，牙关紧闭，腹痛吐泻，四肢发麻。

【注意】孕妇禁用。

Syncope-relieving Tablet

Name of Chinese Phonetic Alphabet Shu Zheng Pian

Formula Gleditsiae Fructus Abnormalis, Asari Radix et Rhizoma, Menthae Haplocalycis Herba, Pogostemonis Herba, Aucklandiae Radix, Angelicae Dahuricae Radix, Saposhnikoviae Radix, Citri Reticulatae Pericarpium, Pinelliae Rhizoma (prepared), Platycodonis Radix, Glycyrrhizae Radix et Rhizoma, Dryopteridis Crassirhizomatis Rhizoma, Alumen (calcined), Realgar and Cinnabaris.

Actions and Indications Dispelling cold, exorcising pestilence, resolving turbidity and inducing resuscitation. It is used for syncope, lockjaw, abdominal pain, vomiting and diarrhea, and numbness of limbs.

Warning It is contraindicated for pregnant women.

暑湿感冒冲剂

【处方】藿香、防风、紫苏叶、佩兰、白芷、苦杏仁、大腹皮、香薷、陈皮、半夏、茯苓。

【功能主治】清暑去湿，芳香化浊。用于外感风寒引起的感冒，胸闷呕吐，腹泻便溏。

Common Cold (Summer-heat-damp) Relieving Soluble Granules

Name of Chinese Phonetic Alphabet Shu Shi Gan Mao Chong Ji

Formula Agastaches Herba, Saposhnikoviae Radix, Perillae Folium, Eupatorii Herba, Angelicae Dahuricae Radix, Armeniacae Semen Amarum, Arecae Pericarpium, Moslae Herba, Citri Reticulatae Pericarpium, Pinelliae Rhizoma and Poria.

Actions and Indications Clearing summer-heat and dispelling dampness, resolving turbidity. It is used for common cold marked by chest distress, vomiting, diarrhea and sloppy stool due to exogenous wind-cold.

景天三七糖浆

【处方】本品为景天三七制成的糖浆。

【功能主治】止血。用于各种出血病症。

Alpine Stonecrop* Syrup

Name of Chinese Phonetic Alphabet Jing Tian San Qi Tang Jiang

Formula Sedi Aizoon Herba.

Actions and Indications Relieving bleeding. It is indicated for various hemorrhagia.

*景天三七

黑锡丹

【处方】黑锡、硫黄、川楝子、胡芦巴、木香、附子（制）、肉豆蔻、补骨脂、沉香、小茴香、阳起石、肉桂。

【功能主治】升降阴阳，坠痰定喘。用于真元亏惫，上实下虚，痰壅气喘，胸腹冷痛。

Galenite* Pill

Name of Chinese Phonetic Alphabet Hei Xi Dan

Formula Plumbum, Sulfur, Toosendan Fructus, Trigonellae Semen, Aucklandiae Radix, Aconiti Lateralis Radix Preparata, Myristicae Semen, Psoraleae Fructus, Aquilariae Lignum Resinatum, Foeniculi Fructus, Tremolitum and Cinnamomi Cortex.

Actions and Indications Upraising and downbearing *yin* and *yang*, downbearing phlegm and calming dyspnea. It is used for dyspnea, cold-pain of the chest and abdomen due to depletion of genuine *qi*, upper excess and lower deficiency.

*黑锡

锁阳固精丸

【处方】锁阳、肉苁蓉（蒸）、巴戟天（制）、补骨脂（盐炒）、菟丝子、杜仲（炭）、八角茴香、韭菜子、芡实（炒）、莲子、莲须、牡蛎（煅）、龙骨（煅）、鹿角霜、熟地黄、山茱萸（制）、牡丹皮、山药、茯苓、泽泻、知母、黄柏、牛膝、大青盐。

【功能主治】温肾固精。用于肾虚滑精，腰膝酸软，眩晕耳鸣，四肢无力。

Cynomorium* Bolus for Arresting Emission

Name of Chinese Phonetic Alphabet Suo Yang Gu Jing Wan

Formula Cynomorii Caulis Carnosus, Cistanches Caulis Carnosus (steamed), Morindae Officinalis Radix (prepared), Psoraleae Fructus (fried with salt), Cuscutae Semen, Eucommiae Cortex (carbonated), Anisi Stellati Fructus, Allii Tuberosi Semen, Euryales Semen (fried), Nelumbinis Semen, Nelumbinis Stamen, Ostreae Concha (calcined), Draconis Os (calcined), Cervi Cornu Degelatinatum, Rehmanniae Radix Praeparata, Corni Fructus (prepared), Moutan Cortex, Dioscoreae Rhizoma, Poria, Alismatis Rhizoma, Anemarrhenae Rhizoma, Phellodendri Chinensis Cortex, Achyranthis Bidentatae Radix and Halitum.

Actions and Indications Warming the kidney, arresting emission. It is used for spermatorrhea, soreness and weakness of the waist and knees, vertigo, tinnitus and weakness of extremities due to deficiency of the kidney.

*锁阳

筋骨草胶囊

【处方】本品为筋骨草经加工制成的胶囊剂。

【功能主治】清热解毒，止咳，祛痰，平喘。用于急、慢性支气管炎，肺脓疡。

【注意】孕妇慎服。

Ciliate Bugle* Capsule for Relieving Bronchitis

Name of Chinese Phonetic Alphabet Jin Gu Cao Jiao Nang

Formula Ajugae Herba.

Actions and Indications Clearing heat and detoxicating, relieving cough and dyspnea, dispelling phlegm. It is indicated for acute, chronic bronchitis and pulmonary abscess.

Warning It should be used carefully for pregnant women.

*筋骨草

智托洁白丸

【处方】寒水石、矮紫堇、诃子、兔耳草、木香、蜂蜜等。

【功能主治】清胃热，制酸，止咳。用于慢性胃炎，胃痛，呕吐酸水，咳嗽，音哑，呼吸不畅。

Zhituo Jiebai Pill for Relieving Gastritis

Name of Chinese Phonetic Alphabet Zhi Tuo Jie Bai Wan

Formula Gypsum Rubrum, Corydalis Pygmaeae Herba, Chebulae Fructus, Pecteilidis Susannae Radix, Aucklandiae Radix, Mel, etc.

Actions and Indications Clearing stomach-heat, antiacid, relieving cough. It is indicated for chronic gastritis, stomachache, acid vomitus, cough, hoarseness and difficult breathing.

舒心糖浆

【处方】丹参、北沙参、黄柏、龙骨、牡蛎。

【功能主治】活血散瘀，养阴益气，定悸除烦，用于心悸、怔忡，心烦失眠。

Heart-soothing Syrup

Name of Chinese Phonetic Alphabet Shu Xin Tang Jiang

Formula Salviae Miltiorrhizae Radix et Rhizoma, Glehniae Radix, Phellodendri Chinensis Cortex, Draconis Os and Ostreae Concha.

Actions and Indications Activating blood, dissipating stasis, nourishing *yin*, tonifying *qi*, relieving palpitation and vexation. It is used for palpitation, fearful throbbing, vexation and insomnia.

舒肝丸

【处方】川楝子、延胡索（醋制）、白芍（酒炒）、片姜黄、木香、沉香、豆蔻、砂仁、厚朴（姜制）、陈皮、枳壳（炒）、茯苓、朱砂。

【功能主治】舒肝和胃，理气止痛。用于肝郁气滞，胸胁胀满，胃脘疼痛，嘈杂呕吐，嗳气反酸。

【注意】孕妇慎用。

Liver-soothing Bolus

Name of Chinese Phonetic Alphabet Shu Gan Wan

Formula Toosendan Fructus, Corydalis Rhizoma (prepared with vinegar), Paeoniae Radix Alba (fried with wine), Wenyujin Rhizoma Concisum, Aucklandiae Radix, Aquilariae Lignum Resinatum, Amomi Fructus Rotundus, Amomi Fructus, Magnoliae Officinalis Cortex (prepared with ginger), Citri Reticulatae Pericarpium, Aurantii Fructus (fried), Poria and Cinnabaris.

Actions and Indications Soothing the liver and harmonizing the stomach, regulating *qi* and alleviating pain. It is used for fullness in hypochondrium, stomach duct pain, gastric upset, vomiting, eructation and acid regurgitation due to liver depression and stagnation of *qi*.

Warning It should be used carefully for pregnant women.

舒肝止痛丸

【处方】柴胡、当归、白芍、赤芍、白术（炒）、薄荷、甘草、生姜、香附（醋制）、郁金 、延胡索（醋制）、川楝子、木香、陈皮、半夏（制）、黄芩、川芎、莱菔子（炒）。

【功能主治】舒肝理气，和胃止痛。用于肝胃不和，肝气郁结，胸胁胀满，呕吐酸水，脘腹疼痛。

【注意】孕妇慎用。

Liver-soothing and Pain-alleviating Pill

Name of Chinese Phonetic Alphabet Shu Gan Zhi Tong Wan

Formula Bupleuri Radix, Angelicae Sinensis Radix, Paeoniae Radix Alba, Paeoniae Radix Rubra, Atractylodis Macrocephalae Rhizoma (fried), Menthae Haplocalycis Herba, Glycyrrhizae Radix et Rhizoma, Zingiberis Rhizoma Recens, Cyperi Rhizoma (prepared with vinegar), Curcumae Radix, Corydalis Rhizoma (prepared with vinegar), Toosendan Fructus, Aucklandiae Radix, Citri Reticulatae Pericarpium, Pinelliae Rhizoma (prepared), Scutellariae Radix, Chuanxiong Rhizoma and Raphani Semen (fried).

Actions and Indications Soothing the liver, regulating *qi*, harmonizing the stomach and alleviating pain. It is used for hypochondriac fullness, acid vomiting and abdominal pain due to disharmony of the liver and stomach, and stagnation of liver-*qi*.

Warning It should be used carefully for pregnant women.

舒肝平胃丸

【处方】厚朴（姜炙）、陈皮、枳壳（麸炒）、法半夏、苍术、甘草（蜜炙）、槟榔（炒焦）。

【功能主治】舒肝，消滞。用于胸胁胀满，倒饱嘈杂，呕吐酸水，胃脘疼痛，食滞不消。

【注意】孕妇忌服。

Liver-soothing and Stomach-pacifying Pill

Name of Chinese Phonetic Alphabet Shu Gan Ping Wei Wan

Formula Magnoliae Officinalis Cortex (prepared with ginger), Citri Reticulatae Pericarpium, Aurantii Fructus (fried with bran), Pinelliae Rhizoma Praeparatum, Atractylodis Rhizoma, Glycyrrhizae Radix et Rhizoma (prepared with honey) and Arecae Semen (charred).

Actions and Indications Soothing the liver and removing food stagnation. It is used for hypochondriac fullness, gastric upset, acid vomiting, pain in stomach duct and dyspepsia.

Warning It is contraindicated for pregnant women.

舒肝和胃丸

【处方】香附（醋制）、白芍、佛手、木香、郁金、白术（炒）、陈皮、柴胡、广藿香、甘草（蜜炙）、莱菔子、槟榔（炒焦）、乌药。

【功能主治】平肝舒郁，和胃止痛。用于两肋胀满，食欲不振，呕吐，胃脘疼痛，大便失调。

Liver-soothing and Stomach-harmonizing Bolus

Name of Chinese Phonetic Alphabet Shu Gan He Wei Wan

Formula Cyperi Rhizoma (prepared with vinegar), Paeoniae Radix Alba, Citri Sarcodactylis Fructus, Aucklandiae Radix, Curcumae Radix, Atractylodis Macrocephalae Rhizoma (fried), Citri Reticulatae Pericarpium, Bupleuri Radix, Pogostemonis Herba, Glycyrrhizae Radix et Rhizoma (prepared with honey), Raphani Semen, Arecae Semen (charred) and Linderae Radix.

Actions and Indications Pacifying the liver, relieving depression, harmonizing the stomach, alleviating pain. It is used for hypochondriac fullness, poor appetite, vomiting, pain in stomach duct and disorder of bowels movement.

舒肝健胃丸

【处方】厚朴（姜制）、香附（醋制）、白芍（麸炒）、柴胡（醋制）、青皮（醋炒）、香橼、陈皮、檀香、豆蔻、枳壳、鸡内金（炒）、槟榔、延胡索（醋炒）、五灵脂（醋制）、牵牛子（炒）。

【功能主治】疏肝开郁，导滞中和。用于肝胃不和引起的胃脘胀痛，胸胁满闷，呕吐吞酸，腹胀便秘。

【注意】孕妇忌服。

Liver-soothing and Stomach-fortifying Pill

Name of Chinese Phonetic Alphabet Shu Gan Jian Wei Wan

Formula Magnoliae Officinalis Cortex (prepared with ginger), Cyperi Rhizoma (prepared with vinegar), Paeoniae Radix Alba (fried with bran), Bupleuri Radix (prepared with vinegar), Citri Reticulatae Pericarpium Viride (prepared with vinegar), Citri Fructus, Citri Reticulatae Pericarpium, Santali Albi Lignum, Amomi Fructus Rotundus, Aurantii Fructus, Galli Gigerii Endothelium Corneum (fried), Arecae Semen, Corydalis Rhizoma (prepared with vinegar), Trogopterori Faeces (prepared with vinegar) and Pharbitidis Semen (fried).

Actions and Indications Soothing the liver, relieving depression, reducing stagnation. It is used for fullness and pain of stomach duct, hypochondriac fullness and depression, vomiting, acid regurgitation, abdominal fullness and constipation due to disharmony of the liver and stomach.

Warning It is contraindicated for pregnant women.

舒肝理气丸

【处方】青木香、姜半夏、陈皮、延胡索（制）、玫瑰花、山楂、香附（炒）、柴胡、丹参、甘草、广藿香。

【功能主治】舒肝理气，解郁。用于胸胁胀闷，气郁不舒。

【注意】服药期间忌饮酒，忌食辛辣厚味。

Liver-soothing and *Qi*-regulating Pill

Name of Chinese Phonetic Alphabet Shu Gan Li Qi Wan

Formula Aristolochiae Radix, Pinelliae Rhizoma cum Zingibere Praeparatum et Alumine, Citri Reticulatae Pericarpium, Corydalis Rhizoma (prepared), Rosae Rugosae Flos, Crataegi Fructus, Cyperi Rhizoma (prepared), Bupleuri Radix, Salviae Miltiorrhizae Radix et Rhizoma, Glycyrrhizae Radix et Rhizoma and Pogostemonis Herba.

Actions and Indications Soothing the liver, regulating *qi*, relieving depression. It is used for hypochondriac fullness and depression due to stagnation of *qi*.

Warning During medication, wine, pungent and greasy diet are prohibited.

舒冠片

【处方】制何首乌、川芎、黄精（制）、丹参、淫羊藿、红花、五灵脂（醋制）。

【功能主治】养阴活血，益气温阳。用于防治冠心病，心绞痛，动脉粥样硬化，高脂血症及抗血栓。

Preventing Coronary Heart Disease Tablet

Name of Chinese Phonetic Alphabet Shu Guan Pian

Formula Polygoni Multiflori Radix Praeparata, Chuanxiong Rhizoma, Polygonati Rhizoma (prepared), Salviae Miltiorrhizae Radix et Rhizoma, Epimedii Folium, Carthami Flos and Trogopterori Faeces (prepared with vinegar).

Actions and Indications Nourishing *yin*, activating blood, tonifying *qi*, warming *yang*. It is used for preventing coronary heart disease, angina pectoris, atherosclerosis, hyperlipemia and anti-thrombosis.

舒眠胶囊

【处方】酸枣仁、柴胡、白芍、僵蚕、合欢花、蝉蜕、灯心草。

【功能主治】疏肝解郁，宁心安神。用于肝郁伤身所致的失眠症。症见失眠多梦，精神抑郁或急躁易怒，胸胁苦满或胸膈不畅，口苦目眩，舌边尖略红，苔白或微黄，脉弦。

Peaceful Sleep Capsule

Name of Chinese Phonetic Alphabet Shu Mian Jiao Nang

Formula Ziziphi Spinosae Semen, Bupleuri Radix, Paeoniae Radix Alba, Bombyx Batryticatus, Albiziae Flos, Cicadae Periostracum and Junci Medulla.

Actions and Indications Soothing the liver, releasing depression, tranquilizing the mind. It is indicated for insomnia manifested as insomnia, profuse dreaming, depression of spirit, impatience, querulousness, fullness and oppression in chest and hypochondrium, bitter taste in the mouth, dizzy vision, slight red in the margin and tip of tongue, white or slightly yellow tongue fur and string-like pulse.

舒胸胶囊

【处方】三七、红花、川芎。

【功能主治】活血，祛瘀，止痛。用于瘀血阻滞，胸痹心痛；跌打损伤，瘀血肿痛；冠心病、心绞痛、心律失常、软组织挫伤。

【注意】孕妇慎用，热证所致淤血忌用。

Chest-soothing Capsule

Name of Chinese Phonetic Alphabet Shu Xiong Jiao Nang

Formula Notoginseng Radix et Rhizoma, Carthami Flos and Chuanxiong Rhizoma.

Actions and Indications Activating blood, dispelling stasis, alleviating pain. It is used for chest impediment syndrome and cardialgia due to blood-stasis; injury due to fall and strike; swelling and pain due to blood-stasis; also used for coronary heart disease, angina pectoris, arrhythmia and soft tissue injury.

Warning It should be used carefully for pregnant women and is contraindicated for cases with blood-stasis of heat syndrome.

舒筋定痛酒

【处方】乳香（醋炙）、没药（醋炙）、当归、红花、延胡索（醋炙）、香附（醋炙）、骨碎补、血竭、自然铜（煅醋淬）。

【功能主治】舒筋活血，散瘀止痛。用于跌打损伤，扭伤，血瘀肿痛。

【注意】孕妇、肝功能异常及对酒精过敏者忌用；高血压、心脏病患者慎服。

Medicated Wine for Relieving Traumatic Injury

Name of Chinese Phonetic Alphabet Shu Jin Ding Tong Jiu

Formula Olibanum (prepared with vinegar), Myrrha (prepared with vinegar), Angelicae Sinensis Radix, Carthami Flos, Corydalis Rhizoma (prepared with vinegar), Cyperi Rhizoma (prepared with vinegar), Drynariae Rhizoma, Draconis Sanguis and Pyritum (calcined and quenched by vinegar).

Actions and Indications Relaxing sinews, activating blood, dissipating stasis, alleviating pain. It is used for traumatic injury and sprain marked by swelling, pain and blood-stasis.

Warning It is contraindicated for pregnant women, disorder of hepatic function and hypersensitivity of alcohol. The preparation should be used cautiously for cases with hypertension, heart disease.

舒筋活血片

【处方】红花、香附（制）、狗脊（制）、香加皮、络石藤、伸筋草、泽兰叶、槲寄生、鸡血藤、自然铜（煅）。

【功能主治】舒筋活络，活血散瘀。用于筋骨疼痛，肢体拘挛，腰背酸痛，跌打损伤。

【注意】孕妇忌服。

Sinew-relaxing and Blood-activating Tablet

Name of Chinese Phonetic Alphabet Shu Jin Huo Xue Pian

Formula Carthami Flos, Cyperi Rhizoma (prepared), Cibotii Rhizoma(prepared), Periplocae Cortex, Trachelospermi Caulis et Folium, Lycopodii Herba, Lycopi Folium, Visci Herba, Spatholobi Caulis and Pyritum (calcined).

Actions and Indications Relaxing sinews, activating collaterals, activating blood, dissipating stasis. It is used for ostealgia, spasm of limbs, soreness and pain of the waist and back, traumatic injury.

Warning It is contraindicated for pregnant women.

舒筋活血定痛散

【处方】乳香（醋炙）、没药（醋炙）、当归、香附（醋炙）、延胡索（醋炙）、血竭、红花、骨碎补、自然铜（煅醋淬）。

【功能主治】舒筋活血，散瘀止痛。用于跌打损伤，闪腰岔气，伤筋动骨，血瘀肿痛。

【注意】孕妇忌服。

Sinew-relaxing and Pain-relieving Powder

Name of Chinese Phonetic Alphabet Shu Jin Huo Xue Ding Tong San

Formula Olibanum (prepared with vinegar), Myrrha (prepared with vinegar), Angelicae Sinensis Radix, Cyperi Rhizoma (prepared with vinegar), Corydalis Rhizoma (prepared with vinegar), Draconis Sanguis, Carthami Flos, Drynariae Rhizoma and Pyritum (calcined and quenched by vinegar).

Actions and Indications Relaxing sinews, activating blood, dissipating stasis, alleviating pain. It is used for traumatic injury, sudden lumbar sprain with swelling, pain and blood-stasis.

Warning It is contraindicated for pregnant women.

猴头健胃灵胶囊

【处方】猴头菌培养物浸膏、海螵蛸、延胡索（制）、白芍（制）、香附（制）。

【功能主治】舒肝和胃，理气止痛。用于因肝胃不和导致的慢性胃炎及胃、十二指肠溃疡。

Mycelium Hedgehog* Extract Capsule

Name of Chinese Phonetic Alphabet Hou Tou Jian Wei Ling Jiao Nang

Formula Hericii Erinacei Mycelium Extractum, Sepiae Endoconcha, Corydalis Rhizoma (prepared), Paeoniae Radix Alba (perpaerd) and Cyperi Rhizoma (perpaerd).

Actions and Indications Soothing the liver, harmonizing the stomach, regulating *qi* and alleviating pain. It is indicated for chronic gastritis and gastric and duodenal ulcer due to disharmony of the liver and stomach.

* 猴头菌菌丝体

猴头菌片

【处方】猴头菌菌丝体。

【功能主治】益气养血，扶正培本。用于气血病症引起的胃溃疡、十二指肠溃疡、慢性胃炎、萎缩性胃炎。

Mycelium Hedgehog* Tablet

Name of Chinese Phonetic Alphabet Hou Tou Jun Pian

Formula Hericii Erinacei Mycelium.

Actions and Indications Tonifying *qi* and blood, supporting healthy *qi* and strengthening body resistance. It is indicated for gastric ulcer, duodenal ulcer, chronic gastritis and atrophic gastritis due to dual deficiency of *qi* and blood.

*猴头菌菌丝体

痢必灵片

【处方】苦参、白芍、木香。

【功能主治】清热利湿。用于湿热泻痢，热泻，腹痛。

Dysentery-relieving Tablet

Name of Chinese Phonetic Alphabet Li Bi Ling Pian

Formula Sophorae Flavescentis Radix, Paeoniae Radix Alba and Aucklandiae Radix.

Actions and Indications Clearing heat and draining dampness. It is indicated for dysentery due to damp-hcat; diarrhca and abdominal pain.

痢特敏片

【处方】仙鹤草与翻白草的浸膏粉、甲氧苄氨嘧啶。

【功能主治】清热解毒，抗菌止痢。用于急性痢疾、肠炎与腹泻属湿热证者。

【注意】可引起白细胞及血小板减少；孕妇禁用，肝、肾功能不全者慎用；虚寒型痢疾、泄泻患者勿用。

Powerful Tablet for Relieving Dysentery

Name of Chinese Phonetic Alphabet Li Te Min Pian

Formula Agrimoniae Herba and Potentillae Discoloris Herba (powder of dried extract) and Methoxybenzyl Aminopyrimidine.

Actions and Indications Clearing heat and detoxicating, antisepsis and relieving dysentery. It is indicated for acute dysentery, enteritis and diarrhea, attributive to damp-heat syndrome.

Warning The preparation can cause decrease of white cell and platelet. It is contraindicated for pregnant women and should be used carefully for cases with hepatic and renal insufficiency. It is contraindicated for cases with dysentery of deficiency-cold type and diarrhea.

痛风定胶囊

【处方】黄柏、秦艽、赤芍、车前子等。

【功能主治】清热祛风除湿，活血通络定痛。主治痹病中的湿热证。症见关节红肿热痛，伴有发热，汗出不解，口渴喜饮，心烦不安，小便黄，舌质红，苔黄腻，脉滑数。

【注意】服药后不宜立即饮茶；孕妇慎用。

Alleviating Gout Capsule

Name of Chinese Phonetic Alphabet Tong Feng Ding Jiao Nang

Formula Phellodendri Chinensis Cortex, Gentianae Macrophyllae Radix, Paeoniae Radix Rubra, Plantaginis Semen, etc.

Actions and Indications Clearing heat and dispelling wind and dampness, activating blood and dredging collaterals, alleviating pain. It is used for damp-heat syndrome of impediment, manifested as red, swelling and pain of the joints, accompanied by fever, sweating, thirst with the desire to drink, vexation, yellow urine, red tongue, yellow and slimy fur, slippery and rapid pulse.

Warning Patients should not drink tea after medication and it should be used carefully for pregnant women.

痛血康胶囊

【处方】重楼、草乌、金铁锁、化血丹等。

【功能主治】止血镇痛，活血化瘀。用于跌打损伤，外伤出血，以及胃十二指肠溃疡、炎症引起的轻度出血。

【注意】服药期间忌食蚕豆、鱼类及酸冷食物；在医生指导下内服；心、肝、肾功能有严重损害者，不可内服。

Paris* Capsule for Relieving Bleeding

Name of Chinese Phonetic Alphabet Tong Xue

Kang Jiao Nang

Formula Paridis Rhizoma, Aconiti Kusnezoffii Radix, Psammosilenes Radix, Ligulariae Lapathifoliae Radix et Folium, etc.

Actions and Indications Relieving bleeding, settling pain, activating blood and resolving stasis. It is used for injury due to fall and strike; traumatic bleeding, mild hemorrhage due to gastroduodenal ulcer and inflammation.

Warning During medication, broad bean, fish, sour and cold foods should be avoided; during oral medication, patients should follow physician's advice; it is contraindicated for oral use in cases with severe cardial, hepatic or renal dysfunction.

* 重楼

痛经口服液

【处方】当归、川芎、白芍、香附（制）、乌药。

【功能主治】行气活血，调经止痛。用于气滞血瘀引起痛经症的经前、经期腹部胀痛或痉挛性疼痛，以及经期伴头痛。

Dysmenorrhea-relieving Oral Liquid

Name of Chinese Phonetic Alphabet Tong Jing Kou Fu Ye

Formula Angelicae Sinensis Radix, Chuanxiong Rhizoma, Paeoniae Radix Alba, Cyperi Rhizoma (prepared) and Linderae Radix.

Actions and Indications Promoting *qi* moving, activating blood, regulating menstruation, alleviating pain. It is used for premenstrual abdominal pain or spasmodic pain, abdominal pain during menstrual period, or headache during menstrual period due to *qi*-stagnation and blood-stasis.

痛经宝冲剂

【处方】红花、当归、肉桂、三棱、莪术、丹参、五灵脂、木香、延胡索（醋制）。

【功能主治】温经化瘀，理气止痛。用于妇女痛经。

Dysmenorrhea-relieving Soluble Granules

Name of Chinese Phonetic Alphabet Tong Jing Bao Chong Ji

Formula Carthami Flos, Angelicae Sinensis Radix, Cinnamomi Cortex, Sparganii Rhizoma, Curcumae Rhizoma, Salviae Miltiorrhizae Radix et Rhizoma, Trogopterori Faeces, Aucklandiae Radix and Corydalis Rhizoma (prepared with vinegar).

Actions and Indications Warming meridians, resolving stasis, regulating *qi*, alleviating pain. It is indicated for dysmenorrhea.

湿毒清胶囊

【处方】地黄、当归、丹参、蝉蜕、苦参、白鲜皮、甘草、黄芩、土茯苓。

【功能主治】养血润燥，化湿解毒，祛风止痒。用于皮肤瘙痒症属血虚证。

Relieving Cutaneous Pruritus Capsule

Name of Chinese Phonetic Alphabet Shi Du Qing Jiao Nang

Formula Rehmanniae Radix, Angelicae Sinensis Radix, Salviae Miltiorrhizae Radix et Rhizoma, Cicadae Periostracum, Sophorae Flavescentis Radix, Dictamni Cortex, Glycyrrhizae Radix et Rhizoma, Scutellariae Radix and Smilacis Glabrae Rhizoma.

Actions and Indications Nourishing blood and moistening dryness, resolving dampness and detoxicating, dispelling wind and relieving itching. It is indicated for cutaneous pruritus attributed to blood-deficiency syndrome.

湿热痹冲剂

【处方】苍术、忍冬藤、地龙、连翘、黄柏、薏苡仁、防风、川牛膝、粉萆薢、桑枝、防己、威灵仙。

【功能主治】祛风除湿，清热消肿，通络定痛。

用于湿热痹证，其症状为肌肉或关节红肿热痛，有沉重感，步履艰难，发热，口渴不欲饮，小便黄。

Relieving Damp-heat Impediment Syndrome Soluble Granules

Name of Chinese Phonetic Alphabet Shi Re Bi Chong Ji

Formula Atractylodis Rhizoma, Lonicerae Japonicae Caulis, Pheretima, Forsythiae Fructus, Phellodendri Chinensis Cortex, Coicis Semen, Saposhnikoviae Radix, Cyathulae Radix, Dioscoreae Hypoglaucae Rhizoma, Mori Ramulus, Stephaniae Tetrandrae Radix and Clematidis Radix et Rhizoma.

Actions and Indications Dispelling wind and dampness, clearing heat and dispersing swelling, dredging collaterals, and alleviating pain. It is indicated for damp-heat impediment syndrome, manifested as red, swelling and pain of the muscle or joint, heavy sensation of the body, difficulty in walk, fever, thirst without desire to drink and yellow urine.

温肾全鹿丸

【处方】人参、鹿角胶、补骨脂（盐炒）、黄柏、巴戟天（制）、锁阳、川牛膝、五味子（醋炙）、小茴香（盐炒）、老鹳草膏、鹿茸、菟丝子、杜仲（炭）、黄芪（蜜炙）、香附（醋炙）、牛乳、大青盐、龙眼肉、冬虫夏草、秋石、楮实子、鹿角、茯苓、胡芦巴（炒）、鹿鞭、天冬、麦冬、狗肾、熟地黄、甘草、牛膝、琥珀、鲜鹿肉（带骨）、没药（醋炙）、益母草膏、枸杞子、党参、鹿尾、肉苁蓉（酒炙）、远志肉（甘草水炙）、花椒、覆盆子、紫河车、川芎、白术（麸炒）、当归、陈皮、沉香、红花、地黄、木香、砂仁、续断、黄芩、山药、木瓜、酸枣仁、酸枣仁（炒）、桑白皮（蜜炙）。

【功能主治】温肾固精，益气养血。用于肾阳虚弱，气血亏损引起的头晕健忘，目暗耳鸣，腰膝酸软，倦怠嗜卧，阳痿滑精，宫寒带下，滑胎小产。

Deer Bolus for Warming Kidney

Name of Chinese Phonetic Alphabet Wen Shen Quan Lu Wan

Formula Ginseng Radix et Rhizoma, Cervi Cornus Colla, Psoraleae Fructus (fried with salt), Phellodendri Chinensis Cortex, Morindae Officinalis Radix (prepared), Cynomorii Caulis Carnosus, Cythulae Radix, Schisandrae Chiensis Fructus (prepared with vinegar), Foeniculi Fructus (fried with salt), Geranii Herba Extractum, Cervi Cornu Pantotrichum, Cuscutae Semen, Eucommiae Cortex (carbonated), Astragali Radix (prepared with honey), Cyperi Rhizoma (prepared with vinegar), Vaccae Lac, Halitum, Longan Arillus, Cordyceps, Hominis Urinea Sedimentum et Sal Praeparata, Broussonetiae Fructus, Cervi Cornu, Poria, Trigonellae Semen (fried), Cervi Penis, Asparagi Radix, Ophiopogonis Radix, Canis Ren, Rehmanniae Radix Praeparata, Glycyrrhizae Radix et Rhizoma, Achyranthis Bidentatae Radix, Succinum, Cervi Caro Dulcis (bearing with bone), Myrrha (prepared with vinegar), Leonuri Extractum, Lycii Fructus, Codonopsis Radix, Cervi Cauda, Cistanches Caulis Carnosus (prepared with wine), Polygalae Radix (demotus lignum prepared with licorice root water), Zanthoxyli Pericarpium, Rubi Fructus, Hominis Placenta, Chuanxiong Rhizoma, Atractylodis Macrocephalae Rhizoma (fried with bran), Angelicae Sinensis Radix, Citri Reticulatae Pericarpium, Aquilariae Lignum Resinatum, Carthami Flos, Rehmanniae Radix, Aucklandiae Radix, Amomi Fructus, Dipsaci Radix, Scutellariae Radix, Dioscoreae Rhizoma, Chaenomelis Fructus, Ziziphi Spinosae Semen, Ziziphi Spinosae Semen (fried) and Mori Cortex (prepared with honey).

Actions and Indications Warming the kidney, arresting essence, tonifying *qi* and nourishing blood. It is use for dizziness, amnesia, dim eyesight, tinnitus, soreness and weakness of the waist and knees, tiredness, somnolence, impotence, spermatorrhea, uterus-coldness, white vaginal discharge and habitual abortion due to deficiency of kidney-*yang* and depletion of *qi* and blood.

温胃舒胶囊

【处方】党参、附子（制）、黄芪（炙）、肉桂、山药、肉苁蓉（制）、白术（炒）、山楂（炒）、乌梅、砂仁、陈皮、补骨脂。

【功能主治】扶正固本，温胃养胃，行气止痛。用于慢性萎缩性胃炎、慢性胃炎所引起的胃脘冷痛，腹胀，嗳气，纳差，畏寒，无力。

【注意】胃大出血时忌用。

Chronic-gastritis-relieving Capsule

Name of Chinese Phonetic Alphabet Wen Wei Shu Jiao Nang

Formula Codonopsis Radix, Aconiti Lateralis Radix Praeparata, Astragali Radix (prepared), Cinnamomi Cortex, Dioscoreae Rhizoma, Cistanches Caulis Carnosus (prepared), Atractylodis Macrocephalae Rhizoma (fried), Crataegi Fructus (fried), Mume Fructus, Amomi Fructus, Citri Reticulatae Pericarpium and Psoraleae Fructus.

Actions and Indications Reinforcing the healthy *qi*, warming and nourishing the stomach, moving *qi*, alleviating pain. It is indicated for chronic atrophic gastritis and chronic gastritis marked by cold pain in stomach duct, abdominal fullness, eructation, anorexia, fear of cold and fatigue.

Warning It is contraindicated for massive hemorrhage of the stomach.

渴乐宁胶囊

【处方】本品为黄芪、地黄等经加工制成的胶囊剂。

【功能主治】益气养阴生津。用于气阴两虚型消渴病（非胰岛素依赖型糖尿病），症见口渴多饮，五心烦热，乏力多汗，心慌气短。

Relieving Non-insulin-dependent Diabetes Capsule

Name of Chinese Phonetic Alphabet Ke Le Ning Jiao Nang

Formula Astragali Radix, Rehmanniae Radix, etc.

Actions and Indications Tonifying *qi* and nourishing *yin* to promote fluid-engendering. It is indicated for non-insulin-dependent diabetes attributed to dual deficiency of *qi* and *yin*, and manifested as thirst, polydipsia, vexing heat in the chest, palms and soles, fatigue, hyperhidrosis, fluster and shortness of breath.

溃平宁冲剂

【处方】大黄浸膏、白及、延胡索粗碱。

【功能主治】止血，止痛，收敛。用于胃溃疡、十二指肠溃疡，合并上消化道出血症。

Relieving Gastric Ulcer Soluble Granules

Name of Chinese Phonetic Alphabet Kui Ping Ning Chong Ji

Formula Rhei Extractum, Bletillae Rhizoma and Corydaline.

Actions and Indications Relieving bleeding, alleviating pain and astringing. It is indicated for gastric ulcer, duodenal ulcer complicated with hemorrhage of upper digestive tract.

溃疡宁胶囊

【处方】青黛、象牙屑、蚕茧（炭）、人指甲（滑石烫）、珍珠、珍珠层粉、牛黄、冰片。

【功能主治】清热解毒，生肌止痛。用于十二指肠球部溃疡，胃溃疡，糜烂性胃炎属胃热肝郁证者。

【注意】服药后不再进食进水。忌食辛辣物。

Relieving Gastric Ulcer Capsule

Name of Chinese Phonetic Alphabet Kui Yang Ning Jiao Nang

Formula Indigo Naturalis, Elephantis Frustillum, Bombycis Incunabulum (carbonated), Hominis Unguis (scalded with talc), Margarita, Margaritae Concha Strati Pulvis, Bovis Calculus and Borneolum Syntheticum.

Actions and Indications Clearing heat and detoxicating, promoting tissue regeneration and alleviating pain. It is indicated for duodenal bulbar ulcer, gastric ulcer, erosive gastritis attributive to stomach-heat and liver depression syndrome.

Warning Foods and water are prohibited after medication. Pungent foods are prohibited.

溃疡胶囊

【处方】瓦楞子、鸡蛋壳、陈皮、枯矾、水红花子、珍珠粉、仙鹤草。

【功能主治】制酸止痛，生肌收敛。用于胃脘疼痛，呕恶反酸，胃及十二指肠溃疡。

Gastric and Duodenal Ulcer Relieving Capsule

Name of Chinese Phonetic Alphabet Kui Yang Jiao Nang

Formula Arcae Concha, Galli Ovi Chorion, Citri Reticulatae Pericarpium, Alumen Usta, Polygoni Orientalis Fructus, Magaritae Pulvis and Agrimoniae Herba.

Actions and Indications Antiacid, alleviating pain, promoting tissue regeneration, astringent. It is used for stomach duct pain, vomiting, nausea, acid regurgitation, gastric and duodenal ulcer.

滋心阴口服液

【处方】本品为麦冬、赤芍、北沙参、三七等药经加工制成的口服液。

【功能主治】滋养心阴，活血止痛。用于心悸、失眠，五心烦热，少苔质红，脉细数等心阴不足型胸痹心痛。

Oral Liquid of Enriching Heart

Name of Chinese Phonetic Alphabet Zi Xin Yin Kou Fu Ye

Formula Ophiopogonis Radix, Paeoniae Radix Rubra, Glehniae Radix, Notoginseng Radix et Rhizoma, etc.

Actions and Indications Enriching heart-*yin*, activating blood and alleviating pain. It is indicated for chest impediment syndrome and cardialgia due to insufficiency of heart-*yin* and marked by palpitation, insomnia, vexing heat in the chest, palms and soles, red tongue with few tongue fur, fine and rapid pulse.

滋肾育胎丸

【处方】菟丝子、砂仁、熟地黄、人参、桑寄生、阿胶（炒）、何首乌、艾叶、巴戟天、白术、党参、鹿角霜、枸杞子、续断、杜仲。

【功能主治】补肾健脾，益气培元，养血安胎，强壮身体。用于脾肾两虚，冲任不固所致的滑胎，对习惯性流产和先兆性流产有防治作用。

【注意】孕妇禁房事。

Nourishing Kidney Pill for Preventing Abortion

Name of Chinese Phonetic Alphabet Zi Shen Yu Tai Wan

Formula Cuscutae Semen, Amomi Fructus, Rehmanniae Radix Praeparata, Ginseng Radix et Rhizoma, Taxilli Herba, Asini Corii Colla (fried), Polygoni Multiflori Radix, Artemisiae Argyi Folium, Morindae Officinalis Radix, Atractylodis Macrocephalae Rhizoma, Codonopsis Radix, Cervi Cornu Degelatinatum, Lycci Fructus, Dipsaci Radix and Eucommiae Cortex.

Actions and Indications Tonifying the kidney and fortifying the spleen, enriching source *qi*, nourishing blood, preventing abortion. It is indicated for preventing and treating the habitual abortion, threatened abortion due to dual deficiency of the spleen and kidney, and insecurity of the thoroughfare and conception vessels.

Warning Sexual intercourse is prohibited for pregnant women.

普乐安胶囊

【处方】本品为油菜花花粉经加工制成的胶囊。

【功能主治】补肾固本。用于肾气不固，腰膝酸软，尿后余沥或失禁，及慢性前列腺炎，前列腺增生具有上述症候者。

Tonifying Kidney Capsule for Relieving Prostatitis

Name of Chinese Phonetic Alphabet Pu Le An Jiao Nang

Formula Brassicae Campestris Pollen.

Actions and Indications Tonifying the kidney. It is used for soreness and weakness of the waist and knees, dripping urination or urinary incontinence, and also used for chronic prostatitis and hyperplasia of prostate with the above mentioned symptoms.

寒热痹冲剂

【处方】桂枝、防风、白芍、知母、附子、干姜、麻黄、白术、甘草、地龙。

【功能主治】散寒清热，和营定痛。用于肌肉关节疼痛，以及风湿和类风湿性关节炎见上述证候者。

Relieving Cold-heat Impediment Soluble Granules

Name of Chinese Phonetic Alphabet Han Re Bi Chong Ji

Formula Cinnamomi Ramulus, Saposhnikoviae Radix, Paeoniae Radix Alba, Anemarrhenae Rhizoma, Aconiti Lateralis Radix Praeparata, Zingiberis Rhizoma, Ephedrae Herba, Atractylodis Macrocephalae Rhizoma, Glycyrrhizae Radix et Rhizoma and Pheretima.

Actions and Indications Dissipating cold and clearing heat, harmonizing the nutrient and alleviating pain. It is indicated for pain of muscles and joints, and rheumatic or rheumatoid arthritis with the above mentioned symptoms.

寒湿痹片

【处方】附子（制）、制川乌、黄芪、桂枝、麻黄、白术（炒）、当归、白芍、威灵仙、木瓜、细辛、甘草（制）。

【功能主治】祛寒除湿，温通经络。用于肢体关节疼痛，疲困或肿胀，局部畏寒，风湿性关节炎。

【注意】孕妇忌服，身热高热者禁用。

Relieving Cold-damp Impediment Tablet

Name of Chinese Phonetic Alphabet Han Shi Bi Pian

Formula Aconiti Lateralis Radix Praeparata, Aconiti Radix Cocta, Astragali Radix, Cinnamomi Ramulus, Ephedrae Herba, Atractylodis Macrocephalae Rhizoma (fried), Angelicae Sinensis Radix, Paeoniae Radix Alba, Clematidis Radix et Rhizoma, Chaenomelis Fructus, Asari Radix et Rhizoma and Glycyrrhizae Radix et Rhizoma (prepared).

Actions and Indications Dispelling cold and dampness, warming and dredging meridians and collaterals. It is indicated for pain of the limbs and joints, tiredness or swelling, local fear of cold and rheumatic arthritis.

Warning It is contraindicated for pregnant women and cases with high fever.

强力天麻杜仲胶囊

【处方】天麻、羌活、制草乌、当归、附子（制）、独活、藁本、川牛膝、玄参、地黄、槲寄生、杜仲（盐制）。

【功能主治】散风活血，舒筋止痛。用于中风引起的筋脉掣痛，肢体麻木，行走不便，腰腿酸痛，头痛头昏。

Gastrodia* and Gutta-percha-tree** Capsule

Name of Chinese Phonetic Alphabet Qiang Li Tian Ma Du Zhong Jiao Nang

Formula Gastrodiae Rhizoma, Notopterygii Rhizoma et Radix, Aconiti Kusnezoffii Radix Cocta, Angelicae Sinensis Radix, Aconiti Lateralis Radix Praeparata, Angelicae Pubescentis Radix, Ligustici Rhizoma et Radix, Cyathulae Radix, Scrophulariae

Radix, Rehmanniae Radix, Visci Herba and Eucommiae Cortex (prepared with salt).

Actions and Indications Dissipating wind, activating blood, relaxing sinews, alleviating pain. It is used for pain of sinews, numbness of extremities, difficult walking, soreness and pain of the waist and legs, headache and dizziness due to apoplexy.

* 天麻 ** 杜仲

强力枇杷露

【处方】枇杷叶、罂粟壳、百部、白前、桑白皮、桔梗、薄荷脑。

【功能主治】养阴敛肺，镇咳祛痰。用于久咳劳嗽，支气管炎。

Loquat Leaf* Oral Liquid

Name of Chinese Phonetic Alphabet Qiang Li Pi Pa Lu

Formula Eriobotryae Folium, Papaveris Pericarpium, Stemonae Radix, Cynanchi Stauntonii Rhizoma et Radix, Mori Cortex, Platycodonis Radix and Menthol.

Actions and Indications Nourishing *yin*, constraining the lung, relieving cough, dispelling phlegm. It is indicated for chronic cough, bronchitis.

* 枇杷叶

强心丸

【处方】当归、紫河车、阿胶、牡蛎（煅）、熟地黄、麦冬、党参、白芍、黄芩、陈皮、龙骨（煅）、枸杞子、龙眼肉、酸枣仁（炒）、蒺藜（盐炙）、女贞子（酒炙）、地锦草、鹿角霜、黄芪（蜜炙）、白术（麸炒）、地黄、天冬、远志（甘草炙）、丹参、石斛、人参、黄柏、甘草（蜜炙）、乌梅、何首乌、菟丝子、木蝴蝶、仙鹤草、五味子（醋炙）、墨旱莲、茯神、柴胡、肉桂、白附片、磁朱丸、玉竹、知母。

【功能主治】滋阴补气，强心安神。用于气血虚弱，虚火上升引起的健忘失眠，心跳气短，惊悸不安，遗精盗汗，目暗耳鸣，腰酸腿软，午后发热，肢体倦怠。

【注意】孕妇忌服。

Cardiotonic Pill

Name of Chinese Phonetic Alphabet Qiang Xin Wan

Formula Angelicae Sinensis Radix, Hominis Placenta, Asini Corii Colla, Ostreae Concha (calcined), Rehmanniae Radix Praeparata, Ophiopogonis Radix, Codonopsis Radix, Paeoniae Radix Alba, Scutellariae Radix, Citri Reticulatae Pericarpium, Draconis Os (calcined), Lycii Fructus, Longan Arillus, Ziziphi Spinosae Semen (fried), Tribuli Fructus (prepared with salt), Ligustri Lucidi Fructus (prepared with wine), Euphorbiae Humifusae Herba, Cervi Cornu Degelatinatum, Astragali Radix (prepared with honey), Atractylodis Macrocephalae Rhizoma (fried with bran), Rehmanniae Radix, Asparagi Radix, Polygalae Radix (prepared with licorice root), Salviae Miltiorrhizae Radix et Rhizoma, Dendrobii Caulis, Ginseng Radix et Rhizoma, Phellodendri Chinensis Cortex, Glycyrrhizae Radix et Rhizoma (prepared with honey), Mume Fructus, Polygoni Multiflori Radix, Cuscutae Semen, Oroxyli Semen, Agrimoniae Herba, Schisandrae Chinensis Fructus (prepared with vinegar), Ecliptae Herba, Poria Sclerotium Circum Pini Radicem, Bupleuri Radix, Cinnamomi Cortex, Typhonii Rhizoma (sliced), Magnetitum and Cinnabaris Pill, Polygonati Odorati Rhizoma and Anemarrhenae Rhizoma.

Actions and Indications Enriching *yin*, tonifying *qi*, cardiotonic and tranquilizing the mind. It is indicated for amnesia, insomnia, palpitation, shortness of breath, restlessness, nocturnal emission, night sweating, dim vision, tinnitus, soreness of the waist and weakness of the legs, afternoon fever and tiredness due to dual deficiency of *qi* and blood and deficiency-fire flaming upward.

Warning It is contraindicated for pregnant women.

强阳宝肾丸

【处方】淫羊藿（羊油炙）、阳起石、肉苁蓉、胡芦巴（盐水炙）、补骨脂（盐水炙）、五味子（醋制）、沙苑子、蛇床子、覆盆子、韭菜子、芡实（麸炒）、肉桂、小茴香（盐水炙）、茯苓、远志（甘草制）。

【功能主治】补肾壮阳。用于肾阳不足引起的精神疲倦，阳痿遗精，腰酸腿软，腰腹冷痛。

Tonifying Kidney-*yang* Bolus

Name of Chinese Phonetic Alphabet Qiang Yang Bao Shen Wan

Formula Epimedii Folium (prepared with sheep suet), Tremolitum, Cistanches Caulis Carnosus, Trigonellae Semen (prepared with salt water), Psoraleae Fructus (prepared with salt water), Schisandrae Chinensis Fructus (prepared with vinegar), Astragali Complanati Semen, Cnidii Fructus, Rubi Fructus, Allii Tuberosi Semen, Euryales Semen (fried with bran), Cinnamomi Cortex, Foeniculi Fructus (prepared with salt water), Poria and Polygalae Radix (prepared with licorice root).

Actions and Indications Tonifying kidney-*yang*. It is used for lassitude of spirit, impotence, nocturnal emission, soreness of the waist and weakness of the legs, cold-pain of waist and abdomen due to insufficiency of kidney-*yang*.

强肝糖浆

【处方】茵陈、板蓝根、当归、白芍、丹参、郁金、黄芪、党参、泽泻、黄精、地黄、山药、山楂、六神曲、秦艽、甘草。

【功能主治】清热利湿，补脾养血，益气解郁。用于慢性肝炎，早期肝硬化，脂肪肝，中毒性肝炎。

Strengthening Liver Syrup

Name of Chinese Phonetic Alphabet Qiang Gan Tang Jiang

Formula Artemisiae Scopariae Herba, Isatidis Radix, Angelicae Sinensis Radix, Paeoniae Radix Alba, Salviae Miltiorrhizae Radix et Rhizoma, Curcumae Radix, Astragali Radix, Codonopsis Radix, Alismatis Rhizoma, Polygonati Rhizoma, Rehmanniae Radix, Dioscoreae Rhizoma, Crataegi Fructus, Medicata Massa Fermentata, Gentianae Macrophyllae Radix and Glycyrrhizae Radix et Rhizoma.

Actions and Indications Clearing heat and draining dampness, tonifying the spleen and nourishing blood, replenishing *qi* to relieve depression. It is indicated for chronic hepatitis, early stage of cirrhosis, fatty liver and toxic hepatitis.

强肾片

【处方】鹿茸、山药、山茱萸、熟地黄、枸杞子、丹参、补骨脂、牡丹皮、桑椹、益母草、茯苓、泽泻、杜仲（炙）、人参茎叶总皂苷。

【功能主治】补肾填精，益气壮阳，扶正固本。用于肾虚水肿、腰痛、遗精、阳痿、早泄。亦可用于属肾虚证的慢性肾炎和久治不愈的肾盂肾炎。

Tonifying Kidney Tablet

Name of Chinese Phonetic Alphabet Qiang Shen Pian

Formula Cervi Cornu Pantotrichum, Dioscoreae Rhizoma, Corni Fructus, Rehmanniae Radix Praeparata, Lycii Fructus, Salviae Miltiorrhizae Radix et Rhizoma, Psoraleae Fructus, Moutan Cortex, Mori Fructus, Leonuri Herba, Poria, Alismatis Rhizoma, Eucommiae Cortex (prepared) and Total Saponin of Ginseng Folium et Caulis.

Actions and Indications Tonifying the kidney and nourishing essence, replenishing *qi* and strengthening *yang*, reinforcing and securing the healthy *qi*. It is indicated for edema, lumbago, spermatorrhea, impotence and prospermia due to kidney-deficiency; also for chronic nephritis and pyelonephritis attributive to kidney-deficiency syndrome.

强筋英雄丸

【处方】制川乌、制草乌、石斛、半夏（制）、川牛膝、天南星（制）、党参、木瓜、钩藤、续断、陈皮、制马钱子。

【功能主治】祛风除痰，强筋壮骨。用于瘫痪，筋骨疼痛，风湿麻木，腰膝萎软。

【注意】孕妇忌用。

Powerful Pill for Strengthening Bone

Name of Chinese Phonetic Alphabet Qiang Jin Ying Xiong Wan

Formula Aconiti Radix Cocta, Aconiti Kusnezoffii Radix Cocta, Dendrobii Caulis, Pinelliae Rhizoma (prepared), Cyathulae Radix, Arisaematis Rhizoma (prepared), Codonopsis Radix, Chaenomelis Fructus, Uncariae Ramulus cum Uncis, Dipsaci Radix, Citri Reticulatae Pericarpium and Strychni Semen Praeparata.

Actions and Indications Dispelling wind and eliminating phlegm, strengthening sinews and bone. It is indicated for paralysis, ostealgia, numbess and wilting of the waist and knees.

Warning It is contraindicated for pregnant women.

疏风定痛丸

【**处方**】马钱子（制）、麻黄、乳香（醋制）、没药（醋制）、千年健、自然铜（煅）、地枫皮、桂枝、牛膝、木瓜、甘草、杜仲（盐水制）、防风、羌活、独活。

【**功能主治**】祛风散寒，活血止痛。用于风寒湿痹，四肢麻木，腰腿疼痛，跌打损伤，瘀血作痛。

【**注意**】体弱者慎服，孕妇忌服。

Relieving Impediment Syndrome Bolus

Name of Chinese Phonetic Alphabet Shu Feng Ding Tong Wan

Formula Strychni Semen (prepared), Ephedrae Herba, Olibanum (prepared with vinegar), Myrrha (prepared with vinegar), Homalomenae Rhizoma, Pyritum (calcined), Illicii Cortex, Cinnamomi Ramulus, Achyranthis Bidentatae Radix, Chaenomelis Fructus, Glycyrrhizae Radix et Rhizoma, Eucommiae Cortex (prepared with salt water), Saposhnikoviae Radix, Notopterygii Rhizoma et Radix and Angelicae Pubescentis Radix.

Actions and Indications Dispelling wind and cold, activating blood and alleviating pain. It is used for wind-cold-damp impediment syndrome, marked by numbness of the limbs, pain of the waist and legs, traumatic injury and pain due to blood-stasis.

Warning It should be used carefully for physical debility and is contraindicated for pregnant women.

疏血通注射液

【**处方**】水蛭、地龙。

【**功能主治**】活血化瘀、通经活络。用于瘀血阻络所致的缺血性中风病中经络急性期，症见半身不遂、口舌歪斜、语言謇涩。适用于急性期脑梗塞见上述表现者。

【**注意**】为避免发生过敏反应，使用前应做皮试。

Injection of Leech* and Earthworm**

Name of Chinese Phonetic Alphabet Shu Xue Tong Zhu She Ye

Formula Hirudo and Pheretima.

Actions and Indications Activating blood, resolving stasis, dredging meridians and activating collaterals. It is indicated for acute stage of ischemic stroke due to stagnation of blood-stasis in collaterals, and manifested as hemiparalysis, deviated eyes and mouth, dysphasia, and also used for acute stage of cerebral infarction with the above mentioned manifestations.

Warning For preventing the allergic reaction, the skin test should be applied first.

* 水蛭 ** 地龙

疏痛安涂膜剂

【**处方**】透骨草、伸筋草、红花、薄荷脑。

【**功能主治**】舒筋活血，消肿止痛。用于头面部神经痛，面神经麻痹，急、慢性软组织损伤。

【**注意**】外用药。

Relieving Facial Neuralgia Pigmentum

Name of Chinese Phonetic Alphabet Shu Tong An Tu Mo Ji

Formula Speranskiae Tuberculatae Herba,

Lycopodii Herba, Carthami Flos and Menthol.

Actions and Indications Relaxing sinews, activating blood, reducing swelling, alleviating pain. It is used for facial neuralgia, facial paralysis, acute, chronic soft tissue injury.

Warning It is for external use only.

十三画

感冒丸

【处方】麻黄、紫苏叶、苦杏仁、薄荷、前胡、金银花、石膏、菊花、黄芩、甘草、桔梗、桑叶。

【功能主治】清热止咳，宣肺平喘。用于感冒，头痛发热、鼻流清涕，咳嗽，气逆喘急。

Common-cold-relieving Bolus

Name of Chinese Phonetic Alphabet Gan Mao Wan

Formula Ephedrae Herba, Perillae Folium, Armeniacae Semen Amarum, Menthae Haplocalycis Herba, Peucedani Radix, Lonicerae Japonicae Flos, Gypsum Fibrosum, Chrysanthemi Flos, Scutellariae Radix, Glycyrrhizae Radix et Rhizoma, Platycodonis Radix and Mori Folium.

Actions and Indications Clearing heat and relieving cough, diffusing the lung to calm panting. It is indicated for common cold, marked by headache, fever, clear nasal discharge, cough, dyspnea.

感冒止咳糖浆

【处方】柴胡、金银花、葛根、青蒿、连翘、黄芩、桔梗、苦杏仁、薄荷脑。

【功能主治】清热解表，止咳化痰。用于感冒发热，头痛鼻塞，伤风咳嗽，咽喉肿痛，四肢怠倦，流行性感冒。

Common-cold-relieving Syrup

Name of Chinese Phonetic Alphabet Gan Mao Zhi Ke Tang Jiang

Formula Bupleuri Radix, Lonicerae Japonicae Flos, Puerariae Lobatae Radix, Artemisiae Annuae Herba, Forsythiae Fructus, Scutellariae Radix, Platycodonis Radix, Armeniacae Semen Amarum and Menthol.

Actions and Indications Clearing heat and releasing the exterior, relieving cough and resolving phlegm. It is indicated for common cold, marked by fever, headache, nasal congestion, cough, sore-throat, tiredness of the limbs, and also used for influenza.

感冒软胶囊

【处方】羌活、麻黄、桂枝、荆芥穗、防风、白芷、川芎、石菖蒲、葛根、薄荷、当归、苦杏仁、黄芩、桔梗。

【功能主治】散风解热。用于外感风寒引起的头痛身热，鼻塞流涕，恶寒无汗，骨节酸痛，咽喉肿痛。

Relieving Common Cold Soft Capsule

Name of Chinese Phonetic Alphabet Gan Mao Ruan Jiao Nang

Formula Notopterygii Rhizoma et Radix, Ephedrae Herba, Cinnamomi Ramulus, Schizonepetae Spica, Saposhnikoviae Radix, Angelicae Dahuricae Radix, Chuanxiong Rhizoma, Acori Tatarinowii Rhizoma, Puerariae Lobatae Radix, Menthae Haplocalycis Herba, Angelicae Sinensis Radix, Armeniacae Semen Amarum, Scutellariae Radix and Platycodonis Radix.

Actions and Indications Dispersing wind and releasing heat. It is used for headache and fever, stuffy nose, rhinorrhea, aversion to cold, anhidrosis, soreness and pain of the bones and joints and sore-throat due to exogenous wind-cold.

感冒退热冲剂

【处方】大青叶、板蓝根、连翘、拳参。

【功能主治】清热解毒。用于上呼吸道感染，急性扁桃体炎，咽喉炎。

Common Cold (Exterior Excess Type) Relieving Soluble Granules

Name of Chinese Phonetic Alphabet Gan Mao Tui Re Chong Ji

Formula Isatidis Folium, Isatidis Radix, Forsythiae Fructus and Bistortae Rhizoma.

Actions and Indications Clearing heat and detoxicating. It is indicated for upper respiratory infection, acute tonsillitis and laryngopharyngitis.

感冒清热口服液

【处方】荆芥穗、薄荷、防风、苦地丁、紫苏叶、葛根、桔梗、苦杏仁、白芷、柴胡、芦根。

【功能主治】疏风散寒，解表清热。用于风寒感冒，头痛发热，恶寒身痛，鼻流清涕，咳嗽咽干。

Relieving Common Cold Oral Liquid

Name of Chinese Phonetic Alphabet Gan Mao Qing Re Kou Fu Ye

Formula Schizonepetae Spica, Menthae Haplocalycis Herba, Saposhnikoviae Radix, Corydalis Bungeanae Herba, Perillae Folium, Puerariae Lobatae Radix, Platycodonis Radix, Armeniacae Semen Amarum, Angelicae Dahuricae Radix, Bupleuri Radix and Phragmitis Rhizoma.

Actions and Indications Dispersing wind and dissipating cold, releasing the exterior, clearing heat. It is used for common cold (wind-cold) type, marked by headache, fever, aversion to cold, generalized pain, clear nasal discharge, cough, dry throat.

感冒舒冲剂

【处方】大青叶、连翘、荆芥、防风、薄荷、牛蒡子、桔梗、白芷、甘草。

【功能主治】疏风清热，发表宣肺。用于感冒所致的头痛体困，发热恶寒，鼻塞流涕，咳嗽咽痛等症。

Soluble Granules for Relieving Common Cold

Name of Chinese Phonetic Alphabet Gan Mao Shu Chong Ji

Formula Isatidis Folium, Forsythiae Fructus, Schizonepetae Herba, Saposhnikoviae Radix, Menthae Haplocalycis Herba, Arctii Fructus, Platycodonis Radix, Angelicae Dahuricae Radix and Glycyrrhizae Radix et Rhizoma.

Actions and Indications Dispersing wind and clearing heat, effusing exterior and diffusing the lung. It is indicated for common cold, marked by headache, tiredness, fever, aversion to cold, nasal congestion, rhinorrhea, cough and sore-throat.

雷公藤浸膏片

【处方】本品为雷公藤提取物制成的片剂。

【功能主治】具有抗炎及免疫抑制作用。用于治疗类风湿性关节炎。

【注意】本品有一定的毒副作用，孕妇忌用，肝肾功能不全者慎用或忌用。

Tablet of Tripterygium* Extract

Name of Chinese Phonetic Alphabet Lei Gong Teng Jin Gao Pian

Formula Tripterygii Wilfordii Extractum.

Actions and Indications The preparation possesses the effect of anti-inflammation and immunosuppression. It is indicated for rheumatoid arthritis.

Warning This product has some toxic and side effects. It should be used carefully or contraindicated for pregnant women and cases with insufficiency of the liver and kidney.

* 雷公藤

雷龙片

【处方】附子（制）、肉桂、狗脊、淫羊藿、黑豆。

【功能主治】补肾壮阳，温经益气，强筋健骨。用于腰膝酸软，疲劳无力，心悸气短。主要用于大运动量消耗引起的疲乏无力，四肢末梢发冷等“肾阳虚”症候群。

【注意】阴虚阳亢者及外感热证者禁用。

Leilong Tablet for Strengthening Sinews and Bone

Name of Chinese Phonetic Alphabet Lei Long Pian

Formula Aconiti Lateralis Radix Praeparata, Cinnamomi Cortex, Cibotii Rhizoma, Epimedii Folium and Sojae Semen Nigrum.

Actions and Indications Tonifying kidney-*yang*, warming the meridians, tonifying *qi*, strengthening the sinews and bone. It is used for soreness and weakness of the waist and knees, tiredness, fatigue, palpitation and shortness of breath. It is mainly used for tiredness, terminal cold of limbs due to heavy load and deficiency of kidney-*yang* syndrome.

Warning It is contraindicated for *yin*-deficiency with *yang* hyperactivity and heat-syndrome with external contraction.

蛾苓丸

【处方】本品为雌性蚕蛾等经加工制成的水丸。

【功能主治】扶正培元，健脾安神，补肝壮肾。用于淋证（男性前列腺肥大）及妇女更年期综合征。

Silkworm Imago* Pill

Name of Chinese Phonetic Alphabet E Ling Wan

Formula Bombycis Imagine Foeminei.

Actions and Indications Supporting healthy *qi*, fortifying the spleen, tranquilizing the mind and tonifying the liver and kidney. It is indicated for prostatic hyperplasia, menopausal syndrome.

*家蚕

蜂蜡素胶囊

【处方】蜂蜡素。

【功能主治】健脾益胃、化浊除痰、调理血脂。用于高脂血症属痰浊阻遏证者。

【注意】孕妇慎用。

Myricin* Capsule for Relieving Hyperlipemia

Name of Chinese Phonetic Alphabet Feng La Su Jiao Nang

Formula Myricin.

Actions and Indications Fortifying the spleen and nourishing the stomach, resolving turbidity and eliminating phlegm, regulating blood-lipid. It is indicated for hyperlipemia attributive to stagnation of phlegm turbidity.

Warning It should be used carefully for pregnant women.

*蜂蜡素

嗣育保胎丸

【处方】黄芪、党参、茯苓、鹿茸粉、白术（麸炒）、甘草、当归、川芎、白芍、熟地黄、阿胶、桑寄生、菟丝子、艾叶（炭）、荆芥穗、厚朴（姜炙）、枳壳（去瓤麸炒）、川贝母、羌活。

【功能主治】补气养血，安胎保产。用于孕妇气血不足引起的恶心呕吐，腰酸腹痛，足膝浮肿，胎动不安，屡经流产。

Abortion-preventing Bolus

Name of Chinese Phonetic Alphabet Si Yu Bao Tai Wan

Formula Astragali Radix, Codonopsis Radix, Poria, Cervi Cornu Pantotrichum Pulvis, Atractylodis Macrocephalae Rhizoma (fried with bran), Glycyrrhizae Radix et Rhizoma, Angelicae Sinensis Radix, Chuanxiong Rhizoma, Paeoniae Radix Alba, Rehmanniae Radix Praeparata, Asini Corii Colla, Taxilli Herba, Cuscutae Semen, Artemisiae Argyi Folium (carbonated), Schizonepetae Spica, Magnoliae Officinalis Cortex (prepared with ginger), Aurantii Fructus (removed pulp and fried with bran), Fritillariae Cirrhosae Bulbus and Notopterygii

Rhizoma et Radix.

Actions and Indications Tonifying *qi* and nourishing blood, preventing abortion. It is used for nausea, vomiting, soreness of the waist, abdominal pain, edema of the feet, excessive fetal movement and abortion due to dual insufficiency of *qi* and blood.

锡类散

【**处方**】象牙屑、青黛、人指甲（滑石粉制）、壁钱炭、珍珠、冰片、牛黄。

【**功能主治**】解毒化腐。用于咽喉糜烂肿痛。

Xi Lei Powder for Laryngeal Erosion

Name of Chinese Phonetic Alphabet Xi Lei San

Formula Elephantis Frustillum, Indigo Naturalis, Hominis Unguis (prepared with talc powder), Uroctea Carbonisatus, Margarita, Borneolum Syntheticum and Bovis Calculus.

Actions and Indications Detoxicating and removing necrosis. It is used for laryngeal erosion, sore-throat.

愈三消胶囊

【**处方**】黄芪、地黄、熟地黄、麦冬、天冬、玄参、五味子、淫羊藿（制）、丹参、红花、当归、黄连、红参、鹿茸、知母、党参、天花粉。

【**功能主治**】养阴生津，益气活血。用于轻、中Ⅱ度型糖尿病属气阴两虚兼血瘀者，症见口渴喜饮，易饥多食，疲倦乏力，自汗盗汗，舌质暗，有瘀斑，脉细数。

【**注意**】孕妇忌服；阴虚火旺者不宜使用。

Relieving Diabetes Capsule

Name of Chinese Phonetic Alphabet Yu San Xiao Jiao Nang

Formula Astragali Radix, Rehmaniae Radix, Rehmanniae Radix Praeparata, Ophiopogonis Radix, Asparagi Radix, Scrophulariae Radix, Schisandrae Chinensis Fructus, Epimedii Folium (prepared), Salviae Miltiorrhizae Radix et Rhizoma, Carthami Flos, Angelicae Sinensis Radix, Coptidis Rhizoma, Ginseng Radix et Rhizoma Rubra, Cervi Cornu Pantotrichum, Anemarrhenae Rhizoma, Codonopsis Radix and Trichosanthis Radix.

Actions and Indications Nourishing *yin*, promoting fluid-engendering, tonifying *qi* and activating blood. It is indicated for mild and middle degree diabetes attributed to dual deficiency of *qi* and *yin* associated with blood-stasis, and manifested as thirst, polydipsia, polyphagia, tiredness, fatigue, spontaneous sweating, night sweating, dull tongue with ecchymosis, fine and rapid pulse.

Warning It is contraindicated for pregnant women, and *yin*-deficiency with effulgent fire.

愈风宁心片

【**处方**】本品为葛根经加工制成的浸膏片。

【**功能主治**】解痉止痛，增强脑及冠脉血流量。用于高血压头晕，头痛，颈项疼痛，冠心病，心绞痛，神经性头痛，早期突发性耳聋。

Dizziness-relieving Tablet

Name of Chinese Phonetic Alphabet Yu Feng Ning Xin Pian

Formula Puerariae Lobatae Radix (extract).

Actions and Indications Relaxing spasm, alleviating pain, increasing cerebral and coronary artery blood flow. It is indicated for dizziness and headache due to hypertension; and also used for pain of neck, coronary heart disease, angina pectoris and early stage of sudden deafness.

愈伤灵胶囊

【**处方**】土鳖虫、红花、自然铜（煅）、冰片、续断、三七、黄瓜子（炒）、当归、落新妇提取物。

【**功能主治**】活血散瘀，消肿止痛。用于跌打挫伤，筋骨瘀血肿痛，亦可用于骨折的辅助治疗。

Relieving Traumatic Contusion Capsule

Name of Chinese Phonetic Alphabet Yu Shang Ling Jiao Nang

Formula Eupolyphaga seu Steleophaga, Carthami Flos, Pyritum (calcined), Borneolum Syntheticum, Dipsaci Radix, Notoginseng Radix et Rhizoma, Cucumidis Sativi Semen (fried), Angelicae Sinensis Radix and Astilbes Chinensis Herba (extract).

Actions and Indications Activating blood, dissipating stasis, reducing swelling, alleviating pain. It is used for traumatic injury and contusion marked by swelling, pain and blood-stasis, and also used as a supplemental treatment of fracture.

愈带丸

【处方】当归、白芍、芍药花、熟地黄、艾叶（炒炭）、棕榈炭、蒲黄（炒）、百草霜、鸡冠花、香附（醋炙）、木香、知母、黄柏、牛膝、干姜（微炒）、肉桂（炒焦）、甘草（蜜炙）。

【功能主治】益气调经，散寒止带。用于气虚血亏、子宫湿寒引起的经血不调、赤白带下、凝滞腹痛、腰腿酸软、骨蒸潮热、头晕耳鸣。

【注意】忌食生冷油腻；孕妇忌服。

Leucorrhea-recovering Pill

Name of Chinese Phonetic Alphabet Yu Dai Wan

Formula Angelicae Sinensis Radix, Paeoniae Radix Alba, Paeoniae Lactiflorae Flos, Rehmanniae Radix Praeparata, Artemisiae Argyi Folium (carbonated), Trachycarpi Petiolus Carbonisatus, Typhae Pollen, (fried), Gramen Fumi Carbonisatus, Celosiae Cristatae Flos, Cyperi Rhizoma (prepared with vinegar), Aucklandiae Radix, Anemarrhenae Rhizoma, Phellodendri Chinensis Cortex, Achyranthis Bidentatae Radix, Zingiberis Rhizoma (slightly fried), Cinnamomi Cortex (charred) and Glycyrrhizae Radix et Rhizoma (prepared with honey).

Actions and Indications Tonifying *qi*, regulating menstruation, dissipating cold and arresting leucorrhea. It is used for irregular menstruation, red and white vaginal discharge, abdominal pain, soreness and weakness of the waist and legs, tidal fever, dizziness and tinnitus due to dual deficiency of *qi* and blood, and uterus-coldness.

Warning It is contraindicated for pregnant women, and uncooked and oily foods should be avoided.

腰肾膏

【处方】肉苁蓉、八角、茴香、熟地黄、补骨脂、淫羊藿、蛇床子、牛膝、续断、甘草、杜仲、菟丝子、枸杞子、车前子、小茴香、附子、五味子、乳香、没药、丁香、锁阳、樟脑、冰片、薄荷油、肉桂油、水杨酸甲酯、枫香脂稠膏、盐酸苯海拉明。

【功能主治】温肾助阳，强筋壮骨，祛风止痛。用于肾虚性腰膝酸痛，肌肉酸痛，亦可用于夜尿、遗精、早泄、阳痿。

【注意】孕妇慎用。

Strengthening Sinews and Bone Plaster

Name of Chinese Phonetic Alphabet Yao Shen Gao

Formula Cistanches Caulis Carnosus, Anisi Stellati Fructus, Rehmanniae Radix Praeparata, Psoraleae Fructus, Epimedii Folium, Cnidii Fructus, Achyranthis Bidentatae Radix, Dipsaci Radix, Glycyrrhizae Radix et Rhizoma, Eucommiae Cortex, Cuscutae Semen, Lycii Fructus, Plantaginis Semen, Foeniculi Fructus, Aconiti Lateralis Radix Praeparata, Schisandrae Chinensis Fructus, Olibanum, Myrrha, Caryophylli Flos, Cynomorri Caulis Carnosus, Camphora, Borneolum Syntheticum, Menthae Haplocalycis Oleum, Cinnamomi Oleum, Methylsalicylate, Liguidamburm (thick extract) and Diphenhydramine Hydrochloride.

Actions and Indications Warming kidney-*yang*, strengthening the sinews and bone, dispelling wind and alleviating pain. It is used for soreness and pain of the waist, knees and muscle due to deficiency of the kidney, and also used for frequent urination at night, nocturnal emission, ejaculatio praecox and impotence.

Warning It should be used carefully for pregnant women.

腰椎痹痛丸

【处方】桂枝、千年健、五加皮、桃仁、骨碎补、赤芍、防风、独活、绵萆薢、防己、威灵仙、制草乌、桑寄生、秦艽、红花、海风藤、白芷、续断、当归。

【功能主治】壮筋骨，益气血，舒筋活络，祛风除湿，通痹止痛。用于治疗实证腰痛。

【注意】感冒发热者勿服。

Relieving Lumbar Vertebrae Impediment Pill

Name of Chinese Phonetic Alphabet Yao Zhui Bi Tong Wan

Formula Cinnamomi Ramulus, Homalomenae Rhizoma, Acanthopanacis Cortex, Persicae Semen, Drynariae Rhizoma, Paeoniae Radix Rubra, Saposhnikoviae Radix, Angelicae Pubescentis Radix, Dioscoreae Spongiosae Rhizoma, Stephaniae Tetrandrae Radix, Clematidis Radix et Rhizoma, Aconiti Kusnezoffii Radix Cocta, Taxilli Herba, Gentianae Macrophyllae Radix, Carthami Flos, Piperis Kadsurae Caulis, Angelicae Dahuricae Radix, Dipsaci Radix and Angelicae Sinensis Radix.

Actions and Indications Strengthening sinews and bone, nourishing *qi* and blood, activating collaterals, dispelling wind and dampness, relaxing impediment and alleviating pain. It is indicated for lumbago of excess pattern.

Warning It is contraindicated for cases with common cold and fever.

腰痛片

【处方】杜仲叶（盐炒）、补骨脂（盐炒）、续断、当归、白术（炒）、牛膝、肉桂、乳香（制）、狗脊（制）、赤芍、泽泻、土鳖虫（酒炒）。

【功能主治】强腰补肾，活血止痛。用于肾虚腰痛，腰肌劳损。

【注意】阴虚火旺，有实热者忌用。

Relieving Lumbago Tablet

Name of Chinese Phonetic Alphabet Yao Tong Pian

Formula Eucommiae Folium (fried with salt), Psoraleae Fructus (fried with salt), Dipsaci Radix, Angelicae Sinensis Radix, Atractylodis Macrocephalae Rhizoma (fried), Achyranthis Bidentatae Radix, Cinnamomi Cortex, Olibanum (prepared), Cibotii Rhizoma(prepared), Paeoniae Radix Rubra, Alismatis Rhizoma and Eupolyphaga seu Steleophaga (fried with wine).

Actions and Indications Strengthening the waist, tonifying the kidney, activating blood, alleviating pain. It is indicated for lumbago and lumbar muscle strain due to deficiency of the kidney.

Warning It is contraindicated for *yin*-deficiency with effulgent fire and excess heat.

腰痛宁胶囊

【处方】马钱子粉（制）、土鳖虫、川牛膝、甘草、麻黄、乳香、没药、全蝎、僵蚕、苍术。

【功能主治】消肿止痛，疏散寒邪，温经通络。用于腰椎间盘突出症、腰椎增生症、坐骨神经痛、腰肌劳损、腰肌纤维炎、慢性风湿性关节炎。

【注意】孕妇及小孩禁服。

Relieving Prolapse of Lumbar Intervertebral Disc Capsule

Name of Chinese Phonetic Alphabet Yao Tong Ning Jiao Nang

Formula Strychni Semen Pulvis (prepared), Eupolyphaga seu Steleophaga, Cyathulae Radix, Glycyrrhizae Radix et Rhizoma, Ephedrae Herba, Olibanum, Myrrha, Scorpio, Bombyx Batryticatus and Atractylodis Rhizoma.

Actions and Indications Reducing swelling, alleviating pain, dissipating cold, warming meridians, dredging collaterals. It is indicated for prolapse of lumbar intervertebral disc, lumbar hyperplasia, sciatica, lumbar muscle strain, lumbar muscle fibrositis, chronic rheumatic arthritis.

Warning It is contraindicated for children and pregnant women.

腰腿痛丸

【处方】麻黄、红参、豹骨（制）、羌活、木瓜、乳香（制）、甘草、地枫皮、防风、马钱子粉、鹿茸、牛膝、独活、鸡血藤、没药（制）、千年健、杜仲炭。

【功能主治】强筋壮骨，舒筋活血。用于气血双亏，风寒湿痹，外邪侵袭所致的腰腿酸软，肢体麻木等症。

【注意】孕妇忌服。

Strengthening Sinews and Bone Bolus

Name of Chinese Phonetic Alphabet Yao Tui Tong Wan

Formula Ephedrae Herba, Ginseng Radix et Rhizoma Rubra, Pardi Os (prepared), Notopterygii Rhizoma et Radix, Chenomelis Fructus, Olibanum (prepared), Glycyrrhizae Radix et Rhizoma, Illicii Cortex (prepared), Saposhnikoviae Radix, Strychni Semen Pulvis, Cervi Cornu Pantotrichum, Achyranthis Bidentatae Radix, Angelicae Pubescentis Radix, Spatholobi Caulis, Myrrha (prepared), Homalomenae Rhizoma and Eucommiae Cortex Carbonisatus.

Actions and Indications Strengthening the sinews and bone, activating blood. It is indicated for wind-cold-damp impediment syndrome due to dual depletion of *qi* and blood; soreness and weakness of the waist and legs and numbness of limbs due to invasion of external pathogen.

Warning It is contraindicated for pregnant women.

腮腺宁糊剂

【处方】芙蓉叶、白芷、大黄、乳香（醋炙）、苎麻根、赤小豆、薄荷油。

【功能主治】散瘀解毒，消肿止痛。用于腮腺炎，红肿热痛。

【注意】外用药，切勿入口。

Parotitis-relieving Paste

Name of Chinese Phonetic Alphabet Sai Xian Ning Hu Ji

Formula Hibisci Mutabilis Folium, Angelicae Dahuricae Radix, Rhei Radix et Rhizoma, Olibanum (prepared with vinegar), Boehmeriae Niveae Radix, Vignae Semen and Menthae Haplocalycis Oleum.

Actions and Indications Dissipating stasis and detoxicating, dispersing swelling and relieving pain. It is used for parotitis with red, swelling and causalgia.

Warning The product is applied for external use only.

腮腺炎片

【处方】蓼大青叶、板蓝根、连翘、蒲公英、夏枯草、牛黄。

【功能主治】清热解毒，消肿散结。用于腮腺炎。

Parotitis-relieving Tablet

Name of Chinese Phonetic Alphabet Sai Xian Yan Pian

Formula Polygoni Tinctorii Folium, Isatidis Radix, Forsythiae Fructus, Taraxaci Herba, Prunellae Spica and Bovis Calculus.

Actions and Indications Clearing heat and detoxicating, dispersing swelling and dissipating mass. It is indicated for parotitis.

腹可安片

【处方】扭肚藤、火炭母、车前草、救必应、石榴皮。

【功能主治】清热利湿，收敛止痛。用于急性胃肠炎、消化不良引起的腹痛、腹泻、呕吐。

Abdomen-soothing Tablet

Name of Chinese Phonetic Alphabet Fu Ke An

Pian

Formula Jasmini Amplexicaulis Folium, Polygoni Chinensis Herba, Plantaginis Herba, Ilicis Rotundae Cortex and Granati Pericarpium.

Actions and Indications Clearing heat and draining dampness, astringing and relieving pain. It is indicated for abdominal pain, diarrhea and vomiting due to acute gastroenteritis and dyspepsia.

雏凤精

【处方】砂仁、肉桂、牡丹皮、九节菖蒲、沉香、黄芪、甘草、人参、鹿茸、莲须、白芍、补骨脂、覆盆子、枸杞子、泽泻、熟地黄、肉苁蓉、山药、当归、牛膝、茯苓、锁阳、狗鞭、淫羊藿（羊油炙）、杜仲、羊外肾、羊鞭、鸡胎。

【功能主治】温肾壮阳，补气生血。用于气虚贫血，腰酸背痛，四肢乏力，头晕耳鸣，神衰失眠，心慌心跳，肾亏泻滑，记忆力减退，食欲不振及妇女宫冷，月经不调症。

Tonifying Kidney-*yang* Oral Liquid

Name of Chinese Phonetic Alphabet Chu Feng Jing

Formula Amomi Fructus, Cinnamomi Cortex, Moutan Cortex, Anemones Altaicae Rhizoma, Aquilariae Lignum Resinatum, Astragali Radix, Glycyrrhizae Radix et Rhizoma, Ginseng Radix et Rhizoma, Cervi Cornu Pantotrichum, Nelumbinis Stamen, Paeoniae Radix Alba, Psoraleae Fructus, Rubi Fructus, Lycii Fructus, Alismatis Rhizoma, Rehmanniae Radix Praeparata, Cistanches Caulis Carnosus, Dioscoreae Rhizoma, Angelicae Sinensis Radix, Achyranthis Bidentatae Radix, Poria, Cynomorii Caulis Carnosus, Canis Testis et Penis, Epimedii Folium (prepared with sheep suet), Eucommiae Cortex, Carprinus Testis, Caprinus Testis et Penis and Galli Foetus.

Actions and Indications Warming kidney-*yang*, tonifying *qi* and blood. It is indicated for anemia due to *qi*-deficiency, soreness of the waist, backache, weakness of the limbs, fatigue, dizziness, tinnitus, insomnia, fluster, palpitation, spermatorrhea, hypomnesis, poor appetite, uterus-coldness, irregular menstruation.

解郁安神冲剂

【处方】柴胡、大枣、石菖蒲、半夏（制）、白术（炒）、浮小麦、远志（制）、甘草（炙）、栀子（炒）、百合、胆南星、郁金、龙齿、酸枣仁（炒）、茯苓、当归。

【功能主治】疏肝解郁，安神定志。用于情志不舒，肝郁气滞等精神刺激所致的心烦、焦虑、失眠、健忘、更年期症候群，神经官能症。

Depressing-releasing Soluble Granules

Name of Chinese Phonetic Alphabet Jie Yu An Shen Chong Ji

Formula Bupleuri Radix, Jujubae Fructus, Acori Tatarinowii Rhizoma, Pinelliae Rhizoma (prepared), Atractylodis Macrocephalae Rhizoma (fried), Tritici Aestivi Fructus Natantia, Polygalae Radix (prepared), Glycyrrhizae Radix et Rhizoma (prepared), Gardeniae Fructus (fried), Lilii Bulbus, Arisaema cum Bile, Curcumae Radix, Draconis Dens, Ziziphi Spinosae Semen (fried), Poria and Angelicae Sinensis Radix.

Actions and Indications Soothing the liver, releasing depression, tranquilizing the mind. It is used for vexation, worry, insomnia, amnesia, menopausal syndrome and neurosis due to emotional upset and stagnation of liver-*qi*.

解毒生肌膏

【处方】紫草、当归、白芷、甘草、乳香（醋制）、轻粉。

【功能主治】活血散瘀，消肿止痛，解毒拔脓，祛腐生肌。用于创面感染，Ⅱ度烧伤。

Tissue Regeneration Plaster

Name of Chinese Phonetic Alphabet Jie Du Sheng Ji Gao

Formula Arnebiae Radix, Angelicae Sinensis

Radix, Angelicae Dahuricae Radix, Glycyrrhizae Radix et Rhizoma, Olibanum (prepared with vinegar) and Calomelas.

Actions and Indications Activating blood and dissipating stasis, dispersing swelling and relieving pain, detoxicating, draining pus, removing necrosis and promoting tissue regeneration. It is used for wound infection and II degree burn.

解热清肺糖浆

【处方】桑白皮、紫苏叶、前胡、紫菀、枳壳、鱼腥草、甘草、黄芩、土牛膝。

【功能主治】清热解毒，祛痰止咳，宣肺利咽。用于风热感冒，发热头痛，咽痛，咳嗽。

Syrup for Relieving Common Cold

Name of Chinese Phonetic Alphabet Jie Re Qing Fei Tang Jiang

Formula Mori Cortex, Perillae Folium, Peucedani Radix, Asteris Radix et Rhizoma, Aurantii Fructus, Houttuyniae Herba, Glycyrrhizae Radix et Rhizoma, Scutellariae Radix and Achyranthis Bidentatae Radix.

Actions and Indications Clearing heat and detoxicating, dispelling phlegm and relieving cough, diffusing the lung and soothing the throat. It is indicated for common cold due to wind-heat, marked by fever and headache, sore-throat and cough.

新生化冲剂

【处方】当归、川芎、桃仁、红花、甘草（炙）、干姜（炭）、益母草。

【功能主治】活血，祛瘀，止痛。用于产后恶露不行，少腹疼痛，也可试用于上节育环后引起的阴道流血，月经过多。

Lochiostasis-relieving Soluble Granules

Name of Chinese Phonetic Alphabet Xin Sheng Hua Chong Ji

Formula Angelicae Sinensis Radix, Chuanxiong Rhizoma, Persicae Semen, Carthami Flos, Glycyrrhizae Radix et Rhizoma (prepared), Zingiberis Rhizoma (carbonated) and Leonuri Herba.

Actions and Indications Activating blood, dispelling stasis, alleviating pain. It is used for lochiostasis marked by pain in lower abdomen or trial for cases with vaginal bleeding and hypermenorrhea due to application of contraceptive ring.

新血宝胶囊

【处方】鸡血藤、黄芪、大枣、当归、白术、陈皮、硫酸亚铁。

【功能主治】补血益气，健脾和胃。用于消化道出血，痔疮出血，月经过多，尤其适用于妊娠及偏食所致的缺铁性贫血。

【注意】宜饭后服，忌与茶、咖啡及含鞣酸类药物服用。

New Blood Treasure Capsule

Name of Chinese Phonetic Alphabet Xin Xue Bao Jiao Nang

Formula Spatholobi Caulis, Astragali Radix, Jujubae Fructus, Angelicae Sinensis Radix, Atractylodis Macrocephalae Rhizoma, Citri Reticulatae Pericarpium and Ferrous Sulfate.

Actions and Indications Tonifying *qi* and blood, fortifying the spleen and harmonizing the stomach. It is indicated for hemorrhage of digestive tract, hemorrhoidal bleeding, hypermenorrhea, especially for hypoferric anemia due to diet partiality and during gestational period.

Warning It should be taken after meal and avoided to be taken with tea, cafe and tannic medicine simultaneously.

新雪颗粒

【处方】磁石、石膏、滑石、寒水石、硝石、玄明粉、栀子、竹叶卷心、升麻、穿心莲、珍珠层粉、沉香、牛黄、冰片。

【功能主治】清热解毒。用于各种热性病之发热，如扁桃体发炎、上呼吸道炎、气管炎、感冒所引起的高热以及温热病之烦热不解。

Heat-clearing and Detoxifying Granules

Name of Chinese Phonetic Alphabet Xin Xue Ke Li

Formula Magnetitium, Gypsum Fibrosum, Talcum, Gypsum Rubrum, Nitrum, Natrii Sulfas Exsiccatus, Gardeniae Fructus, Lingnaniae Chungii Folium Involutus Juevenalis, Cimicifugae Rhizoma, Andrographis Herba, Margaritae Concha Strati Pulvis, Aquilariae Lignum Resinatum, Bovis Calculus and Borneolum Syntheticum.

Actions and Indications Clearing heat and detoxifying. It is indicated for high fever due to various febrile diseases such as tonsillitis, inflammation of upper respiratory tract, trachitis and common cold, high fever and heat vexation of warm-heat disease.

新癀片

【处方】肿节风、三七、人工牛黄、猪胆汁膏、肖梵天花、珍珠层粉、红曲、吲哚美辛、水牛角浓缩粉。

【功能主治】清热解毒，活血化瘀，消肿止痛。用于热毒瘀血所致的咽喉肿痛，牙痛，胁痛，黄疸，无名肿毒。

【注意】胃及十二指肠溃疡者、肾功能不全者及孕妇慎用；有消化道出血史者忌用。

Xin Huang Tablet

Name of Chinese Phonetic Alphabet Xin Huang Pian

Formula Sarcandrae Herba, Notoginseng Radix et Rhizoma, Bovis Calculus Artifactus, Suillus Bilis Extractum, Urenae Lobatae Radix seu Herba, Margaritae Concha Strati Pulvis, Oryzae Fructus Monascus, Indomethacin and Bubali Cornu Pulvis Concentratio.

Actions and Indications Clearing heat and detoxicating, activating blood and resolving stasis, dispersing swelling and relieving pain. It is indicated for sore-throat, toothache, hypochondriac pain, jaundice, pain and swelling of unknown origin due to heat-toxin and blood-stasis.

Warning It should be used cautiously for cases with gastric and duodenal ulcer, renal insufficiency and pregnant women. It is contraindicated for cases with disgestive tract bleeding history.

痹祺胶囊

【处方】马钱子（调制粉）、地龙、党参、茯苓、白术、甘草、川芎、丹参、三七、牛膝。

【功能主治】益气养血，祛风除湿，活血止痛。用于气血不足，风湿瘀阻，肌肉关节酸痛，关节肿大，僵硬变形或肌肉萎缩，气短乏力；风湿、类风湿性关节炎，腰肌劳损，软组织挫伤属上述证候者。

【注意】高血压病患者、孕妇忌服。

Bi Qi Capsule for Relieving Rheumatism

Name of Chinese Phonetic Alphabet Bi Qi Jiao Nang

Formula Strychni Semen (powder), Pheretima, Codonopsis Radix, Poria, Atractylodis Macrocephalae Rhizoma, Glycyrrhizae Radix et Rhizoma, Chuanxiong Rhizoma, Salviae Miltiorrhizae Radix et Rhizoma, Notoginseng Radix et Rhizoma and Achyranthis Bidentatae Radix.

Actions and Indications Tonifying *qi* and nourishing blood, dispelling wind and dampness, activating blood and alleviating pain. It is used for aching pain of the muscles and joints, arthrocele, stiffness and deformation of the joints, or muscle atrophy, shortness of breath and fatigue due to insufficiency of *qi* and blood, wind-damp-stasis, rheumatism and rheumatoid arthritis, lumbar muscle strain, soft tissue sprain with the above mentioned symptoms.

Warning It is contraindicated for pregnant women and cases with hypertension.

瘀血痹冲剂

【处方】乳香（炙）、威灵仙、红花、丹参、没药（炙）、川牛膝、川芎、当归、姜黄、香附（炙）、黄芪（炙）。

【功能主治】活血化瘀，通络定痛。用于瘀血阻络的痹证。症见肌肉关节疼痛剧烈，多呈刺痛感，部位固定不移，痛处拒按，可有硬节或瘀斑。

Blood-stasis-resolving Soluble Granules

Name of Chinese Phonetic Alphabet Yu Xue Bi Chong Ji

Formula Olibanum (prepared), Clematidis Radix et Rhizoma, Carhami Flos, Salviae Miltiorrhizae Radix et Rhizoma, Myrrha (prepared), Cyathulae Radix, Chuanxiong Rhizoma, Angelicae Sinensis Radix, Curcumae Longae Rhizoma, Cyperi Rhizoma (prepared) and Astragali Radix (prepared).

Actions and Indications Activating blood, resolving stasis, dredging collaterals, settling pain. It is used for impediment syndrome due to blood-stasis and manifested as fixed and stabbing pain of muscles and joints, tenderness, scleroma and ecchymosis in pain spots.

痰咳净散

【处方】桔梗、咖啡因、远志、冰片、苦杏仁、五倍子、甘草。

【功能主治】通窍顺气，消炎镇咳，促进排痰。用于急慢性支气管炎、咽喉炎、肺气肿等引起的咳嗽多痰、气促、气喘。

Dispelling Phlegm and Relieving Cough Powder

Name of Chinese Phonetic Alphabet Tan Ke Jing San

Formula Platycodonis Radix, Caffeine, Polygalae Radix, Borneolum Syntheticum, Armeniacae Semen Amarum, Galla Chinensis and Glycyrrhizae Radix et Rhizoma.

Actions and Indications Dredging nasal orifice and downbearing *qi*, antiphlogistic and relieving cough, expectorating phlegm. It is indicated for cough with profuse phlegm, shortness of breath and dyspnea due to acute, chronic bronchitis, laryngopharyngitis and pulmonary emphysema.

满山白糖浆

【处方】本品为满山白经提取制成的糖浆剂。

【功能主治】祛痰止咳。用于急、慢性支气管炎。

Syrup of Savatier Monochasma* for Relieving Bronchitis

Name of Chinese Phonetic Alphabet Man Shan Bai Tang Jiang

Formula Monochasmae Savatieri Herba.

Actions and Indications Dispelling phlegm and relieving cough. It is indicated for acute, chronic bronchitis.

* 满山白

溶栓胶囊

【处方】本品为地龙经加工制成的胶囊。

【功能主治】清热定惊，通络，利尿。用于肢体麻木，半身不遂，高血压症。

【注意】有严重出血患者慎用。

Prepared Earthworm* Capsule

Name of Chinese Phonetic Alphabet Rong Shuan Jiao Nang

Formula Pheretima.

Actions and Indications Clearing heat, settling fright, dredging collaterals, inducing diuresis. It is indicated for numbness of limbs, hemiparalysis and hypertension.

Warning It should be used cautiously for cases with severe hemorrhage.

* 地龙

裸花紫珠片

【处方】本品为裸花紫珠浸膏片。

【功能主治】消炎，解毒，收敛，止血。用于细菌感染引起的炎症，急性传染性肝炎，呼吸道和消化道出血。

Nakeflower Beautyberry* Tablet

Name of Chinese Phonetic Alphabet Luo Hua Zi Zhu Pian

Formula Callicarpae Nudiflorae Ramulus et Folium (extract).

Actions and Indications Counteracting inflammation, detoxifying, astringent, relieving bleeding. It is used for inflammation due to bacterial infection, acute infective hepatitis, respiratory and digestive tracts bleeding.

* 裸花紫珠

障眼明片

【处方】石菖蒲、决明子、肉苁蓉、葛根、青葙子、党参、蔓荆子、枸杞子、车前子、白芍、山茱萸、甘草、菟丝子、升麻、蕤仁(去内果皮)、菊花、密蒙花、川芎、黄精、熟地黄、黄柏、黄芪。

【功能主治】补益肝肾，退翳明目。用于初期及中期老年性白内障。

Improving Cataract Tablet

Name of Chinese Phonetic Alphabet Zhang Yan Ming Pian

Formula Acori Tatarinowii Rhizoma, Cassiae Semen, Cistanches Caulis Carnosus, Puerariae Lobatae Radix, Celosiae Semen, Codonopsis Radix, Viticis Fructus, Lycii Fructus, Plantaginis Semen, Paeoniae Radix Alba, Corni Fructus, Glycyrrhizae Radix et Rhzoma, Cuscutae Semen, Cimicifugae Rhizoma, Prinsepiae Nux (removed endocarp), Chrysanthemi Flos, Buddlejae Flos, Chuanxiong Rhizoma, Polygonati Rhizoma, Rehmanniae Radix Praeparata, Phellodendri Chinensis Cortex and Astragali Radix.

Actions and Indications Tonifying the liver and kidney, removing the nebula to improve vision. It is indicated for senile initial or middle stage of cataract.

障翳散

【处方】丹参、红花、茺蔚子、青葙子、决明子、蝉蜕、没药、黄芪、昆布、海藻、关木通、炉甘石、牛胆干膏、羊胆干膏、珍珠、琥珀、冰片、麝香、硼砂、海螵蛸、黄连素、核黄素、山药、无水硫酸钙、荸荠粉。

【功能主治】行滞祛瘀，退障消翳。用于老年性白内障及角膜翳。

Nebula-removing Powder

Name of Chinese Phonetic Alphabet Zhang Yi San

Formula Salviae Miltiorrhizae Radix et Rhizoma, Carthami Flos, Leonuri Fructus, Celosiae Semen, Cassiae Semen, Cicadae Periostracum, Myrrha, Astragali Radix, Laminariae seu Eckloniae Thallus, Sargassum, Aristochiae Manshuriensis Caulis, Calamina, Bovis Bilis Extractum, Carprinus Fel Extractum, Margarita, Succinum, Borneolum Syntheticum, Moschus, Borax, Sepiae Endoconcha, Berberine, Riboflavin, Dioscoreae Rhizoma, Anhydrous Calcium Sulfate and Eleocharitis Cormus Dulcis Pluvis.

Actions and Indications Moving stagnation and dispelling stasis, removing nebula to improve vision. It is used for senile cataract and corneal nebula.

十四画

静灵口服液

【处方】本品为熟地黄、山药、茯苓、牡丹皮、泽泻、远志、龙骨、女贞子等药经加工制成的口服液。

【功能主治】滋阴潜阳，宁神益智。用于儿童多动症，见有注意力涣散，多动多语，容易冲动，学习困难，舌质红，脉细数等肾阴不足，肝阳偏旺者。

【注意】忌辛辣刺激食物，外感发热暂停服用。

Tranquilizing Oral Liquid

Name of Chinese Phonetic Alphabet Jing Ling Kou Fu Ye

Formula Rehmanniae Radix Praeparata, Dioscoreae Rhizoma, Poria, Moutan Cotex, Alismatis Rhizoma, Polygalae Radix, Draconis Os and Ligustri Lucidi Fructus, etc.

Actions and Indications Enriching *yin* and subduing *yang*, tranquilizing the mind. It is used for children hyperkinesis manifested as distractibility, hyperactivity, verbose, impulse, learning difficulty, red tongue body and fine and rapid pulse due to insufficiency of kidney-*yin* and ascendant hyperactivity of liver-*yang*.

Warning Pungent and irritant foods are prohibited, suspend medication for cases with fever.

槟榔四消丸

【处方】槟榔、大黄（酒炒）、牵牛子（炒）、猪牙皂（炒）、香附（醋制）、五灵脂（醋炒）。

【功能主治】消食导滞，行气。用于食积痰饮，消化不良，脘腹胀满，嗳气吞酸，大便秘结。

【注意】孕妇忌服。

Betel Nut* Pill for Digestion-promoting

Name of Chinese Phonetic Alphabet Bing Lang Si Xiao Wan

Formula Arecae Semen, Rhei Radix et Rhizoma (fried with wine), Pharbitidis Semen (fried), Gleditsiae Fructus Abnormalis (fried), Cyperi Rhizoma (prepared with vinegar) and Trogopterori Faeces (fried with vinegar).

Actions and Indications Promoting digestion and removing food stagnation, moving *qi*. It is used for food stagnation, phlegm-fluid retention, dyspepsia, abdominal distention and fullness, eructation and acid regurgitation, constipation.

Warning It is contraindicated for pregnant women.

* 槟榔

截疟七宝丸

【处方】常山、草果、槟榔、厚朴（姜炙）、青皮（醋炙）、陈皮、甘草。

【功能主治】行气化滞，除湿截疟。用于疟疾、胸胁满闷，不思饮食，肢体酸痛，寒热交作。

【注意】忌食生冷油腻。

Seven Medicinals Pill for Checking Malaria

Name of Chinese Phonetic Alphabet Jie Nue Qi Bao Wan

Formula Dichroae Radix, Tsaoko Fructus, Arecae Semen, Magnoliae Officinalis Cortex (prepared with ginger), Citri Reticulartae Pericarpium Viride (prepared with vinegar), Citri Reticulatae Pericarpium and Glycyrrhizae Radix et Rhizoma.

Actions and Indications Moving *qi* and improving stagnation, dispelling dampness and checking malaria. It is indicated for malaria, chest and hypochondriac fullness and oppression, anorexia, aching pain of the limbs and body, alternating chills and fever.

Warning Uncooked, cold and oily foods are prohibited.

磁朱丸

【处方】磁石（煅）、朱砂、六神曲（炒）。

【功能主治】镇心，安神，明目。用于心肾阴虚，心阳偏亢，心悸失眠，耳鸣，视物昏花。

Magnetite* and Cinnabar** Pill

Name of Chinese Phonetic Alphabet Ci Zhu Wan

Formula Magnetitum (calcined), Cinnabaris and Medicata Massa Fermentata (fried).

Actions and Indications Tranquilizing the mind,

inproving vision. It is used for palpitation, insomnia, tinnitus and blurred vision due to dual *yin*-deficiency of the heart and kidney, and hyperactivity of heart-*yang*.

*磁石 **朱砂

豨桐丸

【处方】臭梧桐叶、豨莶草。

【功能主治】祛风湿，止痛。用于四肢麻痹，骨节疼痛，风湿性关节炎。

【注意】忌食猪肝，羊血。

Siegesbeckia* and Hairy Clerodendron** Pill for Relieving Ostealgia

Name of Chinese Phonetic Alphabet Xi Tong Wan

Formula Clerodendri Trichotomi Folium and Siegesbeckiae Herba.

Actions and Indications Dispelling wind and dampness, alleviating pain. It is indicated for paralysis of the limbs, ostealgia and rheumatic arthritis.

Warning Pig liver and goat blood are prohibited.

*豨莶草 **臭梧桐

豨莶丸

【处方】本品为豨莶草制成的蜜丸。

【功能主治】祛风湿，通经络，清热解毒。用于风湿痹症，骨节疼痛，四肢麻木及中风手足不遂。

Siegesbeckia* Bolus for Cold-damp Impediment Syndrome

Name of Chinese Phonetic Alphabet Xi Xian Wan

Formula Siegesbeckiae Herba.

Actions and Indications Dispelling wind-damp, dredging meridians and collaterals, clearing heat and detoxicating. It is used for cold-damp impediment syndrome, marked by ostealgia, numbness of the limbs due to apoplexy.

*豨莶草

稳心颗粒剂

【处方】党参、黄精、三七、琥珀、甘松 。

【功能主治】益气养阴，定悸复脉，活血化瘀。用于气阴两虚兼心脉郁阻引起的心悸不宁，气短乏力，头晕，胸闷胸痛。适用于心律失常，室性早搏，房性早搏等见上述症状者。

【注意】孕妇慎用。

Relieving Arrhythmia Soluble Granules

Name of Chinese Phonetic Alphabet Wen Xin Ke Li Ji

Formula Codonopsis Radix, Polygonati Rhizoma, Notoginseng Radix et Rhizoma, Succinum and Nardostachyos Radix et Rhizoma.

Actions and Indications Tonifying *qi* and nourishing *yin*, relieving palpitation, restoring normal pulse beat, activating blood and resolving stasis. It is indicated for palpitation, shortness of breath, fatigue, dizziness, chest distress and pain due to dual deficiency of *qi* and *yin* and heart vessel obstruction. It is also used for arrhythmia, ventricular or atrial premature beat with the above mentioned symptoms.

Warning It should be used carefully for pregnant women.

鼻炎口服液

【处方】本品为苍耳子、辛夷、防风、连翘、野菊花、五味子、桔梗、白芷、知母、荆芥、甘草等药经加工制成。

【功能主治】祛风宣肺，清热解毒。用于急、慢性鼻渊。

Rhinitis-relieving Oral Liquid

Name of Chinese Phonetic Alphabet Bi Yan Kou Fu Ye

Formula Xanthii Fructus, Magnoliae Flos, Saposhnikoviae Radix, Forsythiae Fructus, Chrysanthemi

Indici Flos, Schisandrae Chinensis Fructus, Platycodonis Radix, Angelicae Dahuricae Radix, Anemarrhenae Rhizoma, Schizonepetae Herba, Glycyrrhizae Radix et Rhizoma, etc.

Actions and Indications Dispelling wind and diffusing the lung, clearing heat and detoxicating. It is indicated for acute, chronic sinusitis.

鼻炎片

【处方】苍耳子、辛夷、防风、连翘、野菊花、五味子、桔梗、白芷、知母、荆芥、黄柏、甘草。

【功能主治】祛风宣肺，清热解毒。用于急、慢性鼻炎。

Rhinitis-relieving Tablet

Name of Chinese Phonetic Alphabet Bi Yan Pian

Formula Xanthii Fructus, Magnoliae Flos, Saposhnikoviae Radix, Forsythiae Fructus, Chrysanthemi Indici Flos, Schisandrae Chinensis Fructus, Platycodonis Radix, Angelicae Dahuricae Radix, Anemarrhenae Rhizoma, Schizonepetae Herba, Phellodendri Chinensis Cortex and Glycyrrhizae Radix et Rhizoma.

Actions and Indications Dispelling wind and diffusing the lung, clearing heat and detoxicating. It is indicated for acute, chronic rhinitis.

鼻炎康片

【处方】鼻炎康水提干浸膏、当归干浸膏、猪胆汁、黄芩提取物、麻黄粉、薄荷油、扑尔敏。

【功能主治】清热解毒，宣肺通窍，消肿止痛。用于急、慢性鼻炎，过敏性鼻炎。

【注意】用药期间不宜驾驶车辆、管理机器及高空作业等。

Relieving Rhinitis Tablet

Name of Chinese Phonetic Alphabet Bi Yan Kang Pian

Formula Biyangkang (extract), Angelicae Sinensis Radix (extract), Suillus Bilis, Scutellariae (extract), Ephedrae Pulvis, Menthae Haplocalycis Oleum and Chlorpheniramine.

Actions and Indications Clearing heat and detoxicating, diffusing the lung and dredging the orifices, dispersing swelling and releving pain. It is indicated for acute, chronic rhinitis, allergic rhinitis.

Warning During medication, driving, administering machine and high altitude work are prohibited.

鼻炎糖浆

【处方】苍耳子、辛夷、野菊花、金银花、茜草。

【功能主治】祛风宣肺，清热解毒，通窍止痛。用于鼻塞鼻渊，通气不畅，流涕黄浊，嗅觉不灵，头痛，眉棱骨痛。

Rhinitis-relieving Syrup

Name of Chinese Phonetic Alphabet Bi Yan Tang Jiang

Formula Xanthii Fructus, Magnoliae Flos, Chrysanthemi Indici Flos, Lonicerae Japonicae Flos and Rubiae Radix.

Actions and Indications Dispelling wind and diffusing the lung, clearing heat and detoxicating, dredging the orifices, alleviating pain. It is indicated for nasal congestion and sinusitis, marked by yellow and turbid nasal discharge, hyposmia, headache, supraorbital bone pain.

鼻咽灵片

【处方】山豆根、茯苓、天花粉、蛇泡勒、麦冬、半枝莲、玄参、石上柏、党参、白花蛇舌草。

【功能主治】清热解毒，软坚散结，益气养阴。用于胸膈风热，痰火郁结，热毒上攻，耗气伤津之证。其症状常见口干，咽痛，声嘶头痛，鼻塞，流脓涕或涕中带血。也用于治疗急、慢性咽喉炎，口腔炎，鼻咽炎及鼻咽癌放疗、化疗辅助治疗。

【注意】忌食辛辣及油炸食物。

Soothing Nasal Pharynx Tablet

Name of Chinese Phonetic Alphabet Bi Yan Ling Pian

Formula Sophorae Tonkinensis Radix et Rhizoma, Poria, Trichosanthis Radix, Rubi Parvifolii Herba, Ophiopogonis Radix, Scutellariae Barbatae Herba, Scrophulariae Radix, Selaginellae Doederleinii Herba, Codonopsis Radix and Hedyotis Diffusae Herba.

Actions and Indications Clearing heat and detoxicating, softening hardness and dissipating mass, tonifying *qi* and nourishing *yin*. It is used for stagnation of phlegm-fire, heat-toxin attacking upward and consumption of *qi* and fluid syndrome, manifested as dryness in the mouth, sore-throat, dry throat, hoarseness, headache, nasal congestion, rhinorrhea or nasal blood-stained discharge, also for acute and chronic laryngopharyngitis, stomatitis, nasopharyngitis and adjuvant treatment of nasopharyngeal carcinoma with radiotherapy and chemotherapy.

Warning Pungent and fried foods are prohibited.

鼻咽清毒冲剂

【处方】野菊花、苍耳子、重楼、蛇泡勒、两面针、夏枯草、龙胆、党参。

【功能主治】清热解毒，消炎散结。用于鼻咽部慢性炎症，咽喉肿痛以及鼻咽癌放射治疗后分泌物增多。

Nasopharyngeal Detoxicating Soluble Granules

Name of Chinese Phonetic Alphabet Bi Yan Qing Du Chong Ji

Formula Chrysanthemi Indici Flos, Xanthii Fructus, Paridis Rhizoma, Rubi Parvifolii Herba, Zanthoxyli Radix, Prunellae Spica, Gentianae Radix et Rhizoma and Codonopsis Radix.

Actions and Indications Clearing heat and detoxicating, counteracting inflammation and dissipating mass. It is indicated for chronic pharyngitis, sore-throat and profuse secretion after radiotherapy of nasopharyngeal carcinoma.

鼻通丸

【处方】苍耳子（炒）、辛夷 、白芷、鹅不食草、薄荷、黄芩、甘草。

【功能主治】清风热，通鼻窍。用于外感风热或风寒化热，鼻塞流涕，头痛流泪，慢性鼻炎。

Soothing Nasal Cavity Bolus

Name of Chinese Phonetic Alphabet Bi Tong Wan

Formula Xanthii Fructus (fried), Magnoliae Flos, Angelicae Dahuricae Radix, Centipedae Herba, Menthae Haplocalycis Herba, Scutellariae Radix and Glycyrrhizae Radix et Rhizoma.

Actions and Indications Clearing wind-heat, soothing nasal cavity. It is indicated for nasal congestion, rhinorrhea, headache, lacrimation and chronic rhinitis due to exogenous wind-heat or wind-cold transforming into heat.

鼻渊舒胶囊

【处方】辛夷、苍耳子、栀子、黄芩、黄芪、川芎、柴胡、细辛、薄荷、茯苓、白芷、桔梗。

【功能主治】清热解毒，疏风排脓，通鼻窍。用于鼻窦炎、慢性鼻炎。

Sinusitis-relieving Capsule

Name of Chinese Phonetic Alphabet Bi Yuan Shu Jiao Nang

Formula Magnoliae Flos, Xanthii Fructus, Gardeniae Fructus, Scutellariae Radix, Astragali Radix, Chuanxiong Rhizoma, Bupleuri Radix, Asari Radix et Rhizoma, Menthae Haplocalycis Herba, Poria, Angelicae Dahuricae Radix and Platycodonis Radix.

Actions and Indications Clearing heat and detoxicating, dispersing wind and discharging pus, soothing nasal cavity. It is indicated for sinusitis, chronic rhinitis.

鼻窦炎口服液

【处方】辛夷、荆芥、薄荷、桔梗、柴胡、苍耳子、白芷、川芎、黄芩、栀子、茯苓、川木通、黄芪、龙胆。

【功能主治】通利鼻窍。用于鼻塞不通，流黄浊涕，慢性鼻炎，鼻窦炎。

Sinusitis-relieving Oral Liquid

Name of Chinese Phonetic Alphabet Bi Dou Yan Kou Fu Ye

Formula Magnoliae Flos, Schizonepetae Herba, Menthae Haplocalycis Herba, Platycodonis Radix, Bupleuri Radix, Xanthii Fructus, Angelicae Dahuricae Radix, Chuanxiong Rhizoma, Scutellariae Radix, Gardeniae Fructus, Poria, Clematidis Armandii Caulis, Astragali Radix and Gentianae Radix et Rhizoma.

Actions and Indications Dredging the nasal orifice. It is indicated for nasal congestion, yellow and turbid nasal discharge, chronic rhinitis, sinusitis.

慢支固本冲剂

【处方】黄芪、白术、当归、防风。

【功能主治】补肺健脾，固表和血。用于慢性支气管炎非急性发作期，症见乏力自汗，恶风寒，咳嗽、咯痰，易感冒，食欲不振。

【注意】慢性支气管炎急性发作或咳喘较重者不适用。

Chronic Bronchitis Relieving Soluble Granules

Name of Chinese Phonetic Alphabet Man Zhi Gu Ben Chong Ji

Formula Astragali Radix, Atractylodis Macrocephalae Rhizoma, Angelicae Sinensis Radix and Saposhnikoviae Radix.

Actions and Indications Tonifying the lung and fortifying the spleen, securing the superfices and harmonizing blood. It is indicated for non-acute attack of chronic bronchitis due to deficiency of lung-*qi*, manifested as fatigue, spontaneous sweating, aversion to wind and cold, cough, spitting phlegm, easiness to catch common cold and anorexia.

Warning It is not suitable for cases with acute attack of chronic bronchitis or severe cough and asthma.

慢性肾炎液

【处方】黄芪、淫羊藿、桂枝、地黄等。

【功能主治】益气温阳，利湿化瘀。用于肺脾气虚，脾肾阳虚所致的水肿，头晕，乏力，纳差以及慢性肾炎见上述证候者。

Relieving Chronic Nephritis Liquid

Name of Chinese Phonetic Alphabet Man Xing Shen Yan Ye

Formula Astragali Radix, Epimedii Folium, Cinnamomi Ramulus, Rehmanniae Radix, etc.

Actions and Indications Tonifying *qi* and warming *yang*, draining dampness and resolving stasis. It is indicated for edema, dizziness, fatigue, anorexia due to *qi*-deficiency of the lung and spleen, *yang*-deficiency of the spleen and kidney; and chronic nephritis with the above mentioned symptoms.

滴耳油

【处方】核桃油、黄柏、五倍子、薄荷油、冰片。

【功能主治】清热解毒，消肿止痛。用于肝经湿热上攻，耳鸣，耳内生疮，肿痛刺痒，破流脓水。

Ear Drop Oils

Name of Chinese Phonetic Alphabet Di Er You

Formula Juglandis Oleum, Phellodendri Chinensis Cortex, Galla Chinensis, Menthae Haplocalycis Oleum and Borneolum Syntheticum.

Actions and Indications Clearing heat and detoxicating, dispersing swelling and relieving pain. It is used for tinnitus, sore in the ears, swelling, stabbing pain and itching and otopyosis due to upward attack of damp-heat in the liver meridian.

精制冠心软胶囊

【处方】丹参、赤芍、川芎、红花、降香。

【功能主治】活血化瘀。用于心血瘀阻之冠心病、心绞痛。

Relieving Coronary Heart Disease Soft Capsule

Name of Chinese Phonetic Alphabet Jing Zhi Guan Xin Ruan Jiao Nang

Formula Salviae Miltiorrhizae Radix et Rhizoma, Paeoniae Radix Rubra, Chuanxiong Rhizoma, Carthami Flos and Dalbergiae Odoriferae Lignum.

Actions and Indications Activating blood, resolving stasis. It is indicated for coronary heart disease and angina pectoris due to blood-stasis.

精制银翘解毒胶囊

【处方】扑热息痛、桔梗、连翘、淡豆豉、甘草、淡竹叶、金银花、牛蒡子、荆芥穗、薄荷脑。

【功能主治】清热散风，解表退热。用于流行性感冒，发热，四肢酸软，头痛咳嗽，咽喉肿痛，温毒发颐。

Refined Honeysuckle Flower* and Weeping Forsythia** Capsule

Name of Chinese Phonetic Alphabet Jing Zhi Yin Qiao Jie Du Jiao Nang

Formula Paracetamol, Platycodonis Radix, Forsythiae Fructus, Sojae Semen Praeparatum, Glycyrrhizae Radix et Rhizoma, Lophatheri Herba, Lonicerae Japonicae Flos, Arctii Fructus, Schizonepetae Spica and Menthol.

Actions and Indications Clearing heat and dispersing wind, releasing the exterior and defervesce. It is indicated for influenza, marked by fever, soreness and weakness of the limbs, headache, cough, sore-throat, suppurative parotitis.

* 金银花 ** 连翘

精黄片

【处方】大黄等。

【功能主治】祛瘀，泻火，止血。用于胃、十二指肠溃疡引起的出血症。

【注意】出血量大且出血速度快，伴有全身症状者不宜使用。

Rhubarb* Tablet

Name of Chinese Phonetic Alphabet Jing Huang Pian

Formula Rhei Radix et Rhizoma, etc.

Actions and Indications Dispelling stasis, purging fire, relieving bleeding. It is indicated for hemorrhage due to gastric and duodenal ulcer.

Warning It is contraindicated for cases with rapid and massive bleeding complicated with general symptoms.

* 大黄

赛金化毒散

【处方】乳香（制）、黄连、没药（制）、甘草、川贝母、赤芍、雄黄、冰片、天花粉、牛黄、大黄、珍珠、大黄（酒炒）。

【功能主治】清热解毒。用于小儿毒火内热，口疮、咽炎、咳嗽、便秘。

Infant *Sai Jin* Detoxifing Powder

Name of Chinese Phonetic Alphabet Sai Jin Hua Du San

Formula Olibanum (prepared), Coptidis Rhizoma, Myrrha (prepared), Glycyrrhizae Radix et Rhizoma, Fritillariae Cirrhosae Bulbus, Paeoniae Radix Rubra, Realgar, Borneolum Syntheticum, Trichosanthis Radix, Bovis Calculus, Rhei Radix et Rhizoma, Margarita and Rhei Radix et Rhizoma (fried with wine).

Actions and Indications Clearing heat and detoxicating. It is used for infantile aphthae, pharyngitis, cough and constipation due to internal heat and heat-toxin.

赛胃安胶囊

【处方】石膏、冰片。

【功能主治】止血，消炎，收敛，促进肉芽新生，使溃疡面愈合。用于胃、十二指肠溃疡，急、慢性胃炎，食管炎，口腔炎。

【注意】服药期间忌服碱性药物；本品应空腹服用，使该药接触溃疡面机会较多，愈合更快。

Stomach-calming Capsule

Name of Chinese Phonetic Alphabet Sai Wei An Jiao Nang

Formula Gypsum Fibrosum and Borneolum Syntheticum.

Actions and Indications Relieving bleeding, antiphlogistic, astringing, promoting regeneration of granulation, healing ulcer. It is indicated for gastric ulcer, duodenal ulcer, acute or chronic gastritis, esophagitis, stomatitis.

Warning Alkaline drugs should be prohibited during medication; it should be taken in empty stomach, in order to increase its possibility to contact the ulcer area for healing faster.

赛霉安散

【处方】石膏、冰片。

【功能主治】清热止血，收敛祛湿，化腐生肌。用于口、鼻、喉黏膜溃疡、发炎、出血，牙周溃疡，刀伤、慢性溃疡，子宫颈糜烂，阴道炎，痔疮，肛瘘，褥疮。也可作新生婴儿脐粉。

【注意】勿与水混合使用。

Sai Mei An Powder

Name of Chinese Phonetic Alphabet Sai Mei An San

Formula Gypsum Fibrosum and Borneolum Syntheticum.

Actions and Indications Clearing heat and relieving bleeding, astringing and dispelling dampness, removing necrosis and promoting tissue regeneration. It is used for mucosal ulcer of the mouth, nose and throat, inflammation, bleeding, peridental ulcer, cutting and chronic ulcer, cervical erosion, vaginitis, hemorrhoid, anal fistula, bedsore, and it is also used as umbilical powder for newborn.

Warning The preparation is prohibited from being mixed with water.

蜜炼川贝枇杷膏

【处方】川贝母、枇杷叶、桔梗、陈皮、水半夏、北沙参、五味子、款冬花、杏仁水、薄荷脑。

【功能主治】清热润肺，止咳平喘，理气化痰。适用于肺燥之咳嗽，痰多，胸闷，咽喉痛痒，声音沙哑。

Honeyed Sichuan Fritillary* and Loquat Leaf** Soft Extract

Name of Chinese Phonetic Alphabet Mi Lian Chuan Bei Pi Pa Gao

Formula Fritillariae Cirrhosae Bulbus, Eriobotryae Folium, Platycodonis Radix, Citri Reticulatae Pericarpium, Pinelliae Cordatae Tuber, Glehniae Radix, Schisandrae Chinensis Fructus, Farfarae Flos, Armeniacae Semen Amarum (water solution) and Menthol.

Actions and Indications Clearing heat, moistening the lung, relieving cough and dyspnea, regulating *qi*, resolving phlegm. It is used for cough with profuse phlegm, chest distress, throat itching and hoarseness due to lung-dryness.

* 川贝 ** 枇杷叶

嫦娥加丽丸

【处方】人参、当归、川芎、丹参、赤芍、淫羊藿、韭菜子、蛇床子、薏苡仁、蟾酥。

【功能主治】补肾益气，养血活血，调经赞育。用于肾阳虚损，更年期综合征，月经紊乱，痛经，功能性不孕症，性欲减退等症。

【注意】孕妇及肾阴虚者忌服。

Goddess Pill for Menopausal Syndrome

Name of Chinese Phonetic Alphabet Chang E Jia Li Wan

Formula Ginseng Radix et Rhizoma, Angelicne Sinensis Radix, Chuanxiong Rhizoma, Salviae Miltiorrhizae Radix et Rhizoma, Paeoniae Radix Rubra, Epimedii Folium, Allii Tuberosi Semen, Cnidii Fructus, Coicis Semen and Bufonis Venenum.

Actions and Indications Tonifying the kidney and *qi*, nourishing and activating blood, regulating menstruation. It is indicated for menopausal syndrome, menstrual disorder, dysmenorrhea, functional sterility and sexual hypoesthesia due to deficiency of kidney-*yang*.

Warning It is contraindicated for pregnant women and cases with *yin*-deficiency of the kidney.

熊胆开明片

【处方】熊胆粉、石决明、菊花、枸杞子、泽泻等。

【功能主治】清肝泄热，滋阴明目。用于瞳神紧小症，症见目赤肿痛，羞明流泪，视物模糊以及急性虹膜睫状体炎见以上证候者。

Tablet of Bear Gall* for Miosis

Name of Chinese Phonetic Alphabet Xiong Dan Kai Ming Pian

Formula Ursi Fel Pulvis, Haliotidis Concha, Chrysanthemi Flos, Lycii Fructus, Alismatis Rhizoma, etc.

Actions and Indications Clearing the liver-heat, nourishing *yin* and improving vision. It is indicated for miosis manifested as conjunctival congestion, photophobia, lacrimation, blurred vision and acute iridocyclitis with the above mentioned symptoms.

* 熊胆

熊胆胶囊

【处方】本品为熊胆制成的胶囊。

【功能主治】清热，解毒，利胆，明目，解痉。用于惊风抽搐，黄疸，咽喉肿痛。

Bear Gall* Capsule

Name of Chinese Phonetic Alphabet Xiong Dan Jiao Nang

Formula Ursi Fel.

Actions and Indications Clearing heat, detoxicating, soothing the gallbladder, improving eyesight, relaxing spasm. It is indicated for convulsive spasm, jaundice, sore-throat.

* 熊胆

熊胆救心丸

【处方】熊胆、蟾酥、冰片、麝香、人参、珍珠、牛黄、猪胆膏、水牛角浓缩粉。

【功能主治】强心益气，芳香开窍。用于心气不足所指的胸痹心痛，胸闷气短和心悸。

【注意】小儿及孕妇忌服。

Cardiotonic Pill of Bear Gall*

Name of Chinese Phonetic Alphabet Xiong Dan Jiu Xin Wan

Formula Ursi Fel, Bufonis Venenum, Borneolum Syntheticum, Moschus, Ginseng Radix et Rhizoma, Margarita, Bovis Calculus, Suillus Fel Extractum and Bubali Cornu Pulvis Concentratio.

Actions and Indications Cardiotonic, tonifying *qi*, inducing resuscitation. It is indicated for chest impediment, heart pain, chest distress, shortness of breath and palpitation due to insufficiency of heart-*qi*.

Warning It is contraindicated for children and pregnant women.

* 熊胆

熊胆痔灵膏

【处方】熊胆、冰片、炉甘石（煅）、珍珠母、蛋黄油、凡士林等。

【功能主治】清热解毒，消肿止痛，敛疮生肌，止痒，止血。用于内外痔，痔漏，肠风下血，直肠炎，肛窦炎及内痔手术止血。

Bear Gall* Ointment for Hemorrhoid

Name of Chinese Phonetic Alphabet Xiong Dan Zhi Ling Gao

Formula Ursi Fel, Borneolum Syntheticum, Calamina (calcined), Margaritifera Concha, Ovi Luteum Oleum, Vaseline, etc.

Actions and Indications Clearing heat and detoxicating, dispersing swelling and alleviating pain, astringing and promoting tissue regeneration, relieving itching and bleeding. It is indicated for internal and external hemorrhoid, internal hemorrhoid and anal fistula, hematochezia, proctitis, anal sinusitis and relieving bleeding during surgery of internal hemorrhoid.

*熊胆

缩泉丸

【处方】山药、益智（盐炒）、乌药。

【功能主治】补肾缩尿。用于肾虚之小便频数，夜卧遗尿。

Urination-reducing Pill

Name of Chinese Phonetic Alphabet Suo Quan Wan

Formula Dioscorcac Rhizoma, Alpiniac Oxyphyllae Fructus (fried with salt) and Linderae Radix.

Actions and Indications Tonifying the kidney, reducing urination. It is used for frequent urination and enuresis at night due to deficiency of the kidney.

十五画

增光片

【处方】党参、石菖蒲、茯苓、泽泻、五味子、麦冬、枸杞子、当归、牡丹皮、远志（甘草水制）。

【功能主治】补气益血，滋养肝肾，明目安神，增加视力。用于治疗近视眼。

Promoting Vision Tablet

Name of Chinese Phonetic Alphabet Zeng Guang Pian

Formula Codonopsis Radix, Acori Tatarinowii Rhizoma, Poria, Alismatis Rhizoma, Schisandrae Chinensis Fructus, Ophiopogonis Radix, Lycii Fructus, Angelicae Sinensis Radix, Moutan Cortex and Polygalae Radix (prepared with licorice root water).

Actions and Indications Tonifying *qi* and, enriching and nourishing the liver and kidney, calming the mind and improving visual acuity. It is indicated for the treatment of myopia.

橡皮生肌膏

【处方】橡皮（制）、血余炭、龟甲、地黄、当归、石膏、蜂蜡、炉甘石。

【功能主治】止痛生肌，消炎。用于褥疮、烧伤及大面积创面感染的后期治疗。

Sawtooth Oak* Plaster for Promoting Tissue Regeneration

Name of Chinese Phonetic Alphabet Xiang Pi Shcng Ji Gao

Formula Querci Acutissimae Cortex (prepared), Crinis Carbonisatus, Testudinis Carapax et Plastrum, Rehmanniae Radix, Angelicae Sinensis Radix, Gypsum Fibrosum, Cera Flava and Calamina.

Actions and Indications Relieving pain and promoting tissue regeneration, counteracting inflammation. It is used for late treatment of bedsore, burn and wound infection of extensive surface.

*橡皮

镇心痛口服液

【处方】党参、三七、延胡索（醋炙）、地龙、薤白、肉桂、葶苈子（炒）、冰片、薄荷脑。

【功能主治】益气活血，祛痰通络，宽胸止痛。适用于气虚血瘀痰阻型胸痹，症见胸痛、胸闷、心悸、气短、乏力、舌暗有瘀斑、苔白腻、脉弦细，及冠心病、心绞痛见上述证候者。

【注意】孕妇慎用。

Chest-soothing Oral Liquid

Name of Chinese Phonetic Alphabet Zhen Xin Tong Kou Fu Ye

Formula Codonopsis Radix, Notoginseng Radix et Rhizoma, Corydalis Rhizoma (prepared with vinegar), Pheretima, Allii Macrostemonis Bulbus, Cinnamomi Cortex, Lepidii Semen (fried), Borneolum Syntheticum and Menthol.

Actions and Indications Tonifying *qi*, activating blood, dispelling phlegm, dredging collaterals, soothing the chest, alleviating pain. It is used for chest impediment syndrome manifested as chest pain and distress, palpitation, shortness of breath, fatigue, purple tongue with ecchymosis, whitish and greasy tongue fur, string-like and fine pulse due to deficiency of *qi*, blood-stasis and stagnation of phlegm, and also used for coronary heart disease, angina pectoris with the above mentioned symptoms.

Warning It should be used cautiously for pregnant women.

镇咳宁糖浆

【处方】甘草流浸膏、桔梗酊、盐酸麻黄碱、桑白皮酊。

【功能主治】镇咳祛痰。用于伤风咳嗽，支气管炎，哮喘。

【注意】冠心病、心绞痛和甲状腺功能亢进患者慎用。

Settling Cough Syrup

Name of Chinese Phonetic Alphabet Zhen Ke Ning Tang Jiang

Formula Glycyrrhizae Extractum, Platycodonis Tincturae, Ephedrine Hydrochloride and Tinctura Mori Cortex.

Actions and Indications Settling cough and dispelling phlegm. It is indicated for cough due to common cold; bronchitis and asthma.

Warning It should be used carefully for cases with coronary heart disease, angina pectoris and hyperthyroidism.

镇脑宁胶囊

【处方】本品为川芎、藁本、细辛、白芷、水牛角浓缩粉、丹参、猪脑粉等经加工制成的胶囊剂。

【功能主治】息风通络。用于内伤头痛，伴有恶心，呕吐，视物不清，肢体麻木，头昏，耳鸣及高血压，动脉硬化，血管神经性头痛。

Headache-relieving Capsule

Name of Chinese Phonetic Alphabet Zhen Nao Ning Jiao Nang

Formula Chuanxiong Rhizoma, Ligustici Rhizoma et Radix, Asari Radix et Rhizoma, Angelicae Dahuricae Radix, Bubali Cornu Pulvis Concentratio, Salviae Miltiorrhizae Radix et Rhizoma, Suillus Encephalon Pulvis, etc.

Actions and Indications Extinguishing wind, dredging collaterals. It is used for headache due to internal damage accompanied with nausea, vomiting, poor vision, numbness of limbs, dizziness, tinnitus and also used for hypertension, arteriosclerosis, angioneurotic headache.

瘢痕止痒软化膏

【处方】复方五倍子浸膏、冰片、薄荷脑、樟脑、水杨酸甲酯。

【功能主治】活血，除湿止痒。用于灼伤或手术后的增殖性瘢痕。

【注意】孕妇慎用。

Soft Ointment for Hyperplastic Scar

Name of Chinese Phonetic Alphabet Ban Hen

Zhi Yang Ruan Hua Gao

Formula Galla Chinensis Extractum, Borneolum Syntheticum, Menthol, Camphora and Methyl Salicylate.

Actions and Indications Activating blood, eliminating dampness and relieving itching. It is used for hyperplastic scar after burn or operation.

Warning It should be used cautiously for pregnant women.

糊药

【处方】苍术（炒）、厚朴（炒）、陈皮、枳实（炒）、山楂（焦）、麦芽（炒）、六神曲（炒）、槟榔（炒）、草果（炒）、酒药（炒）、麦饼（炒）、糯米饭（炒）、鸡内金（炒）、甘草（炒）。

【功能主治】开胃消食，理气，化滞。用于消化不良，停食反胃，嗳腐吞酸，脘腹胀痛，腹泻。

【注意】体弱者慎用。

Medicinal Pasty for Appetite-improving

Name of Chinese Phonetic Alphabet Hu Yao

Formula Atractylodis Rhizoma (fried), Magnoliae Officinalis Cortex (fried), Citri Reticulatae Pericarpium, Aurantii Fructus Immaturus (fried), Crataegi Fructus (charred), Hordei Fructus Germinatus (fried), Medicata Massa Fermentata (fried), Arecae Semen (fried), Tsaoko Fructus (fried), Vine-fermentum (fried), Trici Aestivi Massa Pulvis (fried), Oryzae Glutinosae Fructus (cooked rice), Galli Gigerii Enthothelium Corneum (fried) and Glycyrrhizae Radix et Rhizoma (fried).

Actions and Indications Increasing appetite and promoting digestion, regulating *qi*, dispersing stagnation. It is used for dyspepsia, stagnant food, food regurgitation, eructation, acid regurgitation, abdominal distention and pain and diarrhea.

Warning It is contraindicated for general debility.

鹤草芽栓

【处方】仙鹤草。

【功能主治】杀虫，驱虫止痛。用于绦虫病，表现为腹痛、腹泻、呕吐，或大便可见白色长寸许的节片，消瘦，纳食不香。

【注意】局部有皮肤病者慎用。

Hairyvein Agrimonia* Suppository for Expelling Cestode

Name of Chinese Phonetic Alphabet He Cao Ya Shuan

Formula Agrimoniae Herba.

Actions and Indications Expelling and killing worms, relieving pain. It is used for cestodiasis, manifested as abdominal pain, diarrhea, vomiting, proglottis in stool, emaciation and poor appetitie.

Warning It is contraindicated for cases with topical dermatosis.

* 仙鹤草

鹤蟾片

【处方】仙鹤草、干蟾皮、猫爪草、浙贝母、生半夏、鱼腥草、天冬、人参、葶苈子。

【功能主治】解毒除痰，凉血祛瘀，消癥散结。用于原发性支气管癌，能够改善患者的主观症状体征，提高患者体质。

Hairyvein Agrimonia* and Toad Skin** Tablet for Relieving Primary Bronchogenic Carcinoma

Name of Chinese Phonetic Alphabet He Chan Pian

Formula Agrimoniae Herba, Bufonis Cutis, Ranunculi Ternati Radix, Fritillariae Thunbergii Bulbus, Pinelliae Rhizoma, Houttuyniae Herba, Asparagi Radix, Ginseng Radix et Rhizoma and Lepidii Semen.

Actions and Indications Detoxicating and eliminating phlegm, cooling blood and dispelling stasis, eliminating mass. It is indicated for primary bronchogenic carcinoma, and can improve patients' subjective symptoms and signs, and promote the patients' constitution.

* 仙鹤草 ** 干蟾皮

十六画

橘红化痰丸

【处方】橘红、锦灯笼、川贝母、苦杏仁（炒）、罂粟壳、五味子、白矾、甘草。

【功能主治】滋阴清肺，敛肺止咳，化痰平喘。用于肺肾阴虚，咳嗽，气促喘急，咽干舌红，胸膈满闷。

Satsuma Orange Exocarp* Bolus for Resolving Phlegm

Name of Chinese Phonetic Alphabet Ju Hong Hua Tan Wan

Formula Citri Exocarpium Rubrum, Physalis Calyx seu Fructus, Fritillariae Cirrhosae Bulbus, Armeniacae Semen Amarum (fried), Papaveris Pericarpium, Schisandrae Chinensis Fructus, Alumen and Glycyrrhizae Radix et Rhizoma.

Actions and Indications Enriching *yin* and clearing lung-heat, astringing the lung to relieve cough, resolving phlegm and calming dyspnea. It is indicated for cough, shortness of breath, dry throat and red tongue and chest upset due to *yin*-deficiency of the lung and kidney.

* 橘红

橘红片

【处方】化橘红、陈皮、半夏（制）、茯苓、甘草、桔梗、苦杏仁、紫苏子（炒）、紫菀、款冬花、瓜蒌皮、浙贝母、地黄、麦冬、石膏。

【功能主治】清肺，化痰，止咳。用于咳嗽痰多，痰不易出，胸闷口干。

Huazhou Pummelo Peel* Tablet for Relieving Productive Cough

Name of Chinese Phonetic Alphabet Ju Hong Pian

Formula Citri Grandis Exocarpium, Citri Reticulatae Pericarpium, Pinelliae Rhizoma (prepared), Poria, Glycyrrhizae Radix et Rhizoma, Platycodonis Radix, Armeniacae Semen Amarum, Perillae Fructus (fried), Asteris Radix et Rhizoma, Farfarae Flos, Trichosanthis Pericarpium, Fritillariae Thunbergii Bulbus, Rehmanniae Radix, Ophiopogonis Radix and Gypsum Fibrosum.

Actions and Indications Clearing lung-heat, resolving phlegm and relieving cough. It is indicated for cough with profuse phlegm, difficult expectoration, oppression in the chest and dry mouth.

* 化橘红

橘红梨膏

【处方】化橘红、梨、川贝母、天冬、麦冬、苦杏仁、枇杷叶、五味子。

【功能主治】养阴清肺，止咳化痰。用于肺胃阴虚，口干咽燥，久咳痰少。

Huazhou Pummelo Peel* and Pear Soft Extract

Name of Chinese Phonetic Alphabet Ju Hong Li Gao

Formula Citri Grandis Exocarpium, Pyri Fructus, Fritillariae Cirrhosae Bulbus, Asparagi Radix, Ophiopogonis Radix, Armeniacae Semen Amarum, Eriobotryae Folium and Schisandrae Chinensis Fructus.

Actions and Indications Nourishing *yin*, clearing lung-heat, relieving cough, resolving phlegm. It is used for dry mouth and throat and chronic cough with few productive due to dual *yin*-deficiency of the lung and stomach.

* 化橘红

橘红痰咳液

【处方】化橘红、百部（蜜炙）、茯苓、半夏（制）、白前、甘草、苦杏仁、五味子。

【功能主治】理气祛痰，润肺止咳。用于治疗感冒，支气管炎、咽喉炎引起的痰多咳嗽，气喘。

Huazhou Pummelo Peel* Oral Liquid for Reducing Productive Cough

Name of Chinese Phonetic Alphabet Ju Hong Tan Ke Ye

Formula Citri Grandis Exocarpium, Stemonae Radix (prepared with honey), Poria, Pinelliae Rhizoma (prepared), Cynanchi Stauntonii Rhizoma et Radix, Glycyrrhizae Radix et Rhizoma, Armeniacae Semen Amarum and Schisandrae Chinensis Fructus.

Actions and Indications Regulating *qi* and dispelling phlegm, moistening the lung and relieving cough. It is indicated for cough with profuse phlegm and dyspnea due to common cold, bronchitis and laryngopharyngitis.

* 化橘红

醒脑再造丸

【处方】黄芪、淫羊藿、石菖蒲、红参、三七、地龙、当归、红花、粉防己、赤芍、桃仁（炒）、石决明、天麻、仙鹤草、槐花（炒）、白术（炒）、胆南星、葛根、玄参、黄连、连翘、泽泻、川芎、枸杞子、全蝎（去钩）、制何首乌、决明子、沉香、白附子（制）、细辛、木香、僵蚕（炒）、猪牙皂、冰片、珍珠（豆腐制）、大黄。

【功能主治】化痰醒脑，祛风活络。用于神志不清，语言謇涩，口角流涎，肾虚痿痹，筋骨酸痛，手足拘挛，半身不遂及脑血栓形成的恢复期和后遗症。

【注意】孕妇忌服。

Mind-enlivening Pill

Name of Chinese Phonetic Alphabet Xing Nao Zai Zao Wan

Formula Astragali Radix, Epimedii Folium, Acori Tatarinowii Rhizoma, Ginseng Radix et Rhizoma Rubra, Notoginseng Radix et Rhizoma, Pheretima, Angelicae Sinensis Radix, Carthami Flos, Stephaniae Tetrandrae Radix, Paeoniae Radix Rubra, Persicae Semen (fried), Haliotidis Concha, Gastrodiae Rhizoma, Agrimoniae Herba, Sophorae Flos (fried), Atractylodis Macrocephalae Rhizoma (fried), Arisaema cum Bile, Puerariae Lobatae Radix, Scrophulariae Radix, Coptidis Rhizoma, Forsythiae Fructus, Alismatis Rhizoma, Chuanxiong Rhizoma, Lycii Fructus, Scorpio (removed hook), Polygoni Multiflori Radix Praeparata, Cassiae Semen, Aquilariae Lignum Resinatum, Typhonii Rhizoma (prepared), Asari Radix et Rhizoma, Aucklandiae Radix, Bombyx Batryticatus (fried), Gleditsiae Fructus Abnormalis, Borneolum Syntheticum, Margarita (prepared with bean curd) and Rhei Radix et Rhizoma.

Actions and Indications Resolving phlegm, enlivening the mind, dispelling wind, activating collaterals. It is used for unconsciousness, dysphasia, salivation, flaccidity syndrome, soreness and pain of the sinews and bone, spasm of extremities, convalescent period and sequela of hemiparalysis and cerebral thrombosis.

Warning It is contraindicated for pregnant women.

醒脑降压丸

【处方】黄芩、黄连、郁金、栀子、玄精石、珍珠母、辛夷、零陵香、朱砂、雄黄、冰片。

【功能主治】通窍醒脑，清心镇静，抗热消炎。用于高血压，言语不清，痰涎壅盛。

【注意】孕妇及肠胃溃疡者忌服。

Hypertension-relieving Pill

Name of Chinese Phonetic Alphabet Xing Nao Jiang Ya Wan

Formula Scutellariae Radix, Coptidis Rhizoma, Curcumae Radix, Gardeniae Fructus, Selenitum, Margaritifera Concha, Magnoliae Flos, Lysimachiae Foenum-graeci Herba, Cinnabaris, Realgar and Borneolum Syntheticum.

Actions and Indications Dredging orifices, enlivening the mind, clearing heart-fire, tranquilizing the mind, clearing heat, counteracting inflammation. It is used for hypertension, alalia and excessive phlegm.

Warning It is contraindicated for pregnant women and cases with gastrointestinal ulcer.

醒脑静注射液

【处方】麝香、郁金、冰片、栀子。

【功能主治】清热泻火，凉血解毒，开窍醒脑。用于流行性乙型脑膜炎，肝昏迷，热入营血，内陷心包，高热烦躁，神昏谵语，舌绛脉数。

Heat-clearing and Detoxifying Injection

Name of Chinese Phonetic Alphabet Xing Nao Jing Zhu She Ye

Formula Moschus, Curcumae Radix, Borneolum Syntheticum and Gardeniae Fructus.

Actions and Indications Clearing heat, purging fire, cooling blood and detoxifying, inducing resuscitation. It is indicated for epidemic encephalitis B, hepatic coma, high fever, vexation, coma, delirious speech, crimson tongue and rapid pulse due to heat entering nutrient and blood aspects and heat inward invading the pericardium.

醒消丸

【处方】雄黄、麝香、乳香（制）、没药（制）。

【功能主治】活血消肿，止痛。用于痈疽肿毒。

【注意】孕妇禁用。

Xing Xiao Pill

Name of Chinese Phonetic Alphabet Xing Xiao Wan

Formula Realgar, Moschus, Olibanum (prepared) and Myrrha (prepared).

Actions and Indications Activating blood and dispersing swelling, relieving pain. It is used for abscess and deep-rooted boil.

Warning It is contraindicated for pregnant women.

薯蓣丸

【处方】山药、人参、白术（麸炒）、茯苓、甘草、地黄、当归、白芍、川芎、阿胶、六神曲（麸炒）、大豆黄卷、大枣（去核）、苦杏仁（去皮、炒）、桂枝、柴胡、防风、干姜、桔梗、白蔹、麦冬。

【功能主治】调理脾胃，益气和营。用于气血两虚，脾肺不足所致之虚劳，胃脘痛，痹症，闭经，月经不调。

Chinese Yam* Pill

Name of Chinese Phonetic Alphabet Shu Yu Wan

Formula Dioscoreae Rhizoma, Ginseng Radix et Rhizoma, Atractylodis Macrocephalae Rhizoma (fried with bran), Poria, Glycyrrhizae Radix et Rhizoma, Rehmanniae Radix, Angelicae Sinensis Radix, Paeoniae Radix Alba, Chuanxiong Rhizoma, Asini Corii Colla, Medicata Massa Fermentata (fried with bran), Sojae Semen Germinatum, Jujubae Fructus (removed nucleus), Armeniacae Semen Amarum (removed coat and fried), Cinnamomi Ramulus, Bupleuri Radix, Saposhnikoviae Radix, Zingiberis Rhizoma, Platycodonis Radix, Ampelopsis Radix and Ophiopogonis Radix.

Actions and Indications Regulating the spleen and stomach, tonifying *qi* and harmonizing nutrient. It is indicated for consumptive disease, stomach duct pain, impediment syndrome, amenorrhea and irregular menstruation due to dual deficiency of *qi* and blood.

* 薯蓣

癃闭通胶囊

【处方】穿山甲（砂烫）、肉桂。

【功能主治】活血软坚，温阳利水。适用于血瘀凝聚、膀胱气化不利所致癃闭，见有排尿不畅、夜尿频多、尿细无力、淋漓不尽或尿频、尿急。或用于早期良性前列腺增生见有上述证候者。

Alleviating Difficult Urination Capsule

Name of Chinese Phonetic Alphabet Long Bi Tong Jiao Nang

Formula Manis Squama (scalded by sand) and Cinnamomi Cortex.

Actions and Indications Activating blood and

softening mass, warming *yang* and inducing diuresis. It is indicated for difficult urination due to stagnation of blood-stasis and inhibited *qi* of the bladder, manifested as difficult urination, frequency of nocturia, dribbling urine, frequency of micturition, urgency of urination, also for early stage of benign hyperplasia of prostate with the above mentioned symptoms.

癃闭舒胶囊

【处方】补骨脂、益母草、金钱草、海金沙、琥珀、山慈菇。

【功能主治】温肾化气，清热通淋，活血化瘀，散结止痛。用于肾气不足，湿热瘀阻之癃闭所致尿频尿急，尿赤尿痛，尿细如线，小腹拘急疼痛，腰膝酸软。前列腺增生有以上证候者也可应用。

Relieving Difficult Urination Capsule

Name of Chinese Phonetic Alphabet Long Bi Shu Jiao Nang

Formula Psoraleae Fructus, Leonuri Herba, Lysimachiae Herba, Lygodii Spora, Succinum and Cremastrae seu Pleiones Pseudobulbus.

Actions and Indications Warming the kidney and resolving *qi*, clearing heat and relieving strangury, activating blood and resolving stasis, dispersing mass and alleviating pain. It is indicated for frequency of micturition, urgency of urination, dark urine and urodynia, thready urine, spasm and pain in the lower abdomen, aching and wilting of the waist and knee due to insufficiency of kidney-*qi*, obstruction of damp-heat, also for hyperplasia of prostate with the above mentioned symptoms.

癃清片

【处方】金银花、黄柏、白花蛇舌草、牡丹皮、泽泻等。

【功能主治】清热解毒，凉血通淋。用于热淋所致的尿频、尿痛、腰痛、小腹坠胀。

【注意】体虚胃寒者不宜服用。

Relieving Difficult Urination Tablet

Name of Chinese Phonetic Alphabet Long Qing Pian

Formula Lonicerae Japonicae Flos, Phellodendri Chinensis Cortex, Hedyotis Diffusae Herba, Moutan Cortex, Alismatis Rhizoma, etc.

Actions and Indications Clearing heat and detoxicating, cooling blood and relieving strangury. It is indicated for frequency of micturition, urodynia, lumbago, distention in the lower abdomen due to heat strangury.

Warning It is not suitable for cases with debility and stomach cold.

糖脉康颗粒

【处方】黄芪、地黄、丹参、牛膝、麦冬、黄精等。

【功能主治】养阴清热，活血化瘀，益气固肾。用于糖尿病气阴两虚兼血瘀所致的倦怠乏力，气短懒言，自汗盗汗，五心烦热，口渴喜饮，胸中闷痛，肢体麻木或刺痛，便秘，舌质红少津，舌体胖大，苔薄，或舌黯有瘀斑，脉弦细或细数，或沉涩，以及Ⅱ型糖尿病及并发症见有上述证候者。

【注意】孕妇慎服。

Relieving Diabetes Granules

Name of Chinese Phonetic Alphabet Tang Mai Kang Ke Li

Formula Astragali Radix, Rehmanniae Radix, Salviae Miltiorrhizae Radix et Rhizoma, Achyranthis Bidentatae Radix, Ophiopogonis Radix, Polygonati Rhizoma, etc.

Actions and Indications Nourishing *yin*, clearing heat, activating blood and resolving stasis, tonifying *qi* and securing the kidney. It is indicated for diabetes attributed to dual deficiency of *qi* and *yin* associated with blood-stasis, and manifested as tiredness, fatigue, shortness of breath, indolent speaking, spontaneous sweating, night sweating, vexing heat in the chest, palms and soles, thirst, polydipsia, chest distress and pain, numbness or stabbing pain of limbs, constipation, red tongue with few fluid, enlarged tongue, thin tongue fur or dull tongue with ecchymosis, string like and fine or fine and rapid pulse or sunken and rough pulse. And also used for Ⅱ type diabetes and its complications with the above mentioned symptoms.

Warning It should be used carefully for pregnant women.

潞党参膏滋

【处方】本品为潞党参经加工制成的煎膏剂。

【功能主治】补中益气，健脾益肺，滋补强壮，增强人体免疫能力。用于脾肺虚弱，气短心悸，食少便溏，虚喘咳嗽。主治脾虚型小儿泄泻，妇产科贫血，慢性胃炎，慢性肾炎及放化疗后脾肺气虚。

【注意】不宜与藜芦同用。

Bellflower* Soft Extract

Name of Chinese Phonetic Alphabet Lu Dang Shen Gao Zi

Formula Codonopsis Radix.

Actions and Indications Tonifying the middle and *qi*, fortifying the spleen and tonifying the lung, tonifying and strengthening diathesis, enhancing body immunity. It is used for shortness of breath and palpitation, poor appetite and sloppy stool due to deficiency of the spleen and lung; dyspnea, cough and children diarrhea due to deficiency of the spleen; anemia of obstetrics, and chronic gastritis, chronic nephritis, *qi*-deficiency of the spleen and lung after radiotherapy and chemotherapy.

Warning It is not suitable to be used together with black falsehellebore**.

* 党参 ** 藜芦

避瘟散

【处方】檀香、零陵香、白芷、香榧草、姜黄、玫瑰花、甘松、丁香、木香、麝香、冰片、朱砂、薄荷脑 。

【功能主治】祛暑，开窍止痛。用于夏季暑邪引起的头目眩晕，头痛鼻塞，恶心，呕吐，晕车晕船。

Relieving Summer-heat Powder

Name of Chinese Phonetic Alphabet Bi Wen San

Formula Santali Albi Lignum, Lysimachiae Foenum-graeci Herba, Angelicae Dahuricae Radix, Eragrostidis Tenellae Herba, Curcumae Longae Rhizoma, Rosae Rugosae Flos, Nardostachyos Radix et Rhizoma, Caryophylli Flos, Aucklandiae Radix, Moschus, Borneolum Syntheticum, Cinnabaris and Menthol.

Actions and Indications Dispelling summer-heat, opening the orifices and relieving pain. It is used for headache, vertigo, nasal congestion, nausea, vomiting, car sickness and naupathia due to summer-heat pathogen.

十七画

藏青果冲剂

【处方】本品为西青果制成的冲剂。

【功能主治】清热，利咽、生津。用于急、慢性咽炎，慢性喉炎，慢性扁桃体炎。

Myrobalan* Soluble Granules

Name of Chinese Phonetic Alphabet Zang Qing Guo Chong Ji

Formula Chebulae Fructus.

Actions and Indications Clearing heat, soothing throat, engendering fluid. It is used for acute, chronic pharyngitis, chronic laryngitis and chronic tonsillitis.

* 藏青果

黛蛤散颗粒

【处方】青黛、蛤壳。

【功能主治】清肝利肺，降逆除烦。用于肝肺实热，头晕耳鸣，咳嗽吐衄，肺痿肺痈，咽膈不利，口渴心烦。

Indigo* and Clam Shell** Soluble Granules for Relieving Dizziness

Name of Chinese Phonetic Alphabet Dai Ge San Ke Li

Formula Indigo Naturalis and Meretricis Concha.

Actions and Indications Clearing liver-fire and soothing the lung, directing *qi* downward and relieving vexation. It is indicated for dizziness and tinnitus, cough and hematemesis, lung atrophy, lung abscess, discomfort in the throat, thirst and vexation due to excess heat of the liver and lung.

*青黛 **蛤壳

十八画

礞石滚痰丸

【处方】金礞石（煅）、沉香、黄芩、大黄。

【功能主治】降火逐痰。用于实热顽痰，发为癫狂惊悸，或咳喘痰稠，大便秘结。

【注意】孕妇忌服。

Mica-schist* Pill for Dispelling Phlegm

Name of Chinese Phonetic Alphabet Meng Shi Gun Tan Wan

Formula Micae Lapis Aureus (calcined), Aquilariae Lignum Resinatum, Scutellariae Radix and Rhei Radix et Rhizoma.

Actions and Indications Downbearing fire and dispelling phlegm. It is indicated for stubborn phlegm of excess heat syndrome, manifested as epilepsy, fright palpitation, or cough with thick phlegm, constipation.

Warning It is contraindicated for pregnant women.

*金礞石

鹭鸶咯丸

【处方】麻黄、苦杏仁、石膏、甘草、细辛、紫苏子（炒）、芥子（炒）、牛蒡子（炒）、瓜蒌皮、射干、青黛、蛤壳、天花粉、栀子（姜炙）、牛黄。

【功能主治】宣肺，化痰，止咳。用于百日咳，痰浊阻肺，咳嗽，痰鸣气促，咽干声哑。

Lu Si Ka Pill for Relieving Pertussis

Name of Chinese Phonetic Alphabet Lu Si Ka Wan

Formula Ephedrae Herba, Armeniacae Semen Amarum, Gypsum Fibrosum, Glycyrrhizae Radix et Rhizoma, Asari Radix et Rhizoma, Perillae Fructus (fried), Sinapis Semen (fried), Arctii Fructus (fried), Trichosanthis Pericarpium, Belamcandae Rhizoma, Indigo Naturalis, Meretricis Concha, Trichosanthis Radix, Gardeniae Fructus (prepared with ginger) and Bovis Calculus.

Actions and Indications Diffusing the lung, resolving phlegm and relieving cough. It is indicated for pertussis, stagnation of phlegm turbidity in the lung, cough, wheezing sound and shortness of breath, dry throat and hoarseness.

十九画

藿香正气丸

【处方】广藿香、紫苏叶、白芷、白术（炒）、陈皮、姜半夏、厚朴（姜制）、茯苓、桔梗、甘草、大腹皮、大枣、生姜。

【功能主治】解表，化湿，理气，和中。用于外感风寒，内伤湿滞，头痛昏重，胸膈痞闷，脘腹胀痛，呕吐泄泻。

Cablin Potchouli* Pill for Regulating *Qi*

Name of Chinese Phonetic Alphabet Huo Xiang Zheng Qi Wan

Formula Pogostemonis Herba, Perillae Folium, Angelicae Dahuricae Radix, Atractylodis Macrocephalae Rhizoma (fried), Citri Reticulatae Pericarpium, Pinelliae Rhizoma Praeparatum cum Zingibere et Alumine, Magnoliae Officinalis Cortex (prepared with ginger), Poria, Platycodonis Radix, Glycyrrhizae Radix et Rhizoma, Arecae Pericarpium, Jujubae Fructus and Zingiberis Rhizoma Recens.

Actions and Indications Releasing the exterior, resolving dampness, regulating *qi*, harmonizing the middle. It is indicated for headache, dizziness, chest distress, abdominal distention and pain, vomiting and diarrhea due to exogenous wind-cold, stagnation of internal dampness.

* 广藿香

藿胆丸

【处方】广藿香叶、猪胆浸膏。

【功能主治】清热化浊，宣通鼻窍。用于风寒化热，胆火上攻引起的鼻塞欠通，鼻渊头痛。

Huodan Pill

Name of Chinese Phonetic Alphabet Huo Dan Wan

Formula Pogostemonis Folium and Suillus Fel Extractum.

Actions and Indications Clearing heat and resolving turbidity, soothing the nasal orifice. It is indicated for nasal congestion, sinusitis and headache due to wind-cold transforming into heat and gallbladder fire flaming upward.

蟾酥注射液

【处方】本品为蟾酥经加工制成的灭菌水溶液。

【功能主治】清热解毒。用于急性、慢性化脓性感染，亦可作为抗肿瘤辅助用药。

Toad Venom* Injection

Name of Chinese Phonetic Alphabet Chan Su Zhu She Ye

Formula Bufonis Venenum.

Actions and Indications Clearing heat and detoxicating. It is used for actue or chronic pyogenic infection. It can also be used as an adjuvant medicine for anti-tumor.

* 蟾酥

癣灵药水

【处方】土荆皮、黄柏、白鲜皮、徐长卿、苦参、石榴皮、洋金花、南天仙子、地肤子、樟脑。

【功能主治】清热除湿，杀虫止痒，有较强的抗真菌作用。用于脚癣、手癣、体癣、股癣。

Medicated Aqua for Tinea

Name of Chinese Phonetic Alphabet Xuan Ling Yao Shui

Formula Pseudolaricis Cortex, Phellodendri Chinensis Cortex, Dictamni Cortex, Cynanchi Paniculati Radix et Rhizoma, Sophorae Flavescentis Radix, Granati Pericarpium, Daturae Flos, Hygrophilae Salicifoliae Semen, Kochiae Fructus and Camphora.

Actions and Indications Clearing heat and dispelling dampness, killing worms and relieve itching, anti-fungi. It is indicated for tinea pedis, tinea manuum, tinea corporis, tinea cruris.

癣湿药水

【处方】土荆皮、蛇床子、大枫子、百部、防风、当归、凤仙透骨草、侧柏叶、吴茱萸、花椒、蝉蜕、斑蝥。

【功能主治】祛风除湿，杀虫止痒。用于鹅掌风，灰指甲，湿癣，脚癣。

【注意】切忌入口，严防触及眼、鼻、口腔等黏膜处。

Medicated Aqua for Exudative Dermatitis

Name of Chinese Phonetic Alphabet Xuan Shi Yao Shui

Formula Pseudolaricis Cortex, Cnidii Fructus, Hydnocarpi Anthelmintici Semen, Stemonae Radix, Saposhnikoviae Radix, Angelicae Sinensis Radix, Impatientis Balsaminae Herba, Platycladi Cacumen, Euodiae Fructus, Zanthoxyli Pericarpium, Cicadae Periostracum and Mylabris.

Actions and Indications Dispelling wind and dampness, killing worms and relieving itching. It is indicated for tinea manuum, tinea of the nail, exudative dermatitis and tinea pedis.

Warning It is contraindicated for oral use. It cannot be touched by the mucosas of the eyes, nose and mouth.

二十画

獾油

【处方】獾油、冰片。

【功能主治】清热解毒，消肿止痛。用于烧伤、烫伤、皮肤肿痛。

Badger Fat*

Name of Chinese Phonetic Alphabet Huan You

Formula Melis Adeps and Borneolum Syntheticum.

Actions and Indications Clearing heat and detoxicating, dispersing swelling and relieving pain. It is used for burn, scald and swelling and pain of skin.

* 獾油

二十一画

麝香风湿胶囊

【处方】制川乌、全蝎、地龙（酒洗）、黑豆（炒）、蜂房（酒洗）、麝香、乌梢蛇（去头酒浸）。

【功能主治】祛风除湿，活络镇痛。用于风寒湿痹，关节疼痛，手足拘挛。

【注意】孕妇忌服。

Musk* Capsule for Relieving Wind-damp Impediment Syndrome

Name of Chinese Phonetic Alphabet She Xiang Feng Shi Jiao Nang

Formula Aconiti Radix Cocta, Scorpio, Pheretima (washed by wine), Sojae Semen Nigrum (fried), Vespae Nidus (washed by wine), Moschus and Zaocys (removed head, immerged in wine).

Actions and Indications Dispelling wind and dampness, activating collaterals and alleviating pain. It is indicated for wind-cold-damp impediment syndrome, marked by arthralgia, spasm of the hands and feet.

Warning It is contraindicated for pregnant women.

* 麝香

麝香壮骨膏

【处方】麝香、薄荷脑、水杨酸甲酯、豹骨、硫酸、软骨素、冰片、盐酸苯海拉明、樟脑等。

【功能主治】镇痛，消炎。用于风湿痛，关节痛，腰痛，神经痛，肌肉酸痛，扭伤，挫伤。

【注意】孕妇慎用。

Musk* Plaster for Strengthening Bone

Name of Chinese Phonetic Alphabet She Xiang Zhuang Gu Gao

Formula Moschus, Menthol, Methyl Salicylate, Pardi Os, Chondroitin Sulfuric Acid, Borneolum Syntheticum, Diphenhydramine Hydrochloride, Camphora, etc.

Actions and Indications Settling pain and antiphlogistic. It is indicated for rheumatalgia, arthralgia, lumbago, neuralgia, aching pain of muscle, sprain, contusion.

Warning It should be used carefully for pregnant women.

* 麝香

麝香抗栓胶囊

【处方】麝香、羚羊角、三七、天麻、全蝎、乌梢蛇、红花、地黄、大黄、葛根、川芎、僵蚕、黄芪、地龙、赤芍、胆南星、当归、豨莶草、忍冬藤、鸡血藤、络石藤、水蛭（烫）。

【功能主治】通络活血，醒脑散瘀。用于中风，半身不遂，言语不清，头昏目眩。

【注意】孕妇慎用。

Musk* Capsule for Reliving Apoplexy

Name of Chinese Phonetic Alphabet She Xiang Kang Shuan Jiao Nang

Formula Moschus, Saigae Tataricae Cornu, Notoginseng Radix et Rhizoma, Gastrodiae Rhizoma, Scorpio, Zaocys, Carthami Flos, Rehmanniae Radix, Rhei Radix et Rhizoma, Puerariae Lobatae Radix, Chuanxiong Rhizoma, Bombyx Batryticatus, Astragali Radix, Pheretima, Paeoniae Radix Rubra, Arisaema cum Bile, Angelicae Sinensis Radix, Siegesbeckiae Herba, Lonicerae Japonicae Caulis, Spatholobi Caulis, Trachelospermi Caulis et Folium and Hirudo (scalded).

Actions and Indications Dredging collaterals, activating blood, enlivening the mind, dissipating stasis. It is indicated for apoplexy, hemiparalysis, alalia, dizziness and dizzy vision.

Warning It should be used cautiously for pregnant women.

* 麝香

麝香保心丸

【处方】本品由麝香、人参、苏合香、蟾酥等药经加工制成。

【功能主治】芳香温通，益气强心。用于心肌缺血引起的心绞痛，胸闷及心肌梗死。

【注意】孕妇禁用。

Musk* Pill for Strengthening Heart

Name of Chinese Phonetic Alphabet She Xiang Bao Xin Wan

Formula Moschus, Ginseng Radix et Rhizoma, Styrax, Bufonis Venenum, etc.

Actions and Indications Tonifying *qi*, strengthening the heart. It is indicated for angina pectoris due to myocardial ischemia; chest distress and myocardial infarction.

Warning It is contraindicated for pregnant women.

* 麝香

麝香祛风湿油

【处方】麝香、血竭、乳香、没药、水杨酸甲酯、桉油、薄荷脑、桂皮油、丁香罗勒油、樟脑、冰片、颠茄浸膏、麝香草脑、盐酸苯海拉明。

【功能主治】祛风湿，活血，镇痛，消肿。用于风湿痛，筋骨痛，关节痛，腰腿酸痛，坐骨神经痛以及跌打肿痛。

【注意】孕妇慎用。

Musk* Oils for Dispelling Rheumatalgia

Name of Chinese Phonetic Alphabet She Xiang Qu Feng Shi You

Formula Moschus, Draconis Sanguis, Olibanum, Myrrha, Methyl Salicylate, Eucalypti Oleum, Menthol, Cinnamomi Oleum, Ocimi Basilici Oleum, Camphora, Borneolum Syntheticum, Belladonnae Extractum, Thymol and Diphenhydramine Hydrochloride.

Actions and Indications Dispelling wind and dampness, activating blood and relieving pain, dispersing swelling. It is indicated for rheumatalgia, ostealgia, arthralgia, soreness and pain of the waist and legs, sciatica and traumatic injury.

Warning It should be used carefully for pregnant women.

* 麝香

麝香舒活精

【处方】樟脑、冰片、薄荷脑、麝香酊、红花酊、三七酊、血竭酊、地黄酊。

【功能主治】活血散瘀，消肿止痛。用于运动损伤，急、慢性软组织损伤；骨折肿痛及脱位愈合后的关节肿痛，风湿痛。

【注意】孕妇慎用。

Musk* Tincture

Name of Chinese Phonetic Alphabet She Xiang

Shu Huo Jing

Formula Camphora, Borneolum Syntheticum, Menthol, Moschus Tinctura, Carthami Flos Tinctura, Notoginseng Tinctura, Draconis Sanguis Tinctura and Rehmanniae Tinctura.

Actions and Indications Activating blood, dissipating stasis, dispersing swelling, alleviating pain. It is uesd for sport injury, acute or chronic soft tissue injury, swelling due to fracture, arthralgia after healed dislocation and rheumatalgia.

Warning It should be used carefully for pregnant women.

* 麝香

麝香镇痛膏

【处方】麝香、生川乌、水杨酸甲酯、颠茄流浸膏、辣椒、红茴香根、樟脑。

【功能主治】散寒，活血，镇痛。用于风湿性关节痛，关节扭伤。

Musk* Plaster for Relieving Rheumatic Arthralgia

Name of Chinese Phonetic Alphabet She Xiang Zhen Tong Gao

Formula Moschus, Aconiti Radix, Methylsalicylate, Belladonnae Extractum, Capsici Fructus, Illicii Lanceolati Radix and Camphora.

Actions and Indications Dissipating cold, activating blood, relieving pain. It is indicated for rheumatic arthralgia and sprain of joints.

* 麝香

麝珠明目滴眼液

【处方】麝香、珍珠、冰片、冬虫夏草、石决明、炉甘石、黄连、黄柏、大黄、蛇胆、猪胆膏、荆芥、紫苏叶。

【功能主治】消翳明目。用于老年性初、中期白内障。

【注意】治疗过程中如局部出现炎症反应，立即停药。

Musk* and Pearl** Eye Drops

Name of Chinese Phonetic Alphabet She Zhu Ming Mu Di Yan Ye

Formula Moschus, Margarita, Borneolum Syntheticum, Cordyceps, Haliotidis Concha, Calamina, Coptidis Rhizoma, Phellodendri Chinensis Cortex, Rhei Radix et Rhizoma, Naja Fel, Suillus Fel Extractum, Schizonepetae Herba and Perillae Folium.

Actions and Indications Removing the nebula to improve vision. It is indicated for senile initial or middle stage of cataract.

Warning In case the topical inflammation occurred, suspended the medicine immediately.

* 麝香 ** 珍珠

癫痫康胶囊

【处方】天麻、石菖蒲、僵蚕、胆南星、川贝母、丹参、远志、全蝎、麦冬、淡竹叶、生姜、琥珀、人参、冰片、人工牛黄。

【功能主治】镇惊息风，化痰开窍，滋阴活血。用于痰迷心窍、心神失养、肝风内动、神昏抽搐。

Relieving Epilepsy Capsule

Name of Chinese Phonetic Alphabet Dian Xian Kang Jiao Nang

Formula Gastrodiae Rhizoma, Acori Tatarinowii Rhizoma, Bombyx Batryticatus, Arisaema cum Bile, Fritillariae Cirrhosae Bulbus, Salviae Miltiorrhizae Radix et Rhizoma, Polygalae Radix, Scorpio, Ophiopogonis Radix, Lophatheri Herba, Zingiberis Rhizoma Recens, Succinum, Ginseng Radix et Rhizoma, Borneolum Syntheticum and Bovis Calculus Artifactus.

Actions and Indications Settling fright and extinguishing wind, resolving phlegm and opening the orifices, enriching *yin* and activating blood. It is indicated for loss of consciousness and spasm due to phlegm clouding the pericardium, inadequate nourishment of the heart and internal stirring of liver-wind.

附录一　中成药英文名称检索表

Appendix I: Key of Chinese Patent Medicines Names in English

A

B

C

D

E

F

G

H

I

J

K

L

M

N

O

P

Q

R

S

T

U

V

W

X

Y

Z

附录二 中药学名检索表
Appendix Ⅱ: Key of Scientific Names of Chinese Medicinals

说明：

1.按中药名称首字笔画多少排序。

2.第一行标示中药名称及其拉丁文药材名称；第二行为中药的药用部（英文）及其原植（动）物的学名；矿物药只标示名称。

3.凡有＊号者，均出自《中华人民共和国药典》。

4.下列中药，偶见同一药物而名称不同者。

一画

一点红 *Duchesneae Indicae Herba*
herb of *Duchesnea indica* (Andr.) Focke 蛇莓

二画

十大功劳叶 *Mahoniae Folium*
leaf of *Mahoniae bealei* (Fort.) Carr. 阔叶十大功劳

七叶莲 *Schefflerae Arboricolae Radix*
root of *Schefflera arboricola* Hayata 鹅掌藤

七叶一枝花 *Paridis Rhizoma*
rhizome of *Paris polyphylla* Smith var. *chinensis* (Franch.) Hara 七叶一枝花

丁香＊ *Caryophylli Flos*
alabastrum of *Eugenia caryophyllata* Thunb. 丁香

丁香油 *Caryophylli Oleum*
flower oil of *Eugenia caryophyllata* Thunb. 丁香

丁香罗勒油 *Ocimi Basilici Oleum*
herb oil of *Ocimum basilicum* L. 罗勒

丁公藤＊ *Erycibes Caulis*
stem of *Ericibe obtusifolia* Benth. 丁公藤

丁茄根 *Solani Surattensis Radix*
root of *Solanum surattense* Burm. f. 丁茄

丁香蓼 *Ludwigiae Prostratae Herba*
herb of *Ludwigia prostrate* Roxb. 丁香蓼

丁癸草 *Zorniae Diphyllae Herba*
herb of *Zornia diphylla* Pers. 丁癸草

八角枫根 *Alangii Radix*
root of *Alangium chinense* (Lour.) Harms 八角枫

八角茴香＊ *Anisi Stellati Fructus*
fruit of *Illicum verum* Hook. f. 八角茴香

八角茴香油 *Anisi Stellati Oleum*
oil of *Illicum verum* Hook. f. 八角茴香

人工牛黄＊ *Bovis Calculus Artifactus*
artificial bezoar

人工麝香 *Moschus Artifactus*
artificial musk

人参＊ *Ginseng Radix et Rhizoma*
root and rhizome of *Panax ginseng* C. A. Mey. 人参

人参须 *Ginseng Radix Fibrosa*

fibrous root of *Panax ginseng* C. A. Mey. 人参

人参粉 *Ginseng Pulvis*
powder of *Panax ginseng* C. A. Mey. 人参

人指甲 *Hominis Unguis*
finger nail

儿茶 * *Catechu*
twig extract of *Acacia catechu* (L. f.) Willd 儿茶

九节茶 *Sarcandrae Herba*
herb of *Sarcandra glabra* (Thunb.) Nakai 草珊瑚

九节菖蒲 *Anemones Altaicae Rhizoma*
rhizome of *Anemone altaica* Fisch. 阿尔泰银莲花

九里香 * *Murrayae Folium et Cacumen*
leaf and tender twig of *Murraya exotica* L. 九里香

九层风 *Spatholobi Caulis*
stem of *Spatholobus suberectus* Dunn 密花豆

九层塔 *Ocimi Basilici Herba*
herb of *Ocimum basilicum* L. 罗勒

九香虫 * *Aspongopus*
insect of *Aspongopus chinensis* Dallas 九香虫

了哥王 *Wikstroemiae Indicae Caulis et Folium*
stem and leaf of *Wikstroemia indica* (L.) C. A. Mey. 了哥王

了刁竹 *Cynanchi Paniculati Radix et Rhizoma*
root and rhizome of *Cynanchum paniculatum* (Bge.) Kitag. 徐长卿

三画

三七 * *Notoginseng Radix et Rhizoma*
root and rhizome of *Panax notoginseng* (Burk.) F. H. Chen 三七

三七茎叶 *Notoginseng Caulis et Folium*
stem and leaf of *Panax notoginseng* (Burk.) F. H. Chen 三七

三七浸膏 *Notoginseng Extractum*
extract of *Panax notoginseng* (Burk.) F. H. Chen 三七

三叉苦 *Euodiae Leptae Folium*
leaf of *Euodia lepta* (Spr.) Merr. 三叉苦

三棱 * *Sparganii Rhizoma*
tuber of *Sparganium stoloniferum* Buch.-Ham. 黑三棱

干姜 * *Zingiberis Rhizoma*
dried rhizome of *Zingiber officinale* Rosc. 姜

干漆 * *Toxicodendri Resina*
resin of *Toxicodendron vernicifluum* (Stokes) F. A. Barkl. 漆树

干蟾皮 *Bufonis Cutis*
dried skin of *Bufo bufo gargarizans* Cantor 中华大蟾蜍

土大黄 *Rumicis Nepalensis Radix*
root of *Rumex nepalensis* Spreng. 尼泊尔酸模

土木香 * *Inulae Radix*
root of *Inula helenium* L. 土木香

土贝母 * *Bolbostemmae Rhizoma*
tuber of *Bolbostemma paniculatum* (Maxim.) Franquet 土贝母

土牛膝 *Achyranthis Bidentatae Radix*
root of *Achyranthes bidentata* Bl. 牛膝

土田七 *Stahlianthi Involucrati Rhizoma*
rhizome of *Stahlianthus involucratus* (King ex Bak.) Craib. 土田七

土细辛 *Tylophorae Ovatae Radix et Rhizoma*
root and rhizome of *Tylophora ovata* (Lindl.) Hook. ex Steud. 娃儿藤

土荆皮 * *Pseudolaricis Cortex*
root-bark of *Pseudolarix amabilis* (Nelson) Rehd. 金钱松

土荆芥 *Chenopodii Ambrosioidis Herba*
herb of *Chenopodium ambrosioides* L.土荆芥

土茯苓 * *Smilacis Glabrae Rhizoma*
rhizome of *Smilax glabra* Roxb. 光叶菝葜

土鳖虫 * *Eupolyphaga seu Steleophaga*
insect of *Eupolyphaga sinensis* Walker 地鳖 or *Steleophaga plancyi* (Boleny)冀地鳖

大枣 * *Jujubae Fructus*
fruit of *Ziziphus jujube* Mill. 枣

大黄 * *Rhei Radix et Rhizoma*
root and rhizome of *Rheum officinale* Baill. 药用大黄

大黄粉 *Rhei Pulvis*
powder of *Rheum officinale* Baill. 药用大黄

大黄浸膏 *Rhei Extractum*
extract of *Rheum officinale* Baill. 药用大黄

大蒜 * *Allii Sativi Bulbus*
bulb of *Allium sativum* L. 大蒜

大蓟 * *Cirsii Japonici Herba*
herb of *Cirsium japonicum* Fisch. ex DC. 蓟

大力王 *Cardui Crispi Herba*

herb of *Carduus crispus* L. 飞廉
大风子 *Hydnocarpi Anthelmintici Semen*
seed of *Hydnocarpus anthelminticus* Pier. 大风子
大风子油 *Hydnocarpi Anthelmintici Semen Oleum*
seed oil of *Hydnocarpus anthelminticus* Pier. 大风子
大风艾 *Blumae Balsamiferae Folium et Ramulus*
leaf and tender twig of *Bluma balsamifera* (L.) DC. 艾纳香
大血藤 * *Sargentodoxae Caulis*
stem of *Sargentodoxa cuneata* (Oliv.) Rehd. et Wils. 大血藤
大红袍 *Myrsines Africanae Herba*
herb of *Myrsine africana* L.铁仔
大青叶 * *Isatidis Folium*
leaf of *Isatis indigotica* Fort.菘蓝
大青盐 *Halitum*
大罗伞 *Clerodendri Serrati Herba*
herb of *Clerodendron serratum* (L.) Spr. 三对节
大腹皮 * *Arecae Pericarpium*
pericarp of *Areca catechu* L. 槟榔
大叶紫珠 * *Callicarpae Macrophyllae Folium*
root or leaf of *Callicarpa macrophylla* Vahl. 大叶紫珠
大豆黄卷 * *Sojae Semen Germinatum*
dried sprout of *Glycine max* (L.) Merr. 大豆
山柰 * *Kaempferiae Rhizoma*
rhizome of *Kaempferia galanga* L. 山柰
山药 * *Dioscoreae Rhizoma*
rhizome of *Dioscorea opposita* Thunb. 薯蓣
山姜 *Alpiniae Japonicae Rhizoma seu Herba*
rhizome or herb of *Alpinia japonica* (Thunb.) Miq. 山姜
山楂 * *Crataegi Fructus*
fruit of *Crataegus pinnatifida* Bge. 山楂
山楂叶 **Crataegi Folium*
leaf of *Crataegus pinnatifida* Bge. 山楂
山白芷 *Inulae Cappae Radix*
root of *Inula cappa* (Buch.-Ham.) DC. 羊耳菊
山豆根 * *Sophorae Tonkinensis Radix et Rhizoma*
root and rhizome of *Sophora tonkinensis* Gagnep. 越南槐
山豆根浸膏 *Sophorae Tonkinensis Extractum*
extract of *Sophora tonkinensis* Gagnep. 越南槐
山芝麻 *Helicteris Angustifoliae Herba*
herb of *Helicteres angustifolia* L. 山芝麻
山芝麻浸膏 *Helicteris Angustifoliae Extractum*
extract of *Helicteres angustifolia* L. 山芝麻
山茱萸 * *Corni Fructus*
fruit of *Cornus officinalis* Sieb. et Zucc. 山茱萸
山绿茶 *Camelliae Sinensis Folium Gemmae*
leaf of *Camellia sinensis* Kuntze 茶
山慈菇 * *Cremastrae seu Pleiones Pseudobulbus*
pseudobulb of *Cremastra appendiculata* (D.Don.) Makino 杜鹃兰or *Pleione bulbocodioides* (Franch.) Rolfe 独蒜兰
山橘叶 *Fortunellae Hindsii Folium*
leaf of *Fortunella hindsii* (Champ.) Swingle 山橘
山羊血粉 *Caprinus Sanguis Pulvis*
blood powder of *Capra hircus* Linnaeus 山羊
千斤拔 *Flemingiae Philippinensis Radix*
root of *Flemingia philippinensis* Merr. et Rolfe 蔓性千斤拔
千年健 * *Homalomenae Rhizoma*
rhizome of *Homalomena occulta* (Lour.) Schott 千年健
千里光 *Senecionis Scandentis Herba*
herb of *Senecio scandens* Buch.-Ham. 千里光
千金子霜 * *Euphorbiae Semen Pulveratum*
seed preparation of *Euphorbia lathyris* L. 续随子
川乌 * *Aconiti Radix*
axial root of *Aconitum carmichaeli* Debx. 乌头
制川乌 * *Aconiti Radix Cocta*
prepared axial root of *Aconitum carmichaeli* Debx. 乌头
川芎 * *Chuanxiong Rhizoma*
rhizome of *Lingusticum chuanxiong* Hort. 川芎
川木通 * *Clematidis Armandii Caulis*
stem of *Clematis armandii* Franch. 小木通
川贝母 * *Fritillariae Cirrhosae Bulbus*
bulb of *Fritillaria cirrhosa* D. Don 川贝母
川贝母浸膏 *Fritillariae Cirrhosae Extractum*
extract of *Fritillaria cirrhosa* D. Don 川贝母
川牛膝 * *Cyathulae Radix*
root of *Cyathula officinalis* Kuan 川牛膝
川明参 *Changii Radix*
root of *Changium smyrnioides* Wolff 明党参
川射干 * *Iridis Tectori Rhizoma*
rhizome of *Iris tectorum* Maxim. 鸢尾
川楝子 * *Toosendan Fructus*

fruit of *Melia toosendan* Sieb. et Zucc. 川楝

广枣 * *Choerospondiatis Fructus*

fruit of *Choerospondias axillaris* (Roxb.) Burtt et Hill 南酸枣

广木香 *Saussureae Lappae Radix*

root of *Saussurea lappa* Clarke 云木香

广防己 *Aristolochiae Fangchi Radix*

root of *Aristolochia fangchi* Y. C. Wu ex L. D. Chou et S. M. Hwang 广防己

广金钱草 * *Desmodii Styracifolii Herba*

herb of *Desmodium styracifolium* (Osb.) Merr. 广金钱草

广藿香 * *Pogostemonis Herba*

herb of *Pogostemon cablin* (Blanco) Benth.广藿香

广藿香叶 *Pogostemonis Folium*

leaf of *Pogostemon cablin* (Blanco) Benth.广藿香

广东土牛膝 *Eupatorii Chinensis Radix*

root of *Eupatorium chinense* L. 华泽兰

广东紫珠浸膏 *Callicarpae Kwangtungensis Extractum*

extract of *Callicarpa kwangtungensis* Chun 广东紫珠

女贞子 * *Ligustri Lucidi Fructus*

fruit of *Ligustrum lucidum* Ait.女贞

小麦 *Tritici Aestivi Fructus*

fruit of *Triticum aestivum* L. 小麦

小蓟 * *Cirsii Herba*

herb of *Cirsium setosum* (Willd.) MB. 刺儿菜

小罗伞 *Ardisiae Punctatae Herba*

herb of *Ardisia punctata* Lindl. 山血丹

小茴香 * *Foeniculi Fructus*

fruit of *Foeniculum vulgare* Mill. 茴香

小檗皮 *Berberidis Amurensis Cortex*

bark of *Berberis amurensis* Rupr. 黄芦木

马勃 * *Lasiosphaera seu Calvatia*

sporocarp of *Lasiosphaera fenzlii* Reich. 脱皮马勃 or *Calvatia gigantea* (Batsh ex Pers.)Lloyd 大马勃

马蓝 *Baphicacanthi Cusiae Rhizoma et Radix*

rhizome and root of *Baphicacanthus cusia* Bremek. 马蓝

马兰草 *Wedeliae Chinensis Herba seu Radix*

herb or root of *Wedelia chinensis* (Osbeck) Merr. 蟛蜞菊

马尾连 *Thalictri Rhizoma et Radix*

rhizome and root of *Thalictrum foliolosum* DC. 多叶唐松草

马尿泡 *Pedicularidis Resupinatae Folium seu Radix*

leaf or root of *Pedicularis resupinata* L. 返顾马先蒿

马齿苋 * *Portulacae Herba*

herb of *Portulaca oleracea* L. 马齿苋

马兜铃 * *Aristolochiae Fructus*

fruit of *Aristolochia debilis* Sieb. et Zucc. 马兜铃

马钱子 * *Strychni Semen*

seed of *Strychnos nux-vomica* L. 马钱

马钱子粉 * *Strychni Semen Pulveratum*

seed powder of *Strychnos nux-vomica* L. 马钱

四画

云芝 * *Coriolus*

sporocarp of *Coriolus versicolor* (L.ex Fr.) Quel 彩绒革盖菌

天冬 * *Asparagi Radix*

root tuber of *Asparagus cochinchinensis* (Lour.) Merr. 天冬

天麻 * *Gastrodiae Rhizoma*

tuber of *Gastrodia elata* Bl. 天麻

天名精 *Carpesii Abrotanoidis Radix et Folium*

root and leaf of *Carpesium abrotanoides* L. 天名精

天花粉 * *Trichosanthis Radix*

root of *Trichosanthes kirilowii* Maxim. 栝楼

天竺黄 * *Bambusae Concretio Silicea*

culm secretion of *Bambusa textilis* McClure 青皮竹

天南星 * *Arisaematis Rhizoma*

tuber of *Arisaema erubescens* (Wall.) Schott 天南星

天葵子 * *Semiaquilegiae Radix*

root of *Semiaquilegia adoxoides* (DC.) Mak. 天葵

木瓜 * *Chaenomelis Fructus*

fruit of *Chaenomeles speciosa* (Sweet)Nakai 贴梗海棠

木香 * *Aucklandiae Radix*

root of *Aucklandia lappa* Decne. 木香

木贼 *Equiseti Hiemalis Herba**

aerial part of *Equisetum hiemale* L. 木贼

木通 * *Akebiae Caulis*

stem of *Akebia quinata* (Thunb.) Decne. 木通

木棉皮 *Gossampini Cortex*

bark of *Gossampinus malabarica* DC. Merr. 木棉

木棉花 * *Gossampini Flos*
flower of *Gossampinus malabarica* DC. Merr. 木棉
木蝴蝶 * *Oroxyli Semen*
seed of *Oroxylum indicum* (L.) Vent. 木蝴蝶
木鳖子 * *Momordicae Semen*
seed of *Momordica cochinchinensis* (Lour.) Spreng. 木鳖
瓦楞子 * *Arcae Concha*
shell of *Arca subcrenata* Lischke 毛蚶
王不留行 * *Vaccariae Semen*
seed of *Vaccaria segetalis* (Neck.) Garcke 麦蓝菜
五加皮 * *Acanthopanacis Cortex*
root-bark of *Acanthopanax gracilistylus* W. W. Smith 细柱五加
五灵脂 *Trogopterori Faeces*
feces of *Trogopterus xanthipes* Milne-Edwards复齿鼯鼠
五灵脂膏 *Trogopterori Extractum*
feces extract of *Trogopterus xanthipes* Milne-Edwards 复齿鼯鼠
五味子 * *Schisandrae Chinensis Fructus*
fruit of *Schisandra chinensis* (Trucz.) Baill.五味子
五味子浸膏 *Schisandrae Chinensis Extractum*
extract of *Schisandra chinensis* (Trucz.) Baill.五味子
五味藤 *Securidacae Inappendiculatae Radix*
root of *Securidaca inappendiculata* Hassk. 蝉翼藤
五倍子 * *Galla Chinensis*
gall of *Rhus chinensis* Mill. 盐肤木
五倍子浸膏 *Galla Chinensis Extractum*
extract of *Galla chinensis* Mill. 盐肤木
五指毛桃 *Fici Simplicissimae Radix*
root of *Ficus simplicissima* Lour. 粗叶榕
五脉绿绒蒿 *Meconopsidis Quintuplinerviae Flos*
flower of *Meconopsis quintuplinervia* Reg. 五脉绿绒蒿
车前子 * *Plantaginis Semen*
seed of *Plantago asiatica* L. 车前
车前草 * *Plantaginis Herba*
herb of *Plantago asiatica* L. 车前
丰城鸡血藤 *Millettiae Dielsianae Caulis*
stem of *Millettia dielsiana* Harms 香花岩豆藤
太子参 * *Psedostellariae Radix*
root of *Psedostellaria heterophlla* (Miq.) Pax ex Pax et Hoffm. 孩儿参

化血丹 *Radix et Folium Ligulariae Lapathifoliae*
root and leaf of *Ligularia lapathifolia* (Franch.) Hand.-Mazz. 牛蒡叶橐吾
化香树 *Folium Platycaryae Strobilaceae*
leaf of *Platycarya strobilacea* Sieb.et Zucc. 化香树
化香树果序 *Infructescentia Platycaryae Strobilaceae*
infructescence of *Platycarya strobilacea* Sieb.et Zucc. 化香树
化橘红 * *Citri Grandis Exocarpium*
exocarp of *Citrus grandis var. tomentosa* Hort. 化州柚
手参 *Gymnadeniae Tuber*
tuber of *Gymnadenia conopsea* (L.) R. Br. 手参
毛冬青 *Ilecis Pubescentis Radix*
root of *Ilex pubescens* Hook. et Arn. 毛冬青
毛老虎 *Inulae Cappae Herba*
herb of *Inula cappa* (Buch.-Ham.) DC. 羊耳菊
毛诃子 * *Terminaliae Belliricae Fructus*
fruit of *Terminalia bellirica* (Gaertn.) Roxb. 毗黎勒
毛鸡 *Centropodis Sinensis Caro*
meat of *Centropus sinensis* (Stephens) 褐翅鸦鹃
牛心 *Bovis Cor*
heart of *Bos taurus domesticus* Gmelin 黄牛
牛至 *Origani Vulgaris Herba*
herb of *Origanum vulgare* L. 牛至
牛乳 *Vaccae Lac*
milk of *Bos taurus domesticus* Gmelin 黄牛
牛胆 *Bovis Fel*
gall of *Bos taurus domesticus* Gmelin 黄牛
牛胆汁 *Bovis Bilis*
bile of *Bos taurus domesticus* Gmelin 黄牛
牛胆粉 *Bovis Fel Pulvis*
gall powder of *Bos taurus domesticus* Gmelin 黄牛
牛胆干膏 *Bovis Bilis Extractum*
bile extract of *Bos taurus domesticus* Gmelin 黄牛
牛黄 * *Bovis Calculus*
bezoar of *Bos taurus domesticus* Gmelin 黄牛
牛膝 * *Achyranthis Bidentatae Radix*
root of *Achyranthes bidentata* Bl. 牛膝
牛鞭 *Bovis Testis et Penis*
testes and penis of *Bos taurus domesticus* Gmelin 黄牛
牛髓 *Bovis Medulla Spinalis*
spinal cord of *Bos taurus domesticus* Gmelin 黄牛
牛大力 *Millettiae Speciosae Radix*

root of *Millettia speciosa* Champ. 牛大力藤
牛白藤 *Hedyotidis Hedyotideae Caulis et Folium*
stem and leaf of *Hedyotis hedyotidea* (DC.) Merr. 牛白藤
牛耳枫 *Daphniphylli Calycini Radix*
root of *Daphniphyllum calycinum* Benth. 牛耳枫
牛尾蕨 *Smilacis Nipponicae Rhizoma et Radix*
rhizome and root of *Smilax nipponica* Miq. 白背牛尾菜
牛尾藤 *Emiliae Sonchifoliae Herba*
herb of *Emilia sonchifolia* (L.) DC. 一点红
牛蒡子 * *Arctii Fructus*
fruit of *Arctium lappa* L. 牛蒡
升麻 * *Cimicifugae Rhizoma*
rhizome of *Cimicifuga foetida* L. 升麻
升华硫 *Sublimed Sulfur*
片姜黄 * *Wenyujin Rhizoma Concisum*
rhizome of *Curcuma wenyujin* Y.H. Chen et C. Ling 温郁金
片仔癀粉 *Pian Zai Huang Pulvis*
powder of *Pian Zai Huang*
乌鸡 *Galli Caro cum Osse Nigro*
whole body of *Gallus gallus domesticus* Brisson 乌骨鸡
乌药 * *Linderae Radix*
root tuber of *Lindera aggregate* (Sims) Kosterm. 乌药
乌药干浸膏 *Linderae Extractum*
extract of *Lindera aggregate* (Sims) Kosterm.乌药
乌梅 * *Mume Fructus*
fruit of *Prunus mume* (Sieb.) Sieb. et Zucc.梅
乌梢蛇 * *Zaocys*
dried body of *Zaocys dhumnades* (Cantor) 乌梢蛇
勾儿茶 *Berchemiae Floribundae Radix*
root of *Berchemia floribunda* (Wall.) Brongn. 多花勾儿茶
丹参 * *Salviae Miltiorrhizae Radix et Rhizoma*
root and rhizome of *Salvia miltiorrhiza* Bge. 丹参
风藤 *Fici Martini Radix et Caulis*
root and stem of *Ficus martini* Levl. et Vant. 爬藤榕
凤尾草 *Pteridis Multifidae Herba*
herb of *Pteris multifida* Poir. 井栏边草
凤凰衣 *Ovi Follicularis Membrana*
hen egg's inner shell membrane of *Gallus gallus domesticus* Brisson 家鸡
凤仙透骨草 *Impatientis Balsaminae Herba*
herb of *Impatiens balsamina* L. 凤仙花
六神曲 *Medicata Massa Fermentata*
方儿茶 *Catechu Extractum*
extract of *Acacia catechu* (L .f.) Willd. 儿茶
火炭母 *Polygoni Chinensis Herba*
herb of *Polygonum chinense* L. 火炭母
火麻仁 * *Cannabis Semen*
seed of *Cannabis sativa* L. 大麻
巴豆霜 * *Crotonis Semen Pulveratum*
seed preparation of *Croton tiglium* L. 巴豆
巴戟天 * *Morindae Officinalis Radix*
root of *Morinda officinalis* How 巴戟天
水龙 *Jussiaeae Repentis Herba*
herb of *Jussiaea repens* L.水龙
水蛭 * *Hirudo*
dried body of *Whitmania pigra* Whitman 蚂蟥
水飞蓟 * *Silybi Fructus*
fruit of *Silybum marianum* (L.) Gaertn 水飞蓟
水牛角 * *Bubali Cornu*
horn of *Bubalus bubalis* Linnaeus 水牛
水牛角浓缩粉 *Bubali Cornu Pulvis Concentratio*
horn powder of *Bubalus bubalis* Linnaeus 水牛
水田七 *Taccae Tuber*
tuber of *Tacca plantaginea* (Hance) Drake 裂果薯
水半夏 *Pinelliae Cordatae Tuber*
tuber of *Pinellia cordata* N. E. Br. 心叶半夏
水团花 *Adinae Piluliferae Herba*
herb of *Adina pilulifera* (Lam.) Franch. ex Drake 水团花
水线草 *Hedyotis Corymbosae Herba*
herb of *Hedyotis corymbosa* (L.) Lam. 伞房花耳草
水柏枝 *Myricariae Germanicae Ramulus*
twig of *Myricaria germanica* (L.) Desv. 水柏枝
水翁花 *Cleistocalycis Operculati Flos Immaturus*
immature flower of *Cleistocalyx operculatus* (Roxb.) Merr. et Perry 水翁
水红花子 * *Polygoni Orientalis Fructus*
fruit of *Polygonum orientale* L. 红蓼

五画

功劳木 * *Mahoniae Caulis*

stem of *Mahonia bealei* (Fort.) Carr. 阔叶十大功劳
功劳叶 *Mahoniae Folium*
leaf of *Mahonia bealei* (Fort.) Carr. 阔叶十大功劳
艾叶 * *Artemisiae Argyi Folium*
leaf of *Artemisia argyi* Levl. et Vant. 艾
艾叶炭 *Artemisiae Argyi Folium Carbanisatus*
carbonated leaf of *Artemisia argyi* Levl. et Vant. 艾
平贝母 * *Fritillariae Ussuriensis Bulbus*
bulb of *Fritillaria ussuriensis* Maxim. 平贝母
平贝母浸膏 *Fritillariae Ussuriensis Extractum*
extract of *Fritillaria ussuriensis* Maxim. 平贝母
玉竹 * *Polygonati Odorati Rhizoma*
rhizome of *Polygonatum odoratum* (Mill.) Druce 玉竹
玉米须 *Zeae Maydis Stylus*
style of *Zea mays* L. 玉蜀黍
玉叶金花 *Mussaendae Erosae Folium*
leaf of *Mussaenda erosa* Champ. 楠藤
甘松 * *Nardostachyos Radix et Rhizoma*
root and rhizome of *Nardostachys chinensis* Batal. 甘松
甘草 * *Glycyrrhizae Radix et Rhizoma*
root and rhizome of *Glycyrrhiza uralensis* Fisch. 甘草
甘草流浸膏 *Glycyrrhizae Extractum*
extract of *Glycyrrhiza uralensis* Fisch. 甘草
甘遂 * *Kansui Radix*
root tuber of *Euphorbia kansui* T. N. Liou ex T. P. Wang 甘遂
布渣叶 * *Microctis Folium*
leaf of *Microcos paniculata* L. 布渣叶
石韦 * *Pyrrosiae Folium*
leaf of *Pyrrosia lingua* (Thunb.) Farwell 石韦
石耳 *Umbilicariae Esculentae Carpophorum*
carpophore of *Umbilicaria esculenta* (Miyoshi) Minks 石耳
石斛 * *Dendrobii Caulis*
stem of *Dendrobium nobile* Lindl. 金钗石斛
石蜡 *Paraffin*
石膏 * *Gypsum Fibrosum*
石燕 *Spiriferis Fossilia*
fossil shell of *Cyrtiospirifer sinensis* (Graban) 中华弓石燕
石上柏 *Selaginellae Doederleinii Herba*
herb of *Selaginella doederleinii* Hieron 深绿卷柏
石决明 * *Haliotidis Concha*
shell of *Haliotis diversicolor* Reeve 杂色鲍
石南藤 *Photiniae Serrulatae Herba*
herb of *Photinia serrulata* Lindl. 石楠
石菖蒲 * *Acori Tatarinowii Rhizoma*
rhizome of *Acorus tatarinowii* Schott 石菖蒲
石菖蒲油 *Oleum Acori Tatarinowii*
oil of *Acorus tatarinowii* Schott 石菖蒲
石菖蒲浸膏 *Acori Tatarinowii Extractum*
extract of *Acorus tatarinowii* Schott 石菖蒲
石榴子 *Granati Fructus*
fruit of *Punica granatum* L. 石榴
石榴皮 * *Granati Pericarpium*
pericarp of *Punica granatum* L. 石榴
龙齿 *Draconis Dens*
teeth of *Stegodon orientalis* Owen 东方剑齿象
龙骨 *Draconis Os*
bone of *Stegodon orientalis* Owen 东方剑齿象
龙胆 * *Gentianae Radix et Rhizoma*
root and rhizome of *Gentiana scabra* Bge. 龙胆
龙胆花 *Gentianae Flos*
flower of *Gentiana scabra* Bge. 龙胆
龙葵 *Solani Nigri Herba*
herb of *Solanum nigrum* L. 龙葵
龙眼肉 * *Longan Arillus*
aril of *Dimocarpus longan* Lour. 龙眼
北豆根 * *Menispermi Rhizoma*
rhizome of *Menispermum dauricum* DC. 蝙蝠葛
北沙参 * *Glehniae Radix*
root of *Glehnia littoralis* Fr. Schmidt ex Miq. 珊瑚菜
北败酱 *Sonchi Arvensis Herba*
herb of *Sonchus arvensis* L. 野苦苣菜
北细辛 *Asari Mandshurici Herba*
herb of *Asarum heterotropoides* Fr. Schmidt var. *mandshuricum* (Maxim.) Kitag. 北细辛
北瓜清膏 *Cucurbitae Kintogae Extractum*
extract of *Cucurbita pepo* L. var. *kintoga* Mak. 北瓜
叶下珠 *Phyllanthi Urinariae Herba*
herb of *Phyllanthus urinaria* L. 叶下珠
田螺壳 *Cipangopaludinae Concha*
shell of *Cipangopaludina chiesnsis*(Gray.) 中华圆田螺
四块瓦 *Chloranthi Herba*
herb of *Chloranthus henryi* Hemsl. 宽叶金粟兰
四季青 * *Ilicis Chinensis Folium*
leaf of *Ilex chinensis* Sims 冬青

seed powder of *Trichosanthes kirilowii* Maxim. 栝楼

汉桃叶 *Schefflerae Arboricolae Radix seu Folium*
root or leaf of *Schefflera arboricola* Hoyata 鹅掌藤

玄参 * *Scrophulariae Radix*
root of *Scrophularia ningpoensis* Hemsl. 玄参

玄明粉 * *Natrii Sulfas Exsiccatus*

玄精石 *Selenitum*

半夏 * *Pinelliae Rhizoma*
tuber of *Pinellia ternata* (Thunb.) Breit. 半夏

半夏曲 *Pinelliae Massa Fermentata*
femented mass with *Pinellia ternata* (Thunb.) Breit. 半夏

法半夏 * *Pinelliae Rhizoma Praeparatum*
licorice root prepared *Pinellia ternata* (Thunb.) Breit. 半夏

姜半夏* *Pinelliae Rhizoma Praeparatum cum Zingibere et Alumine*
ginger prepared *Pinellia ternata* (Thunb.) Breit. 半夏

清半夏* *Pinelliae Rhizoma Praeparatum cum Alumine*
alum prepared *Pinellia ternata* (Thunb.) Breit. 半夏

半边莲 * *Lobeliae Chinensis Herba*
herb of *Lobelia chinensis* Lour. 半边莲

半枝莲 * *Scutellariae Barbatae Herba*
herb of *Scutellaria barbata* D. Don 半枝莲

丝绵 *Bombycis Incunabulum*
silk cocoon of *Bombyx mori* Linnaeus 家蚕

丝瓜络 * *Luffae Fructus Retinervus*
vegetable sponge of *Luffa cylindrica* (L.) Roem. 丝瓜

母丁香 * *Caryophylli Fructus*
fruit of *Eugenia caryophyllata* Thunb. 丁香

六画

地龙 * *Pheretima*
dried body of *Pheretima aspergillum* (E. Perrier) 参环毛蚓

地黄 * *Rehmanniae Radix*
root tuber of *Rehmannia glutinosa* Libosch. 地黄

地菍 *Melastomatis Dodecandri Herba*
herb of *Melastoma dodecandrum* Lour. 地菍

地榆 * *Sanguisorbae Radix*
root of *Sanguisorba officinalis* L. 地榆

地榆炭 *Sanguisorbae Radix Carbonisatus*
carbonated *Sanguisorba officinalis* L. 地榆

地耳草 *Hyperici Japonici Herba*
herb of *Hypericum japonicum* Thunb. 地耳草

地枫皮 * *Illicii Cortex*
bark of *Illicium difengpi* K. I. B. et K. I. M. 地枫皮

地肤子 * *Kochiae Fructus*
fruit of *Kochia scoparia* (L.) Schrad. 地肤

地骨皮 * *Lycii Cortex*
root-bark of *Lycium chinensis* Mill. 枸杞

地胆草 *Elephantopi Herba*
herb of *Elephantopus scaber* L. 地胆草

地桃花 *Urenae Lobatae Radix seu Herba*
root or herb of *Urena lobata* L. 地桃花

地锦草 * *Euphorbiae Humifusae Herba*
herb of *Euphorbia humifusa* Willd. 地锦

芋头 *Colocasiae Esculentae Tuber*
tuber of *Colocasia esculenta* Schott 芋

芍药花 *Paeoniae Lactiflorae Flos*
flower of *Paeonia lactiflora* Pall. 芍药

芒硝 * *Natrii Sulfas*

芒果叶干浸膏 *Mangiferae Indicae Folium Extractum*
leaf extract of *Mangifera indica* L. 芒果

芝麻壳 *Sesami Pericarpium*
pericarp of *Sesamum indicum* L. 脂麻

老鹳草 * *Geranii Herba*
herb of *Geranium wilfordii* Maxim. 老鹳草

西瓜霜 * *Mirabilitum Praeparatum*
prepared pericarp of *Citrullus lanatus* (Thunb.) Matsum. et Nakai 西瓜

西红花 * *Croci Stigma*
stigma of *Crocus sativus* L. 番红花

西青果 * *Chebulae Fructus Immaturus*
fruit of *Terminalia chebula* Retz. 诃子

西河柳 * *Tamaricis Cacumen*
twig of *Tamarix chinensis* Lour. 柽柳

西洋参 * *Panacis Quinquefolii Radix*
root of *Panax quinquefolium* L. 西洋参

百合 * *Lilii Bulbus*
bulb of *Lilium brownii* F.E.Brown var. *viridulum* Baker 百合

百草霜 *Gramen Fumi Carbonisatus*

百部 * *Stemonae Radix*
root tuber of *Stemona sessilifolia* (Miq.) Miq. 直立

百部

百部流浸膏 *Stemonae Extractum*

root tuber extract of *Stemona sessilifolia* (Miq.) Miq. 直立百部

过江龙 *Lycopodii Complanati Herba*

herb of *Lycopodium complanatum* L. 地刷子石松

过塘蛇 *Jussiaeae Repentis Herba*

herb of *Jussiaea repens* L. 水龙

当归 * *Angelicae Sinensis Radix*

root of *Angelica sinensis* (Oliv.) Diels 当归

当归干浸膏 *Angelicae Sinensis Extractum*

extract of *Angelica sinensis* (Oliv.) Diels 当归

当归尾 *Angelicae Sinensis Radix Cauda*

root tail of *Angelica sinensis* (Oliv.) Diels 当归

当药 * *Swertiae Herba*

herb of *Swertia Pseudochinensis* Hara 瘤毛獐牙菜

光明盐 *Sal*

光慈菇 *Tulipae Edulis Bulbus*

bulb of *Tulipa edulis* (Miq.) Bak. 老鸦瓣

虫草菌 *Cordyceps Fungus*

fungus of *Cordyceps sinensis* (Berk.) Sacc. 冬虫夏草菌

肉桂 * *Cinnamomi Cortex*

bark of *Cinnamomum cassia* Presl 肉桂

肉桂油 *Cinnamomi Oleum*

oil of *Cinnamomum cassia* Presl 肉桂

肉豆蔻 * *Myristicae Semen*

seed of *Myristica fragrans* Houtt. 肉豆蔻

肉苁蓉 * *Cistanches Caulis Carnosus*

fleshy stem of *Cistanche deserticola* Y. C. Ma 肉苁蓉

竹叶 *Phyllostachydis Henonis Folium*

leaf of *Phyllostachys nigra* (Lodd. ex Lindl.) Munro var. *henonis*（Mitf.）Stapf ex Rendle 毛金竹

竹沥 *Phyllostachydis Henonis Succus*

culm juice of *Phyllostachys nigra* (Lodd. ex Lindl.) Munro var. *henonis*（Mitf.）Stapf ex Rendle 金毛竹

竹茹 * *Bambusae Caulis in Taenias*

culm medium of *Bambusae tuldoides* Munro 青秆竹

竹黄 *Shiraiae Bambusicolae Stroma*

stroma of *Shiraia bambusicola* P. Henn. 肉座菌（真菌）

竹节香附 *Anemones Raddeanae Rhizoma*

rhizome of *Anemone raddeana* Reg. 多被银莲花

竹叶卷心 *Lingnaniae Chungii Folium Involutus Juvenalis*

rolled juvenile leaf of *Lingnania chungii* McClure 粉单竹

竹叶柴胡 *Bupleuri Radix*

root of *Bupleurum chinense* DC. 柴胡

丢了棒 *Claoxyli Polot Radix et Folium*

root and leaf of *Claoxylon polot* (Burm. f.) Merr. 白桐树

朱砂 * *Cinnabaris*

朱砂根 * *Ardisiae Crenatae Radix*

root of *Ardisia crenata* Sims. 朱砂根

朱砂粉 *Cinnabaris Pulvis*

伏龙肝 *Terra Flava Usta*

伊贝母 * *Fritillariae Pallidiflorae Bulbus*

bulb of *Fritillaria pallidiflora* Schrenk 伊犁贝母

延胡索 * *Corydalis Rhizoma*

tuber of *Corydalis yanhusuo* W. T. Wang 延胡索

延胡索浸膏 *Corydalis Extractum*

extract of *Corydalis yanhusuo* W. T. Wang 延胡索

自然铜 * *Pyritum*

血竭 * *Draconis Sanguis*

fruit resin of *Daemonorops draco* Bl. 麒麟竭

血余炭 * *Crinis Carbonisatus*

全蝎 * *Scorpio*

dried body of *Buthus martensii* Karch 东亚钳蝎

合欢皮 * *Albiziae Cortex*

bark of *Albizia julibrissin* Durazz. 合欢

合欢花 * *Albiziae Flos*

inflorescence of *Albizia julibrissin* Durazz. 合欢

合欢藤 *Albiziae Caulis*

stem of *Albizia julibrissin* Durazz. 合欢

伞梗虎耳草 *Saxifragae Umbellulatae Herba*

herb of *Saxifraga umbellulata* HK. f. ex Thoms. 小伞虎耳草

刘寄奴 *Artemisiae Anomalae Herba*

herb of *Artemisia anomala* S. Moore 奇蒿

灯心草 * *Junci Medulla*

stem pith of *Juncus effuses* L. 灯心草

灯盏细辛 * *Erigerontis Herba*

herb of *Erigeron breviscapus* (Vant.) Hand.-Mazz. 短葶飞蓬

灯盏细辛浸膏 *Erigerontis Extractum*

extract of *Erigeron breviscapus* (Vant.) Hand.-Mazz. 短葶飞蓬

决明子 * *Cassiae Semen*

seed of *Cassia obtusifolia* L. 决明
冰片 * *Borneolum Syntheticum*
borneol
江南卷柏 *Selaginellae Moellendorfii Herba*
herb of *Selaginella moellendorfii* 江南卷柏
守宫 *Gekko Chinensis*
whole body of *Gekko chinensis* Gray 中国壁虎
安息香 * *Benzoinum*
resin of *Styrax tonkinensis* (Pierre) Craib ex Hart. 白花树
关木通 *Aristolochiae Manshuriensis Caulis*
woody stem of *Aristolochia manshuriensis* Kom. 关木通
关白附 *Aconiti Coreani Radix*
root of *Aconitum coreanum* (Levl.) Raipaics 黄花乌头
羊毛脂 *Lanolinum*
羊肝 *Caprinus Jecur*
liver of *Capra hircus* Linnaeus 山羊
羊角 *Caprinus Cornu*
horn of *Capra hircus* Linnaeus 山羊
羊肾 *Caprinus Ren*
kidney of *Capra hircus* Linnaeus 山羊
羊骨 *Caprinus Os*
bone of *Capra hircus* Linnaeus 山羊
羊胆 *Caprinus Fel*
gall of *Capra hircus* Linnaeus 山羊
羊胆汁 *Caprinus Bilis*
bile of *Capra hircus* Linnaeus 山羊
羊胆干膏 *Caprinus Fel Extractum*
gall extract of *Capra hircus* Linnaeus 山羊
羊鞭 *Caprinus Testis et Penis*
testes and penis of *Capra hircus* Linnaeus 山羊
羊开口 *Akebiae Fructus*
fruit of *Akebia quinata* (Houtt.) Decne. 木通
羊外肾 *Caprinus Testis*
testes of *Capra hircus* Linnaeus 山羊
羊耳菊 *Inulae Cappae Herba*
herb of *Inula cappa* (Buch.-Ham.) DC. 羊耳菊
米醋 *Oryzi-Acetum*
vinegar
寻骨风 *Aristolochiae Mollissimae Rhizoma seu Herba*
rhizome or herb of *Aristolochia mollissima* Hance 绵毛马兜铃
阳起石 *Tremolitum*
阴行草 *Siphonostegiae Chinensis Herba*
herb of *Siphonostegia chinensis* Benth. 阴行草
防己 * *Stephaniae Tetrandrae Radix*
root of *Stephania tetrandra* S. Moore 粉防己
防风 * *Saposhnikoviae Radix*
root of *Saposhnikovia divaricata* (Turcz.) Schischk. 防风
红曲 *Oryzae Fructus Monascus*
Monascus purpureus Went (fungus) parasitized on *Fructus Oryzae Sativae*
红花 * *Carthami Flos*
flower of *Carthamus tinctorius* L. 红花
红参 * *Ginseng Radix et Rhizoma Rubra*
prepared root and rhizome of *Panax ginseng* C. A. Mey. 人参
红茶 *Camelliae Sinensis Folium Gemmae Fermentatio*
black tea
红粉 * *Hydrargyri Oxydum Rubrum*
红藤 *Sargentodoxae Caulis*
stem of *Sargentodoxa cuneata* (Oliv.) Rehd. et Wils. 大血藤
红大戟 * *Knoxiae Radix*
tuber of *Knoxia valerianoides* Thorel et Pitard 红大戟
红杜仲 *Parabarii Micranthi Caulis seu Radix*
stem or root of *Parabarium micranthum* (A. DC.) Pier. 杜仲藤
红豆蔻 * *Galangae Fructus*
fruit of *Alpinia galanga* Willd. 大高良姜
红根草 *Lysimachiae Cletheroidis Radix seu Herba*
root or herb of *Lysimachia clethroides* Duby 珍珠草
红景天 * *Rhodiolae Crenulatae Radix et Rhizoma*
root and rhizome of *Rhodiola crenulata* (Hook. f. et Thoms.) H. Ohba 大花红景天
红茴香根 *Illicii Lanceolati Radix*
root of *Illicium lanceolatum* A. C. Smith 莽草
红花夹竹桃 *Nerii Indici Folium seu Cortex*
leaf or bark of *Nerium indicum* Mill. 夹竹桃

七画

麦冬 * *Ophiopogonis Radix*
root tuber of *Ophiopogon japonicum* (Thunb.) Ker-Gawl. 麦冬

麦芽 * *Hordei Fructus Germinatus*
germinant fruit of *Hordeum vulgare* L. 大麦
麦饼 *Trici Aestivi Massa Pulvis*
powder cake of *Triticum aestivum* L. 小麦
远志 * *Polygalae Radix*
root of *Polygala tenuifolia* Willd. 远志
远志肉 *Polygalae Radix (Demotus Lignum)*
removed heart wood of *root from Polygala tenuifolia* Willd. 远志
远志流浸膏 *Polygalae Extractum*
extract of *Polygala tenuifolia* Willd. 远志
杜仲 * *Eucommiae Cortex*
bark of *Eucommia ulmoides* Oliv. 杜仲
杜仲叶 * *Eucommiae Folium*
leaf of *Eucommia ulmoides* Oliv. 杜仲
杜仲炭 *Eucommiae Cortex Carbonisatus*
carbonated *Eucommia ulmoides* Oliv. 杜仲
芒果 *Mangiferae Indicae Fructus*
fruit of *Mangifera indica* L. 杧果
芒果叶浸膏 *Mangiferae Indicae Folium Extractum*
leaf extract of *Mangifera indica* L. 杧果
杨梅根 *Myricae Rubrae Radix*
root of *Myrica rubra* (Lour.) Sieb. et Zucc. 杨梅
豆蔻 * *Amomi Fructus Rotundus*
fruit of *Amomum kravanh* Pierre ex Gagnep. 白豆蔻
豆豉姜 *Litseae Cubebae Radix et Rhizoma*
root and rhizome of *Litsea cubeba* (Lour.) Pers. 山鸡椒
声色草 *Polycarpaeae Corymbosae Herba*
herb of *Polycarpaea corymbosa* (L.) Lam. 白鼓钉
芙蓉叶 *Hibisci Mutabilis Folium*
leaf of *Hibiscus mutabilis* L. 木芙蓉
芫花 * *Genkwa Flos*
flower bud of *Daphne genkwa* Sieb. et Zucc. 芫花
芫花枝条 *Genkwa Ramulus*
twig of *Daphne genkwa* Sieb. et Zucc. 芫花
芫荽果 *Coriandri Sativi Fructus*
fruit of *Coriandrum sativum* L. 芫荽
芜荑 *Ulmi Macrocarpae Fructus*
fruit of *Ulmus macrocarpa* Hance 大果榆
芸香 *Cymbopogonis Distantis Herba*
herb of *Cymbopogon distans* (Nees) Wats. 芸香草
芸香浸膏 *Cymbopogonis Distantis Extractum*
extract of *Cymbopogon distans* (Nees) Wats. 芸香草
苣胜子 *Lactucae Sativae Semen*
seed of *Lactuca sativa* L. 莴苣
花椒 * *Zanthoxyli Pericarpium*
pericarp of *Zanthoxylum bungeanum* Maxim. 花椒
花生衣 *Arachidis Hypogaea Testae*
external seed coat of *Arachis hypogaea* L. 落花生
花锚草 *Haleniae Corniculatae Herba*
herb of *Halenia corniculata* (L.) Cornaz. 花锚
花蕊石 * *Ophicalcitum*
芥子 * *Sinapis Semen*
seed of *Sinapis alba* L. 白芥
苍术 * *Atractylodis Rhizoma*
rhizome of *Atractylodes chinensis* (DC.) Koidz. 北苍术
苍耳子 * *Xanthii Fructus*
fruit of *Xanthium sibiricum* Patr. 苍耳
芡实 * *Euryales Semen*
seed of *Euryale ferox* Salisb. 芡
苎麻根 *Boehmeriae Niveae Radix*
root of *Boehmeria nivea* (L.) Gaud. 苎麻
芦荟 * *Aloe*
leaf juice of *Aloe ferox* Miller 好望角芦荟
芦根 * *Phragmitis Rhizoma*
rhizome of *Phragmites communis* Trin. 芦苇
苏木 * *Sappan Lignum*
heart wood of *Caesalpinia sappan* L. 苏木
苏合香 * *Styrax*
resin of trunk of *Liquidambar orientalis* Mill. 苏合香树
赤芍 * *Paeoniae Radix Rubra*
root of *Paeonia lactiflora* Pall. 芍药
赤小豆 * *Vignae Semen*
seed of *Vigna umbellata* Ohwi et Ohashi 赤小豆
赤石脂 * *Halloysitum Rubrum*
赤茯苓 *Poria Rubra*
pink sclerotium of *Poria cocos* (Schw.) Wolf 茯苓
杏仁水 *Armeniacae Aqua Amarum*
decocted water with seed of *Prunus armeniaca* L. 杏
两头尖 * *Anemones Raddeanae Rhizoma*
rhizome of *Anemone raddeana* Reg. 多被银莲花
两面针 * *Zanthoxyli Radix*
root of *Zanthoxylum nitidum* (Roxb.) DC. 两面针
扶芳藤 *Euonymi Fortunei Caulis seu Folium*
stem or leaf of *Euonymus fortunei* (Turcz.) Hand.-

Mazz. 扶芳藤
扯根菜 *Lysimachiae Clethroidis Radix seu Herba*
root or herb of *Lysimachia clethroides* Duby 珍珠菜
扭肚藤 *Jasmini Amplexicaulis Folium*
leaf of *Jasminum amplexicaule* Buch-Ham. 扭肚藤
连翘 * *Forsythiae Fructus*
fruit of *Forsythia suspensa* (Thunb.) Vahl 连翘
连钱草 * *Glechomae Herba*
herb of *Glechoma longituba* (Nakai) Kupr. 活血丹
坚龙胆 *Gentianae Radix et Rhizoma*
root and rhizome of *Gentiana rigescens* Franch. 滇龙胆
坚龙胆浸膏 *Gentianae Extractum*
extract of *Gentiana rigescens* Franch. 滇龙胆
肖梵天花 *Urenae Lobatae Radix seu Herba*
root or herb of *Urena lobata* L. 肖梵天花
吴茱萸 * *Euodiae Fructus*
fruit of *Euodia rutaecarpa* (Juss.) Benth. 吴茱萸
岗松 *Baeckeae Frutescentis Herba*
herb of *Baeckea frutescens* L. 岗松
岗梅 *Ilicis Asprellae Folium seu Radix*
leaf or root of *Ilex asprella* (Hook. et Arn.) Champ. ex Benth. 秤星树
牡蛎 * *Ostreae Concha*
shell of *Ostrea talienwhanensis* Crosse 大连湾牡蛎
牡丹皮 * *Moutan Cortex*
root-bark of *Paeonia suffruticosa* Andr. 牡丹
何首乌 * *Polygoni Multiflori Radix*
root tuber of *Polygonum multiflorum* Thunb. 何首乌
伸筋草 * *Lycopodii Herba*
herb of *Lycopodium japonicum* Thunb. 石松
伸筋藤 *Tinosporae Sinensis Caulis*
stem of *Tinospora sinensis* (Lour.) Merr. 中华青牛胆
佛手 * *Citri Sarcodactylis Fructus*
fruit of *Citrus medica* L.var. *sarcodactylis* Swingle 佛手
皂矾 *Melanteritum*
皂荚 *Gleditsiae Fructus*
fruit of *Gleditsia sinensis* Lam. 皂荚
皂角刺 * *Gleditsiae Spina*
spine of *Gleditsia sinensis* Lam. 皂荚
返魂草 *Senecionis Cannabifolii Herba*
herb of *Senecio cannabifolius* Less. 麻叶千里光
余甘子 * *Phyllanthi Fructus*
fruit of *Phyllanthus emblica* L. 余甘子
谷芽 * *Setariae Fructus Germinatus*
sprout of *Setaria italica* (L.) Beauv. 粟
谷精草 * *Eriocauli Flos*
capitulum of *Eriocaulon buergerianum* Koern. 谷精草
龟甲 * *Testudinis Carapax et Plastrum*
shell and plastron of *Chinemys reevesii* (Gray) 乌龟
龟甲胶 * *Testudinis Carapacis et Plastri Colla*
shell and plastron glue of *Chinemys reevesii* (Gray) 乌龟
辛夷 * *Magnoliae Flos*
flower bud of *Magnolia biondii* Pamp. 望春花
沙棘 * *Hippophae Fructus*
fruit of *Hippophae rhamnoides* L. 沙棘
沙苑子 * *Astragali Complanati Semen*
seed of *Astragalus complanatus* R. Br. 扁茎黄芪
没药 * *Myrrha*
resin of *Commiphora myrrha* Engl. 没药树
沉香 * *Aquilariae Lignum Resinatum*
resiniferous wood of *Aquilaria sinensis* (Lour.) Gilg 白木香
羌活 * *Notopterygii Rhizoma et Radix*
rhizome and root of *Notopterygium incisum* Ting ex H. T. Chang 羌活
诃子 * *Chebulae Fructus*
fruit of *Terminalia chebula* Retz. 诃子
补骨脂 * *Psoraleae Fructus*
fruit of *Psoralea corylifolia* L. 补骨脂
灵芝 * *Ganoderma*
sporocarp of *Ganoderma lucidum* (Leyss. ex Fr.) Karst. 赤芝
灵猫香 *Zibethum*
secretion of *Viverra zibetha* Linnaeus 大灵猫
阿胶 * *Asini Corii Colla*
ass-hide gelatin of *Equus asinus* Linnaeus 驴
阿魏 * *Ferulae Resina*
resin of *Ferula sinkiangensis* K. M. Shen 新疆阿魏
陈皮 * *Citri Reticulatae Pericarpium*
pericarp of *Citrus reticulata* Blanco 橘
陈皮流浸膏 *Citri Reticulatae Extractum*
extract of *Citrus reticulata* Blanco 橘
附子 * *Aconiti Lateralis Radix Praeparata*
lateral root of *Aconitum carmichaeli* Debx. 乌头

忍冬藤 * *Lonicerae Japonicae Caulis*
stem of *Lonicera japonica* Thunb. 忍冬
鸡肠 *Galli Intestina*
intestine of *Gallus gallus domesticus* Brisson 家鸡
鸡胎 *Galli Foetus*
fetus of *Gallus gallus domesticus* Brisson 家鸡
鸡骨 *Galli Os*
bone of *Gallus gallus domesticus* Brisson 家鸡
鸡内金 * *Galli Gigerii Endothelium Corneum*
inner wall of gizzard of *Gallus gallus domesticus* Brisson 家鸡
鸡矢藤 *Paederiae Scandentis Herba et Radix*
herb and root of *Paederia scandens* (Lour.) Merr. 鸡矢藤
鸡血藤 * *Spatholobi Caulis*
stem of *Spatholobus suberectus* Dunn 密豆花
鸡骨草 * *Abri Herba*
herb of *Abrus cantoniensis* Hance 广州相思子
鸡骨香 *Crotonis Crassifolii Radix*
root of *Croton crassifolius* Geisel. 鸡骨香
鸡胆浸膏 *Galli Fel Extractum*
gall extract of *Gallus gallus domesticus* Brisson 家鸡
鸡冠花 * *Celosiae Cristatae Flos*
inflorescence of *Celosia cristata* L. 鸡冠花
鸡蛋壳 *Galli Ovi Chorion*
egg shell of *Gallus gallus domesticus* Brisson 家鸡
鸡蛋参 *Codonopsis Convolvulaceae Radix*
root of *Codonopsis convolvulacea* Kurz 鸡蛋参
驴皮 *Asini Corium*
fur of *Equus asinus* Linnaeus 驴
驴肾 *Asini Ren*
kidney of *Equus asinus* Linnaeus 驴
驴鞭 *Asini Testis et Penis*
testes and penis of *Equus asinus* Linnaeus 驴

八画

玫瑰花 * *Rosae Rugosae Flos*
flower bud of *Rosa rugosa* Thunb. 玫瑰
青皮 * *Citri Reticularae Pericarpium Viride*
pericarp of *Citrus reticulata* Blanco 橘
青果 * *Canarii Fructus*
fruit of *Canarium album* Rauesch. 橄榄
青蒿 * *Artemisiae Annuae Herba*
herb of *Artemisia annua* L. 黄花蒿
青黛 * *Indigo Naturalis*
prepared mass of *Baphicacanthus cusia* (Nees) Bremek. 马蓝
青木香 *Aristolochiae Radix*
root of *Aristolochia debilis* Sieb. et Zucc. 马兜铃
青风藤 * *Sinomenii Caulis*
stem of *Sinomenium acutum* (Thunb.) Rehd. et Wils. 青藤
青叶胆 * *Swertiae Mileensis Herba*
herb of *Swertia mileensis* T. N. Ho. et W. L. Shih 青叶胆
青葙子 * *Celosiae Semen*
seed of *Celosia argentea* L. 青葙
青礞石 * *Chloriti Lapis*
枇杷叶 * *Eriobotryae Folium*
leaf of *Eriobotrya japonica* (Thunb.) Lindl. 枇杷
板栗壳 *Cupula Castaneae Mollissimae*
cup of *Castanea mollissima* Bl. 栗
板蓝根 * *Isatidis Radix*
root of *Isatis indigotica* Fort. 菘蓝
松香 *Pini Resina*
resin of *Pinus massoniana* Lamb. 马尾松
松塔 *Pini Strobilus*
cone of *Pinus massoniana* Lamb. 马尾松
松节油 *Terebinthinae Oleum*
枫香脂 * *Liquidambaris Resina*
resin of *Liquidambar formosana* Hance 枫香树
枫荷桂 *Sassafratis Tzumu Radix*
root of *Sassafras tzumu* (Hemsl.) Hemsl. 擦木
枫树叶 *Liquidambaris Folium*
leaf of *Liquidambar formosana* Hance 枫香树
刺五加* *Acanthopanacis Senticosi Radix et Rhizoma seu Caulis*
root and rhizome or stem of *Acanthopanax senticosus* (Rupr. et Maxim.) Harms 刺五加
刺五加浸膏 *Acanthopanacis Senticosi Extractum*
extract of *Acanthopanax senticosus* (Rupr. et Maxim.) Harms 刺五加
刺玫果 *Rosae Davuricae Fructus*
fruit of *Rosa davurica* Pall. 刺玫蔷薇
刺猬皮 *Erinacei Corium*
hide of *Erinaceus europaeus* Linnaeus 普通刺猬
苦木 * *Picrasmae Ramulus et Folium*

twig and leaf of *Picrasma quassioides* (D. Don) Benn. 苦木

苦参 * *Sophorae Flavescentis Radix*

root of *Sophora flavescens* Ait. 苦参

苦玄参 * *Picriae Herba*

herb of *Picria felterrae* Lour. 苦玄参

苦地丁 * *Corydalis Bungeanae Herba*

herb of Corydalis bungeana Turcz. 紫堇

苦豆草 *Astragali Melilotoidis Herba*

herb of *Astragalus melilotoides* Pall. 草木樨状黄芪

苦杏仁 * *Armeniacae Semen Amarum*

seed of *Prunus armeniaca* L. 杏

苦楝皮 * *Meliae Cortex*

bark of *Melia azedarach* L. 楝

苘麻子 * *Abutili Semen*

seed of *Abutilon theophrastii* Medic. 苘麻

茅膏菜 *Droserae Peltatae Herba*

herb of *Drosera peltata* Smith 茅膏菜

郁金 * *Curcumae Radix*

root tuber of *Curcuma wenyujin* Y.H. Chen et C. Ling 温郁金

郁李仁 * *Pruni Semen*

seed of *Prunus japonica* Thunb. 郁李

虎杖 * *Polygoni Cuspidati Rhizoma et Radix*

rhizome and root of *Polygonum cuspidatum* Sieb et Zucc. 虎杖

虎刺 *Damnacanthi Indici Herba seu Radix*

herb or root of *Damnacanthus indicus* Gaertn. f. 虎刺

虎骨 *Tigris Os*

bone of *Panthera tigris* Linnaeus 虎

败酱草 *Patriniae Herba*

herb of *Patrinia villosa* Juss. 白花败酱

岩白菜素 *Bergenin*

昆布 * *Laminariae seu Eckloniae Thallus*

thallus of *Laminaria japonica* Aresch. 海带 or *Ecklonia kurome* Okam.昆布

昆明山海棠 *Tripterygii Hypoglauci Cortex*

root-bark of *Tripterygium hypoglaucum* (Levl.) Hutch. 昆明雷公藤

罗汉果 * *Siraitiae Fructus*

fruit of *Siraitia grosvenori* (Swingle) C. Jeffrey ex A. M. Lu et Z. Y. Zhang 罗汉果

罗勒油 *Ocimi Basilici Oleum*

oil of *Ocimum basilicum* L. 罗勒

罗布麻叶 * *Apocyni Veneti Folium*

leaf of *Apocynum venetum* L. 罗布麻

垂盆草 * *Sedi Herba*

herb of *Sedum sarmentosum* Bunge 垂盆草

知母 * *Anemarrhenae Rhizoma*

rhizome of *Anemarrhena asphodeloides* Bge. 知母

使君子 * *Quisqualis Fructus*

fruit of *Quisqualis indica* L. 使君子

使君子仁 *Quisqualis Semen*

seed of *Quisqualis indica* L. 使君子

侧柏叶 * *Platycladi Cacumen*

twig tip and leaf of *Platycladus orientalis* (L.) Franco 侧柏

佩兰 * *Eupatorii Herba*

aerial part of *Eupatorium fortunei* Turcz. 佩兰

乳香 * *Olibanum*

resin of *Boswellia carterii* Birdw. 乳香树

金橘 *Fortunellae Fructus*

fruit of *Fortunella margarita* (Lour.) Swingle 金橘

金不换 *Stephaniae Sinicae Radix*

root of *Stephania sinica* Diels 汝兰

金牛草 *Polygalae Telephioidis Herba*

herb of *Polygala telephioides* Willd. 小花远志

金刚藤 *Smilacis Bockii Rhizoma*

rhizome of *Smilax bockii* Warb. 西南菝葜

金针菇 *Collybiae Sporocarpium*

sporocarp of *Collybia velutipes* (Curt. ex Fr.) Quel. 金钱菌（真菌）

金沙藤 *Lygodii Flexuosi Herba*

herb of *Lygodium flexuosum* (L.) Sw. 曲轴海金沙

金荞麦 * *Fagopyri Dibotryis Rhizoma*

rhizome of *Fagopyrum dibotrys* (D.Don) Hara 金荞麦

金果榄 * *Tinosporae Radix*

root of *Tinospora capillipes* Gagnep. 金果榄

金莲花 *Trollii Flos*

flower of *Trollius chinensis* Bge. 金莲花

金钱草 * *Lysimachiae Herba*

herb of *Lysimachia christinae* Hance 过路黄

金铁锁 * *Psammosilenes Radix*

root of *Psammosilene tunicoides* W. C. Wu et C. Y. Wu 金铁锁

金银花 * *Lonicerae Japonicae Flos*

flower of *Lonicera japonica* Thunb. 忍冬

金银花叶 *Lonicerae Japonicae Folium*

leaf of *Lonicera japonica* Thunb. 忍冬
金樱子 * *Rosae Laevigatae Fructus*
fruit of *Rosa laevigata* Michx. 金樱子
金樱子清膏 *Rosae Laevigatae Extractum*
extract of *Rosa laevigata* Michx. 金樱子
金樱根 *Rosae Laevigatae Radix*
root of *Rosa laevigata* Michx. 金樱子
金礞石 * *Micae Lapis Aureus*
金钱白花蛇 * *Bungarus Parvus*
dried body of *Bungarus multicinctus* Blyth 银环蛇
狗肾 *Canis Ren*
kidney of *Canis familiaris* Linnaeus 狗
狗骨 *Canis Os*
bone of *Canis familiaris* Linnaeus 狗
狗骨胶 *Canis Os Colla*
bone glue of *Canis familiaris* Linnaeus 狗
狗脊 * *Cibotii Rhizoma*
rhizome of *Cibotium barometz* (L.) J. Sm. 金毛狗脊
狗鞭 *Canis Testis et Penis*
testes and penis of *Canis familiaris* Linnaeus 狗
兔心 *Cuniculi Cor*
heart of *Oryctolagus cuniculus* domesticus (Gmelin) 兔
兔耳草 *Pecteilidis Susannae Radix*
root of *Pecteilis susannae* (L.) Raf. 白蝶兰
肿节风 * *Sarcandrae Herba*
herb of *Sarcandra glabra* (Thunb.) Nakai 草珊瑚
鱼鳔 *Piscis Colla*
swim-bladder of *Pseudosciaena crocea* (Richardson) 大黄鱼
鱼腥草 * *Houttuyniae Herba*
aerial part of *Houttuynia cordata* Thunb. 蕺菜
炙甘草* *Glycyrrhizae Radix et Rhizoma Praeparata cum Melle*
prepared with honey of *Glycyrrhiza uralensis* Fisch. 甘草
京墨 *Chinese Ink*
京大戟 * *Euphorbiae Pekinensis Radix*
root of *Euphorbia pekinensis* Rupr. 大戟
夜交藤 *Polygoni Multiflori Caulis*
stem of *Polygonum multiflorum* Thunb. 何首乌
夜明砂 *Vespertilionis Faeces*
feces of *Vespertilio supelans* Thomas 蝙蝠
闹羊花 * *Rhododendri Mollis Flos*
flower of *Rhododendron molle* G. Don 羊踯躅
炉甘石 * *Calamina*
油松节 * *Pini Lignum Nodi*
node of *Pinus tabulaeformis* Carr. 油松
油菜花花粉 *Brassicae Campestris Pollen*
pollen of *Brassica campestris* L. 油菜
泽兰 * *Lycopi Herba*
aerial part of *Lycopus lucidus* Turcz. var. *hirtus* Regel 地瓜儿苗
泽兰叶 *Lycopi Folium*
leaf of *Lycopus lucidus* Turcz. var. *hirtus* Regel地瓜儿苗
泽泻 * *Alismatis Rhizoma*
tuber of *Alisma orientalis* (Sam.) Juzep. 泽泻
单面针 *Zanthoxyli Dissiti Fructus seu Semen*
fruit or seed of *Zanthoxylum dissitum* Hemsl. 蚬壳花椒
卷柏 * *Selaginellae Herba*
herb of *Selaginella tamariscina* (Beauv.) Spring 卷柏
建曲 *Medicata Massa Fermentata*
降香 * *Dalbergiae Odoriferae Lignum*
heart wood of *Dalbergia odorifera* T. Chen 降香檀
降香油 *Dalbergiae Odoriferae Oleum*
oil of *Dalbergia odorifera* T. Chen 降香檀
细辛 * *Asari Radix et Rhizoma*
root and rhizome of *Asarum heterotropoides* Fr. Schmidt var. *mandshuricum* (Maxim.) Kitag. 北细辛
细辛油.*Asari Oleum*
oil of *Asarum heterotropoides* Fr. Schmidt var. *mandshuricum* (Maxim.) Kitag. 北细辛
细梗胡枝子 *Lespedezae Virgatae Herba*
herb of *Lespedeza virgata* (Thunb.) DC. 细梗胡枝子

九画

玳瑁 *Eretmochelydis Carapax*
carapax of *Eretmochelys imbricata* (Linnaeus) 玳瑁
玳瑁粉 *Eretmochelydis Carapax Pulvis*
carapax powder of *Eretmochelys imbricata* (Linnaeus) 玳瑁
珍珠 * *Margarita*
pearl of *Pteria martensii*(Dunker) 马氏珍珠贝
珍珠母 * *Margaritifera Concha*
shell of *Hyriopsis cumingii* (Lea) 三角帆蚌

珍珠香 *Aucklandiae Radix*
root of *Aucklandia lappa* Decne. 木香
珍珠粉 *Margaritae Pulvis*
pearl powder of *Pteria martensii* (Dunker) 马氏珍珠贝
珍珠液 *Margaritae Liquidum*
liquid of *Pteria martensii* (Dunker) 马氏珍珠贝
珍珠层粉 *Margaritae Concha Strati Pulvis*
shell layer powder of *Pteria martensii* (Dunker) 马氏珍珠贝
珊瑚 *Corallii Japonici Sceletus Calx*
lime skeleton of *Corallium japonicum* Kishinouye 桃色珊瑚
枯矾 *Alumen Usta*
枳壳 * *Aurantii Fructus*
fruit of *Citrus aurantium* L. 酸橙
枳实 * *Aurantii Fructus Immaturus*
immature fruit of *Citrus aurantium* L. 酸橙
柏子仁 * *Platycladi Semen*
seed of *Platycladus orientalis* (L.) Franco 侧柏
栀子 * *Gardeniae Fructus*
fruit of *Gardenia jasminoides* Ellis 栀子
栀子浸膏 *Gardeniae Extractum*
extract of *Gardenia jasminoides* Ellis 栀子
枸杞子 * *Lycii Fructus*
fruit of *Lycium barbarum* L. 宁夏枸杞
柳枝 *Salicis Babylonicae Ramulus*
twig of *Salix babylonica* L. 垂柳
柿蒂 * *Kaki Calyx*
calyx of *Diospyros kaki* Thunb. 柿
柿霜 *Kaki Fructus Pulveratum*
powder on fruit of *Diospyros kaki* Thunb. 柿
胡芦巴 * *Trigonellae Semen*
seed of *Trigonella foenum-graecum* L. 胡芦巴
胡黄连 * *Picrohizae Rhizoma*
rhizome of *Picrorhiza scrophulariiflora* Pennell 胡黄连
胡椒 * *Piperis Fructus*
fruit of *Piper nigrum* L. 胡椒
胡颓子 *Elaeagni Pungentis Fructus*
fruit of *Elaeagnus pungens* Thunb. 胡颓子
胡颓子叶 *Elaeagni Pungentis Folium*
leaf of *Elaeagnus pungens* Thunb. 胡颓子
荆芥 * *Schizonepetae Herba*
aerial part of *Schizonepeta tenuifolia* Briq. 荆芥
荆芥穗 * *Schizonepetae Spica*
spike of *Schizonepeta tenuifolia* Briq. 荆芥
南沙参 * *Adenophorae Radix*
root of *Adenophora stricta* Miq. 沙参
南天仙子 *Hygrophilae Salicifoliae Semen*
seed of *Hygrophila salicifolia* (Vahl) Ness 水蓑衣
南五味子 * *Schisandrae Sphenantherae Fructus*
fruit of *Schisandra sphenanthera* Rehd. et Wils. 华中五味子
南板蓝根 * *Baphicacanthis Cusiae Rhizoma et Radix*
rhizome and root of *Baphicacanthus cusia* (Nees) Bremek. 马蓝
茜草 * *Rubiae Radix et Rhizoma*
rhizome and root of *Rubia cordifolia* L. 茜草
荜茇 * *Piperis Longi Fructus*
fruit of *Piper longum* L. 荜茇
荜茇油 *Piperis Longi Fructus Oleum*
fruit oil of *Piper longum* L. 荜茇
荜澄茄 * *Litseae Fructus*
fruit of *Litsea cubeba* (Lour.) Pers. 山鸡椒
草乌 * *Aconiti Kusnezoffii Radix*
root-tuber of *Aconitum kusnezoffii* Reichb. 北乌头
制草乌 * *Aconiti Kusnezoffii Radix Cocta*
prepared root-tuber of *Aconitum kusnezoffii* Reichb. 北乌头
草果 * *Tsaoko Fructus*
fruit of *Amomum tsaoko* Crevost et Lemaire 草果
草豆蔻 * *Alpiniae Katsumadai Semen*
seed of *Alpinia katsumadai* Hayata. 草豆蔻
草河车 *Paridis Rhizoma*
rhizome of *Paris polyplyllum* Smith var. *yunnanensis* (Franch.) Hand.-Mazz. 云南重楼
草珊瑚 *Sarcandrae Herba*
herb of *Sarcandra glabra* (Thunb.) Nakai 草珊瑚
草珊瑚浸膏 *Sarcandrae Extractum*
extract of *Sarcandra glabra* (Thunb.) Nakai 草珊瑚
茵陈 * *Artemisiae Scopariae Herba*
herb of *Artemisia scoparia* Waldst. et Kit. 滨蒿
茴香 *Foeniculi Fructus*
fruit of *Foeniculum vulgare* Mill. 茴香
茴香油 *Foeniculi Oleum*
fruit oil of *Foeniculum vulgare* Mill. 茴香
茯苓 * *Poria*
sclerotium of *Poria cocos* (Schw.) Wolf 茯苓（真菌）

茯苓皮 * *Poriae Cutis*
Exoperidium Poriae cocos (Schw.) Wolf 茯苓
茯神 *Poria Sclerotium Circum Pini Radicem*
sclerotium of *Poria cocos* (Schw.) Wolf around the pine root
茶叶 *Camelliae Sinensis Folium Gemmae*
leaf-bud of *Camellia sinensis* O. Ktze. 茶
茺蔚子 * *Leonuri Fructus*
fruit of *Leonurus japonicus* Houtt. 益母草
荔枝核 * *Litchi Semen*
seed of *Litchi chinensis* Sonn. 荔枝
砂仁 * *Amomi Fructus*
fruit of *Amomum villosum* Lour. 阳春砂
砂仁叶油 *Amomi Folium Oleum*
leaf oil of *Amomum villosum* Lour. 阳春砂
牵牛子 * *Pharbitidis Semen*
seed of *Pharbitis nil* (L.) Choisy 裂叶牵牛
厚朴 * *Magnoliae Officinalis Cortex*
bark or root-bark of *Magnolia officinalis* Rehd. et Wils. 厚朴
威灵仙 * *Clematidis Radix et Rhizoma*
root and rhizome of *Clematis chinensis* Osbeck 威灵仙
轻粉 * *Calomelas*
鸦胆子油 *Bruceae Fructus Oleum*
fruit oil of *Brucea javanica* (L.) Merr. 鸦胆子
韭菜子 * *Allii Tuberosi Semen*
seed of *Allium tuberosum* Rottl. 韭菜
虾蟆草 *Plantaginis Herba*
herb of *Plantago asiatica* L. 车前
虻虫 *Tabanus*
female body of *Tabanus budda* Portshinsky 布虻
蚂蚁 *Formica Fusca*
whole body of *Formica fusca* L. 黑蚁
蚂蟥 *Hirudo*
dried body of *Whitmania pigra* Whitman 蚂蟥
骨碎补 * *Drynariae Rhizoma*
rhizome of *Drynaria fortunei* (Kunze) J. Sm. 槲蕨
秋石 *Hominis Urinae Sedimentum et Sal Praeparata*
prepared human urine sediment and salt
钩藤 * *Uncariae Ramulus cum Uncis*
twig with hook of *Uncaria rhynchophylla* (Miq.) Jacks. 钩藤
香附 * *Cyperi Rhizoma*
rhizome of *Cyperus rotundus* L. 莎草
香菇 *Lentini Edodis Sporocarpium*
sporocarp of *Lentinus edodes* (Berk.) Sing. 香蕈
香樟 *Cinnamomi Camphorae Radix*
root of *Cinnamomum camphora* (L.) Presl 樟
香墨 *Chinese Ink*
香橼 * *Citri Fructus*
fruit of *Citrus medica* L. 枸橼
香薷 * *Moslae Herba*
aerial part of *Mosla chinensis* Maxim. 石香薷
香白芷 *Angelicae Dahuricae Radix*
root of *Angelica dahurica* (Fisch.ex Hoffm.) Benth. et Hook. f. 白芷
香加皮 * *Periplocae Cortex*
root-bark of *Periploca sepium* Bge. 杠柳
香茶菜 *Rabdosiae Glaucocalycis Herba*
herb of *Rabdosia japonica* (Burm. f.) Hara var. *glaucocalyx* (Maxim.) Hara 蓝萼
香榧草 *Eragrostidis Tenellae Herba*
herb of *Eragrostis tenella* (L.) Beauv. 乱草
重楼 * *Paridis Rhizoma*
rhizome of *Paris polyplyllum* Smith var. *yunnanensis* (Franch.) Hand.-Mazz. 云南重楼
禹余粮 * *Limonitum*
鬼针草 *Bidentis Bipinnatae Herba*
herb of *Bidens bipinnata* L. 鬼针草
鬼画符 *Breyniae Fruticosae Folium*
leaf of *Breynia fruticosa* (L.) Hook. f. 黑面神
食盐 *Sal*
独活 * *Angelicae Pubescentis Radix*
root of *Angelica pubescens* Maxim. f. biserrata Shan et Yuan 重齿毛当归
独一味 * *Lamiophlomis Herba*
herb of *Lamiophlomis rotata* (Benth.) Kudo独一味
胆南星 * *Arisaema cum Bile*
ox or pig bile prepared with rhizome of *Arisaema erubescens* (Wall.) Schott 天南星
胖大海 * *Sterculiae Lychnophorae Semen*
seed of *Sterculia lychnophora* Hance 胖大海
急性子 * *Impatientis Semen*
seed of *Impatiens balsamina* L. 凤仙花
炮姜 * *Zingiberis Rhizoma Praeparatum*
prepared rhizome of *Zingiber officinale* Rosc.姜
洋金花 * *Daturae Flos*
flower of *Datura metel* L. 白花曼陀罗
洋葱头 *Allii Cepae Bulbus*

bulb of *Allium cepa* L. 洋葱

前胡 * *Peucedani Radix*

首乌藤 * *Polygoni Multiflori Caulis*

stem of *polygonum multiflorum* Thunb.何首乌

穿山龙 * *Dioscoreae Nipponicae Rhizoma*

rhizome of *Dioscorea nipponica* Makino 穿龙薯蓣

穿山甲 * *Manis Squama*

scale of *Manis pentadactyla* Linnaeus 穿山甲

穿心莲 * *Andrographis Herba*

aeril part of *Andrographis paniculata* (Burm f.) Nees 穿心莲

穿心莲叶 *Andrographis Folium*

leaf of *Andrographis paniculata* (Burm f.) Nees 穿心莲

穿心莲浸膏 *Andrographis Extractum*

extract of *Andrographis paniculata* (Burm f.) Nees 穿心莲

穿破石 *Cudraniae Radix*

root of *Cudrania cochinchinensis* (Lour.) Kudo et Masam. 构棘

穿壁风 *Piperis Hancei Caulis et Folium*

stem and leaf of *Piper hancei Maxim.* 山蒟

姜皮 *Zingiberis Rhizomatis Epidermis*

rhizome epidermis of *Zingiber officinale* Rosc. 姜

姜黄 * *Curcumae Longae Rhizoma*

rhizome of *Curcuma longa* L. 姜黄

祖师麻 *Daphnes Giraldii Cortex*

bark of *Daphne giraldii* Nitsche 黄瑞香

神曲 *Medicata Massa Fermentata*

络石藤 * *Trachelospermi Caulis et Folium*

stem and leaf of *Trachelospermum jasminoides* (Lindl.) Lem. 络石

绞股蓝 *Gynostemmae Pentaphylli Herba*

herb of *Gynostemma pentaphyllum* (Thunb.) Mak. 绞股蓝

十画

蚕茧 *Bombycis Incunabulum*

silk cocoon of *Bombyx mori* Linnaeus 家蚕

蚕砂 *Bombycis Feculae*

silkworm feces of *Bombyx mori* Linnaeus 家蚕

蚕蛾 *Bombycis Imagine Femineus*

imago of *Bombyx mori* Linnaeus 家蚕

蚕蛹 *Bombycis Pupa*

chrysalis of *Bombyx mori* Linnaeus 家蚕

秦艽 * *Gentianae Macrophyllae Radix*

root of *Gentiana macrophylla* Pall. 秦艽

秦皮 * *Fraxini Cortex*

bark of *Fraxinus chinensis* Roxb. 白蜡树

桂皮油 *Cinnamomi Oleum*

bark oil of *Cinnamomum cassia* Presl 肉桂

桂枝 * *Cinnamomi Ramulus*

tender twig of *Cinnamomum cassia* Presl 肉桂

桔梗 * *Platycodonis Radix*

root of *Platycodon grandiflorus* (Jacq.) A. DC. 桔梗

桔梗流浸膏 *Platycodonis Extractum*

extract of *Platycodon grandiflorus* (Jacq.) A. DC. 桔梗

桃仁 * *Persicae Semen*

seed of *Prunus persica* (L.) Batsch 桃

桃枝 * *Persicae Ramulus*

twig of *Prunus persica* (L.) Batsch 桃

桃金娘根 *Rhodomyrti Tomentosae Radix*

root of *Rhodomyrtus tomentosa* (Ait.) Hassk. 桃金娘

核桃仁 * *Juglandis Semen*

seed of *Juglans regia* L. 胡桃

核桃油 *Juglandis Oleum*

seed oil of *Juglans regia* L.胡桃

核桃楸皮 *Juglandis Mandshuricae Cortex*

bark of *Juglans mandshurica* Maxim. 胡桃楸

桉叶 *Eucalypti Folium*

leaf of *Eucalyptus globulus* Labill. 蓝桉

桉油 *Eucalypti Oleum*

leaf oil of *Eucalyptus globulus* Labill.蓝桉

荸荠 *Eleocharitis Dulcis Cormus*

corm of *Eleocharis dulcis* (Burm. f.) Trin. ex Henschel 荸荠

荸荠粉 *Eleocharitis Cormus Dulcis Pulvis*

corm powder of *Eleocharis dulcis* (Burm. f.) Trin. ex Henschel 荸荠

莱阳梨 *Pyri Fructus*

fruit of *Pyrus bretschneideri* Rehd. 白梨 (Laiyang pear)

莱菔子 * *Raphani Semen*

seed of *Raphanus sativus* L. 萝卜

莲子 * *Nelumbinis Semen*

dried body of *Hippocampus kuda* Bleeker 大海马

海龙 * *Syngnathus*

dried body of *Solenognathus hardwickii* (Gray) 刁海龙

海胆 *Echinoideae Osseus Concha*

bony shell of *Hemicentrotus pulcherrimus* (A. Agassiz) 马粪海胆

海星 *Asterias*

dried body of *Asterias rollestoni* Bell 罗氏海盘车

海藻 * *Sargassum*

algae of *Sargassum pallidum* (Turn.) C. Ag. 海蒿子

海风藤 * *Piperis Kadsurae Caulis*

stem of *Piper kadsura* (Choisy) Ohwi 风藤

海金沙 * *Lygodii Spora*

spore of *Lygodium japonicum* (Thunb.) Sw. 海金沙

海金沙藤 *Lygodii Caulis*

stem of *Lygodium japonicum* (Thunb.) Sw. 海金沙

海桐皮 *Erythrinae Orientalis Cortex*

bark of *Erythrina variegate* L. var. *orientalis* (L.) Merr. 刺桐

海螵蛸 * *Sepiae Endoconcha*

inner shell of *Sepiella maindroni* de Rochebrune 无针乌贼

浮萍 * *Spirodelae Herba*

herb of *Spirodela polyrrhiza* (L.) Schleid. 紫萍

浮小麦 *Tritici Aestivi Fructus Natantia*

blighted fruit of *Triticum aestivum* L. 小麦

浮海石 *Pumex*

粉防己 *Stephaniae Tetrandrae Radix*

root of *Stephania tetrandra* S. Moore 粉防己

粉萆薢 * *Dioscoreae Hypoglaucae Rhizoma*

rhizome of *Dioscorea hypoglauca* Palibin 粉背薯蓣

益母草 * *Leonuri Herba*

aerial part of *Leonurus japonicus* Houtt. 益母草

益母草干浸膏 *Leonuri Extractum*

extract of *Leonurus japonicus* Houtt. 益母草

益智 * *Alpiniae Oxyphyllae Fructus*

fruit of *Alpinia oxyphylla* Miq. 益智

宽筋藤 *Cissi Hexangularis Caulis*

stem of *Cissus hexangularis* Pl. 翅茎白粉藤

拳参 * *Bistortae Rhizoma*

rhizome of *Polygonum bistorta* L. 拳参

桑叶 * *Mori Folium*

leaf of *Morus alba* L. 桑

桑枝 * *Mori Ramulus*

tender twig of *Morus alba* L. 桑

桑椹 * *Mori Fructus*

fruit of *Morus alba* L. 桑

桑椹浸膏 *Mori Fructus Extractum*

fruit extrct of *Morus alba* L. 桑

桑白皮 * *Mori Cortex*

root-bark of *Morus alba* L. 桑

桑寄生 * *Taxilli Herba*

twig bearing with leaf of *Taxillus chinensis* (DC.) Danser 桑寄生

桑螵蛸 * *Mantidis Ootheca*

egg-case of *Tenodera sinensis* Saussure 大刀螂

通草 * *Tetrapanacis Medulla*

pith of *Tetrapanax papyriferus* (Hook.) K. Koch 通脱木

十一画

梅花 * *Mume Flos*

flower bud of *Prunus mume* (Sieb.) Sieb. et Zucc. 梅

菥蓂 *Thlaspis Herba*

herb of *Thlaspi arvense* L. 菥蓂

菝葜 * *Smilacis Chinae Rhizoma*

rhizome of *Smilax china* L. 菝葜

菟丝子 * *Cuscutae Semen*

seed of *Cuscuta chinensis* Lam. 菟丝子

菊花 * *Chrysanthemi Flos*

capitulum of *Chrysanthemum morifolium* Ramat. 菊

黄米 *Panici Miliacei Fructus*

fruit of *Panicum miliaceum* L. 稷

黄杨木 *Buxi Sinicae Ramulus*

twig of *Buxus sinica* (Rehd. et Wils.) Cheng 黄杨

黄芩 * *Scutellariae Radix*

root of *Scutellaria baicalensis* Georgi 黄芩

黄芪 * *Astragali Radix*

root of *Astragalus membranaceus*（Fisch.）Bge. var. *mongholicus* (Bge.) Hsiao 蒙古黄芪

黄芪干浸膏 *Astragali Extractum*

extract of *Astragalus membranaceus*（Fisch.）Bge. var. *mongholicus* (Bge.) Hsiao 蒙古黄芪

黄连 * *Coptidis Rhizoma*

rhizome of *Coptis chinensis* Franch. 黄连

黄连须 *Coptidis Radix Fibrosae*
fibrous root of *Coptis chinensis Franch.* 黄连
黄柏 * *Phellodendri Chinensis Cortex*
bark of *Phellodendron chinense* Schneid. 黄皮树
黄精 * *Polygonati Rhizoma*
rhizome of *Polygonatum sibiricum* Red. 黄精
黄藤 * *Fibraureae Caulis*
stem of *Fibraurea recisa* Pierre. 黄藤
黄瓜子 *Cucumidis Sativi Semen*
seed of *Cucumis sativus* L. 黄瓜
黄药子 *Dioscoreae Bulbiferae Rhizoma*
tuber of *Dioscorea bulbifera* L. 黄独
黄毛耳草 *Hedyotis Chrysotrichae Herba*
herb of *Hedyotis chrysotricha* (Palib.) Merr. 金毛耳草
黄杜鹃根 *Rhododendri Mollis Radix*
root of *Rhododendron molle* G. Don 羊踯躅
硇砂 *Sal Ammoniacum*
雪胆 *Hemsleyae Radix*
root-tuber of *Hemsleya amabilis* Diels 小蛇莲
雪莲 *Saussureae Herba*
herb of *Saussurea medusa* Maxim. 水母雪兔子
雪莲花 *Saussureae Herba cum Flos*
herb with flower of *Saussurea medusa* Maxim. 水母雪兔子
雪上一枝蒿 *Aconiti Kongboensis Radix*
root of *Aconitum kongboense* Lauener 工布乌头
接骨木 *Sambuci Williamsii Ramulus*
twig of *Sambucus williamsii* Hance 接骨木
救必应 * *Ilicis Rotundae Cortex*
bark of *Ilex rotunda* Thunb. 铁冬青
雀肉 *Caro Passeris*
meat of *Passer montanus* (Linnaeus) 麻雀
雀脑 *Passeris Encephalon*
brain of *Passer montanus* (Linnaeus) 麻雀
常山 * *Dichroae Radix*
root of *Dichroa febrifuga* Lour. 常山
眼镜蛇 *Naja*
dried body of *Naja naja* (Linnaeus) 眼镜蛇
蛇胆 *Naja Fel*
gall of *Naja naja* (Linnaeus) 眼镜蛇
蛇胆汁 *Naja Bilis*
bile of *Naja naja* (Linnaeus) 眼镜蛇
蛇蜕 * *Serpentis Periostracum*
slough of *Elaphe taeniurus* Cope 黑眉锦蛇
蛇床子 * *Cnidii Fructus*
fruit of *Cnidium monnieri* (L.) Cuss. 蛇床
蛇含石 *Limonitum*
蛇泡勒 *Rubi Parvifolii Herba*
herb of *Rubus parvifolius* L. 茅莓
野木瓜 * *Stauntoniae Caulis et Folium*
stem and leaf of *Stauntonia chinensis* DC. 野木瓜
野菊花 * *Chrysanthemi Indici Flos*
capitulum of *Chrysanthemum indicum* L. 野菊
悬钩木 *Rubi Corchorifolii Caulis*
stem of *Rubus corchorifolius* L. f. 山莓
铜绿 *Aeruginosum*
银朱 *Mercuric Sulfide*
银环蛇 *Bungarus Multicinctus*
dried body of *Bungarus multicinctus multicinctus* Blyth 银环蛇
银杏叶 * *Ginkgo Folium*
leaf of *Ginkgo biloba* L. 银杏
银柴胡 * *Stellariae Radix*
root of *Stellaria dichotoma* L. var. *lanceolata* Bge. 银柴胡
甜叶菊 *Steviae Rebaudinae Folium*
leaf of *Stevia rebaudina* Bertoni 甜菊
甜瓜子 * *Melo Semen*
seed of *Cucumis melo* L. 香瓜
甜地丁 *Gueldenstaedtiae Multiflorae Herba*
herb of *Gueldenstaedtia multiflora* Bge. 米口袋
梨 *Pyri Fructus*
fruit of *Pyrus bretschneideri* Rehd. 白梨
假蒟叶 *Piperis Sarmentosi Folium*
leaf of *Piper sarmentosum* Roxb. 假蒟
船形乌头 *Aconiti Navicularis Herba*
herb of *Aconitum naviculare* Stapf 船盔乌头
猪血 *Suillus Sanguis*
blood of *Sus scrofa domestica* Brisson 猪
猪苓 * *Polyporus*
sclerotium of *Polyporus umbellatus* (Pers.) Fries 猪苓（真菌）
猪骨 *Suillus Os*
bone of *Sus scrofa domestica* Brisson 猪
猪胆 *Suillus Fel*
gall of *Sus scrofa domestica* Brisson 猪
猪胆汁 *Suillus Bilis*
bile of *Sus scrofa domestica* Brisson 猪
猪胆汁粉 *Suillus Bilis Pulvis*

bile powder of *Sus scrofa domestica* Brisson 猪
猪胆膏 *Suillus Fel Extractum*
gall extract of *Sus scrofa domestica* Brisson 猪
猪腰 *Suillus Ren*
kidney of *Sus scrofa domestica* Brisson 猪
猪牙皂 * *Gleditsiae Fructus Abnormalis*
infertile fruit of *Gleditsia sinensis* Lam. 皂荚
猪脑粉 *Suillus Encephalon Pulvis*
brain powder of *Sus scrofa domestica* Brisson 猪
猪脊髓 *Suillus Spinalis Medulla*
spinal cord of *Sus scrofa domestica* Brisson 猪
猪蹄甲 *Suillus Unguis*
nail of *Sus scrofa domestica* Brisson 猪
猫爪草 * *Ranunculi Ternati Radix*
root of *Ranunculus ternatus* Thunb. 小毛茛
象皮 *Elephantis Corium*
hide of *Elephas maximus* Linnaeus 亚洲象
象牙屑 *Elephantis Frustillum*
ivory scrip of *Elephas maximus* Linnaeus 亚洲象
旋覆花 * *Inulae Flos*
capitulum of *Inula japonica* Thunb. 旋覆花
鹿肉 *Cervi Caro*
meat of *Cervus nippon* Temminck 梅花鹿
鹿血 *Cervi Sanguis*
blood of *Cervus nippon* Temminck 梅花鹿
鹿角 * *Cervi Cornu*
antler of *Cervus nippon* Temminck 梅花鹿
鹿角胶 * *Cervi Cornus Colla*
antler glue of *Cervus nippon* Temminck 梅花鹿
鹿角霜 * *Cervi Cornu Degelatinatum*
deglued antler mass of *Cervus nippon* Temminck 梅花鹿
鹿尾 *Cervi Cauda*
tail of *Cervus nippon* Temminck 梅花鹿
鹿肾 *Cervi Testis et Penis*
testes and penis of *Cervus nippon* Temminck 梅花鹿
鹿茸 * *Cervi Cornu Pantotrichum*
hairy antler of *Cervus nippon* Temminck 梅花鹿
鹿茸粉 *Cervi Cornu Pantotrichum Pulvis*
hairy antler powder of *Cervus nippon* Temminck 梅花鹿
鹿骨 *Cervi Os*
bone of *Cervus nippon* Temminck 梅花鹿
鹿筋 *Cervi Tendo*
sinew of *Cervus nippon* Temminck 梅花鹿
鹿鞭 *Cervi Penis*
penis of *Cervus nippon* Temminck 梅花鹿
鹿心粉 *Cervi Cor Pulvis*
heart powder of *Cervus nippon* Temminck 梅花鹿
鹿衔草 * *Pyrolae Herba*
herb of *Pyrola calliantha* H. Andres 鹿蹄草
麻黄 * *Ephedrae Herba*
herb of *Ephedra sinica* Stapf 草麻黄
麻黄粉 *Ephedrae Pulvis*
powder of *Ephedra sinica* Stapf 草麻黄
麻黄浸膏 *Ephedrae Extractum*
extract of *Ephedra sinica* Stapf 草麻黄
淡竹叶 * *Lophatheri Herba*
herb of *Lophatherum gracile* Brongn. 淡竹叶
淡豆豉 * *Sojae Semen Praeparatum*
fermented *Glycine max* (L.) Merr. 大豆
淫羊藿 * *Epimedii Folium*
leaf of *Epimedium brevicornum* Maxim. 淫羊藿
羚羊角 * *Saigae Tataricae Cornu*
horn of *Saiga tatarica* Linnaeus 赛加羚羊
羚羊角粉 *Saigae Tataricae Cornu Pulvis*
horn powder of *Saiga tatarica* Linnaeus 赛加羚羊
断节参 *Cynanchi Wallichii Radix*
root of *Cynanchum wallichii* Wight 昆明杯冠藤
断血流 * *Clinopodii Herba*
aerial part of *Clinopodium chinensis* (Benth.) O. Kuntze 风轮菜
密蒙花 * *Buddlejae Flos*
flower of *Buddleja officinalis* Maxim. 密蒙花
蛋黄油 *Ovi Luteum Oleum*
oil of egg yolk of *Gallus gallus domesticus* Brisson 家鸡
续断 * *Dipsaci Radix*
root of *Dipsacus asperoides* C. Y. Cheng et T. M. Ai 川续断
绿豆 *Phaseoli Radiati Semen*
seed of *Phaseolus radiatus* L. 绿豆
绿豆粉 *Phaseoli Radiati Pulvis*
seed powder of *Phaseolus radiatus* L.绿豆
绿茶叶 *Camelliae Sinensis Folium Gemmae*
green tea
绿绒蒿 *Meconopsis Integrifoliae Herba*
herb of *Meconopsis integrifolia* (Maxim.) Franch. 全缘绿绒蒿

绵萆薢 *Dioscoreae Spongiosae Rhizoma*
rhizome of *Dioscorea spongiosa* J. Q. Xi M. Mizuno et W. L.Zhao 绵萆薢
绵马贯众 * *Dryopteridis Crassirhizomatis Rhizoma*
rhizome of *Dryopteris crassirhizoma* Nakai 粗茎鳞毛蕨

十二画

琥珀 *Cutis Succinum*
琥珀粉 *Succini Pulvis*
斑蝥 * *Mylabris*
dried body of *Mylabris phalerata* Pallas 南方大斑蝥
楮实子 * *Broussonetiae Fructus*
fruit of *Broussonetia papyrifera* (L.) Vent. 构树
棉花根 *Gossypii Radix*
root of *Gossypium herbaceum* L. 草棉
棕榈 * *Trachycarpi Petiolus*
petiole of *Trachycarpus fortunei* (Hook. f.) H. Wendl. 棕榈
棕榈炭 *Trachycarpi Petiolus Carbonisatus*
carbonated petiole of *Trachycarpus fortunei* (Hook. f.) H. Wendl. 棕榈
棕榈果 *Trachycarpi Fructus*
fruit of *Trachycarpus fortunei* (Hook. f.) H. Wendl. 棕榈
酢浆草 *Oxalidis Corniculatae Herba*
herb of *Oxalis corniculata* L. 酢浆草
棘豆 *Oxytropis Leptophyllae Radix*
root of *Oxytropis leptophylla* (Pall.) DC. 薄叶棘豆
款冬花 * *Farfarae Flos*
flower bud of *Tussilago farfara* L. 款冬
葛花 *Puerariae Lobatae Flos*
flower of *Pueraria lobata* (Willd.) Ohwi 葛
葛根 * *Puerariae Lobatae Radix*
root of *Pueraria lobata* (Willd.) Ohwi 葛
葡萄干 *Vitis Viniferae Fructus Siccus*
dried fruit of *Vitis vinifera* L. 葡萄
葱 *Allii Fistulosi Folium*
leaf of *Allium fistulosum* L. 大葱
葱白 *Allii Fistulosi Bulbus*
bulb of *Allium fistulosum* L. 大葱
葶苈子 * *Lepidii Semen*
seed of *Lepidium apetalum* Willd. 独行菜
落新妇 *Astilbes Chinensis Herba*
herb of *Astilbe chinensis* (Maxim.) Franch. et Sav. 落新妇
萹蓄 * *Polygoni Avicularis Herba*
aerial part of *Polygonum aviculare* L. 萹蓄
硝石 *Nitrum*
硫黄 * *Sulfur*
雄鸡 *Galli Maris Caro*
meal of male *Gallus gallus domesticus* Brisson 家鸡
雄黄 * *Realgar*
雄黄粉 *Realgar Pulvis*
搜山虎 *Atropanthes Sinensis Radix*
root of *Atropanthe sinensis* (Hemsl.) Pascher 天蓬子
紫草 * *Arnebiae Radix*
root of *Arnebia euchroma* (Royle) Johnst.新疆紫草
紫菀 * *Asteris Radix et Rhizoma*
root and rhizome of *Aster tataricus* L.f 紫菀
紫苏子 * *Perillae Fructus*
fruit of *Perilla frutescens* (L.) Britt. 紫苏
紫苏叶 * *Perillae Folium*
leaf of *Perilla frutescens* (L.) Britt. 紫苏
紫苏叶油 *Perillae Folium Oleum*
leaf oil of *Perilla frutescens* (L.) Britt. 紫苏
紫苏梗 * *Perillae Caulis*
stem of *Perilla frutescens* (L.) Britt. 紫苏
紫河车 * *Hominis Placenta*
human placena of *Homo sapiens* Linnaeus 人
紫荆皮 *Cercis Chinensis Cortex*
bark of *Cercis chinensis* Bge. 紫荆
紫草茸 *Lacca*
secretion of *Laccifer locca* Kerr 紫胶虫
紫珠叶 * *Callicarpae Formosanae Folium*
leaf of *Callicarpa formosana* Rolfe 杜虹花
紫硇砂 *Sal Ammoniacum*
紫花地丁 * *Violae Herba*
herb of *Viola yedoensis* Makino 紫花地丁
蛤壳 * *Meretricis Concha*
shell of *Meretrix meretrix* Linnaeus 文蛤
蛤壳粉 *Meretricis Concha Pulvis*
shell powder of *Meretrix meretrix* Linnaeus 文蛤
蛤蚧 * *Gecko*
dried body of *Gekko gecko* Linnaeus 蛤蚧
蛤蚧粉 *Gecko Pulvis*

power of *Gekko gecko* Linnaeus 蛤蚧
蛴螬 *Holotrichiae Larva*
dried body of *Holotrichia diomphalia* Bates 朝鲜黑金龟子
景天三七 *Sedi Aizoon Herba*
herb of *Sedum aizoon* L. 大三七
黑豆 * *Sojae Semen Nigrum*
soyabean of *Glycine max* (L.) Merr. 大豆
黑矾 *Melanteritum*
黑锡 *Plumbum*
黑木耳 *Auriculariae Sporocarpium*
sporocarp of *Auricularia auricula* (L. ex Hook.) Underw 木耳
黑芝麻 * *Sesami Semen Nigrum*
seed of *Sesamum indicum* L. 脂麻
黑胡椒 *Piperis Fructus Nigrum*
fruit of *Piper nigrum* L. 胡椒
黑老虎根 *Kadsurae Coccineae Radix*
root of *Kadsura coccinea* (Lem.) A. C. Smith 冷饭团
黑种子草 * *Nigellae Semen*
seed of *Nigella glandulifera* Freyn 瘤果黑种草
锁阳 * *Cynomorii Caulis Carnosus*
freshy stem of *Cynomorium songaricum* Rupr. 锁阳
鹅不食草 * *Centipedae Herba*
herb of *Centipeda minima* (L.) A. Br. et Aschers. 鹅不食草
鹅胆干粉 *Anserinus Fel Pulvis*
gall powder of *Anser cygnoides orientalis* (Linnaeus) 家鹅
筋骨草 * *Ajugae Herba*
herb of *Ajuga decumbens* Thunb. 筋骨草
貂心 *Martis Zibellinae Cor*
heart of *Martes zibellina* Linnaeus 紫貂
貂鞭 *Martis Zibellinae Testis et Penis*
testes and penis of *Martes zibellina* Linnaeus 紫貂
番泻叶 * *Sennae Folium*
leaf of *Cassia angustifolia* Vahl 番泻
番石榴叶 *Psidii Guajavae Folium*
leaf of *Psidium guajava* L. 番石榴
猴头菌 *Hericii Erinacei Sporocarpium*
sporocarp of *Hericium erinaceus* (Fr.) Pers. 猴头
猴头菌菌丝体 *Hericii Erinacei Mycelium*
mycelium *Hericium erinaceus* (Fr.) Pers. 猴头
腊梅花 *Chimonanthi Praecocis Flos Immaturus*
immature flower of *Chimonanthus praecox* (L.) Link 腊梅
温郁金 *Curcumae Radix*
root-tuber of *Curcuma wenyujin* Y.H. Chen et C. Ling 温郁金
滑石 * *Talcum*
滑石粉 * *Talci Pulvis*
寒水石 *Gypsum Rubrum*
犀角 *Rhinocerotis Asiatici Cornu*
horn of *Rhinoceros unicornis* Linnaeus 印度犀

十三画

椿皮 * *Ailanthi Cortex*
bark of *Ailanthus altissima* (Mill.) Swingle 臭椿
槐花 * *Sophorae Flos*
flower of *Sophora japonica* L. 槐
槐角 * *Sophorae Fructus*
fruit of *Sophora japonica* L. 槐
槐枝 *Sophorae Ramulus*
twig of *Sophora japonica* L. 槐
榆枝 *Ulmi Pumilae Ramulus*
twig of *Ulmus pumila* L. 榆树
蓝花参 *Wahlenbergiae Margintatae Herba*
herb of *Wahlenbergia margintata* (Thunb.) A. DC. 兰花参
蒺藜 * *Tribuli Fructus*
fruit of *Tribulus terrestris* L. 蒺藜
蓖麻子 * *Ricini Semen*
seed of *Ricinus communis* L. 蓖麻
蒲桃 *Syzygii Jambos Pericarpium*
pericarp of *Syzygium jambos* (L.) Alston 蒲桃
蒲黄 * *Typhae Pollen*
pollen of *Typha angustifolia* L. 水烛香蒲
蒲公英 * *Taraxaci Herba*
herb of *Taraxacum mongolicum* Hand. -Mazz. 蒲公英
蒲公英浸膏 *Taraxaci Extractum*
extract of *Taraxacum mongolicum* Hand. -Mazz. 蒲公英
硼砂 *Borax*
碎骨木 *Ilicis Rotundae Cortex*
bark of *Ilex rotunda* Thunb. 铁冬青
雷丸 * *Omphalia*

sclerotium of *Omphalia lapidescens* Schroet. 雷丸

雷公藤 *Tripterygii Wilfordii Radix Folium seu Flos*

root,leaf or flower of *Tripterygium wilfordii* Hook. f. 雷公藤

零陵香 *Lysimachiae Foenum-graeci Herba*

herb of *Lysimachia foenum-graecum* Hance 灵香草

蜈蚣 * *Scolopendra*

dried body of *Scolopendra subspinipes* mutilans L. Koch 少棘巨蜈蚣

蜂房 * *Vespae Nidus*

honeycomb of *Polites olivaceous* (DeGeer) 果马蜂

蜂蜡 * *Cera Flava*

wax of *Apis mellifera* Linnaeus 意大利蜂

蜂蜜 * *Mel*

honey of *Apis mellifera* Linnaeus 意大利蜂

蜂王浆 *Apis Regis Lac*

royal jelly of *Apis mellifera* Linnaeus 意大利蜂

蜣螂 *Catharsius*

dried body of *Catharsius molossus* Linnaeus 屎壳螂

路路通 * *Liquidambaris Fructus*

infructescence of *Liquidambar formosana* Hance 枫香树

蜀椒 *Zanthoxyli Pericarpium*

pericarp of *Zanthoxylum bungeanum* Maxim. 花椒

矮地茶 * *Ardisiae Japonicae Herba*

herb of *Ardisia japonica* (Thunb.) Blume 紫金牛

矮紫堇 *Corydalis Pygmaeae Herba*

herb of *Corydalis pygmaea* C. Y. Wu et Z. Y. Su 矮紫堇

锦灯笼 * *Physalis Calyx seu Fructus*

calyx or fruit of *Physalis alkekengi* L. var. *franchetii* (Mast.) Makino 酸浆

满山白 *Monochasmae Savatieri Herba*

herb of *Monochasma savatieri* Franch. ex Maxim. 绵毛鹿茸草

满山红 * *Rhododendri Daurici Folium*

leaf of *Rhododendron dauricum* L. 兴安杜鹃

滇紫草 *Onosmae Paniculati Radix*

root of *Onosma paniculatum* Bur. et Franch. 滇紫草

溪黄草 *Rabdosiae Serrae Herba*

herb of *Rabdosia serra* (Maxim.) Hara 溪黄草

裸花紫珠 *Callicarpae Nudiflorae Ramulus et Folium*

twig and leaf of *Callicarpa nudiflora* Hook. et Arn. 裸花紫珠

十四画

榧子 * *Torreyae Semen*

seed of *Torreya grandis* Fort. 榧

槟榔 * *Arecae Semen*

seed of *Areca catechu* L. 槟榔

榕树叶 *Fici Microcarpae Folium*

leaf of *Ficus microcarpa* L. f. 榕树

酸模 *Rumicis Acetosae Radix*

root of *Rumex acetosa* L. 酸模

酸枣仁 * *Ziziphi Spinosae Semen*

seed of *Ziziphus jujuba* Mill var. *spinosa* (Bunge) Hu ex H. F. Chou 酸枣

蔓荆子 * *Viticis Fructus*

fruit of *Vitex trifolia* L. 蔓荆

蔗鸡 *Sacchari Sinensis Gemma*

gemma of *Saccharum sinensis* Roxb. 甘蔗

蔊菜 *Rorippae Indicae Herba seu Flos*

herb or flower of *Rorippa indica* (L.) Hiern 蔊菜

蓼实子 *Polygoni Hydropiperis Fructus*

fruit of *Polygonum hydropiper* L. 水蓼

蓼大青叶 * *Polygoni Tinctorii Folium*

leaf of *Polygonum tinctorium* Ait. 蓼蓝

磁石 * *Magnetitum*

豨莶草 * *Siegesbeckiae Herba*

herb of *Siegesbeckia orientalis* L. 豨莶

蜚蠊 *Blatta*

dried body of *Blatta orientalis* Linnaeus 东方蠊

蜻蜓 *Acestra*

dried body of *Anax parthenope* Selys 大蜻蜓

蝉蜕 * *Cicadae Periostracum*

slough of *Cryptotypana pustulata* Fabricius 黑蚱

罂粟壳 * *Papaveris Pericarpium*

pericarp of *Papaver somniferum* L. 罂粟

罂粟壳浸膏 *Papaveris Pericarpium Extractum*

pericarp extract of *Papaver somniferum* L.罂粟

獐牙菜 *Swertiae Herba*

herb of *Swertia bimaculata* Hook. f. et Thoms. 獐牙菜

辣椒 * *Capsici Fructus*

fruit of *Capsicum frutescens* L. 辣椒

辣椒流浸膏 *Capsici Extractum*
extract of *Capsicum frutescens* L. 辣椒
辣蓼 *Polygoni Flaccidi Herba*
herb of *Polygonum flaccidum* Meisn. 辣蓼
漏芦 * *Rhapontici Radix*
root of *Rhaponticum uniflorum* (L.) DC. 祁州漏芦
熊胆 *Ursi Fel*
gall of *Ursus arctos* Linnaeus 棕熊
熊胆粉 *Ursi Fel Pulvis*
gall powder of *Ursus arctos* Linnaeus 棕熊

十五画

横经席 *Calophylli Membranacei Radix*
root of *Calophylli membranaceum* Gardn. et Champ. 薄叶胡桐
橡皮 *Querci Acutissimae Cortex*
bark of *Quercus acutissima* Carr. 麻栎
槲寄生 * *Visci Herba*
herb of *Viscum coloratum* (Komar.) Nakai 槲寄生
槲叶干浸膏 *Visci Folium Extractum*
leaf extract of *Viscum coloratum* (Komar.) Nakai 槲寄生
樟脑 *Camphora*
樟树根 *Litseae Rubescentis Radix*
root of *Litsea rubescens* Lecomte 红叶木姜子
橄榄核 *Canarii Albi Semen*
seed of *Canarium album* (Lour.) Raeusch. 橄榄
赭石 * *Haematitum*
蕤仁 **Nux Prinsepiae*
nut of *Prinsepia uniflora* Batal. 蕤核
蕲蛇 * *Agkistrodon*
dried body of *Agkistrodon acutus* (Guenther) 五步蛇
蕲蛇肉 *Agkistrodontis Caro*
meat of *Agkistrodon acutus* (Guenther) 五步蛇
暴马子皮 * *Syringae Cortex*
bark of *Syringa reticulata* (Bl.) Hara var. *mandshurica* (Maxim.) Hara 暴马丁香
墨旱莲 * *Ecliptae Herba*
aerial part of *Eclipta prostrata* L. 鳢肠
墨旱莲浸膏 *Ecliptae Extractum*
extrat of *Eclipta prostrata* L. 鳢肠
稻芽 * *Oryzae Fructus Germinatus*
germinated fruit of *Oryza sativa* L.

僵蚕 * *Bombyx Batryticatus*
larva of *Bombyx mori* L. 家蚕 infected by *Beauveria bassiana* (Bals.) Vuill.白僵菌
熟地黄 *Rehmanniae Radix Praeparata*
prepared *Rehmannia glutinosa* Libosch. 地黄
鹤草芽 *Agrimoniae Herba*
aerial part of *Agrimonia pilosa* Ledeb. 龙芽草

十六画

橘叶 *Citri Reticulatae Folium*
leaf of *Citrus reticulata* Blanco 橘
橘红 * *Citri Exocarpium Rubrum*
exocarp of *Citrus reticulata* Blanco 橘
橘络 *Citri Tangerinea Vascular Fascis*
vascular bundle of *Citrus tangerine* Hort. et Tanaka 福橘
橘核 * *Citri Reticulatae Semen*
seed of *Citrus reticulata* Blanco 橘
颠茄流浸膏 *Belladonnae Extractum*
herb extract of *Atropa belladonna* L. 颠茄
薤白 * *Allii Macrostemonis Bulbus*
bulb of *Allium macrostemon* Bge. 小根蒜
薏苡仁 * *Coicis Semen*
seed of *Coix lacryma-jobi* L. var. *mayuen* (Roman.) Stapf 薏苡
薄荷 * *Menthae Haplocalycis Herba*
aerial part of *Mentha haplocalyx* Briq. 薄荷
薄荷油 *Menthae Haplocalycis Oleum*
oil of *Mentha haplocalyx* Briq. 薄荷
螃蟹甲 *Phlomidis Younghusbandii Radix*
root tuber of *Phlomis younghusbandii* Mukerjee 螃蟹甲
壁钱炭 *Uroctea Carbonisatus*
carbonated *Uroctea compactilis* L. Koch 华南壁钱

十七画

檀香 * *Santali Albi Lignum*
heart wood of *Santalum album* L. 檀香
檀香油 *Santali Albi Lignum Oleum*
oil of heart wood of *Santalum album* L. 檀香
藏木香 *Inulae Radix*

root of *Inula helenium* L. 土木香

藏青果 *Chebulae Fructus*

fruit of *Terminalia chebula* Retz. 诃子

藏菖蒲 * *Acori Calami Rhizoma*

rhizome of *Acorus calamus* L. 藏菖蒲

藁本 * *Ligustici Rhizoma et Radix*

rhizome and root of *Ligusticum sinese* Oliv. 藁本

爵床 *Rostellulariae Procumbenstis Herba*

herb of *Rostellularia procumbens* (L.) Ness 爵床

翼首草 * *Pterocephali Herba*

root of *Pterocephalus hookeri* (Clarke) Hoeck匙叶翼首花

十八画

藕节 * *Nelumbinis Nodus Rhizomatis*

rhizome node of *Nelumbo nucifera* Gaertn. 莲

黎芦 *Veratri Radix et Rhizoma*

root and rhizome of *Veratrum nigrum* L. 黑藜芦

覆盆子 * *Rubi Fructus*

fruit of *Rubus chingii* Hu 覆盆子

瞿麦 * *Dianthi Herba*

aerial part of *Dianthus superbus* L. 瞿麦

翻白草 * *Potentillae Discoloris Herba*

herb of *Potentilla discolor* Bge. 翻白草

鹰不扑 *Araliae Armatae Ramulus et Folium*

twig and leaf of *Aralia armata* (Wall.) Seem. 虎刺楤木

十九画

藿香 *Agastaches Herba*

herb of *Agastache rugosa* (Fisch. et Mey.) O. Ktze. 藿香

蘑菇 *Agarici Campestris Sporocarpium*

sporocarp of *Agaricus campestris* L. ex Fr. 蘑菇

蟾皮 *Bufonis Cutis*

skin of *Bufo bufo gargarizans* Cantor 中华大蟾蜍

蟾酥 * *Bufonis Venenum*

skin secretion of *Bufo bufo gargarizans* Cantor 中华大蟾蜍

鳖甲 * *Trionycis Carapax*

carapace of *Trionyx sinensis* Wiegmann 鳖

鳖甲胶 *Trionycis Carapacis Colla*

carapace glue of *Trionyx sinensis* Wiegmann 鳖

二十画

獾油 *Melis Adeps*

fat of *Meles meles* Linnaeus 狗獾

糯米 *Oryzae Glutinosae Fructus*

fruit of *Oryza sativa* L.var. *glutinous* Matsum. 糯稻

糯米饭 *Oryzae Glutinosae Fructus* (cooked rice)

cooked rice of *Oryza sativa* L.var. *glutinous* Matsum. 糯稻

二十一画

麝香 * *Moschus*

secretion of *Moschus berezovskii* Flerov 林麝

附录三 中药英文名称检索表
Appendix Ⅲ: Key of Chinese Medicinal Names in English

一画

一点红 Snake Strawberry

二画

丁香 Clove
人参 Ginseng
九节茶 Glabrous Sarcandra
九里香 Common Jasminorange

三画

三七 Sanchi
三叉苦 Thin Evodia
干蟾皮 Toad Skin
土荆芥 Wormseed
土茯苓 Glabrous Greenbrier
土鳖虫 Ground Beetle
大枫子 Chaulmoogra-tree
大枫子油 Chaulmoogra-tree Oil
大叶紫珠 Large-leaved Callicarpa
大青叶 Woad
大枣 Chinese Date
大黄 Rhubarb
山芝麻 Narrowleaf Screwtree
山羊角 Goat Horn
山豆根 Tonkines Sophora
山药 Chinese Yam
山绿茶 Green Tea
山楂 Chinese Hawthorn
千斤拔 Philippine Flemingia
千里光 Ragwort
川贝母 Sichuan Fritillary
川芎 Chuanxiong Ligusticum
川楝 Szechwan Chinaberry
广枣 Axillary Choerospondias
广藿香 Cablin Potchouli
广金钱草 Snowbellleaf Tickclover
女贞子 Chinese Privet
小茴香 Fonnel
小蓟 Field Thistle
马钱子 Strychnine Seed

四画

天花粉 Trichosanthes Root
天南星 Jackinthepulpit
天麻 Gastrodia
木瓜 Chinese-quince
木香 Common Aucklandia
五味子 Five-flavor-fruit
化香树 Dyetree
化香树果序 Dyetree Infructescence
化橘红 Huazhou Pummelo Peel
毛鸡 Crow Pheasant
牛黄 Bezoar

牛耳枫 Calyx-shaped Daphniphyllum
乌鸡 Silky Chicken
乌梅 Japanese Apricot
乌梢蛇 Garter Snake
丹参 Redroot Sage
火麻仁 Hemp Fimble
水飞蓟 Blessed Thistle
水飞蓟素 Silybin
水团花 Pilular Adina
水蛭 Leech

五画

功劳木 Leatherleaf Mahonia
艾叶 Argy Wormwood
平贝母 Ussuri Fritillary
玉叶金花 Erose Mussaenda
玉竹 Solomon's Seal
甘草 Licorice
石韦 Pyrrosia
石斛 Noble Dendrobium
石榴子 Pomegranate Fruit
石膏 Gypsum
龙骨 Dragon's Bone
龙胆 Scabrous Gentian
龙胆花 Scabrous Gentian Flower
北瓜 Pumpkin
北豆根 Siberian Moonseed
仙鹤草 Hairyvein Agrimony
冬凌草 Blushred Rabdosia
白术 Largehead Atractylodes
白芍 White Peony
白果 Ginkgo Seed
白花蛇舌草 Spreading Hedyotis
汉桃叶 Scandent Schefflera
玄参 Figwort
半夏 Ternate Pinellia
半枝莲 Barbed Skullcap

六画

地龙 Earthworm
地菍 Lesser Melastoma
地黄 Chinese Fox-glove
地榆 Burnet Bloodwort
芋 Taro
芒果 Mango
西瓜霜 Watermelon Mirabilite
西红花 Saffron
西青果 Myrobalan
西洋参 American Ginseng
百合 Lily Bulb
百部 Sessile Stemona
当归 Chinese Angelica
当药 Diluted Swertia
虫草菌 Fungus of Cordyceps
虫草菌丝 Hypha Cordyceps
肉苁蓉 Broomrape
肉桂 Cassia Bark
竹沥 Henon Bamboo Juice
竹黄 Shiraia Bambusicola Stroma
朱砂 Cinnabar
延胡索 Yanhusuo
血竭 Dragon's Blood Palm
全龟 Tortoise
灯盏花素 Breviscapine
灯盏细辛 Erigeron
冰片 Borneol
江南卷柏 Moellendorf 's Spikemoss
羊角 Goat Horn
羊肝 Goat liver
阴行草 Chinese Siphonostegia
防风 Divaricate Saposhnikovia
红花 Safflower
红参 Red Ginseng
红根草 Clethra Loosetrife
红景天 Bigflower Rhodiola

七画

麦冬 Lily-turf
杜仲 Gutta-percha-tree
豆蔻 Krervanh
芙蓉叶 Cottonrose Hibiscus
苍术 Chinese Atractylodes
芦荟 Cape Aloe
苏合香 Storax

扶芳藤 Climbing Euonymus
连翘 Weeping Forsythia
坚龙胆 Rigescent Gentian
牡蛎 Oster Shell
何首乌 Chinese Knotweed
佛手 Finger Citron
皂矾 Melanterite
余甘子 Emblic Myrobalan
龟甲 Tortoise's Shell and Plastron
龟甲胶 Tortoise's Shell and Plastron Glue
辛夷 Biond Magnolia
沙棘 Sand Thorn
沉香 Chinese Eaglewood
羌活 Incised Notopterygium
诃子 Myrobalan
灵芝 Glossy Ganoderma
灵猫香 Civet
阿胶 Ass-hide Gelatin
陈皮 Mardarin Orange Peel
附子 Szechuan Aconite
鸡血藤 Millettia
鸡骨草 Chinese Prayer-beads
鸡胆 Chiken Gall
鸡胆浸膏 Gall Extract of Chicken

八画

青果 Chinese Olive
青黛 Indigo
青风藤 Orientvine
枇杷叶 Loquat leaf
板蓝根 Woad Root
刺五加 Manyprickle Acanthopanax
刺玫果 Dahurian Rose
苦杏仁 Apricot Seed
苦参 Shrubby Sophora
郁金 Turmeric
虎杖 Bushy Knotweed
昆明山海棠 Glaucousback Threewingnut
罗布麻 Dogbane
罗汉果 Grosvenor Siraitia
知母 Common Anemarrhena
侧柏 Chinese Arborvitae
金刚藤 Chinese Greenbrier
金荞麦 Dibotrys Buckwheat
金莲花 Trollius
金钱草 Christina Loosestrife
金银花 Honeysuckle Flower
金礞石 Mica-schist
金樱子 Cherokee Rose
金樱根 Cherokee Rose Root
金橘 Kumquat
狗骨 Dog Bone
肿节风 Glabrous Sarcandra
鱼腥草 Fishword
鱼鳔 Fish Swim-bladder
炉甘石 Smithsonite
泽兰 Shiny Bugleweed
泽泻 Oriental Waterplantain
卷柏 Selaginella
细辛 Chinese Wild Ginger

九画

珍珠 Pearl
珍珠香 Common Aucklandia
珍珠层粉 Shell Inner Layer Powder of Pearl
珊瑚 Coral
柏子 Chinese Arborvitae Seed
栀子 Jasmin
枸杞子 Chinese Wolfberry
荆芥 Fineleaf Schizonepeta
茜草 Indian Madder
茴香 Fennel
南板蓝根 Common Baphicacanthus
毕澄茄 Moutain-pepper
草果 Tsao-ko Amomum
草珊瑚 Glabrous Sarcandra
茵陈 Virgate Wormwood
茯苓 Indian Bread
砂仁 Villous Amomum
厚朴 Magnolia Bark
威灵仙 Chinese Clematis
鸦胆子 Java Brucea
鸦胆子油 Java Brucea Oil
钩藤 Gambir Vine
香附 Nut-grass
香薷 Chinese Mosla

香菇多糖 Lentinan
重楼 Paris
独活 Doubleteeth Pubescent Angelica
独一味 Common Lamiophlomis
胆酸 Cholic Acid
洋金花 Datura
穿山龙 Nippon Yam
穿心莲 Common Andrographis
祖师麻 Girald Daphne
绞股蓝 Fiveleaf Gynostemma
绞股蓝总苷 Gypenosides

十画

蚕蛾 Silkworm Imago
桂枝 Cassia Twig
桔梗 Balloon Flower
莱阳梨 Laiyang Pear
荷叶 Lotus leaf
夏天无 Bending Corydalis
夏枯草 Selfheal
柴胡 Chinese Hare's Ear
党参 Bellflower
钻山风 Oldham Fissistigma
臭灵丹 Wingedtooth Laggera
臭梧桐 Hairy Clerodendron
高良姜 Lesser Galangal
浙贝母 Thunberg Fritillary
海马 Sea Horse
海龙 Pipe Fish
海螵蛸 Cuttle-fish Bone
浮萍 Common Duckmeat
益母草 Chinese Motherwort
桑 White Mulberry
桑叶 White Mulberry Leaf
桑寄生 Chinese Taxillus

十一画

菊花 Chrysanthemum
黄芪 Milkvetch
黄芩 Baical Skullcap
黄连 Golden Thread
黄杨 Chinese Box
黄柏 Chinese Corktree
雪莲 Medusa Saussurea
眼镜蛇 Forest Cobra
蛇胆 Forest Cobra Gall
蛇胆汁 Forest Cobra Bile
野菊花 Wild Chrysanthemum
银杏 Ginkgo
猪苓 Chuling
猪苓多糖 Polypolus Polysaccharide
猪胆浸膏 Hog Gall Extract
麻黄 Chinese Ephedra
鹿角 Deerhorn
鹿角胶 Deerhorn Glue
鹿茸 Pilose Deerhorn
鹿筋 Deer Sinew
羚羊角 Antelope Horn
断血流 Chinese Clinopodium

十二画

琥珀 Amber
斑蝥 Large Blister Beetle
葛根 Lobed Kudzuvine
款冬花 Common Coltsfoot
紫苏 Purple Perilla
紫苏叶 Purple Perilla Leaf
紫苏梗 Purple Perilla Stem
紫河车 Human Placenta
紫珠叶 Taiwan Beautyberry
蛤壳 Clam Shell
蛤蚧 Giant Gecko
黑芝麻 Black Sesame
黑锡 Galenite
景天三七 Alpine Stonecrop
锁阳 Cynomorium
筋骨草 Ciliate Bugle
猴头菌菌丝体 Mycelium Hedgehod

十三画

槐角 Japanese Pagodatree
蒺藜 Caltrop

蒲桃 Roseapple Pericarp
蒲公英 Dandelion
硼砂 Borax
蜂蜡素 Myricin
雷公藤 Tripterygium
满山白 Savatier Monochasma
满山红 Daurian Rhododendron
裸花紫珠 Nakedflower Beautyberry

十四画

槟榔 Betel Nut
酸模 Sour Leek
酸枣仁 Sour Jujube
磁石 Magnetite
豨莶草 Siegesbeckia
蜚蠊 Roach
辣蓼 Smartweed
熊胆 Bear Gall

十五画至二十一画

橡皮 Sawtooth Oak
槲寄生 Colored Mistletoe
暴马子皮 Amur Lilae
墨旱莲 Eclipta
鹤草芽 Hairy Agrimonia
橘红 Satsuma Orange Exocarp
橘核 Satsuma Orange Seed
薯蓣 Common Yam
藏青果 Myrobalan
䗪虫 Ground Beetle
藜芦 Black Falsehellebore
蟾皮 Toad Skin
蟾酥 Toad Venom
鳖甲 Turtle Carapace
獾油 Badger Fat
麝香 Musk

参考文献
References

1. 国家药品监督管理局安全监管司，国家药品监督管理局药品评价中心. 国家基本药物：中成药.北京：人民卫生出版社，2002.

2. 国家药典委员会编. 中华人民共和国药典. 2005 年，一部. 北京：化学工业出版社，2005.

3. 江苏新医学院编. 中药大辞典：上、下册. 上海：上海科学技术出版社，1986.

4. 马其云编. 中国蕨类植物和种子植物名称总汇. 青岛：青岛出版社，2003.

5. 关克俭等. 拉汉英种子植物名称. 北京：科学出版社，1983.

6. Shiu-ying Hu. An Enumeration of Chinese Materia Medica, Second Edition. Hong Kong: The Chinese University Press, 1999.

7. 欧明主编. 汉英中医词典. 广州、香港：广东科技出版社、三联书店（香港）有限公司，1986.

8. 李衍文等. 汉拉英中草药名称辞典. 广州：广东科技出版社，1998.

9. 李衍文主编. 中草药异名词典. 北京：人民卫生出版社，2004.

10. 《中国药用动物志》协作组编. 中国药用动物志：第一册. 天津：天津科学技术出版社，1979.

11. 《中国药用动物志》协作组编. 中国药用动物志：第二册. 天津：天津科学技术出版社，1983.

12. 苏子仁，赖小平主编. 汉英、英汉中草药化学成分词汇：中国中医药出版社，2006.

13. 韩立编. 汉拉英动物药名称. 福州：福建科学技术出版社，1992.

14. 张保国. 矿物药. 北京：中国医药科技出版社，2005.

15. 金魁和主编. 汉英医学大词典. 第 2 版. 北京：人民卫生出版社，2004.

16. John H. Wiersema and Blanca Leon. World Economic Plants: A Standard Reference. London, New York: CRC Press, 1999.

17. 中医药学名词审定委员会. 中医药学名词（Chinese Terms in Traditional Chinese Medicine and Pharmacy）. 北京：科学出版社，2005.

18. World Health Organization Western Pacific Region. WHO International Standard Terminologies on Traditional Medicine in the Western Pacific Region. Manila: 2007.